Shital Gandhi, Dan Farine (Eds.)
Obstetric Medicine

Hot Topics in Perinatal Medicine

Edited by
Joachim W. Dudenhausen

Volume 6

Shital Gandhi, Dan Farine (Eds.)

Obstetric Medicine

The Subspecialty at the intersection of Internal
Medicine and Obstetrics

DE GRUYTER

Editors
Dr. Shital Gandhi
Mount Sinai Hospital
600 University Ave, suite 431
Toronto, ON, Canada M5G 1X5
shital.gandhi@sinaihealth.ca

Dr. Dan Farine
Mount Sinai Hospital
700 University Ave, suite 3914
Toronto, ON, Canada M5G 1Z5
dan.farine@sinaihealth.ca

ISBN 978-3-11-061459-6
e-ISBN (PDF) 978-3-11-061525-8
e-ISBN (EPUB) 978-3-11-061476-3

Library of Congress Control Number: 2021947016

Bibliographic information published by the Deutsche Nationalbibliothek
The Deutsche Nationalbibliothek lists this publication in the Deutsche Nationalbibliografie;
detailed bibliographic data are available on the Internet at http://dnb.d-nb.de.

© 2022 Walter de Gruyter GmbH, Berlin/Boston
Cover image: Comstock/Getty Images
Typesetting: Integra Software Services Pvt. Ltd.
Printing and binding: CPI books GmbH, Leck

www.degruyter.com

I dedicate this book to my parents, Meena and Naresh, and to my partner Rohan for all their support over the years – Shital Gandhi

I dedicate this book to my daughter Tali and her partner Vinicius and to my son Jonathan and his partner Erin – Dan Farine

Contents

List of Contributors —— XXVII

Shital Gandhi, Dan Farine
1   **Introduction** —— 1
1.1   What Is Obstetric Medicine? —— 1
1.2   Why Obstetric Medicine? —— 2

Gali Pariente, Gideon Koren
2   **Approach to Safe Use of Medications in Pregnancy** —— 5
2.1   Introduction —— 5
2.2   Medication Use in Pregnancy —— 5
2.3   Teratogenicity —— 6
2.3.1   Timing of Exposure —— 6
2.3.2   Teratogenic Mechanisms —— 7
2.3.3   Labeling Requirements —— 7
2.4   Drug Pharmacokinetics —— 8
2.4.1   Pregnancy-Induced Pharmacokinetic (PK) Changes of Drugs —— 8
2.4.2   Placental Drug Transfer —— 9
2.5   Drug Pharmacodynamics —— 9
2.5.1   Maternal Drug Actions —— 9
2.5.2   Drugs of Choice —— 10
2.6   Therapeutic Drug Actions in the Fetus —— 13
2.7   Proven Teratogenic Drugs in Humans —— 13
2.7.1   Drugs for Cardiovascular Disorders —— 13
2.7.2   Drugs for Neurological Disorders —— 14
2.7.3   Drugs of Abuse —— 14
2.7.4   Drugs Used for Infection and Inflammation —— 14
2.7.5   Drugs for Nausea and Vomiting —— 15
2.7.6   Other Drugs —— 15
2.8   Drugs in Normal Labor and Delivery —— 16
2.8.1   Pharmacologic Management of Pain During Labor and Delivery —— 16
2.8.2   Drugs for Management of Labor Protraction or Arrest Disorders —— 16
2.9   Conclusion —— 18
     References —— 19

Siobhan Bacon, Ann McNamara
3 **Approach to Diagnostic Imaging in Pregnancy** —— 23
3.1 Introduction —— 23
3.2 Fetal Effects of Radiation: Teratogenicity —— 23
3.3 Fetal Effects of Radiation: Oncogenesis —— 25
3.4 Maternal Effects of Ionizing Radiation —— 25
3.5 Specific Modalities: Non-ionizing Radiation —— 26
3.5.1 Ultrasound —— 26
3.5.2 Magnetic Resonance Imaging (MRI) —— 26
3.6 Specific Modalities: Ionizing Radiation —— 27
3.6.1 Plain Film —— 27
3.6.2 Computed Tomography (CT) —— 27
3.7 Nuclear Imaging: Positron Emission Tomography Scanning Scan —— 27
3.8 Imaging in Particular Clinical Scenarios —— 28
3.8.1 Headache —— 28
3.8.2 Non-obstetric Abdominal Pain —— 29
3.8.3 Suspected Pulmonary Embolism —— 30
3.9 Contrast Agents —— 30
3.9.1 Gadolinium —— 30
3.9.2 Iodinated Contrast —— 31
3.10 How to Reduce Radiation Exposure —— 31
3.11 Lactation —— 32
Conclusion —— 32
Glossary —— 32
References —— 33

Jennifer Yo, Shital Gandhi
4 **Chronic Hypertension** —— 35
4.1 Introduction —— 35
4.2 Definition and Diagnostic Criteria for Hypertensive Disorders in Pregnancy —— 35
4.2.1 Gestational Hypertension —— 35
4.2.2 Preeclampsia —— 36
4.2.3 Chronic Hypertension —— 36
4.2.4 Chronic Hypertension with Superimposed Preeclampsia —— 37
4.2.5 White Coat Hypertension —— 37
4.3 Normal Hemodynamic Changes in Pregnancy —— 37
4.4 Comorbid Conditions —— 38
4.5 Pregnancy Complications in Women with Chronic Hypertension —— 39
4.5.1 Maternal Risks —— 39
4.5.2 Fetal Risks —— 39

4.6   Patient Evaluation —— **39**
4.7   Blood Pressure Measurement —— **40**
4.8   Blood Pressure Target in Pregnancy —— **40**
4.8.1   Management of Non-severe Hypertension
          (BP 140–159/90–110 mmHg) —— **40**
4.8.2   Management of Severe Hypertension (BP ≥ 160/110 mmHg) —— **42**
4.9   Choice of Antihypertensive Agent —— **42**
4.9.1   Sympathetic Nervous System Inhibition —— **43**
4.9.2   Beta-Adrenergic Blockers —— **43**
4.9.3   Calcium Channel Blockers —— **44**
4.9.4   Direct Vasodilators —— **44**
4.9.5   Angiotensin-Converting Enzyme Inhibitors and Angiotensin
          Receptor Antagonists —— **45**
4.10   Management of Postpartum Hypertension —— **45**
          References —— **46**

Laura Berall, Michelle A. Hladunewich
5   Kidney Disease in Pregnancy —— 49
5.1   Introduction —— **49**
5.2   Renal Physiology in Normal Pregnancy and the Diagnosis
          of Kidney Disease —— **49**
5.3   Renal Biopsy in Pregnancy —— **51**
5.4   Acute Kidney Injury in Pregnancy —— **51**
5.5   Pregnancy in Women with Chronic Kidney Disease —— **56**
5.5.1   Prepregnancy Counseling and Optimization —— **56**
5.5.2   Management of CKD in Pregnancy —— **57**
5.5.3   Postpartum Care —— **58**
5.6   Disease-Specific Comments —— **59**
5.6.1   Lupus Nephritis in Pregnancy —— **59**
5.6.2   Diabetic Nephropathy in Pregnancy —— **59**
5.6.3   Hereditary Kidney Disease in Pregnancy —— **60**
5.7   Pregnancy in End-Stage Kidney Disease —— **61**
5.7.1   Pregnancy and Renal Transplant Recipients —— **61**
5.7.2   Pregnancy in Women on Dialysis —— **61**
5.8   Conclusion —— **62**
          References —— **63**

Kelsey McLaughlin, Melanie C. Audette, Sebastian R. Hobson,
John C. Kingdom
6   Preeclampsia —— 69
6.1   Introduction —— **69**
6.2   Preeclampsia Pathogenesis: Stage 1 —— **70**

6.2.1   Abnormal Placentation —— **70**
6.3   Preeclampsia Pathogenesis: Stage 2 —— **71**
6.3.1   Placental-Derived Angiogenic Proteins —— **72**
6.3.2   Systemic Maternal Endothelial Dysfunction —— **72**
6.3.3   Maternal Hemodynamics and Hypertension —— **73**
6.3.4   Glomerular Endotheliosis —— **74**
6.4   Risk Factors for Preeclampsia —— **74**
6.4.1   Genetic Predisposition —— **74**
6.4.2   Pre-Existing Maternal Health —— **75**
6.4.3   Pregnancy History and Characteristics —— **75**
6.5   Clinical Definition of Preeclampsia —— **75**
6.6   Diagnosis of Preeclampsia —— **76**
6.7   Preventative Strategies for Preeclampsia —— **77**
6.7.1   Lifestyle Strategies for Preeclampsia Prevention —— **77**
6.7.2   Therapies for Preeclampsia Prevention —— **77**
6.8   Treatment Options for Established Preeclampsia —— **78**
6.8.1   Expectant Management Versus Delivery —— **79**
6.8.2   Term Preeclampsia (37+ weeks) —— **79**
6.8.3   Late Preterm Preeclampsia (34–37 weeks) —— **79**
6.8.4   Preterm Preeclampsia (<34 weeks) —— **80**
6.8.5   Mode of Delivery —— **80**
6.9   Postpartum Care —— **81**
6.10   Innovations in Preeclampsia —— **83**
6.10.1   Prediction of Preeclampsia —— **83**
6.10.2   Diagnosis and Clinical Management of Preeclampsia —— **83**
6.10.3   Phenotypes of Preeclampsia —— **83**
6.10.4   Therapeutic Strategies —— **83**
6.11   Conclusions —— **84**
          References —— **84**

Omri Zamstein, Eyal Sheiner
7   **Late Consequences of Pregnancy-Associated Hypertensive Disorders —— 91**
7.1   Introduction —— **91**
7.2   Cardiovascular Disease —— **91**
7.3   Diabetes Mellitus —— **94**
7.4   Chronic Kidney Disease —— **94**
7.5   Additional Morbidities Related to Pregnancy-Associated Hypertension —— **95**
7.6   Prognosis of Offspring of Hypertensive Pregnancies —— **95**
7.7   Conclusion —— **96**
          References —— **96**

Harrison Banner, Jack M. Colman, Mathew Sermer
8   Cardiovascular Disease in Pregnancy — 99
8.1   Introduction — 99
8.2   Cardiovascular Physiology and Adaptation to Pregnancy — 99
8.3   Risk Assessment — 100
8.3.1   Maternal Risk — 100
8.3.2   Fetal/Neonatal Risk — 102
8.4   Advanced Cardiac Imaging During Pregnancy — 103
8.5   General Principles for the Management of Patients with Cardiac Disease in Pregnancy — 103
8.5.1   Antepartum Management — 103
8.5.2   Management During Labor and Delivery — 104
8.6   Management of Artificial Heart Valves in Pregnancy — 105
8.6.1   Anticoagulation for Mechanical Heart Valves — 106
8.7   Evaluation and Management of Specific Structural Cardiac Lesions — 107
8.7.1   Volume Overload Lesions: Left-to-Right Shunts — 107
8.7.2   Volume Overload Lesions: Regurgitant Valves — 107
8.7.3   Pressure Overload Lesions (Left Heart): Aortic Stenosis — 108
8.7.4   Pressure Overload Lesions (Left Heart): Mitral Stenosis — 108
8.7.5   Pressure Overload Lesions (Left Heart): Coarctation of the Aorta — 109
8.7.6   Pressure Overload Lesions (Left Heart): Aortopathy — 109
8.7.7   Pressure Overload Lesions (Right Heart): Pulmonary Stenosis — 110
8.7.8   Pressure Overload Lesions (Right Heart): Pulmonary Hypertension — 111
8.8   Arrhythmia — 112
8.8.1   Atrial Arrhythmias — 112
8.8.2   Ventricular Arrhythmias — 112
8.9   Cardiomyopathy and Heart Failure — 113
8.10   Conclusion — 114
           References — 114

Emilie Laflamme, Rachel M. Wald
9   Cardiac Arrest in Pregnancy — 121
9.1   Introduction and Epidemiology — 121
9.2   Etiology of Cardiac Arrest in Pregnancy — 121
9.3   Management of Cardiac Arrest in Pregnancy — 122
9.4   Basic Life Support in Pregnancy — 124
9.5   Advanced Cardiac Life Support in Pregnancy — 124
9.5.1   Airway and Breathing — 124
9.5.2   Circulation — 125

9.6   Perimortem Caesarian Section Delivery —— **125**
9.7   Mechanical Support and Intensive Care Management —— **126**
9.8   Outcomes and Training Perspectives —— **127**
               References —— **127**

Stephanie C. Lapinsky, Stephen E. Lapinsky
10   **Critical Care in Pregnancy** —— **131**
10.1   Introduction —— **131**
10.2   Physiologic Changes in Pregnancy —— **131**
10.3   Critical Illness in Pregnancy —— **133**
10.4   Critical Care Management: ICU Drug Therapy in Pregnancy —— **134**
10.4.1   Catecholamines —— **134**
10.4.2   Sedation, Analgesia, and Neuromuscular Blockade —— **134**
10.5   Ventilatory Support —— **135**
10.5.1   Noninvasive Ventilation —— **135**
10.5.2   Airway Management —— **135**
10.5.3   Mechanical Ventilation —— **135**
10.6   Pregnancy-Specific Conditions Requiring ICU Care —— **136**
10.6.1   Acute Fatty Liver of Pregnancy —— **137**
10.6.2   Amniotic Fluid Embolism —— **137**
10.6.3   Obstetric Hemorrhage —— **138**
10.6.4   Tocolytic Pulmonary Edema —— **139**
10.7   Conditions Not Specific to Pregnancy —— **139**
10.7.1   Acute Respiratory Distress Syndrome in Pregnancy —— **139**
10.7.2   Thyroid Storm —— **139**
10.7.3   Trauma —— **140**
               References —— **141**

Dina Refaat, Mohamed Momtaz
11   **Amniotic Fluid Embolism** —— **145**
11.1   Introduction —— **145**
11.1.1   History —— **145**
11.1.2   Definition —— **146**
11.1.3   Incidence —— **146**
11.2   Risk Factors —— **147**
11.3   Pathophysiology —— **147**
11.4   Clinical Presentations —— **148**
11.5   Diagnosis —— **148**
11.6   Differential Diagnosis —— **149**
11.6.1   Myocardial Infarction —— **149**
11.6.2   Pulmonary Embolism —— **149**
11.6.3   Anesthetic Complications —— **149**

11.6.4   Air Embolism —— 150
11.6.5   Eclampsia —— 150
11.6.6   Transfusion Reactions —— 150
11.6.7   Anaphylactic Shock —— 150
11.7   Management —— 150
11.8   Complications —— 152
11.8.1   Maternal Complications —— 152
11.8.2   Fetal Complications —— 153
            References —— 154

Sam Schulman, Aleksander Makatsariya

12   **Venous Thromboembolism in Pregnancy —— 157**
12.1   Introduction —— 157
12.2   Risk Factors for Venous Thromboembolism —— 157
12.2.1   Physiological Changes in Pregnancy —— 158
12.2.2   Pathology in Pregnancy —— 159
12.2.3   Fetus-Related Risks —— 159
12.2.4   Patient-Related Risk Factors —— 159
12.3   Diagnosis of VTE in Pregnancy —— 161
12.3.1   Deep Vein Thrombosis —— 161
12.3.2   Pulmonary Embolism —— 162
12.3.3   Clinical Prediction —— 162
12.4   Prophylaxis —— 163
12.5   Treatment —— 166
12.5.1   Initiation of Treatment —— 166
12.5.2   Maintenance Therapy —— 167
12.5.3   Around Time of Delivery —— 168
12.6   Investigation for Thrombophilia —— 169
12.7   Conclusions —— 169
            References —— 170

Shaun Yo, John Granton

13   **Pulmonary Hypertension in Pregnancy —— 173**
13.1   Introduction —— 173
13.2   Epidemiology of PAH —— 174
13.3   The Risk of Pregnancy in Patients with PAH —— 174
13.4   Physiological Effects of Pregnancy —— 175
13.5   The Perils of PAH and Pregnancy —— 176
13.6   General Principles and Supportive Therapy in Pregnancy —— 177
13.7   PAH-Targeted Medications in Pregnancy —— 178

13.8   Approach to PAH-targeted Treatment —— **180**
13.9   Peripartum Management —— **182**
13.10   Conclusions —— **183**
            References —— **184**

Alina Blazer, Meyer Balter
14   Asthma in Pregnancy —— 187
14.1   Introduction —— **187**
14.2   Changes in Respiratory Function During Pregnancy —— **187**
14.3   Effects of Pregnancy on Asthma —— **187**
14.3.1   Mechanisms for the Effect of Pregnancy on Maternal Asthma —— **188**
14.4   Effects of Asthma on Pregnancy: Maternal and Fetal
            Outcomes —— **189**
14.5   Treatment of Asthma in Pregnancy: General Principles —— **190**
14.6   Nonpharmacological Management —— **190**
14.7   Pharmacological Management —— **191**
14.7.1   Beta-Agonists —— **191**
14.7.2   Inhaled Corticosteroids —— **192**
14.7.3   Other Asthma Medications —— **192**
14.7.4   Health Behaviors —— **193**
14.8   Treatment of Acute Exacerbations —— **193**
14.9   Labor and Delivery —— **194**
14.10   Asthma Postpartum and Breastfeeding Implications —— **195**
14.11   Conclusion —— **195**
            References —— **195**

Loïc Sentilhes, Hanane Bouchghoul, Aurélien Mattuizzi, Alizée Froeliger,
Hugo Madar
15   Obstetric Hemorrhage —— 199
15.1   Introduction —— **199**
15.2   Definitions and Thresholds for Intervention —— **200**
15.3   Incidence of Postpartum Hemorrhage (PPH) —— **204**
15.4   Causes of Postpartum Hemorrhage (PPH) —— **204**
15.5   Risk Factors for PPH —— **204**
15.6   Prevention of Postpartum Hemorrhage —— **206**
15.6.1   Active Management of the Third Stage of Labor —— **206**
15.6.2   Uterotonics —— **206**
15.6.3   Tranexamic Acid —— **208**
15.6.4   Other Prevention Techniques —— **209**
15.7   Treatment of Postpartum Hemorrhage —— **209**
15.7.1   First-Line Measures —— **211**
15.7.2   Second-Line Measures for Persisting Hemorrhage —— **211**

15.7.3   Third-Line Measures for Refractory Hemorrhage ━━ 217
15.8   After Postpartum Hemorrhage ━━ 219
15.9   Conclusion ━━ 219
          References ━━ 220

Dongmei Sun, Nadine Shehata
16   Anemia in Pregnancy ━━ 225
16.1   Introduction ━━ 225
16.2   Normal Hematological Physiological Changes ━━ 225
16.3   Iron Deficiency Anemia ━━ 225
16.3.1   Diagnosis ━━ 226
16.3.2   Management ━━ 226
16.4   Hemoglobin Disorders in General ━━ 227
16.5   Sickle Cell Disease ━━ 228
16.5.1   Diagnosis ━━ 228
16.5.2   Fetal and Maternal Implications of Sickle Cell Disease ━━ 228
16.5.3   Management ━━ 229
16.6   Thalassemia ━━ 230
16.6.1   Diagnosis ━━ 230
16.6.2   Fetal and Maternal Implications of Thalassemia ━━ 231
16.6.3   Management ━━ 231
16.7   Microangiopathic Hemolytic Anemia in General ━━ 232
16.8   Pregnancy-Associated Microangiopathic Hemolytic Anemia
          Syndromes ━━ 232
16.8.1   HELLP Syndrome ━━ 232
16.8.2   Thrombotic Microangiopathies Associated with MAHA ━━ 233
16.8.3   Thrombotic Thrombocytopenic Purpura ━━ 234
16.8.4   Complement-Mediated Thrombotic Microangiopathy ━━ 234
16.8.5   Management of TTP and HUS ━━ 235
16.8.6   Conclusions ━━ 235
          References ━━ 236

Ann Kinga Malinowski, Emily Delpero
17   Sickle Cell Disease in Pregnancy ━━ 241
17.1   Introduction: Normal Hemoglobin ━━ 241
17.2   Sickle Hemoglobin ━━ 241
17.3   Sickle Cell Trait Versus Sickle Cell Disease ━━ 242
17.4   Pathophysiology of Sickle Cell Disease ━━ 242
17.5   Manifestations of Sickle Cell Disease and Influence
          of Pregnancy ━━ 243
17.5.1   SCD-Related Pain ━━ 243
17.5.2   Chronic Anemia ━━ 244

17.5.3   Cardiac Manifestations —— **244**
17.5.4   Pulmonary Manifestations —— **245**
17.5.4.1   Acute Chest Syndrome (ACS) —— **245**
17.5.4.2   Pulmonary Hypertension (PH) —— **246**
17.5.5   Splenic Manifestations —— **247**
17.5.6   Neurologic Manifestations —— **247**
17.5.7   Renal Manifestations —— **247**
17.5.8   Hepatic Manifestations —— **248**
17.6   Pregnancy Outcomes —— **248**
17.7   Preconception Care —— **249**
17.7.1   Fertility Preservation —— **249**
17.7.2   Determination of Fetal Risk —— **249**
17.7.3   Medical Optimization —— **250**
17.8   Antenatal Care —— **250**
17.8.1   Prenatal Diagnosis —— **250**
17.8.2   Fetal Surveillance —— **251**
17.8.3   Maternal Management —— **251**
17.8.3.1   General Approach —— **251**
17.8.3.2   Prevention of Preeclampsia —— **251**
17.8.3.3   Acute Pain Crisis —— **252**
17.8.3.4   Analgesia during VOE —— **252**
17.8.3.5   The Role of Transfusion —— **253**
17.8.3.6   Intrapartum Care —— **254**
17.8.3.7   Postpartum Care —— **254**
17.9   Newborn Considerations —— **255**
17.9.1   Genetic Testing —— **255**
17.9.2   Neonatal Abstinence Syndrome (NAS) —— **255**
17.10   Conclusion —— **255**
             References —— **256**

Kristin Harris, Mark Yudin
18   Human Immunodeficiency Virus and Pregnancy —— 261
18.1   Introduction —— **261**
18.2   Epidemiology —— **261**
18.3   Prenatal Testing —— **262**
18.4   Maternal and Perinatal Outcomes —— **263**
18.4.1   Maternal Outcomes —— **263**
18.4.2   Fetal Outcomes —— **263**
18.5   Preconception Management —— **264**
18.5.1   Counseling —— **264**
18.5.2   Medications —— **264**
18.5.3   Conception and Fertility Treatment Considerations —— **265**

18.5.4   Immunizations/Infections —— 266
18.6   Pregnancy Management: Antenatal Care —— 266
18.6.1   Schedule of Care —— 266
18.6.2   Antiretroviral Therapy —— 268
18.6.3   Special Circumstance —— 270
18.7   Intrapartum Care —— 270
18.7.1   Mode of Delivery —— 270
18.7.2   Antiretroviral Therapy —— 270
18.7.3   Special Considerations —— 271
18.8   Postpartum Care —— 272
18.8.1   Antiretroviral Therapy —— 272
18.8.2   Infant Feeding —— 272
18.8.3   Infant Care —— 273
18.9   Conclusion —— 274
            References —— 274

Moran Shapira, Yoav Yinon
19   **Congenital Cytomegalovirus Infection —— 281**
19.1   Introduction —— 281
19.2   Congenital CMV Infection —— 281
19.3   Prenatal Diagnosis of Maternal CMV Infection —— 282
19.4   Prenatal Diagnosis of Fetal CMV Infection —— 283
19.5   Prognostic Markers of CMV Disease —— 285
19.5.1   Fetal Imaging —— 285
19.5.2   DNA Counts in Amniotic Fluid —— 285
19.5.3   Fetal Blood Parameters —— 286
19.6   Prevention and Treatment of Intrauterine CMV Infection —— 286
19.6.1   Prevention of Transmission —— 286
19.6.2   Treatment of Intrauterine Infection —— 287
19.6.3   Antiviral Drugs —— 287
19.7   Prevention of Maternal CMV Infection —— 289
19.8   Screening for CMV —— 289
19.9   Conclusion —— 290
            References —— 290

Valentine Faure Bardon, Yves Ville
20   **Fetal Toxoplasmosis —— 297**
20.1   Introduction —— 297
20.2   Maternal Infection —— 297
20.3   Fetal Infection —— 298
20.4   Prognostic Markers of Fetal Infection —— 299
20.4.1   Timing of Maternal Primary Infection (MPI) —— 299

20.4.2   Findings on Imaging —— **300**
20.5   Prognostic Value of Imaging Findings —— **300**
20.5.1   Neurodevelopmental —— **300**
20.5.2   Chorioretinitis —— **301**
20.5.3   Contribution of Fetal Head MRI —— **301**
20.6   Prenatal Treatment —— **301**
20.6.1   Drugs —— **302**
20.6.2   Prevention of Mother-to-Fetus Transmission —— **302**
20.6.3   Antiparasitic Therapy to Reduce Fetal Complications —— **303**
20.7   Neonates Born to women with Toxoplasmosis Infection —— **303**
20.8   Comparison of Various Approaches —— **304**
20.9   Conclusion —— **308**
          References —— **308**

Daniela N. Vasquez, Maria-Teresa Pérez
21   Sepsis in Pregnancy —— 313
21.1   Introduction —— **313**
21.2   Risk Factors —— **313**
21.3   Diagnosis —— **314**
21.4   Sources of Sepsis in Pregnant and Postpartum Patients —— **316**
21.5   Microorganisms Responsible for Maternal Sepsis —— **318**
21.6   Management —— **318**
21.7   Delivery Considerations —— **323**
21.8   Outcomes: Maternal Morbidity and Mortality due to Sepsis —— **324**
21.9   Conclusion —— **324**
          References —— **324**

Mónica Centeno, Diogo Ayres-de-Campos
22   Thyroid Disease in Pregnancy —— 329
22.1   Introduction —— **329**
22.2   Thyroid Physiology During Pregnancy —— **329**
22.2.1   Maternal Thyroid Gland —— **329**
22.2.2   Fetal Thyroid Gland —— **330**
22.3   Hypothyroidism —— **331**
22.3.1   Definition —— **331**
22.3.2   Incidence —— **331**
22.3.3   Etiology —— **331**
22.3.4   Clinical Manifestations —— **331**
22.3.5   Diagnosis —— **332**
22.3.5.1 Hypothyroidism Diagnosed in Pregnancy —— **332**
22.3.6   Complications —— **332**

22.3.7   Management —— **334**
22.4   Iodine Deficiency —— **334**
22.5   Hyperthyroidism —— **335**
22.5.1   Definition and Incidence —— **335**
22.5.2   Etiology —— **335**
22.5.3   Clinical Manifestations —— **335**
22.5.4   Diagnosis —— **335**
22.5.5   Complications —— **336**
22.5.6   Management —— **336**
22.5.7   Management of Fetal and Neonatal Effects —— **337**
22.6   Thyroid Nodules —— **337**
22.7   Thyroid Cancer —— **337**
            References —— **338**

Sawyer Huget-Penner, Denice S. Feig
23   Preexisting Diabetes in Pregnancy —— 343
23.1   Introduction —— **343**
23.2   Maternal Risks of Preexisting Diabetes in Pregnancy —— **343**
23.3   Neonatal Risks of Preexisting Diabetes in Pregnancy —— **345**
23.4   Management of Preexisting Diabetes in Pregnancy —— **347**
23.4.1   Preconception Management —— **347**
23.4.2   Pregnancy Management —— **348**
23.4.3   Antepartum and Intrapartum Monitoring and Management —— **350**
23.5   Conclusion —— **351**
            References —— **351**

Maya Ram, Yariv Yogev
24   Gestational Diabetes Mellitus —— 357
24.1   Introduction —— **357**
24.2   Risk Factors for GDM —— **357**
24.3   Pathophysiology of GDM —— **358**
24.4   The Offspring Point of View —— **363**
24.5   Prevention of Long-Term Effects on the Offspring —— **365**
24.6   Screening and Diagnosis for GDM —— **365**
24.6.1   "Two-Step" Method for Screening —— **367**
24.6.2   "One-Step" Method for Screening —— **368**
24.6.3   Optimal Diagnostic Approach – Evidence-Based —— **368**
24.6.4   Early Pregnancy Testing —— **369**
24.6.5   Repeat Testing —— **370**
24.7   Non-pharmacologic Management —— **370**
24.7.1   Prevention of Gestational Diabetes —— **370**
24.7.2   Lifestyle Intervention —— **370**

24.7.3   Glucose Monitoring and Targets —— **371**
24.8   Pharmacological Treatment —— **372**
24.8.1   Insulin —— **372**
24.8.2   Oral Antidiabetic Medication —— **372**
24.8.2.1   Metformin —— **373**
24.8.2.2   Sulfonylureas —— **373**
24.9   Obstetric Considerations —— **373**
24.10   Postpartum Management and Long-Term Maternal Health —— **374**
            References —— **375**

Haitham Baghlaf, Cynthia Maxwell
25   Obesity and Pregnancy —— 387
25.1   Introduction and Epidemiology —— **387**
25.2   Preconception —— **388**
25.3   First Trimester —— **390**
25.3.1   Maternal Considerations —— **390**
25.3.2   Fetal Considerations —— **391**
25.4   Second Trimester —— **392**
25.4.1   Maternal Considerations —— **392**
25.4.2   Fetal Considerations —— **392**
25.5   Third Trimester —— **392**
25.5.1   Maternal Considerations —— **392**
25.5.2   Fetal Considerations —— **394**
25.5.3   Intrapartum —— **394**
25.6   Postpartum —— **396**
25.7   Conclusion —— **397**
            References —— **397**

Vivian Huang, Geoffrey C. Nguyen
26   Managing Inflammatory Bowel Disease During Pregnancy —— 405
26.1   Background —— **405**
26.2   Prepregnancy and Inflammatory Bowel Disease —— **405**
26.2.1   Voluntary Childlessness —— **405**
26.2.2   IBD Disease Activity —— **405**
26.2.2.1   IBD Medications —— **406**
26.2.2.2   IBD-Related Surgeries —— **406**
26.3   Pregnancy with Inflammatory Bowel Disease —— **406**
26.4   IBD Medications —— **407**
26.4.1   Sulfasalazine and 5-Aminosalicylates —— **407**
26.4.2   Immunomodulators —— **408**
26.4.3   Biologics —— **408**
26.4.4   Small Molecules —— **409**

26.4.5   Corticosteroids —— **409**
26.5   Delivery and Postpartum —— **410**
26.6   Conclusion —— **410**
            References —— **411**

Homero Flores-Mendoza, Harrison Banner, John W. Snelgrove
27   Intrahepatic Cholestasis of Pregnancy —— 413
27.1   Introduction —— **413**
27.2   Etiology —— **413**
27.2.1   Genetics —— **413**
27.2.2   Hormonal —— **414**
27.2.3   Environmental —— **414**
27.2.4   History of Prior Liver Disease —— **414**
27.3   Clinical Manifestations —— **415**
27.4   Diagnosis —— **415**
27.5   Maternal and Fetal Implications —— **418**
27.6   Treatment —— **418**
27.7   Delivery —— **419**
            References —— **420**

Ghaydaa Aldabie, Karen A. Spitzer, Carl A. Laskin
28   Pregnancy and the Rheumatic Diseases —— 423
28.1   Introduction —— **423**
28.2   Rheumatoid Arthritis —— **423**
28.2.1   Effects of RA on Pregnancy —— **423**
28.2.2   Effects of Pregnancy on RA —— **424**
28.3   Management of Rheumatoid Arthritis During Pregnancy —— **424**
28.3.1   Nonsteroidal Anti-inflammatory Drugs —— **424**
28.3.2   Glucocorticoids —— **425**
28.3.3   Conventional Disease-Modifying Antirheumatic Drugs —— **425**
28.3.4   Methotrexate —— **426**
28.3.5   Leflunomide —— **426**
28.3.6   Sulfasalazine —— **427**
28.3.7   Tumor Necrosis Factor Inhibitors (anti-TNF) —— **427**
28.3.8   Injectable Anti-TNF Agents —— **427**
28.3.9   Janus Kinase Pathway Inhibitors —— **427**
28.4   Systemic Lupus Erythematosus —— **428**
28.4.1   Prepregnancy Assessment —— **428**
28.4.2   Disease Activity —— **428**
28.4.3   Medication Review —— **429**
28.4.4   Assessment of Autoantibodies —— **429**
28.5   The Effects of Pregnancy on SLE —— **429**

28.5.1   SLE Flare —— **429**
28.5.2   Renal Disease —— **430**
28.5.3   Preeclampsia —— **430**
28.5.4   The Effects of SLE on Pregnancy —— **431**
28.5.5   Neonatal Lupus —— **431**
28.5.6   Antiphospholipid Antibodies and Pregnancy —— **432**
28.5.7   Advise Against Pregnancy/Early Therapeutic Termination —— **432**
28.5.8   Contraception —— **433**
28.6   Specific Medication Use in the Management of SLE During
            Pregnancy —— **433**
28.6.1   Antimalarials —— **433**
28.6.2   Azathioprine —— **434**
28.6.3   Mycophenolate Mofetil —— **434**
28.6.4   Cyclophosphamide —— **435**
28.7   Conclusion —— **435**
            References —— **436**

Tadeu A. Fantaneanu, Esther Bui
29   Epilepsy and Pregnancy —— 441
29.1   Introduction —— **441**
29.2   Preconception —— **441**
29.2.1   Contraception —— **441**
29.2.2   Preconception Risk Stratification —— **443**
29.2.3   Folate Supplementation —— **445**
29.3   Pregnancy —— **446**
29.3.1   Therapeutic Drug Monitoring —— **446**
29.3.2   Vitamin K Administration —— **446**
29.3.3   Seizures and Emergencies in Pregnancy —— **447**
29.3.4   Labor and Delivery —— **447**
29.4   Postpartum —— **448**
29.4.1   Breastfeeding —— **448**
29.4.2   Safety in the Postpartum period —— **449**
29.5   Conclusion —— **449**
            References —— **450**

Arieh Ingber
30   Specific Dermatoses of Pregnancy —— 453
30.1   Introduction —— **453**
30.2   Polymorphic Eruption of Pregnancy (PEP) —— **453**
30.2.1   Epidemiology —— **453**
30.2.2   Pathogenesis —— **453**

30.2.3   Clinical Presentation —— **454**
30.2.4   Laboratory Tests —— **454**
30.2.5   Histopathology —— **454**
30.2.6   Treatment —— **455**
30.2.7   Prognosis —— **455**
30.3   Pemphigoid Gestationis (PG) —— **455**
30.3.1   Epidemiology —— **455**
30.3.2   Pathogenesis —— **456**
30.3.3   Clinical Presentation —— **456**
30.3.4   Laboratory Tests —— **456**
30.3.5   Histopathology and Immunofluorescence —— **457**
30.3.6   Treatment —— **457**
30.3.7   Prognosis —— **457**
30.4   Impetigo Herpetiformis, also Known as Generalized Pustular
            Psoriasis of Pregnancy —— **458**
30.4.1   Nomenclature —— **458**
30.4.2   Epidemiology —— **458**
30.4.3   Pathogenesis —— **458**
30.4.4   Clinical Presentation —— **459**
30.4.5   Laboratory Investigations —— **459**
30.4.6   Histopathology —— **459**
30.4.7   Treatment —— **459**
30.4.8   Prognosis —— **460**
30.5   Prurigo of Pregnancy (Besnier) —— **460**
30.5.1   Epidemiology —— **460**
30.5.2   Clinical Presentation —— **460**
30.5.3   Laboratory Investigations —— **461**
30.5.4   Histopathology —— **461**
30.5.5   Treatment —— **461**
30.5.6   Prognosis —— **461**
30.6   Pruritic Folliculitis of Pregnancy —— **461**
30.6.1   Epidemiology —— **461**
30.6.2   Pathogenesis —— **462**
30.6.3   Clinical Presentation —— **462**
30.6.4   Laboratory Tests and Histopathology —— **462**
30.6.5   Treatment —— **462**
30.6.6   Prognosis —— **462**
30.7   Linear IgM Dermatosis of Pregnancy —— **463**
30.7.1   Pathogenesis —— **463**
30.7.2   Clinical Presentation —— **463**
30.7.3   Laboratory Tests —— **463**

30.7.4   Histopathology —— 464
30.7.5   Treatment —— 464
30.7.6   Prognosis —— 464
            References —— 464

Christoph Wohlmuth, Taymaa May
31   **Gynecologic Cancer in Pregnancy —— 469**
31.1   Introduction —— 469
31.2   Diagnosis —— 469
31.3   Surgery —— 471
31.4   Systemic Treatment —— 473
31.4.1   Chemotherapy in Pregnancy —— 473
31.4.2   Endocrine Therapy —— 477
31.4.3   Targeted Therapies and Biologic Agents —— 477
31.5   Radiation Therapy —— 477
31.6   Obstetric Management —— 477
31.7   Conclusion —— 478
            References —— 478

Evangelia Vlachodimitropoulou Koumoutsea, Cynthia Maxwell
32   **Maternal and Fetal Malignancies in Pregnancy —— 483**
32.1   Epidemiology —— 483
32.2   Diagnosing Cancer in Pregnancy —— 483
32.2.1   Imaging —— 484
32.2.2   Laboratory Markers —— 484
32.3   Specific Cancers in Pregnancy —— 484
32.3.1   Breast Cancer —— 484
32.3.2   Lymphoma and Leukemia —— 485
32.3.3   Melanoma —— 486
32.4   Targeted Therapies for Certain Malignancies in Pregnancy —— 487
32.4.1   Tamoxifen —— 487
32.4.2   Human Epidermal Growth Factor Receptor 2 (HER2) —— 488
32.4.3   Tyrosine Kinase Inhibitors —— 488
32.4.4   All-Trans Retinoid Acid (ATRA) —— 489
32.4.5   CAR T-Cell Therapy —— 489
32.5   Fetal Tumors —— 490
32.5.1   Sacrococcygeal Teratomas —— 490
32.5.2   Neck Teratomas —— 490
32.6   Counseling for This and Future Pregnancy —— 491

32.7   Conclusion —— **492**
            References —— **493**

Index —— **497**

List of Contributors

Chapter 1
Shital Gandhi
Associate Professor, Medicine
University of Toronto
Canada
shital.gandhi@sinaihealth.ca

Dan Farine
Professor, Obstetrics and Gynecology
University of Toronto
Canada
dfarine@sympatico.ca

Chapter 2
Gideon Koren
Professor, Medicine
Ariel University and Motherisk Israel
Israel
gidiup_2000@yahoo.com

Gali Pariente
Obstetrics and Gynecology
Soroka University Medical Center
Israel
galipa@bgu.ac.il

Chapter 3
Siobhan Bacon
Consultant Endocrinologist
Sligo University Hospital
Ireland
siobhanbacon@gmail.com

Ann McNamara
Consultant Radiologist
Sligo University Hospital
Ireland
ann.mcnamara1@hse.ie

Chapter 4
Jennifer Yo
Department of Nephrology
Monash University
Australia
jennifer.yo@monashhealth.ca

Shital Gandhi
Associate Professor, Medicine
University of Toronto
Canada
shital.gandhi@sinaihealth.ca

Chapter 5
Laura Berall
Consultant Nephrologist
Humber Regional Hospital
Canada
lberall@hrh.ca

Michelle Hladunewich
Professor of Medicine
University of Toronto
Canada
michelle.hladunewich@sunnybrook.ca

Chapter 6
Kelsey McLaughlin
Research Associate, Obstetrics and
Gynecology
University of Toronto
Canada
kelsey.mclaughlin@mail.utoronto.ca

Melanie C. Audette
Resident physician, Obstetrics and
Gynecology
University of Toronto
Canada
m.audette@mail.utoronto.ca

Sebastian R. Hobson
Assistant Professor, Obstetrics and
Gynecology
University of Toronto
Canada
sebastian.hobson@sinaihealth.ca

John C. Kingdom
Professor, Obstetrics and Gynecology
University of Toronto
Canada
john.kingdom@sinaihealth.ca

https://doi.org/10.1515/9783110615258-203

Chapter 7
Eyal Sheiner
Professor, Obstetrics and Gynecoloy
Ben Gurion University
Israel
sheiner@bgu.ac.il

Omri Zamstein
Resident physician, Obstetrics and
Gynecology
Ben Gurion University
Israel
omrizam9@gmail.com

Chapter 8
Harrison Banner
Assistant Professor, Obstetrics and
Gynecology
Western University
Canada
harrison.banner@lhsc.on.ca

Jack Colman
Professor, Medicine
University of Toronto
Canada
jack.colman@sinaihealth.ca

Mathew Sermer
Professor, Obtetrics and Gyneolcogy
University of Toronto
Canada
mathew.sermer@sinaihealth.ca

Chapter 9
Rachel Wald
Associate Professor, Medicine
University of Toronto
Canada
rachel.wald@uhn.ca

Emilie Laflamme
Lecturer, Cardiology
Laval University
Canada
emilie.laflamme@uhn.ca

Chapter 10
Stephen Lapinsky
Professor, Medicine
University of Toronto
Canada
stephen.lapinsky@utoronto.ca

Stephanie Lapinsky
Resident physician, Obstetrics and
Gynecology
University of Toronto
Canada
stephanie.lapinsky@mail.utoronto.ca

Chapter 11
Mohamed Momtaz
Professor, Obstetrics and Gynecology
Cairo University
Egypt
momtaz@hotmail.com

Dina Refaat
Advanced Obstetrics Fellow,
Obstetrics and Gynecology
University of Toronto
Canada
dinadakhly@gmail.com

Chapter 12
Alexander Makatsariya
Professor, Obstetrics and Gynecology
Sechenov University
Russia
gemostasis@mail.ru

Sam Shulman
Professor, Medicine
McMaster University
Canada
schulms@mcmaster.ca

Chapter 13
John Granton
Professor, Medicine
University of Toronto
Canada
john.granton@uhn.ca

Shaun Yo
Consultant Respirologist
Monash University
Australia
shaun.w.yo@gmail.com

Chapter 14
Meyer Balter
Professor, Medicine
University of Toronto
Canada
meyer.balter@sinaihealth.ca

Alina Blazer
Clinical Fellow, Respirology
University of Toronto
Canada
alina.blazer@gmail.com

Chapter 15
Loic Sentilhes
Professor, Obstetrics and Gynecology
Bordeaux University
France
loicsentilhes@hotmail.com

Hanane Bouchghoul
Obstetrics and gynecology
Bordeaux University
France
hanane.bouchghoul@chu-bordeaux.fr

Aurélien Mattuizzi
Obstetrics and Gynecology
Bordeaux University
France
aurelien.mattuizzi@chu-bordeaux.fr

Alizee Froeliger
Obstetrics and Gynecology
Bordeaux University
France
alizee.froeliger@chu-bordeaux.fr

Hugo Madar
Obstetrics and Gynecology
Bordeaux University
France
hugo.madar@chu-bordeaux.fr

Chapter 16
Nadine Shehata
Associate Professor, Medicine
University of Toronto
Canada
nadine.shehata@sinaihealth.ca

Dongmei Sun
Associate Professor, Medicine
Western University
Canada
dongmei.sun@outlook.com

Chapter 17
Ann Kinga Malinowski
Associate Professor, Obstetrics and
Gynecology
University of Toronto
Canada
ann.malinowski@sinaihealthsystem.ca

Emily Delpero
Clinical Fellow, Obstetrics and Gynecology
University of Toronto
Canada
emily.delpero@mail.utoronto.ca

Chapter 18
Mark Yudin
Professor, Obstetrics and Gynecology
University of Toronto
Canada
mark.yudin@unityhealth.to

Kristin Harris
Assistant Professor, Obstetrics and
Gynecology
University of Toronto
Canada
kristin.harris@mail.utoronto.ca

Chapter 19
Yoav Yinon
Associate Professor, Obstetrics and
Gynecology
Tel-Aviv University
Israel
yoav.yinon27@gmail.com

Moran Shapiro
Resident Physician, Obstetrics and
Gynecology
Tel-Aviv University
Israel
shapira.moran@gmail.com

Chapter 20
Yves Ville
Professor, Obstetrics and Gynecology
Paris Descartes University
France
ville.yves@gmail.com

Valentine Faure Bardon
Obstetrics and Gynecology
Paris Descartes University
France
valentine.faure@aphp.fr

Chapter 21
Daniela Vasquez
Associate Professor, Medicine
University of Buenos Aires
Argentina
daniela.vasquez@alumni.utoronto.ca

Maria-Teresa Perez
Editor
Argentina
tereperez1970@gmail.com

Chapter 22
Diogo Ayres-de-Campos
Associate Professor, Obstetrics and
Gynecology
University of Lisbon
Portugal
dayresdecampos@gmail.com

Monica Centeno
Invited Lecturer
University of Lisbon
Portugal
monica.castro.centeno@gmail.com

Chapter 23
Denice Feig
Professor, Medicine
University of Toronto
Canada
denicefeig@gmail.com

Sawyer Huget-Penner
Consulting Endocrinologist
Fraser Health
Canada
sawyerhp@gmail.com

Chapter 24
Yariv Yogev
Professor, Obstetrics and Gynecology
Tel Aviv University
Israel
yarivyogev@hotmail.com

Maya Ram
Obstetrics and Gynecology
Tel Aviv Medical Centre
maya3000@gmail.com

Chapter 25
Cynthia Maxwell
Professor, Obstetrics and Gynecology
University of Toronto
Canada
cynthiadr.maxwell@sinaihealth.ca

Haitham Baghlaf
Clinical Fellow, Maternal Fetal Medicine
University of Toronto
haitham.baghlaf@sinaihealth.ca

Chapter 26
Geoffrey Nguyen
Professor, Medicine
University of Toronto
Canada
geoffrey.nguyen@sinaihealthsystem.ca

Vivian Huang
Assistant Professor, Medicine
University of Toronto
Canada
vivian.huang@sinaihealth.ca

Chapter 27
John Snelgrove
Assistant Professor, Obstetrics and
Gynecology
University of Toronto
Canada
john.snelgrove@sinaihealth.ca

Homero Flores-Mendoza
Clinical Fellow, Maternal Fetal Medicine
University of Toronto
Canada
homero.floresmendoza@sinaihealth.ca

Harrison Banner
Assistant Professor, Obstetrics and
Gynecology
Western University
Canada
harrison.banner@sinaihealth.ca

Chapter 28
Carl Laskin
Associate Professor, Medicine
University of Toronto
Canada
calaskin@gmail.com

Ghaydaa Aldabie
Clinical Fellow, Rheumatology
University of Toronto
Canada
dr.ghaydaa@icloud.com

Karen Spitzer
Research coordinator
Trio Fertility
Canada
kspitzer@triofertility.com

Chapter 29
Esther Bui
Assistant Professor, Medicine
University of Toronto
Canada
esther.bui@uhn.ca

Tadeau Fantaneau
Assistant Professor, Medicine
University of Ottawa
Canada
tad.fantaneanu@gmail.com

Chapter 30
Arieh Ingbar
Professor, Medicine
Hebrew University Israel
Israel
arieh@hadassah.org.il

Chapter 31
Christoph Wohlmuth
Clinical Fellow, Obstetrics and Gynecology
University of Toronto
Canada
christoph.wohlmuth@uhn.ca

Taymaa May
Associate Professor, Obstetrics and
Gynecology
University of Toronto
Canada
taymaa.may@uhn.ca

Chapter 32
Cynthia Maxwell
Professor, Obstetrics and Gynecology
University of Toronto
Canada
cynthiadr.maxwell@sinaihealth.ca

Evangelia Koumoutsea
Clinical Fellow, Maternal Fetal Medicine
Unviersity of Toronto
Canada
evangelia.koumoutsea.11@alumni.ucl.ac.uk

Shital Gandhi, Dan Farine

1 Introduction

1.1 What Is Obstetric Medicine?

Pregnancy is a state of impressive physiologic changes in the body. These changes affect virtually every organ system. Hence, it can be challenging to differentiate between symptoms that are normal for pregnancy versus the development of a superimposed new medical condition. In some cases, women enter into pregnancy with preexisting medical conditions, and so health-care providers need to have an understanding of how pregnancy will affect health in the short-term view of pregnancy, as well as predicting the potential risk of undertaking pregnancy on future health. Finally, health-care providers need to have working knowledge of safety of diagnostic imaging, as well as safety and efficacy of pharmacologic interventions.

Obstetric medicine (OM) is a new field of medicine that meets the evolving need of managing medical issues as they occur in pregnant women. It is perfectly situated at the intersection of obstetrics, internal medicine, subspecialties of internal medicine, primary care, and the allied health disciplines. Health-care providers from all disciplines who are interested in developing expertise in the medical care of pregnant women will benefit from the medical knowledge that is gathered under the umbrella term of OM. "Obstetric internists" are medical physicians who have pursued advanced training in applying their medical knowledge to the pregnant individual. Globally, there are now an increasing number of such specialists, with the development of national and international societies, as well as a medical journal.

The authors in this book reflect the unique mix of general internists, subspecialists of medicine, and experts in maternal–fetal medicine (MFM) that are often brought together to manage patients with complex medical conditions. Each chapter typically addresses the following questions:

1. How does pregnancy affect the underlying medical condition and health of the individual?
2. How does the underlying medical condition impact pregnancy (and fetal) outcomes?
3. Are there any pharmacologic changes necessary?
4. Are there any special considerations necessary for the labor and delivery process, and postpartum?

It is our hope that this resource will be of use to health-care providers dedicated to the management of medical disorders in pregnancy, leading to the skilled care of pregnant individuals.

Shital Gandhi

https://doi.org/10.1515/9783110615258-001

1.2 Why Obstetric Medicine?

In contrast to just needing to have a sound basis in medicine, my subspecialty of Maternal Fetal Medicine (MFM) is residing at the forefront of obstetrics. We are consulted by obstetricians, family doctors, and midwives and are supposed are expected to be in a variety of areas. Three of these areas have evolved into recognized subspecialties: perinatal genetics, fetal medicine, and maternal medicine. The set of skills for each one is different, but generally an MFM specialist has to be very familiar with all three. The set of skills required includes (1) solid clinical acumen, including the care of patients in acute care units; (2) knowledge of fetal anatomy and pathology plus the use of ultrasound (and at times MRI) to evaluate fetal pathology; (3) up-to-date knowledge of genetics in order to perform proper and current genetic diagnosis. All these fields expand exponentially, and there are more than 40,000 relevant papers per year. In addition, obstetrics/gynecology is a surgical discipline. Fetal surgeons have a special set of skills, needing practice, and requiring them to be in the operating room for hours at the time. The perinatologist needs to have working relationships with many specialties and subspecialties. In order to take care of maternal diseases, one needs to be able to understand and to deal with internists and practically all subspecialties of medicine. Neonatology is consulted on essentially all the difficult maternal and fetal cases to plan perinatal care and decide on optimal time of delivery. There is a similar link to most pediatric specialties so the care of the baby is not compromised. In addition, interactions with the pregnant individual have undergone drastic changes recently. Women now have easy access to more information via the internet and social media; at times it can lead them to wrong decisions (e.g., a demand for termination of the pregnancy when the woman and child are relatively well). Usually, they have the right inclination but at times the literature they present to clinicians (as opposed to the usual opposite way) requires extensive discussions. I once had a patient who was upset because I was not aware of a publication she read, although I could discuss the other ten I have read. These issues create pressure in a variety of ways: less than optimal time for reading and updates, pressure on time spent with patients, and the need to be very familiar with practically all specialties and subspecialties.

So why OM? There are a multitude of reasons:
- I usually do not go to Medical Grand Rounds, meetings, or symposia. My colleagues from OM do so, as their primary training is in internal medicine. Their exposure to complex medical issues is often more extensive than ours and our patients benefit from that knowledge.
- Obstetrical patients are often different from those on the internal medicine wards. Our colleagues in OM are aware of pregnancy-related alterations to physiology and incorporate that into the diagnostic and management plans.
- In the past, we often consulted several subspecialists. As you all know, when four physicians are involved, there could be as many as five opinions! The use

of OM allows us to reduce the number of specialties we need to consult and the OM specialists often coordinate the care of the other specialties.

–   Working with the same person(s) on a regular basis allows for better communication among health-care providers as often we have been there before.
–   The patients love the collaboration with one internist (and his/her team). It is also easier when I am told by the patent and/or the family that Dr. Gandhi told them exactly the same thing. If we find that we sing different songs, we have to resolve that as soon as possible.
–   There are OM clinics that can follow the medical issue throughout the pregnancy. The best example is the management of hypertension in pregnancy.
–   Obstetricians and MFM specialist limit their span of care to the duration of pregnancy and 6 weeks postpartum. OM specialists do not and they can follow the patient after the pregnancy.

Those of you who work with OM specialists know that I am right. For those of you who do not, I strongly suggest to give it a try.

Dan Farine

Gali Pariente, Gideon Koren

2 Approach to Safe Use of Medications in Pregnancy

2.1 Introduction

Pregnant women are exposed to a variety of medications that may exert toxic or teratogenic effects. Since the thalidomide disaster in the 1960s, some physicians and pregnant women tend to withhold any medication during pregnancy, although the risk of teratogenic effect from most drugs in therapeutic doses is unproven. Major congenital defects occur in 1–3% of the general population [1]. Of the major defects, about 25% are of genetic origin (genetically inherited diseases, new mutations, and chromosomal abnormalities) and 65% are of unknown etiology (multifactorial, polygenic, spontaneous errors of development and synergistic interactions of teratogens). Only 2–3% of malformations are thought to be associated with drug treatment. The remaining defects are related to other environmental exposures including infectious agents, maternal disease states, mechanical problems, and irradiation [2, 3].

Optimal prescribing in pregnancy is a challenge and should provide maximal safety to the fetus while ensuring therapeutic benefits to the mother. To date, very few drugs are proven teratogens in humans. However, drug-induced malformations are important because they are potentially preventable.

2.2 Medication Use in Pregnancy

Presently, pregnant women frequently take a variety of medications during pregnancy, including prescription and over-the-counter (OTC) agents [4, 5]. During the last three decades, studies have reported a rise in the average number of medications (prescription and nonprescription) used per woman during the first trimester from 1.6 to 2.6 [6]. More recently, from 2006 to 2008, over 80% of women reported using at least one medication during the first trimester and over 90% reported using at least one medication at any point during their pregnancy [6]. Other studies have demonstrated increased rates of use of various OTC medications in the first, second, or third trimesters of pregnancy [7]. While some studies found that the proportion of women receiving at least one prescription medicine increased from the first to third trimester of pregnancy [8, 9], others found that rates of prescription drug use were highest in the first trimester of pregnancy [4, 10]. The most common medications used in pregnancy are nonprescription or OTC medications [7]. A longitudinal study aimed at identifying the medications that are mostly consumed during pregnancy demonstrated that 95.8% of participants took prescription medications, 92.6% self-medicated with OTC

https://doi.org/10.1515/9783110615258-002

medications, and 45.2% used herbal medications. Over time, consumption of OTC medications exceeded prescription medication use [5].

Since the 1960s, a long-term trend of childbearing at an older age has been observed in the United States, such that contemporary birth rates for women aged over 30 years of age are at their highest level [11]. Moreover, over the past few decades, there has been a growing trend of postponing family planning and childbearing to the fifth and even sixth decades of life [12]. These changes are more noticeable in developed countries [13], owing to increasing life expectancy and the widespread use of artificial reproductive technology, including oocyte donation, which makes it possible for postmenopausal women to conceive [14, 15]. The current trend of women to delay childbearing to an older age [16] and the frequency of medical conditions seen during pregnancy among older women, which is dramatically greater than that of younger women [17], result in the reported rise in the use of medications during pregnancy demonstrated in recent studies.

2.3 Teratogenicity

To be considered teratogenic, a candidate substance or process should (1) result in a characteristic set of malformations, indicating selectivity for certain target organs; (2) exert its effects at a particular stage of fetal development, for example, during the limited time period of organogenesis of the target organs; and (3) show a dose-dependent incidence.

2.3.1 Timing of Exposure

The importance of timing of drug exposure has well been documented over the years; the effect produced by a teratogenic agent depends upon the developmental stage in which the conceptus is exposed. Several important phases in human development are recognized [3]:

The "all or none" period is defined as the time from conception until somite formation, which corresponds to the first 17 days after conception. Insults to the embryo in this phase are likely to result in either death and miscarriage, or intact survival. The embryo is undifferentiated, and repair and recovery are possible through multiplication of the still totipotential cells. Consider that exposure to teratogens during the pre-somatic stage usually does not cause congenital malformations unless the agent persists in the body beyond this period [3, 18].

The embryonic period is defined as the time from 18 to 60 days after conception, when the basic steps in organogenesis occur. This is the period of maximum sensitivity to teratogenicity since tissues are differentiating rapidly and damage becomes irreparable. Exposure to teratogenic agents during this period has the greatest likelihood of causing a structural anomaly. The pattern of anomalies produced depends on which systems are differentiating at the time of teratogenic exposure.

The fetal phase is defined as the time from the end of the embryonic stage to term, when growth and functional maturation of formed organs and systems occur. Teratogen exposure in this period will affect fetal growth (e.g., intrauterine growth restriction) and the size or function of an organ, rather than causing gross structural anomalies. The term fetal toxicity is commonly used to describe such an effect.

Long-term effect is the potential effect of psychoactive agents (e.g., antidepressants, antiepileptics, alcohol, and other drugs of abuse) on the developing central nervous system (CNS) which led to the new field of behavioral teratology. In addition, many organ systems continue structural and functional maturation long after birth. Most of the adenocarcinomas associated with first-trimester exposure to diethylstilbestrol occurred many years later.

2.3.2 Teratogenic Mechanisms

The mechanisms by which different drugs exert teratogenic effects are poorly understood and are probably multifactorial. For example, drugs may have a direct effect on maternal tissues with secondary or indirect effects on fetal tissues. Drugs may interfere with the passage of oxygen or nutrients through the placenta and therefore have effects on the most rapidly metabolizing tissues of the fetus. Finally, drugs may have important direct actions on the processes of differentiation in developing tissues [19]. For example, vitamin A (retinol) has been shown to have important differentiation-directing actions in normal tissues. Several vitamin A analogs (isotretinoin and etretinate) are powerful teratogens, suggesting that they alter the normal processes of differentiation [20]. Lastly, deficiency of a critical substance appears to play a role in some types of abnormalities. For example, folic acid supplementation during pregnancy appears to reduce the incidence of neural tube defects [21].

Continued exposure to a teratogen may produce cumulative effects or may affect several organs going through varying stages of development. Chronic consumption of high doses of ethanol during pregnancy, particularly during the first and second trimesters, may result in the fetal alcohol spectrum disorder. In this syndrome, the CNS, growth, and facial development may be affected [22].

2.3.3 Labeling Requirements

The FDA implemented new labeling requirements for pregnancy and breastfeeding for all new drug submissions in the United States as of June 30, 2015. The new format removes the letter-based categorization of risk system (A, B, C, D, X) and provides more complete information pertaining to assessing risk versus benefit of medication use in pregnancy and breastfeeding and in males and females of reproductive potential. Labeling changes for medications submitted on or after June 30, 2001, will be phased in gradually. Medications approved prior to June 30, 2001, will be required to remove the letter category before June 30, 2018, but are not subject to the new narrative labeling requirements. Labeling for nonprescription medications is not affected [23]. Some manufacturers may decide to also follow these FDA labeling requirements in their Canadian product monographs.

2.4 Drug Pharmacokinetics

Most drugs taken by pregnant women can cross the placenta and expose the developing embryo and fetus to their pharmacologic and teratogenic effects. Two critical factors may affect drug impact on the fetus: the mother and the placenta.

2.4.1 Pregnancy-Induced Pharmacokinetic (PK) Changes of Drugs

Most organ systems are affected by substantial anatomical and physiological changes during pregnancy. Such pregnancy-related changes include increased total body water and plasma volume and decreased concentrations of drug-binding proteins (affecting the apparent volume of distribution and clearance rates), decreased gastrointestinal motility and increased gastric pH (impacting absorption), and increased glomerular filtration rate and changes in activity of drug-metabolizing enzymes in the liver (affecting renal and hepatic clearance) [24, 25]. Overall, these changes in physiological indices take place progressively during gestation. The decrease in plasma albumin concentration and altered activity of drug-metabolizing enzymes, together with the increases in total body water, fat compartment, cardiac output, and glomerular filtration rate, are all reported to peak during the third trimester [24, 26].

For some drug classes, many pharmacokinetic (PK) clinical trials during pregnancy have been conducted. However, for most drugs used during pregnancy, there is little or no information available regarding PK changes or dosage requirements during pregnancy. Moreover, it is often unclear if observed PK changes lead to alterations in drug efficacy and/or adverse effect profiles. In their systematic review of the literature, Pariente et al. methodically identified all existing evidence of PK changes of all drugs during pregnancy in the context of clinical significance [27]. All publications of clinical PK studies involving a group of pregnant women with a comparison to nonpregnant participants or nonpregnant population data were eligible to be included in this review. A total of 198 studies involving 121 different medications fulfilled the inclusion criteria. In these studies, commonly investigated drug classes included antiretrovirals (54 studies), antiepileptic drugs (27 studies), antibiotics (23 studies), antimalarial drugs (22 studies), and cardiovascular drugs (17 studies). Reviewed studies were found to vary widely in both design and quality. There were some differences in the stages of pregnancy in which the women were investigated; while some studies reported results from both the second and the third trimesters together, most of the studies provided third trimester results, and a few reported results from all trimesters together or separately. Changes such as reduced half-life, increased clearance rate, and reduced area under the curve in pregnancy have been described for many drugs. These PK changes generally lead to lower drug concentrations in plasma, decreasing maternal target exposure to drug molecules. Nevertheless, the literature review demonstrated a paucity of clinically useful data on whether dose adjustment is necessary for these PK changes.

2.4.2 Placental Drug Transfer

Teratogens must reach the developing conceptus in sufficient amounts to exert their effects. Large molecules with a molecular weight greater than 1,000 (e.g., heparin) do not cross the placenta into the embryonic–fetal bloodstream. Other factors influencing the rate and extent of placental transfer of drugs include protein binding, polarity, lipid solubility, and the existence of specific carrier proteins which may actively eject drugs from the fetus to the mother and placental and fetal drug metabolism.

2.5 Drug Pharmacodynamics

2.5.1 Maternal Drug Actions

The effects of drugs on the reproductive tissues (breast, uterus, etc.) of the pregnant woman are sometimes altered by the endocrine environment appropriate for the stage of pregnancy. Drug effects on other maternal tissues (heart, lungs, kidneys, CNS, etc.) are not changed significantly by pregnancy, although the physiologic context (cardiac output, renal blood flow, etc.) may be altered, requiring the use of drugs that are not needed by the same woman when she is not pregnant. For example, cardiac glycosides and diuretics may be needed for heart failure precipitated by the increased cardiac workload of pregnancy [28], or insulin may be required for control of blood glucose in pregnancy-induced diabetes [29].

2.5.2 Drugs of Choice

The drug of choice is defined as a therapeutic agent that is regarded as being the best to use when treating a particular condition (see Table 2.1). When discussing conditions during pregnancy which require drug treatment, the drug of choice will be a combination of effectiveness to the mother and safety to the fetus.

Table 2.1: Drug of choice during pregnancy [30].

System	Disorder	Drug of choice	Remarks
Cardiovascular	Hypertension	Methyldopa and hydralazine	Alternative: beta blockers – need to monitor fetal growth and newborn for hypoglycemia, bradycardia, and hypotension for first 24–48 h. Calcium channel blockers can be used.
	Anticoagulation	Heparin or low-molecular-weight heparin	Safe, effective. Do not cross the placenta and do not cause fetal anticoagulation.
Respiratory	Asthma	Inhaled bronchodilators: salbutamol, ipratropium bromide, and terbutaline; Inhaled corticosteroids: fluticasone, budesonide, and beclomethasone.	In more severe cases, systemic corticosteroids should be used. Monitor fetal growth and maternal hyperglycemia
	Cough	In cases of allergic rhinitis: antihistamines. Codeine if indicated.	Due to risk of neonatal opioid withdrawal, avoid high doses of codeine near term.
Neuropsychiatric	Anxiety	Benzodiazepines (short-acting lorazepam or oxazepam) for short-term treatment; SSRIs: citalopram, fluoxetine, and sertraline for long-term treatment.	When taken close to term possibility for transient neonatal effect; A questionable small increase in incidence of oral clefts with first trimester use of diazepam.
	Bipolar disorder	Lamotrigine and quetiapine	Lithium is an effective alternative; need to monitor using fetal echocardiography.

Table 2.1 (continued)

System	Disorder	Drug of choice	Remarks
	Depression	Citalopram, fluoxetine, sertraline, and tricyclic antidepressants	A questionable increase in the risk of cardiac malformations observed in some studies, mainly with paroxetine. These are possibly associated with the underlying psychiatric disorder and confounding variables; Neonatal withdrawal may occur when used in third trimester.
	Schizophrenia	Quetiapine, aripiprazole, phenothiazines, and olanzapine	Monitor the woman for metabolic complications (weight gain, hyperglycemia, and hyperlipidemia), especially with second-generation antipsychotics; Watch neonate for possible adverse effects if taken close to term.
	Epilepsy	Lamotrigine, carbamazepine, and levetiracetam	The drug of choice for epilepsy in pregnancy should be the drug that best controls the seizures; monotherapy should be favored. Use the lowest effective dose; Avoid valproic acid when possible, especially in the first trimester. If not possible to avoid, limit dose to <600–1,000 mg/day; With carbamazepine and valproic acid, prescribe peri-conceptual folate supplementation: 5 mg daily po, ideally starting 3 months before trying to conceive and continuing at least until the end of the first trimester.

Table 2.1 (continued)

System	Disorder	Drug of choice	Remarks
	Migraine	Acetaminophen	Other alternatives: NSAIDs and sumatriptan. Avoid NSAIDs in third trimester due to the risk of oligohydramnios and premature closure of ductus arteriosus.
Infection	Bacterial infection	Cephalosporins, clindamycin, erythromycin, and penicillins	Alternatives: aminoglycosides (amikacin, gentamicin, tobramycin), azithromycin, clarithromycin, and quinolones
	Herpetic infection	Acyclovir and valacyclovir	
	Vaginal candidiasis	Vaginal: clotrimazole, miconazole, nystatin Topical azoles are preferred	Alternative: fluconazole single systemic dose of 150 mg.
Gastrointestinal	Diarrhea	Bulk-forming agents (e.g., methylcellulose and psyllium hydrophilic mucilloid)	
	Dyspepsia	Alginic acid compound, antacids (various combinations of aluminum, calcium, and magnesium salts), omeprazole, and ranitidine. Famotidine can also be used.	
	Hemorrhoids	Topical hydrocortisone/ pramoxinetopical lidocaine, topical zinc oxide	
Endocrine	Diabetes mellitus	Insulin Metformin	Strict glycemic control should be achieved before conception and during the first trimester to avoid early pregnancy losses and congenital malformations due to hyperglycemia.

2.6 Therapeutic Drug Actions in the Fetus

Fetal therapeutics is an emerging area in perinatal pharmacology. This involves drug administration, mostly to the pregnant woman, with the fetus as the target for the drug. At present, corticosteroids are used to stimulate fetal lung maturation when preterm birth is expected [31]. Antiarrhythmic drugs have also been given to mothers for treatment of fetal cardiac arrhythmias. Although their efficacy has not yet been established by controlled studies, digoxin, flecainide, procainamide, verapamil, and other antiarrhythmic agents have been shown to be effective in treating fetal arrhythmia [32]. Similarly, it has been shown that maternal use of zidovudine and other HIV drugs substantially decreases transmission of HIV from the mother to the fetus, and use of combinations of three antiretroviral agents can eliminate fetal infection almost entirely [33].

2.7 Proven Teratogenic Drugs in Humans

The following drugs have been extensively studied and were proven with sufficient evidence to have a teratogenic effect in humans [30]. An alternative drug should be used if possible.

2.7.1 Drugs for Cardiovascular Disorders

Angiotensin-converting enzyme inhibitors (ACEIs) and angiotensin II antagonists: Adverse effects relate to hemodynamic effects of ACEIs and angiotensin II antagonists on the fetus. In late pregnancy, ACEI fetopathy includes intrauterine renal insufficiency, neonatal hypotension, oliguria with renal failure, hyperkalemia, complications of oligohydramnios (fetal limb contractures, lung hypoplasia, and craniofacial anomalies), prematurity, intrauterine growth restriction, and fetal death. Regarding first-trimester exposure, the teratogenic risk is questionable of cardiovascular and CNS malformations. Several cohort studies and meta-analyses suggest that the observed risk is associated with the underlying maternal conditions.

Coumarin anticoagulants: First-trimester exposure (6–9 weeks gestation) is associated with fetal warfarin syndrome (nasal hypoplasia and calcific stippling of the epiphyses). Intrauterine growth restriction and developmental delay (CNS damage), eye defects, and hearing loss have also been demonstrated in many studies. Warfarin embryopathy is found in up to one third of the cases where a coumarin derivative was given throughout pregnancy. Coumarin use is also associated with high rate of miscarriage and risk of CNS damage due to hemorrhage if used after the first trimester.

2.7.2 Drugs for Neurological Disorders

Carbamazepine: First-trimester exposure is associated with 1% risk of neural tube defects (10× baseline risk) and an increased risk of cardiovascular malformations. A pattern of malformations similar to the fetal hydantoin syndrome has also been demonstrated.

Hydantoin: Fetal hydantoin syndrome includes craniofacial dysmorphology, anomalies and hypoplasia of distal phalanges and nails, growth restriction, mental deficiency, and cardiac defects.

Valproic acid: First-trimester exposure has been associated with neural tube defects with 1–2% risk of meningomyelocele, primarily lumbar or lumbosacral, cardiovascular malformations, and hypospadias. Fetal valproate syndrome has been delineated by some investigations and includes craniofacial dysmorphology, cardiovascular defects, long fingers and toes, hyperconvex fingernails, and cleft lip. Valproic acid is also a neurobehavioral teratogen.

2.7.3 Drugs of abuse

Ethanol: Fetal alcohol spectrum disorders include four diagnostic categories: fetal alcohol syndrome (FAS), partial FAS, alcohol-related neurodevelopmental disorders, and alcohol-related birth defects. FAS presents as growth impairment, developmental delay, and dysmorphic facies. Cleft palate and cardiac anomalies may occur. Full expression of the syndrome occurs with chronic daily ingestion of 2 g alcohol per kg (8 drinks/day) in about one-third of offspring and partial effects in three-quarters of offspring. Alcohol-related neurodevelopmental disorders are much more common than FAS.

Cocaine: Cocaine abuse has been associated with occurrence of placental abruption, prematurity, fetal loss, decreased birth weight, microcephaly, limb defects, urinary tract malformations, and poorer neurodevelopmental performance. Methodological problems make the findings difficult to interpret. Cocaine abuse is often associated with polydrug abuse, alcohol consumption, smoking, malnutrition, and poor prenatal care. Human epidemiology suggests that cocaine itself is not a gross structural teratogen.

2.7.4 Drugs used for Infection and Inflammation

Tetracycline: Exposure after 17 weeks gestation, when deciduous teeth begin to calcify, has been associated with discoloration of the teeth. Closer to term crowns of permanent teeth may be stained. Oxytetracycline and doxycycline have been associated with a lower incidence of enamel staining.

Folic acid antagonists – aminopterin and methotrexate: Fetal aminopterin–methotrexate syndrome includes CNS defects, craniofacial anomalies, abnormal cranial ossification, abnormalities in first branchial arch derivatives, intrauterine growth restriction, and mental retardation after first-trimester exposure. Maternal dose of methotrexate needed to induce defects is probably above 10 mg/week.

2.7.5 Drugs for Nausea and Vomiting

Thalidomide: Malformations are limited to tissues of mesodermal origin, primarily limbs (reduction defects), ears, cardiovascular system, and gut musculature. The critical period of exposure is 34–50 days after the beginning of the last menstrual period. A single dose of <1 mg/kg has produced the syndrome. Embryopathy is found in about 20% of pregnancies exposed in the critical period.

Diethylstilbestrol: Vaginal clear cell adenocarcinoma has been demonstrated in offspring exposed in utero before 18th week (>90% of the cancers occurred after 14 years of age). High incidence of benign vaginal adenosis has also been shown. There were increased miscarriage rate and preterm delivery. In males exposed in utero , there were no signs of malignancy, but genital lesions were seen in 27% and pathologic changes in spermatozoa in 29%. The drug is not currently available.

2.7.6 Other Drugs

Antineoplastic agents: A significant increase in the incidence of various fetal malformations and early miscarriages occurred following first-trimester exposure.

Misoprostol: First-trimester exposure has been associated with limb defects, Moebius sequence (a congenital facial palsy with impairment of ocular abduction, as a result of dysfunction of cranial nerves VI and VII), and CNS injuries. Absolute teratogenic risk is 1–2%. Uterine contraction inducing activity may cause vascular disruption defects.

Mycophenolate mofetil: First-trimester exposure: ear, eye, and craniofacial malformations, oral clefts, and cardiac, finger, urogenital, gastrointestinal, CNS, and skeletal malformations.

Retinoic acid: Systemic exposure has been shown to be a potent human general and behavioral teratogen. Risk of retinoic acid embryopathy involves craniofacial anomalies, cardiac defects, abnormalities in thymic development, and alterations in CNS development (congenital anomalies in 28% of prospectively ascertained pregnancies that resulted in births). Risk for associated miscarriage is 40%.

2.8 Drugs in Normal Labor and Delivery

The World Health Organization (WHO) defines normal birth as "spontaneous in onset, low-risk at the start of labor and remaining so throughout labor and delivery. The infant is born spontaneously in the vertex position between 37 and 42 completed weeks of pregnancy. After birth, mother and infant are in good condition" [34].

We will discuss the fetal safety perspective of some common drugs used in labor and delivery. Yet, it should be noted that many of the treatment options and usual management of normal delivery have not been studied in clinical trials or the data from clinical trials are insufficient for making strong recommendations regarding the actual management, including medications that are used for pain or augmentation in the setting of labor and delivery. Therefore, the use of these medications during labor and delivery is based upon clinical experience, data from observational studies, and expert opinion [35].

2.8.1 Pharmacologic Management of Pain During Labor and Delivery

Pharmacologic approaches to manage childbirth pain can be broadly classified as either systemic or regional. Systemic administration includes the intravenous, intramuscular, and inhalation routes. Regional analgesic techniques (neuraxial) consist of epidurals, spinals, and combined spinal–epidurals, and are the most popular modalities for analgesia for childbirth (see Table 2.2).

2.8.2 Drugs for Management of Labor Protraction or Arrest Disorders

The Friedman curve [43], the gold standard for rates of cervical dilation and fetal descent during active labor developed 50 years ago, and the norms established from Friedman's data historically had been widely accepted as the standard for assessment of normal labor progression. However, Zhang et al. [44] have proposed a contemporary curve and norms that are different and slower from those cited by Friedman. Labor abnormalities may be related to hypocontractile uterine activity, neuraxial anesthesia, and/or absolute or relative obstruction due to factors such as fetal size/position, or a small maternal bony pelvis. The normal duration of the

Table 2.2: Safety of medications for analgesia during labor and delivery.

Type of analgesia	Medication	Safety
Neuraxial analgesia	Bupivacaine [36, 37]	Systemic bupivacaine treatment of pregnant rats and rabbits interfered with embryo development. This dosing scenario did not represent typical clinical use. Use of bupivacaine for epidural analgesia has been reported without adverse effects.
	Fentanyl [38, 39]	Administration of fentanyl prior to delivery might be associated with neonatal depression. Adverse neonatal effects have also been reported after intravenous or epidural injection of fentanyl, but some investigators have reported not finding detectable neonatal effects after combined spinal epidural analgesia using fentanyl and bupivacaine.
Systemic analgesia	Morphine [40]	Morphine administration to women in labor can be associated with neonatal respiratory depression. Although this effect can occur after administration of any opioid, morphine is believed, based on reports from the 1950s and 1960s, to be more likely to be associated with respiratory depression in the neonate than is meperidine.
	Meperidine [41]	The ability of meperidine to produce respiratory depression and abnormalities in fetal heart tracings at parturition has been noted in a number of reports. The magnitude of these effects will vary with the timing and dose. It is most likely to have observable effects on a neonate when maternal administration occurs between 1 and 4 h before delivery.
	Promethazine [42]	There were conflicting reports on the incidence of neonatal respiratory depression following the administration of promethazine during labor, although the majority of reports did not detect this effect.

latent phase tends to be longer in induced labors than spontaneous labors, but the active phase and second stage have similar durations whether labor is spontaneous or induced [45].

Oxytocin is the only medication approved by the US Food and Drug Administration for labor stimulation in the active phase. It is typically dosed to effect, as predicting a woman's response to a particular dose is not possible [46]. A study has associated the use of oxytocin to labor induction or augmentation with hyperstimulation of the uterus with consequent decreased placental perfusion and fetal impairment [47]. Oxytocin also has antidiuretic hormone activity, which might create clinically important water intoxication if high doses of oxytocin are administered with large volumes of hypotonic fluids [48]. Recent data suggested that maternal oxytocin is not transferred across the placenta [49], supporting an indirect mechanism for this effect. Some studies suggest possible increased incidence of hyperbilirubine-mia in infants prenatally exposed to oxytocin but other studies noted that this outcome might be another effect of induced perinatal hyponatremia, rather than a direct effect of oxytocin [50, 51]. One study suggested a possible relationship between the use of oxytocin in labor and neonatal seizures [52]. However, this study did not adjust for length of labor as prolonged labor typically precedes the administration of oxytocin. One group of investigators reported a relationship between the use of oxytocin for induction or augmentation of labor and the risk of sudden infant death syndrome (SIDS) [53, 54]. This conclusion was based on retrospective reports. In a review of prospective data from the Collaborative Perinatal Project, a convincing association between supplemental oxytocin exposure and SIDS was not evident [55]. While an Australian study evaluating early environmental risk factors associated with attention-deficit/hyperactivity disorder noted a possible protective effect of oxytocin augmentation in female children [56], a Danish study failed to prove such an association [57].

2.9 Conclusion

Since the thalidomide disaster, medicine has been practiced as if every drug were a potential human teratogen when, in fact, fewer than 30 such drugs have been identified, with hundreds of agents proved safe for the unborn. Owing to high levels of anxiety among pregnant women – and because half of the pregnancies in North America are unplanned – every year many thousands of women need counseling about fetal exposure to drugs, chemicals, and radiation. The ability of appropriate counseling to prevent unnecessary abortions has been documented. Clinicians who wish to provide such counsel to pregnant women must ensure that their information is up-to-date and evidence-based, and that the woman understands that the baseline teratogenic risk in pregnancy (i.e., the risk of a neonatal abnormality in the absence of any known teratogenic exposure) is about 3%. It is also critical to address the maternal–fetal risks of the untreated condition if a medication is avoided. Recent studies show serious morbidity in women who discontinued their needed chronic drugs and such morbidity very often surpasses the teratogenic potential of the drug itself.

References

[1] Heinonen OP, Slone D, Shapiro S. Birth Defects and Drugs in Pregnancy. Littleton (MA): Publishing Sciences Group; 1977.
[2] Koren G, Pastuszak A, Ito S. Drugs in pregnancy. N Engl J Med 1998;338(16):1128–1137.
[3] Brent RL, Beckman DA. Environmental teratogens. Bull NY Acad Med 1990;66(2):123–163.
[4] Andrade SE, Gurwitz JH, Davis RL, et al. Prescription drug use in pregnancy. Am J Obstet Gynecol 2004;191(2):398–407.
[5] Glover DD, Amonkar M, Rybeck BF, Tracy TS. Prescription, over-the-counter, and herbal medicine use in a rural, obstetric population. Am J Obstet Gynecol 2003;188(4):1039–1045.
[6] Mitchell AA, Gilboa SM, Werler MM, et al. Medication use during pregnancy, with particular focus on prescription drugs: 1976±2008. Am J Obstet Gynecol 2011;205(1):51e1–8.
[7] Werler MM, Mitchell AA, Hernandez-Diaz S, Honein MA. Use of over-the-counter medications during pregnancy. Am J Obstet Gynecol 2005;193(3 Pt 1):771–777.
[8] Bakker MK, Jentink J, Vroom F, Van Den Berg PB, De Walle HE, De Jong-Van Den Berg LT. Drug prescription patterns before, during and after pregnancy for chronic, occasional and pregnancy-related drugs in the Netherlands. BJOG 2006;113(5):559–568.
[9] Gagne JJ, Maio V, Berghella V, Louis DZ, Gonnella JS. prescription drug use during pregnancy: a population-based study in regione Emilia-Romagna, Italy. Eur J Clin Pharmacol 2008;64(11): 1125–1132.
[10] Olesen C, Steffensen FH, Nielsen GL, De Jong-van Den Berg L, Olsen J, Sorensen HT. Drug use in first pregnancy and lactation: a population-based survey among Danish women. The EUROMAP group. Eur J Clin Pharmacol 1999;55(2):139–144.
[11] Martin JA, Hamilton BE, Ventura SJ, et al. Births: final data for 2009. Natl Vital Stat Rep 2011 Nov;60(1):1–70.
[12] Shan D, Qiu P-Y, Wu Y-X, et al. Pregnancy outcomes in women of advanced maternal age: a retrospective cohort study from China. Sci Rep 2018;8(1):12239.
[13] Carolan M. Maternal age ≥45 years and maternal and perinatal outcomes: a review of the evidence. Midwifery 2013;29(5):479–489.
[14] Krieg SA, Henne MB, Westphal LM. Obstetric outcomes in donor oocyte pregnancies compared with advanced maternal age in in vitro fertilization pregnancies. Fertil Steril 2008;90(1):65–70.
[15] Sheiner E, Shoham-Vardi I, Hershkovitz R, Katz M, Mazor M. Infertility treatment is an independent risk factor for cesarean section among nulliparous women aged 40 and above. Am J Obstet Gynecol 2001;185(4):888–892.
[16] Ventura SJ, Curtin SC, Abma JC, Henshaw SK. Estimated pregnancy rates and rates of pregnancy outcomes for the United States, 1990±2008. Natl Vital Stat Rep 2012;60(7):1–21.
[17] Yogev Y, Melamed N, Bardin R, Tenenbaum-Gavish K, Ben-Shitrit G, Ben-Haroush A. Pregnancy outcome at extremely advanced maternal age. Am J Obstet Gynecol 2010;203(6):558.e1±7.
[18] Adam MP. The all-or-none phenomenon revisited. Birth Defects Res A Clin Mol Teratol 2012;94(8):664–669.
[19] Porter RS, editor. The Merck Manual's Online Medical Library. Whitehouse Station: Merck Research Lab; 2004.
[20] Soprano DR1, Soprano KJ. Retinoids as teratogens. Annu Rev Nutr 1995;15:111.
[21] Copp AJ, Stanier P, Greene ND. Neural tube defects: recent advances, unsolved questions, and controversies. Lancet Neurol 2013 Aug;12(8):799–810.
[22] Bailey BN, Delaney-Black V, Covington CY, et al. Prenatal exposure to binge drinking and cognitive and behavioral outcomes at age 7 years. Am J Obstet Gynecol 2004;191(3):1037.

[23] Mosley JF, Smith LL, Dezan MD. An overview of upcoming changes in pregnancy and lactation labelling information. Pharm Pract (Granada) 2015;13(2):605.

[24] Costantine MM. Physiologic and pharmacokinetic changes in pregnancy. Front Pharmacol 2014;5:65.

[25] Loebstein R, Lalkin A, Koren G. Pharmacokinetic changes during pregnancy and their clinical relevance. Clin Pharmacokinet 1997;33(5):328–343.

[26] Anderson GD. Pregnancy-induced changes in pharmacokinetics: a mechanistic-based approach. Clin Pharmacokinet 2005;44(10):989–1008.

[27] Pariente G, Leibson T, Carls A, Adams-Webber T, Ito S, Koren G. Pregnancy-associated changes in pharmacokinetics: a systematic review. PLoS Med 2016;1, 13(11):e1002160.

[28] Kaye AB, Bhakta A, Moseley AD, et al. J review of cardiovascular drugs in pregnancy. Womens Health (Larchmt). 2018 Nov 8. [Epub ahead of print].

[29] Jovanovic L, Knopp RH, Brown Z, et al. Declining insulin requirement in the late first trimester of diabetic pregnancy. Diabetes Care 2001;24(7):1130.

[30] Koren G. Medication Safety in Pregnancy and Breastfeeding. New York (NY): McGraw-Hill; 2007.

[31] Roberts D, Brown J, Medley N. Dalziel SR Antenatal corticosteroids for accelerating fetal lung maturation for women at risk of preterm birth. Cochrane Database Syst Rev;2017(3): CD004454.

[32] Alsaied T, Baskar S, Fares M, et al. First-line antiarrhythmic transplacental treatment for fetal tachyarrhythmia: a systematic review and meta-analysis. J Am Heart Assoc 2017;6:12.

[33] Centers for Disease Control and Prevention (CDC). Achievements in public health. Reduction in perinatal transmission of HIV infection–United States, 1985–2005. MMWR Morb Mortal Wkly Rep 2006 Jun;55(21):592–597.

[34] Care in normal birth: a practical guide. Technical working group, World Health Organization. Birth 1997 Jun;24(2):121–123.

[35] Berghella V, Baxter JK, Chauhan SP. Evidence-based labor and delivery management. Am J Obstet Gynecol 2008;199(5):445.

[36] Sinatra RS, Eige S, Chung JH, et al. Continuous epidural infusion of 0.05% bupivacaine plus hydromorphone for labor analgesia: an observational assessment in 1830 parturients. Anesth Analg 2002;94(5):1310–1311.

[37] Becker JH, Schaap TP, Westerhuis ME, Van Wolfswinkel L, Visser GH, Kwee A. Intrapartum epidural analgesia and ST analysis of the fetal electrocardiogram. Acta Obstet Gynecol Scand 2011;90(12):1364–1370.

[38] Kumar M, Chandra S, Ijaz Z, Senthilselvan A. Epidural analgesia in labour and neonatal respiratory distress: a case-control study. Arch Dis Child Fetal Neonatal Ed 2014;99(2): F116–9.

[39] Fernando R, Bonello E, Gill P, Urquhart J, Reynolds F, Morgan B. Neonatal welfare and placental transfer of fentanyl and bupivacaine during ambulatory combined spinal epidural analgesia for labour. Anaesthesia 1997;52:517–524.

[40] Eddy NB, Halbach H, Braenden OJ. Synthetic substances with morphine-like effect. Clinical Experience: potency, Side Effects, Addiction Liability. Bull World Health Organ 1957;17 (4–5):569–863.

[41] Ransjo-Arvidson AB, Matthiesen AS, Lilja G, Nissen E, Widstrom AM, Uvnas-Moberg K. Maternal analgesia during labor disturbs newborn behavior: effects on breastfeeding, temperature, and crying. Birth 2001;28:5–12.

[42] Potts CR, Ullery JC. Maternal and fetal effects of obstetric analgesia. Am J Obstet Gynecol 1961;81:1252–1259.

[43] Friedman E. The graphic analysis of labor. Am J Obstet Gynecol 1954;68(6):1568.

[44] Zhang J, Landy HJ, Branch DW, et al. Contemporary patterns of spontaneous labor with normal neonatal outcomes. Obstet Gynecol 2010;116(6):1281.

[45] Janakiraman V, Ecker J, Kaimal AJ. Comparing the second stage in induced and spontaneous labor. Obstet Gynecol 2010;116(3):606.

[46] Satin AJ, Leveno KJ, Sherman ML, McIntire DD. Factors affecting the dose response to oxytocin for labor stimulation. Am J Obstet Gynecol 1992;166(4):1260.

[47] Perlow JH, Wigton T, Hart J, Strassner HT, Nageotte MP, Wolk BM. Birth trauma: a five-year review of incidence and associated perinatal factors. J Reprod Med 1996;41:754–760.

[48] Seifer DB, Sandberg EC, Ueland K, Sladen RN. Water intoxication and hyponatremic encephalopathy from the use of an oxytocin nasal spray. A case report. J Reprod Med 1985 Mar;30(3):225–228.

[49] Patient C, Davison JM, Charlton L, Baylis PH, Thornton S. The effect of labour and maternal oxytocin infusion on fetal plasma oxytocin concentration. Br J Obstet Gynaecol 1999;106: 1311–1313.

[50] Johnson JD, Aldrich M, Angelus P, et al. Oxytocin and neonatal hyperbilirubinemia. Studies of bilirubin production. Am J Dis Child 1984 Nov;138(11):1047–1050.

[51] Leylek OA, Ergur A, Senocak F, et al. Prophylaxis of the occurrence of hyperbilirubinemia in relation to maternal oxytocin infusion with steroid treatment. Gynecol Obstet Invest 1998;46 (3):164–168.

[52] Goodlin RC. Oxytocin may explain neonatal seizures. Am J Obstet Gynecol 1989;161(1):259.

[53] Einspieler C, Kenner T. A possible relation between oxytocin for induct of labor and sudden infant death syndrome (letter). N Engl J Med 1985;313:1660.

[54] Kenner T, Einspieler C. More on oxytocin for induction of labor and sudden infant death syndrome (letter). N Engl J Med 1986;315:193.

[55] Kraus JF, Bulterys M, Greenland S. A nested case-control study of oxytocin and sudden infant death syndrome [letter]. Am J Obstet Gynecol 1992;162:604–605.

[56] Silva D, Colvin L, Hagemann E, Bower C. Environmental risk factors by gender associated with attention-deficit/hyperactivity disorder. Pediatrics 2014;133(1):e14–22.

[57] Henriksen L, Wu CS, Secher NJ, Obel C, Juhl M. Medical augmentation of labor and the risk of ADHD in offspring: a population-based study. Pediatrics 2015;135(3):e672–7.

Siobhan Bacon, Ann McNamara

3 Approach to Diagnostic Imaging in Pregnancy

3.1 Introduction

One in 20 women undergoes an imaging examination using ionizing radiation during her pregnancy. Imaging performed during pregnancy has increased dramatically in the last two decades [1]. Pregnancy is a time of heightened concern for both the mother and treating physician, and the choice of radiological investigation must be carefully considered. In pregnancy, the "ALARA" (as low as reasonably achievable) principle should particularly be applied. In the following sections, we provide an overview of the more pertinent issues that may arise when you are considering referring a pregnant woman for a radiological investigation. It is worth stressing here that, as highlighted by the ACR (American College Radiologists)/ ACOG (American College of Obstetricians and Gynecologists)/SOGC (Society of Obstetricians and Gynaecologists of Canada), if an investigation is deemed essential for the well-being of the mother, it should be performed [2, 3].

We firstly discuss the potential fetal and maternal risks of ionizing radiation and follow with a synopsis of the most relevant imaging modalities in pregnancy and the effect of contrast agents during pregnancy and lactation.

3.2 Fetal Effects of Radiation: Teratogenicity

In terms of risk of teratogenesis from radiation exposure, both timing and dose of ionizing radiation need to be considered. The timing of radiation exposure can be subdivided into the following periods: preimplantation (0–2 weeks postconception), embryogenesis (2–8 weeks postconception), early fetal (8–15 weeks), and late fetal (15–40 weeks). In the preimplantation period, radiation exposure typically results in an "all or none" effect: either death of the embryo, or no effect whatsoever. The period of embryogenesis (2–8 weeks) is highly sensitive to the teratogenic effects of ionizing radiation. In the early fetal period (8–15 weeks), the neuronal cells are rapidly dividing and migrating and as a result the central nervous system can be affected (Table 3.1).

The dose effects of radiation exposure can be classified as deterministic or stochastic. The deterministic effects occur principally above a threshold dose and consist of cell death resulting in potential fetal gross malformation or developmental abnormalities. In comparison, stochastic effects are delayed and manifest only after a period of time following exposure. These effects consist of damage to single cells

https://doi.org/10.1515/9783110615258-003

Table 3.1: Timing of radiation exposure from conception and effect.

Timing of exposure	Effect	Threshold dose
Preimplantation: 0–2 weeks	Death or no consequence	≥50–100 mGy
Embryogenesis: 2–8 weeks	Congenital anomalies	≥200 mGy
Early fetal: 8–15 weeks	Microcephaly Decrease in IQ (by 25 points)	≥200 mGy ≥1,000 mGy
Late fetal: 15–25 weeks 15–38 weeks	Severe mental effects Carcinogenic risk	≥250 mGy ≥100 mGy

and can lead to carcinogenesis. There is no specific threshold radiation level at which a stochastic effect occurs. In this chapter, the unit of absorbed energy referenced is the milligray (mGy). A mGy is equivalent to 0.001 gray. A gray is the dose of one joule of energy absorbed per kilogram of matter.

National and international bodies have issued guidelines that indicate a negligible risk to the fetus for a cumulative radiation dose of <50 mGy [2]. This threshold was selected on the basis of animal studies and large registry data from individuals exposed to radiation in utero. The dose of 50 mGy is conservative but the one that is internationally accepted. Currently, no diagnostic examination reaches this threshold. It is sometimes a useful analogy for the patient to explain radiation dosage relative to environmental radiation exposure such as air travel. One air travel (short flight) results in a radiation exposure of 0.005 mGy, a long flight results in 0.03 mGy. Table 3.2 contains the estimated fetal radiation exposure from various imaging modalities.

Table 3.2: Estimated fetal dose from common imaging modalities (adapted from ACR [15]).

Very low dose (<0.1 mGy)	
Chest X-ray	0.0005–0.01
Head/neck CT	0.001–0.01
Low–moderate dose (0.1–10 mGy)	
Abdominal X-ray	0.1–3
Lumbar spine radiography	1–10

Table 3.2 (continued)

CT chest/CT pulmonary angiography	0.01–0.66
Nuclear medicine (low-dose perfusion only)	0.02–0.2
Nuclear medicine ventilation scan	0.1–0.3
High dose (10–50 mGy)	
Abdominal/pelvic CT	1.3–35
18F PET/CT whole-body scintigraphy	10–35

CT– Computed tomography
PET= Positron Emission Tomography

3.3 Fetal Effects of Radiation: Oncogenesis

The National Radiological Protection Board has adapted an estimated additional risk of childhood cancer of 0.006% per mGy following low-dose irradiation in utero compared to 0.0018% per mGy for radiation exposure shortly after birth. It should be remembered that the baseline risk of childhood cancer is low at 1–2.5 per 1,000. Following exposure to 50 mGy, the risk is 1.1–3 per 1,000 exposed [4]. It also needs to be reiterated that the risk of a missed diagnosis in the mother can be more detrimental than any potential risk from radiation.

3.4 Maternal Effects of Ionizing Radiation

The principal concern with radiation exposure to the mother is the risk of carcinogenicity to the breast, particularly from computed tomography (CT). During pregnancy, the breast is a highly proliferative glandular structure and particularly radiosensitive. The dose delivered by CTPA (CT pulmonary angiography) can represent up to a 150-fold increase in the dose to the breast when compared to perfusion scintigraphy [5]. In the long term, it was estimated that CTPA confers a 14% increased risk over the background risk for breast cancer in pregnant women <40 years of age [6]. However, with modern imaging techniques, the dose delivered to the maternal breast can be reduced to a level that is of negligible health concern to the mother [7, 8]. A recent study by Ray et al. demonstrated no increased incidence of early breast cancer among 5,859 women exposed to thoracic CT in pregnancy. The follow-up period was approximately 6 years. However, despite these reassuring findings, the authors did emphasize that a longer study, duration is essential to determine the safety profile of

CT in pregnancy [9]. The OPTICA study, which is currently in recruitment phase, may offer additional safety data on low-dose CTPA in the pregnant population [10].

3.5 Specific Modalities: Non-ionizing Radiation

3.5.1 Ultrasound

Ultrasound involves the use of sound waves with no ionizing radiation. There have been no adverse effects documented to the fetus with ultrasound and it is deemed safe in pregnancy. There is a theoretical thermal affect to the fetus from ultrasound use. In obstetric ultrasound, the US Food and Drug Administration (FDA) limits the upper limit intensity of the beam to 720 mW/cm^2. Clinicians and pregnant women alike are comfortable with ultrasound usage since it is used routinely in fetal monitoring.

3.5.2 Magnetic Resonance Imaging (MRI)

In a recent study of 4.6 million pregnancies in the USA, there was a high prevalence of MRI usage particularly in the first trimester suggesting inadvertent exposure [11].

MRI as a Non-ionizing form of imaging is preferred in pregnancy. Significant work has proven that MRI offers excellent contrast resolution for evaluation of a wide range of pathology while remaining a safe, radiation-free imaging modality which offers significant advantage over CT. MRI offers reproducible diagnostic imaging which, compared to ultrasound, is not operator dependent. There are disadvantages to MRI, with accessibility being paramount. Many centers do not have access to MRI on a 24 hour basis. MRI costs more than CT and ultrasound. Sainin et al. showed that the technical costs for an ultrasound/CT and MRI at a tertiary academic center were $50, $112, and $266, respectively [12]. From a patient perspective, MRI is more susceptible to motion artifact and requires the woman to remain still for the duration of image acquisition. Due consideration needs to be given to the pregnant state since the enlarged abdomen may not facilitate imaging using standard bore scanner. In addition, if at late gestation, lying supine results in compression of the inferior vena cava and can result in significant hypotension. Thermal and acoustic damage to the fetus is a hypothetical risk of MRI; however, this has not been described in the clinical setting. Moreover, a recent study of 715 neonates exposed to MRI in utero failed to demonstrate any incidence of acoustic damage [13, 14]. MRI of the pregnant woman can be performed at 1.5 or 3 Tesla with no specific recommendations on field strength from national/international bodies. The ACR guidelines recommend MRI usage throughout pregnancy with no restriction in the first trimester [15].

3.6 Specific Modalities: Ionizing Radiation

3.6.1 Plain Film

The British Thoracic Society Guidelines state that a chest radiograph should be undertaken in all patients complaining of a chronic cough (defined as lasting more than 8 weeks). In addition, the guidelines recommend a chest radiograph should be done in patients with a cough who have any one of these atypical symptoms: hemoptysis, breathlessness, fever, chest pain, or weight loss. These associated symptoms should be ruled out by direct questioning and the guidelines should be followed in all patients, including pregnant women [16].

The abdominal X-ray exposes the woman to 35 times the radiation of chest X-ray and is unhelpful largely in diagnosing abdominal pathology. The Royal College of Radiologists recommends the use of an abdominal X ray in the setting of acute abdomen if obstruction, perforation, or if a foreign body is thought to be present [17]. In pregnancy, however, an abdominal X-ray should not be performed.

3.6.2 Computed Tomography (CT)

CT is an extremely useful and commonly used imaging modality in nonpregnant individuals. CT imaging is typically readily available in institutions, and images can be rapidly acquired. Where possible, the pregnant individual should be informed of the potential risk with ionizing radiation. However, the ACOG and ACR both recommend that CT imaging should not be withheld in pregnancy if the clinical scenario dictates [2, 3].

3.7 Nuclear Imaging: Positron Emission Tomography Scanning Scan

Positron Emission Tomography Scanning and PET/CT are now standard of care for the evaluation of malignancies. Fortunately, the occurrence of cancer in pregnancy is low at approximately 1 in 1,000 [18]. There is no formal recommendation by the ACOG, ACR, RCOG UK, or SOGC on the use of PET in pregnancy. To date in the literature, 20 women have been injected with 18F FDG (fluorodeoxyglucose) for clinical indications [19]. These reports show that higher doses of the radioisotope are absorbed in early pregnancy when fetal cells are rapidly proliferating. The estimated dose from 18F FDG PET is between 2 and 5 mGy. Fetal absorbed dose for nuclear medicine studies represent the cumulative effect of external irradiation from both maternal tissues and fetal uptake of radiopharmaceuticals. Nuclear scanning has been enhanced by the addition of hybrid single positron emission computed tomography which allows the simultaneous acquisition of combined multimodality images. There are no studies in pregnancy utilizing such modalities; however, the fetal radiation dose would presumably be greater than any single modality.

3.8 Imaging in Particular Clinical Scenarios

In the following section, we discuss the preferable imaging modalities for common or conditions unique to pregnancy. Headache, non-obstetric abdominal discomfort, and suspected pulmonary embolism will be considered.

3.8.1 Headache

When consenting a woman for radiological imaging of the head, even if using ionizing radiation, one should remember that the fetus will only be exposed to scatter radiation through the mother rather than direct exposure. The differential for a severe secondary headache in pregnancy is broad but includes posterior reversible encephalopathy syndrome (PRES), reversible cerebral vasoconstriction syndrome (RCVS), cerebral venous sinus thrombosis (CVT), intracranial hemorrhage secondary to stroke/arterial dissection. The majority of women presenting with clinical symptoms suggestive of a "secondary" headache will require radiological investigation. We will discuss each entity and preferred imaging modality in the following sections.

PRES is a clinical and radiographic syndrome with a loss of cerebral autoregulation, increased capillary leakage, and consequent vasogenic edema. A non-contrast MRI is the imaging modality of choice. Patchy, parieto-occipital/diffuse hemispheric hyperintensities on T2-weighted and FLAIR sequencing may be noted. The name "PRES" is somewhat a misnomer as it is not always reversible, nor involving the posterior lobes of the brain, nor is the woman always encephalopathic.

RCVS is a clinical and radiographic diagnosis which is associated with reversible, multifocal vasoconstriction in medium- and large-sized blood vessels. The vasospasm, commonly referred to as "beading," can be confirmed using either CTA or MRA. As reversibility is a hallmark of the condition, repeat vascular imaging should be performed 3 months following the event to ensure confirmation of diagnosis and resolution.

CVT is more common in the pregnant state and can have a high morbidity rate if undetected. The gold standard for diagnosis of CVT is digital subtraction angiography which is invasive. MRV enables visualization of the cerebral venous system with a high level of accuracy for diagnosing CVT. Interruption of flow on TOF sequencing is usually indicative of CVT. TOF sequencing avoids the necessity for contrast. A non-contrast CT head can reveal hyperdense thrombus in dural/cortical veins. With contrast, the CT scan can potentially show a "empty delta sign" due to lack of flow causing a triangular filling defect.

In the setting of subarachnoid hemorrhage, MR brain with/without angiography is a safe alternative to CT/CTA for detecting intracranial aneurysms. A study by Sailer et al. demonstrated a pooled sensitivity of 95% and a specificity of 89% for MRI/MRA in detecting such aneurysms [20].

The risk of a stroke in pregnancy is 3-fold higher than that of the young adult population. The recent recommendations for the management of stroke in pregnancy emphasize that if an acute stroke is suspected brain imaging, albeit CT or MR if available, should be performed as a matter of urgency. The authors state that "where immediately available as part of local stroke protocol, MRI of the brain with TOF imaging of blood vessels may be used instead of CT/CTA to visualise the brain and vasculature" [21]. Radiographic findings in pregnancy of an acute/chronic stroke are identical to that of the nonpregnant individual. MRI reveals hyperintense lesions on DWI from the first minutes of stroke onset. CT reveals loss of gray-white matter differentiation, sulcal effacement, and hypodensity of infarcted area. Arterial dissection is best visualized by MRA head/neck during pregnancy. Cross-sectional T1-weighted imaging with fat suppression may show the characteristic crescent-shaped deformity in the wall of the dissected internal carotid artery.

3.8.2 Non-obstetric Abdominal Pain

Ultrasound remains the primary diagnostic tool for evaluation of abdominal pain in pregnancy. However, MRI has become increasingly used as it facilitates better visualization of the visceral organs in certain settings. Accurate visualization of abdominal/pelvic pathology is important in pregnancy as it avoids unnecessary surgical intervention which can be associated with preterm delivery [22]. Appendicitis is the most common non-obstetric cause of abdominal pain necessitating surgery during pregnancy [23]. As a result of the meta-analysis conducted by Eng et al., MRI is recommended as a second-line investigation after an equivocal ultrasound [24].

Ultrasound is the first diagnostic tool employed for urinary tract pathology such as hydronephrosis and nephrolithiasis. While ultrasound is also typically used for accessing gallbladder pathology, MR offers better sensitivity for diagnosing acute cholecystitis (88% vs 65%, respectively). MR allows improved visualization of the bile ducts and thus allows diagnosis of choleodocholithiasis as well as complications such as perforation, abscess formation, and ascending cholangitis. MRI also facilitates better visualization of the pancreas than ultrasound [25]. In a reality, however, ultrasound remains almost exclusively employed for biliary imaging in pregnancy.

In a trauma situation, CT imaging of the abdomen/pelvis is warranted if rapid image acquisition is essential.

3.8.3 Suspected Pulmonary Embolism

In the UK and Ireland, thrombosis and thromboembolism were the most common causes of direct maternal death in the triennium 2013–2015. There is ongoing controversy as to the best imaging modality for detecting pulmonary embolus in pregnancy. A CT pulmonary angiogram uses IV contrast along with computer processing to create tomographic images, with an intraluminal defect being diagnostic of a pulmonary embolus. A V/Q involves radioisotopes being injected and inhaled. Gamma cameras are used to make a two-dimensional image, and a mismatch between ventilated and perfused lung is diagnostic or a "high probability" of a pulmonary embolus.

The concern with regard to CTPA and maternal breast tissue irradiation is discussed in Chapter 11. The fetal radiation dose is similar between CTPA and V/Q when perfusion-only imaging is used. CTPA can identify other chest pathology such as a pneumonia or pulmonary edema. However, the hemodynamic changes of pregnancy result in a higher rate of nondiagnostic scans with CTPA when compared to V/Q (37.5% vs 4%) [26]. A recent survey of 24 sites in the UK representing a population of 15.5 million revealed a similar rate of inadequate or indeterminate CTPA and scintigraphy scans, suggesting initial choice of imaging is best determined by local expertise and resources [27]. The latest published guidelines form the ESC recommend ether perfusion only or CTPA be utilized with the selection being driven by local practice preference [28]. The ESC recommendations on imaging choice for suspected PE are echoed by the RCOG 2015 guidelines [29]. They state that the choice of technique depends on local availability, and individual hospitals should have an agreed protocol. The higher negative predictive value and lower radiation dose to the breast tissue makes perfusion-only imaging attractive if available.

3.9 Contrast Agents

3.9.1 Gadolinium

The use of gadolinium (GAD) in pregnancy as a contrast agent to further characterize lesions with MRI is a matter of much debate. GAD crosses the placenta, enters the fetal circulation, and re-enters on a cyclical basis as the contrast is secreted through the fetal kidney into the amniotic fluid and re-ingested by the fetus. In animal studies, GAD has been shown to be teratogenic at supraphysiological doses. In 2016, Ray et al. reported the outcome of 1.4 million pregnancies exposed to MRI with/without GAD during pregnancy. There was no significant difference between the exposed and nonexposed infant when evaluated for nephrogenic systemic fibrosis-like outcome and no increased risk of congenital anomalies. There were 7 cases of stillbirth among 397 GAD-exposed pregnancies, which represented a 3.7-fold increased relative risk in those exposed to GAD versus nonexposed. A 1.36-fold increased risk for rheumatological, inflammatory, and infiltrative skin disorders was also reported in the offspring exposed in utero. These findings may appear alarming; however, there were a number of cited limitations. Firstly, there was a small number of outcomes in the exposed cohort. There was also a lack of validation of the skin conditions in the newborns and lastly, there was inadequate control for the clinical indication of MRI receipt [30].

The ACR, ACOG, and SOGC recommend that if GAD *is essential* for diagnosis and deferral is inappropriate, then use should proceed with appropriate counseling of the pregnant women [2, 3, 31].

3.9.2 Iodinated Contrast

Intravenous iodinated contrast agents are considered category B drugs using traditional nomenclature by the FDA. In other words, there is no evidence of demonstrable harm in animals but there are no controlled trials in humans. Intravenous contrast can result in maternal anaphylactic reaction and exacerbate renal impairment. Management of a contrast reaction in pregnancy is similar to that in the nonpregnant state with the caveat that the patient should be placed in the left lateral position to alleviate aortocaval compression. Premedication with diphenhydramine and corticosteroids can be used in those at risk of allergic reaction to contrast media. The 2020 ACR manual on contrast media states that iodinated contrast media may be given if the information that it provides cannot be attained without contrast agent (ACR). The previously held theoretical concern regarding fetal thyroid abnormalities has been largely disbanded. In a study by Bourjeily et al., exposure of 343 neonates to iodinated contrast at various gestational ages resulted in normal neonatal thyroxine levels [32].

Women with renal impairment have larger circulation times for contrast and the doses received by the fetus may reach higher levels due to these longer circulation times.

3.10 How to Reduce Radiation Exposure

The dose to the fetus varies with proximity of the uterus to the anatomic location of the scan, the depth of the fetus, thickness of the patient, and the technique utilized. There are various methods that can be employed to reduce the radiation dose to organs not in the direct path of the primary beam. Protocols employed by institutions for implementing a lower dose CT examination include reducing the kilovoltage for a small patient, limiting the field of view, avoiding imaging in multiple phases, using lead shielding/bismuth breast shields to the mother. Modern CT scanners all have dose reduction algorithms which can be appropriately utilized.

For ventilation perfusion scintigraphy (V/Q), performing a perfusion-only image without the ventilation phase can reduce the radiation dose. Newer protocols have also been devised with low-dose perfusion imparting even less radiation to both the fetus and maternal breast without compromising image quality. Hydration and frequent voiding are recommended for reducing fetal exposure to radioisotopes that accumulate in the maternal bladder.

3.11 Lactation

As a general rule, products are considered safe in lactation if the dose that ultimately reaches the infant is <10% of therapeutic dose. For contrast media, 0.5% of dose received by mother is transferred to infant. For GAD, 0.01% of the maternal dose reaches the breast. Therefore, both IV contrast and GAD are safe in lactating mothers. With regard to PET scanning and lactation, a minimal quantity of radioisotope (18F FDG) is secreted in breast milk. However, the lactating breast can accumulate FDG; therefore, the ICRP recommends minimizing contact with the infant for 12 h post scanning to reduce exposure to radiation emitted from the mother. The recommendation is to breastfeed just prior to imaging and use expressed milk for the 12 h [33].

Conclusion

1. The most important point to emphasize when using ionizing imaging in pregnancy is effective communication between all parties involved. To achieve the best outcome for the pregnant woman and her fetus, where possible, a discussion between the primary clinician, radiographer, radiologist, the patient, and her partner should occur. Consistency is paramount among physicians and allied healthcare staff when discussing radiological investigations with the pregnant woman.
2. The guiding principle ALARA, as with all radiological procedures, should be applied.
3. It is worth emphasizing again that, as highlighted by the ACR/ACOG/SOGC, if an investigation is deemed essential for the well-being of the mother, it should be completed.

Glossary

Ionizing radiation: Radiation that consists of X-rays or gamma rays with sufficient energy to cause electrons to detach from atoms/molecules{\hbox)}

MRI/MRA/MRV: Magnetic resonance imaging/magnetic resonance angiography/magnetic resonance venography

CT/CTA/CTV: Computed tomography/computed tomography angiography/computed tomography venography

T1- and T2-weighted imaging: The two basic types of MRI. The timing of radiofrequency pulse sequences serves to optimally display soft tissues, fluid, and blood.

DWI: Diffusion-weighted imaging is based on the random Brownian motion of water molecules within the tissue. In simplified terms, highly cellular tissue has lower diffusion coefficients.

FLAIR: Fluid-attenuated inversion recovery or FLAIR imaging removes the signal from the cerebrospinal fluid making it useful to evaluate diseases of the central nervous system, for example, multiple sclerosis and subarachnoid hemorrhage.2

TOF: Time-of-flight angiography is the non-contrast method for imaging blood vessels. Inflowing blood appears brighter compared to the background tissue.

References

[1]   Ray JG, Schull MJ, Urquia ML, You JJ, Guttmann A, Vermeulen MJ. Major radiodiagnostic imaging in pregnancy and the risk of childhood malignancy: a population-based cohort study in Ontario. PLoS Med 2010;7(9):e1000337.

[2]   Jain C. ACOG committee opinion no. 723: guidelines for diagnostic imaging during pregnancy and lactation. Obstet Gynecol 2019;133(1):186.

[3]   Wieseler KM, Bhargava P, Kanal KM, Vaidya S, Stewart BK, Dighe MK. Imaging in pregnant patients: examination appropriateness. Radiographics 2010;30(5):1215–1229, discussion 30–3.

[4]   Tirada N, Dreizin D, Khati NJ, Akin EA, Zeman RK. Imaging pregnant and lactating patients. Radiographics 2015;35(6):1751–1765.

[5]   Bourjeily G, Paidas M, Khalil H, Rosene-Montella K, Rodger M. Pulmonary embolism in pregnancy. Lancet 2010;375(9713):500–512.

[6]   Cutts BA, Dasgupta D, Hunt BJ. New directions in the diagnosis and treatment of pulmonary embolism in pregnancy. Am J Obstet Gynecol 2013;208(2):102–108.

[7]   Mitchell DP, Rowan M, Loughman E, Ridge CA, MacMahon PJ. Contrast monitoring techniques in CT pulmonary angiography: an important and underappreciated contributor to breast dose. Eur J Radiol 2017;86:184–189.

[8]   Perisinakis K, Seimenis I, Tzedakis A, Damilakis J. Perfusion scintigraphy versus 256-slice CT angiography in pregnant patients suspected of pulmonary embolism: comparison of radiation risks. J Nucl Med 2014;55(8):1273–1280.

[9]   Burton KR, Park AL, Fralick M, Ray JG. Risk of early onset breast cancer among women exposed to thoracic computed tomography in pregnancy or early postpartum. J Thromb Haemost 2018.

[10]   Gillespie C, Foley S, Rowan M, Ewins K, NiAinle F, MacMahon P. The OPTICA study (optimised computed tomography pulmonary angiography in pregnancy quality and safety study): rationale and design of a prospective trial assessing the quality and safety of an optimised CTPA protocol in pregnancy. Thromb Res 2019;177:172–179.

[11]   Bird ST, Gelperin K, Sahin L, et al. First-trimester exposure to gadolinium-based contrast agents: a utilization study of 4.6 million U.S. pregnancies. Radiology 2019;293(1):193–200.

[12]   Saini S, Seltzer SE, Bramson RT, et al. Technical cost of radiologic examinations: analysis across imaging modalities. Radiology 2000;216(1):269–272.

[13]   Jaimes C, Delgado J, Cunnane MB, et al. Does 3-T fetal MRI induce adverse acoustic effects in the neonate? A preliminary study comparing postnatal auditory test performance of fetuses scanned at 1.5 and 3 T. Pediatr Radiol 2019;49(1):37–45.

[14] Strizek B, Jani JC, Mucyo E, et al. Safety of MR Imaging at 1.5 T in Fetuses: A Retrospective Case-Control Study of Birth Weights and the Effects of Acoustic Noise. Radiology 2015;275(2):530–537.

[15] ACR. ACR-SPR practice parameter for imaging pregnant or potentially pregnant adolescents and women with ionizing radiation. American College Radiologists; 2018 [Available from: https://www.acr.org/-/media/ACR/Files/Practice-Parameters/pregnant-pts.pdf.

[16] O'Connor SJ, Verma H, Grubnic S, Rayner CF. Chest radiographs in pregnancy. BMJ 2009;339:b4057.

[17] Remedios D, McCoubrie P. The Royal College of Radiologists guidelines working P. Making the best use of clinical radiology services: a new approach to referral guidelines. Clin Radiol 2007;62(10):919–920.

[18] Hepner A, Negrini D, Hase EA, et al. Cancer during pregnancy: the oncologist overview. World J Oncol 2019;10(1):28–34.

[19] Zanotti-Fregonara P, Chastan M, Edet-Sanson A, et al. New fetal dose estimates from 18F-FDG administered during pregnancy: standardization of dose calculations and estimations with voxel-based anthropomorphic phantoms. J Nucl Med 2016;57(11):1760–1763.

[20] Sailer AM, Wagemans BA, Nelemans PJ, De Graaf R, Van Zwam WH. Diagnosing intracranial aneurysms with MR angiography: systematic review and meta-analysis. Stroke 2014;45(1):119–126.

[21] Ladhani NNN, Swartz RH, Foley N, et al. Canadian stroke best practice consensus statement: acute stroke management during pregnancy. Int J Stroke 2018;13(7):743–758.

[22] Balinskaite V, Bottle A, Sodhi V, et al. The risk of adverse pregnancy outcomes following nonobstetric surgery during pregnancy: estimates from a retrospective cohort study of 6.5 million pregnancies. Ann Surg 2017;266(2):260–266.

[23] Dewhurst C, Beddy P, Pedrosa I. MRI evaluation of acute appendicitis in pregnancy. J Magn Reson Imaging 2013;37(3):566–575.

[24] Eng KA, Abadeh A, Ligocki C, et al. Acute appendicitis: a meta-analysis of the diagnostic accuracy of US, CT, and MRI as second-line imaging tests after an initial US. Radiology 2018;288(3):717–727.

[25] Mervak BM, Altun E, McGinty KA, Hyslop WB, Semelka RC, Burke LM. MRI in pregnancy: indications and practical considerations. J Magn Reson Imaging 2019;49(3):621–631.

[26] Siegel Y, Kuker R, Banks J, Danton G. CT pulmonary angiogram quality comparison between early and later pregnancy. Emerg Radiol 2017;24(6):635–640.

[27] Armstrong L, Gleeson F, Mackillop L, Mutch S, Beale A. Survey of UK imaging practice for the investigation of pulmonary embolism in pregnancy. Clin Radiol 2017;72(8):696–701.

[28] Konstantinides SV, Meyer G, Becattini C et al. ESC Guidelines for the diagnosis and management of acute pulmonary embolism developed in collaboration with the European Respiratory Society (ERS). Eur Heart J 2019:2019.

[29] RCOG. Thrombosis and Embolism during Pregnancy and the Puerperium: Acute Management (green-top Guideline No. 37b) 2015 [Available from: https://www.rcog.org.uk/en/guidelines-research-services/guidelines/gtg37b/.

[30] Ray JG, Vermeulen MJ, Bharatha A, Montanera WJ, Park AL. Association between MRI exposure during pregnancy and fetal and childhood outcomes. JAMA 2016;316(9):952–961.

[31] Patenaude Y, Pugash D, Lim K, et al. The use of magnetic resonance imaging in the obstetric patient. J Obstet Gynaecol Can 2014;36(4):349–363.

[32] Bourjeily G, Chalhoub M, Phornphutkul C, Alleyne TC, Woodfield CA, Chen KK. Neonatal thyroid function: effect of a single exposure to iodinated contrast medium in utero. Radiology 2010;256(3):744–750.

[33] ICRP. Radiation dose to patients from radiopharmaceuticals. Addendum 3 to ICRP Publication 53. ICRP Publication 106. Approved by the Commission in October 2007. Ann ICRP 2008;38(1–2):1–197.

Jennifer Yo, Shital Gandhi
4 Chronic Hypertension

4.1 Introduction

Hypertensive disorders of pregnancy (HDP) complicates 2–8% of pregnancies world-wide [1] and constitutes 16% of maternal deaths in developing nations [1]. The incidence of hypertensive disorders of pregnancy is increasing due to advanced maternal age, obesity, and associated comorbidities such as chronic hypertension and diabetes [2]. HDP has a major effect on fetal and neonatal outcomes including intrauterine growth restriction, placental abruption, preterm delivery, and caesarean birth [3].

4.2 Definition and Diagnostic Criteria for Hypertensive Disorders in Pregnancy

Hypertensive disorders of pregnancy encompass four categories as defined by the International Society for the Study of Hypertension in Pregnancy (ISSHP) and the American Society of Obstetricians and Gynaecologists: gestational hypertension, preeclampsia–eclampsia (discussed in Chapter 6), chronic hypertension, and chronic hypertension with superimposed preeclampsia [4, 5].

The definition of hypertension is a systolic blood pressure (SBP) ≥ 140 mmHg and/or diastolic blood pressure (DBP) ≥ 90 mmHg on two occasions at least 4 hour apart [4, 6]. These thresholds for blood pressure (BP), however, should not be used dogmatically. In fact, older definitions of hypertension in pregnancy required an overall increase in SBP of 30 mmHg, and a diastolic rise of greater than 15 mmHg. For some women, especially those who have low baseline BP prior to pregnancy, it will be more important to follow the change in BP during pregnancy than adhere to strict thresholds. Severe hypertension is further defined as SBP of ≥ 160 mmHg and/or DSP of ≥ 110 mmHg based on an average of at least two measurements confirmed within minutes [4, 6, 7].

4.2.1 Gestational Hypertension

Gestational hypertension is defined as new onset hypertension occurring ≥ 20 weeks gestation in the absence of proteinuria or new signs of end-organ dysfunction with normalization of BP in the postpartum period [3, 5]. The diagnosis of gestational hypertension is more of an exercise of nomenclature than a pragmatic one as the management of gestational hypertension and that of preeclampsia without severe features is similar

https://doi.org/10.1515/9783110615258-004

in many aspects [9]. Both gestational hypertension and preeclampsia without severe features require enhanced surveillance. Indeed, the notion that gestational hypertension is intrinsically less concerning than preeclampsia is incorrect and may not represent a separate entity from preeclampsia [9]. Between 10% and 50% of women with gestational hypertension go on to develop preeclampsia within 1 to 5 weeks following diagnosis [10, 11].

4.2.2 Preeclampsia

Preeclampsia is a placentally mediated hypertensive disorder and is defined as gestational hypertension with one or more of the following: new proteinuria and/or end-organ dysfunctions. The classification of hypertensive disorders of pregnancy and characterization of preeclampsia varies slightly by medical societies. Preeclampsia is discussed in detail in Chapter 6.

4.2.3 Chronic Hypertension

Chronic hypertension complicates 3–5% of pregnancies and needs to be distinguished from gestational hypertension and preeclampsia. Chronic hypertension is defined as hypertension that develops either prepregnancy or at <20 weeks gestation [4]. To establish a diagnosis of chronic hypertension, it is ideal to have knowledge of prepregnancy BP values. However, first diagnosis of chronic hypertension often occurs in the context of pregnancy, as for many women this will be the first time their BP is measured.

The 20-week convention, however, should not be used inflexibly but rather for orientation while maintaining clinical judgment [9]. A woman who had documented normal BP in the beginning of pregnancy and develops de novo hypertension just before 20 weeks (e.g., between 16 and 20 weeks gestation) could have underlying fetoplacental abnormalities such as hydatidiform mole or preterm preeclampsia which should prompt further assessment. Alternatively, she may have developed a new secondary (and non-pregnancy) cause of hypertension, which may require further clinical assessment.

Sometimes the diagnosis of chronic hypertension may only be retrospectively classified once pregnancy has ended. It has also been suggested that hypertension persisting longer than 12 weeks postpartum is due to chronic hypertension [13]. The time, however, for resolution of gestational hypertension or preeclampsia-related hypertension has not been clearly defined. A cohort study of 205 preeclamptic women in the Netherlands found that 39% still had hypertension 12 weeks after delivery. In 50% of these women, it took up to 2 years for BP to normalize [14].

4.2.4 Chronic Hypertension with Superimposed Preeclampsia

Preeclampsia is superimposed when it complicates chronic hypertension. About 20–50% of women with chronic hypertension may develop superimposed preeclampsia [6]. In women with end-organ disease due to hypertension or secondary hypertension, the rate of superimposed preeclampsia has been reported to be as high as 75%.

It can be very difficult to diagnose superimposed preeclampsia, especially if there is preexisting renal impairment and proteinuria. If there is clinical suspicion of preeclampsia, prompt assessment and maternal–fetal medicine referral should be undertaken. Laboratory evidence of HELLP syndrome (Hemolysis, Elevated Liver enzymes, and Low Platelets), such as thrombocytopenia and deranged liver transaminases makes preeclampsia likely. Recently, the advent of biomarkers such as the ratio of soluble FMS-like tyrosine kinase 1 (sFLt-1) to placental growth factor, if available, can often be helpful (see Chapter 6). Evaluation should also include assessment of other factors which may exacerbate BP control such as nonadherence to antihypertensive therapy, and the development of a new secondary cause of hypertension.

4.2.5 White Coat Hypertension

White coat hypertension is defined as hypertension only in the presence of healthcare providers. White coat effect in early pregnancy is common (~30%) [4]. It should not be considered entirely benign, however, as 8% and 40% of such cases will progress to preeclampsia and gestational hypertension, respectively, by the end of pregnancy [15]. A 24 h ambulatory monitor or self-measured home BP may be helpful in these situations, especially with respect to initiation of antihypertensive therapy.

4.3 Normal Hemodynamic Changes in Pregnancy

During normal pregnancy, SBP and DBP typically fall early in gestation and are approximately 5–10 mmHg below baseline in the second trimester, reaching a nadir by 20–22 weeks gestation [16]. BP gradually rises to nonpregnant values by term. This normal physiological decrease in BP is caused by neurohumoral adaptions leading to a decrease in systemic vascular resistance by 30% despite an increase in cardiac output and plasma volume of 30–50% [17–19]. For most women with chronic hypertension, BP will follow this pattern during pregnancy. Thus, previously hypertensive women may become normotensive during pregnancy, and antihypertensives are able to be tapered and sometimes ceased.

4.4 Comorbid Conditions

Chronic hypertension may be primary (or essential) hypertension in the absence of an attributable cause, or secondary hypertension. Most women will have underlying primary (essential) hypertension; however, 10% will have an underlying secondary cause for hypertension (see Table 4.1) [12–20]. While the exact etiology of primary hypertension remains unclear, a number of risk factors includes advancing age, obesity, a strong family history, ethnicity, and high salt diet.

Table 4.1: Causes and screening investigations for secondary causes of hypertension [1].

Secondary hypertension	Investigation (nonpregnant)	Investigations (pregnant)
Chronic kidney disease	Serum creatinine and estimated GFR	Serum creatinine and estimated GFR
Coarctation of the aorta	CT angiography	2D transthoracic echo Magnetic resonance imaging (MRI)
Cushing syndrome or other states of glucocorticoid excess	Dexamethasone suppression test	24 h urinary-free cortisol and late-night salivary cortisol Dexamethasone suppression test is not used during pregnancy due to the risk for false-positive results due to changes in the hypothalamic–pituitary axis in pregnancy [2]
Drug induced	History/drug screening	History/drug screening
Pheochromocytoma	24 h urinary metanephrines and normetanephrines	24 h urinary metanephrines and normetanephrines
Primary aldosteronism and other states of mineralocorticoid excess	Plasma renin activity and plasma aldosterone concentration	Plasma renin activity and plasma aldosterone concentration Due to normal physiologic increases in renin and aldosterone in pregnancy and lack of pregnancy specific ranges, the plasma renin activity and plasma aldosterone concentration can be difficult to interpret
Renovascular hypertension	Doppler flow ultrasound and magnetic resonance angiography	Doppler flow ultrasound and magnetic resonance angiography
Obstructive sleep apnea	Overnight sleep study	Overnight sleep study
Thyroid/parathyroid disease	TSH and serum PTH	Thyroid Stimulating Hormone (TSH) and Parathyroid Hormone (PTH)

4.5 Pregnancy Complications in Women with Chronic Hypertension

4.5.1 Maternal Risks

A population study of nearly 30,000 pregnant women with chronic hypertension demonstrated that maternal mortality and risk of cerebrovascular accidents, pulmonary edema, or renal failure were 5-fold higher than normotensive women [21]. The absolute risk, however, is low in developed countries and most women with mild essential hypertension will have uncomplicated pregnancies. Chronic hypertension is also associated with increased risk of gestational diabetes and postpartum hemorrhage [22]. Up to 20–50% of women with chronic hypertension may develop superimposed preeclampsia [6]. In women with end-organ disease or secondary hypertension, the rate of superimposed preeclampsia has been reported as high as 75%. This is compared to the general population, where the risk of preeclampsia is 3–5%.

4.5.2 Fetal Risks

A large systematic review of maternal and fetal outcomes in chronic hypertension demonstrated that the pooled incidence for low birth weight was approximately 17% and the pooled incidence for preterm delivery was 28% [23]. The rate of stillbirth is also higher in maternal chronic hypertension than in the general population. Women with chronic hypertension have a frequency of placental abruption of 1.56% compared to 0.58% in normotensive women [16].

4.6 Patient Evaluation

Women with chronic hypertension should be evaluated for secondary causes of hypertension (see Table 4.1) when indicated. Ideally, this should occur prior to pregnancy as such an evaluation may involve radiation exposure or require surgical intervention as part of definitive management. Women with chronic hypertension should also be evaluated for evidence of end-organ damage before pregnancy as this may inform maternal fetal risks and allow for individualized risk stratification. This includes serum creatinine and urine albumin/creatinine ratio (ACR) as well as a baseline 12-lead electrocardiograph to assess for left ventricular hypertrophy. A protein/creatinine ratio can be performed instead of an ACR; however, it is less specific for glomerular proteinuria.

Physical examination should include appropriate BP measurement (see below), calculation of body mass index (BMI), and then a focused exam for both the *causes* and *consequences* of hypertension. This would include examining the optic fundi, auscultation for carotid, abdominal, and femoral bruits, and examination of the heart thyroid gland as well as abdomen [12].

4.7 Blood Pressure Measurement

BP should be measured with the woman in the seated position with her feet on the ground and the arm should be at the level of the heart. BP should not be taken with the woman lying supine as the gravid uterus can compress the internal vena cava and provide a false reading. An appropriately sized cuff is imperative and the length should be 1.5 times the circumference of the upper arm [6, 24]. BP cuffs that are too small will result in overestimation. BP should be measured with either a mercury sphygmomanometer, a calibrated aneroid device, or automated BP machine. Mercury sphygmomanometers are the gold standard, however, are often no longer available at many sites. Aneroid devices are commonly used, however, need to be regularly calibrated.

An elevated BP reading should be remeasured at the same visit with at least an interval of 15 min from the first measurement [24]. More than 50% of women with a first BP reading >140/90 mmHg have an underlying white coat effect [15, 25] and should be remeasured several times and the average taken. For women with poorly controlled BP and at risk of preeclampsia, frequent BP monitoring in clinic and at home is often performed.

4.8 Blood Pressure Target in Pregnancy

4.8.1 Management of Non-severe Hypertension (BP 140–159/90–110 mmHg)

The threshold at which antihypertensive therapy is indicated for non-severe hypertension in pregnancy is controversial. It should be emphasized that antihypertensive treatment does not actually prevent or treat preeclampsia; the definitive treatment of preeclampsia begins with delivery. In addition, observational studies and a meta-regression analysis suggested that the treatment of hypertension may adversely affect fetal growth [26].

The international multicenter randomized controlled trial, Control of Hypertension in Pregnancy Study (CHIPS) [27], examined the effects of less tight control (DBP 100 mmHg) compared to tight control (DBP 85 mmHg) on perinatal and maternal outcomes. Of the 987 pregnant women, 75% had chronic hypertension, with the rest having gestational hypertension. There was no difference in the fetal outcomes of mortality or need for admission to high dependency unit, nor was there a difference in serious maternal complications of stroke or renal failure between the two groups. However, there was an increase in the incidence of severe maternal hypertension of BP greater than 160/110 mmHg in the less tight group. One interpretation of the CHIPS Trial is that tight control of BP is not associated with fetal benefit and that there is insufficient evidence to support aiming for lower BP targets. Conversely, tighter BP targets in pregnant women with non-severe hypertension may prevent the development of severe hypertension.

Consequently, clinicians are faced with the challenge of prescribing or continuing antihypertensive agents which may be beneficial for the mother but of unclear benefit for the fetus. Guidelines for the treatment of non-severe hypertension vary among different regions of the world. The ISSHP recommends maintaining BP in the range of 110–140/80–85 mmHg [28]. Hypertension Canada also recommends initiating antihypertensive therapy for SBP $\geq$ 140 mmHg and DBP $\geq$ 90 mmHg in women with chronic hypertension, gestational hypertension, and preeclampsia [24], with a suggested target of DBP = 85 mmHg. In contrast, the American Society of Obstetrics and Gynaecology recommends that BP in women with uncomplicated chronic hypertension be maintained between 120–160/80–105 mm Hg. For women with gestational hypertension or preeclampsia, antihypertensive therapy is not recommended for SBP < 160 mmHg or DBP < 110 mmHg [5].

The authors' practice is to start antihypertensive therapy when the SBP $\geq$ 140 mmHg and DBP $\geq$ 90 mmHg for women with HDP, in keeping with Hypertension Canada Guidelines, with a target SBP 130–140 mmHg and DBP 80–90 mmHg. For women with comorbidities such as underlying renal impairment or cardiovascular disease, aiming for a lower BP target may be appropriate. From a maternal perspective, this practice may minimize episodes of severe hypertension and its associated complications as well as healthcare healthcare resource utilization as a result of repeated visits to triage with severe hypertension.

The most commonly used drugs for treatment of non-severe hypertension are detailed in Table 4.2.

Table 4.2: Commonly used agents to treat non-severe hypertension [3, 4].

Agent	Class	Initial dose	Maximum daily dose	Side effects
Methyldopa	Centrally acting alpha-agonist	250 mg 2 to 3 times per day	3,000 mg	Sedation
Labetalol	Combined alpha- and beta-blocker	100 mg 2 to 3 times per day	2,400 mg	Avoid in women with asthma, decompensated cardiac function and heart block, and bradycardia
Nifedipine extended release	Calcium channel blocker	30–60 mg once daily	120 mg	Edema and headache
Hydralazine	Peripheral vasodilator	10 mg 4 times per day	200 mg	Reflex tachycardia

4.8.2 Management of Severe Hypertension (BP ≥ 160/110 mmHg)

There is a general consensus that this is an urgent indication for treatment to reduce the risk of intracerebral hemorrhage, and treatment decreases the risk of maternal death [8, 29]. Risk of hemorrhagic stroke is increased in pregnancy as a result
of impaired cerebral autoregulation. This alteration in physiology may explain why
some women develop intracranial hemorrhage and cerebral edema despite the lack
of significant hypertension. Of note, a woman with severe hypertension due to
chronic hypertension presenting in early pregnancy (i.e., first trimester) should *not*
be treated in a similar manner to women with preeclampsia with rapid lowering of
BP. Such treatment indeed may be harmful [12, 30]. Reducing severely elevated BP
rapidly in chronic hypertension can result in markedly decreased perfusion to the
brain and potential ischemia or infarction.

Commonly used intravenous and oral antihypertensives used to acutely lower
BP in cases of severe hypertension are listed in Table 4.3. A recent meta-analysis of
24 trials (2,949 women) in which different antihypertensive drugs were compared
for the treatment of severe hypertension in pregnancy did not demonstrate superi-
ority of one of these agents over the other in the acute management of severe hypertension [31].

Table 4.3: Commonly used agents for treatment of BP ≥ 160/110 mmHg [3, 4].

Agent	Dosage	Onset of action	Comments
Nifedipine immediate release	5–10 mg orally, repeat in 20 min if needed	5–10 min	May have precipitous drop in BP Headaches and reflex tachycardia
Hydralazine	5 mg IV or IM, then 5–10 mg IV every 20–40 min	10–20 min	Headaches Can be given as continuous infusion
Labetalol	10–20 mg IV	1–2 min	Avoid in women with asthma, decompensated cardiac function and heart block, and bradycardia

4.9 Choice of Antihypertensive Agent

The drugs most commonly used – methyldopa, labetalol, hydralazine, and nifedipine –
are widely accepted as safe in pregnancy, based on many years of clinical experience,
observational data drawn from large databases, and meta-analyses of small clinical trials. The decision about choice of antihypertensives should take into consideration the

risk–benefit ratio to the patient and fetus, medication side effect profile, availability of medications, clinician experience, and patient preference. Methyldopa, labetalol, and slow-release nifedipine are appropriate first-line agents (Table 4.2) with an acceptable safety profile in pregnancy and recommended by international guidelines [9, 16, 28, 32]. These agents have not been examined in comparative effectiveness trials. For emergent treatment of severe hypertension in preeclampsia, short-acting oral nifedipine, IV hydralazine, or IV labetalol can be used (Table 4.3).

4.9.1 Sympathetic Nervous System Inhibition

Methyldopa is one of the most widely used agents in pregnancy with over 40 years of clinical experience [33]. It is a centrally acting alpha-2-adrenergic agonist pro-drug which is metabolized to alpha-methylnorepinephrine which then lowers arterial pressure by stimulation of central inhibitory alpha-adrenergic receptors. Due to this indirect method of action, BP control is gradual over 6–8 h. Adverse effects that are consequences of central alpha-2-agonism which includes decreased mental alertness, increased sense of fatigue or depression, and xerostomia. Methyldopa is also associated with elevated liver enzymes with reports of hepatitis and hepatic necrosis [35]. Rarely, some patients may also develop Coombs' positive hemolytic anemia with prolonged therapy. While the maximum dose is 3000mg daily, beyond 2000mg, there is less incremental benefit. The authors would recommend adding another agent at this point.

4.9.2 Beta-Adrenergic Blockers

Beta-blockers are commonly used in pregnancy; however, there remain some controversies due to a few small studies suggesting lower birth weight infants. In a meta-analysis and Cochrane review, beta-blockers were associated with an increase in small for gestational age infants [35]. However, this effect may have been exaggerated by the inclusion of one small trial of atenolol use in pregnant women with chronic hypertension which resulted in clinically significant fetal growth restriction [36]. The association of atenolol with intrauterine growth restriction/small for gestational age infants has been further validated in other studies and is thus avoided in pregnancy [37]. Further, beta-blockers may be associated with neonatal bradycardia; however, in a systematic review, labetalol does not seem to cause neonatal heart rate effects [38]. Other potential complications include neonatal hypoglycemia. None of the beta-blockers have been associated with teratogenicity. In a 2013 systematic review, there was no overall increase in major congenital malformations, cleft lip/palate, or neural tube defects [39].

Labetalol is commonly used during pregnancy and has both selective alpha-1-adrenergic and nonselective beta-adrenergic receptor-blocking actions. It has a more rapid onset of action than methyldopa (within 2 h versus 6–8 h). Adverse effects include fatigue, exercise intolerance, peripheral vasoconstriction, sleep disturbance, and bronchoconstriction. As such, labetalol should be avoided in patients with severe asthma as it may precipitate bronchospasm. The maximum dose is 2400 mg daily; however, beyond 1200 mg, there is less incremental benefit. The authors' recommendation would be to add another agent at this point.

4.9.3 Calcium Channel Blockers

Oral nifedipine (short-acting and long-acting) is commonly used for treatment of non-severe as well as severe hypertension in pregnancy. It works by inhibiting the inward inflow of calcium across the L-type slow channels of cellular membranes, thus causing smooth muscle relaxation. Nifedipine has been used to treat hypertension for at least 30 years and appears to be safe and well tolerated [40]. It does not pose teratogenic risks to fetuses exposed in the first trimester [41]. Other calcium channel blockers such as verapamil, diltiazem, and amlodipine have been used in pregnancy but there is very limited published safety data available.

Maternal adverse effects of the calcium channel blockers include tachycardia, palpitations, peripheral edema, headaches, and facial flushing. Orally administered short-acting nifedipine has been reported to be associated with maternal hypotension [42, 43]. In a randomized controlled trial comparing intravenous labetalol with oral nifedipine short acting in 120 women, both agents were effective in controlling BP without adverse maternal or fetal side effects, but nifedipine was found to reduce BP more rapidly [44]. Thus, if oral nifedipine immediate release is used to lower BP in a pregnant patient with preeclampsia and severe hypertension, the authors suggest using small incremental (e.g., 5 mg) doses and titrate to effect.

4.9.4 Direct Vasodilators

Hydralazine relaxes arteriolar smooth muscle, and it is useful as a third- or fourth-line agent for multidrug control of refractory chronic hypertension or intravenously for urgent control in the setting of preeclampsia. Adverse effects include headache, nausea, flushing, or palpitations. Chronic use has been associated with rare immunologic reactions including drug-induced lupus syndrome. Hydralazine has not been shown to be associated with teratogenicity; however, there are case reports of neonatal thrombocytopenia [45]. Due to its side effect profile, hydralazine has been supplanted by other agents with fewer adverse risks. In the management of severe hypertension in pregnancy, hydralazine was associated with more maternal hypotension, caesarean sections, placental abruption and adverse effects on fetal heart rate when compared with nifedipine and labetalol in a meta-analyses of 21 trials [46].

4.9.5 Angiotensin-Converting Enzyme Inhibitors and Angiotensin Receptor Antagonists

Angiotensin-converting enzyme (ACE) inhibitors and angiotensin receptor blockers (ARB) are contraindicated in the second and third trimesters due to toxicity associated with reduced perfusion to the fetal kidneys with resultant fetopathy similar to that observed in Potter's Syndrome (renal tubular dysgenesis, fetal oliguria, oligohydramnios, fetal growth restriction, joint contractures, neonatal anuric renal failure, and calvarial and pulmonary hypoplasia [47–48]). In a more recent study of prospectively ascertained ACE inhibitor and ARB-exposed pregnancies from the databases of six teratology information services demonstrated the rate of fetopathy was 3.2% for ACE inhibitors and 29.2% in ARB. All pregnancies affected with fetopathy were exposed after 20 weeks gestation.

Whether ACE inhibitors or ARBs are associated with fetopathy in the first trimester is controversial. An observational cohort study which included 138 pregnancies exposed to ACE inhibitors or ARBs found no difference in rates of major malformations when compared to disease-matched groups of women with hypertension treated with other antihypertensives or healthy controls [49]. A recent larger cohort study examining first-trimester exposure to ACE inhibitors and ARBs in 4,107 pregnancies found that there was no associated increased risk of major congenital malformations [50]. Regardless, these medications should be discontinued prior to conception or, in the case of unplanned conception, as soon as pregnancy is recognized.

4.10 Management of Postpartum Hypertension

Transient new onset postpartum hypertension can be due to multiple factors including administration of intravenous fluids in women receiving neuraxial anesthesia for labor, administration of nonsteroidal anti-inflammatory agents, mobilization of extravascular fluid postpartum, and ergot derivatives for treatment of postpartum hemorrhage. In previously normotensive women, BP has been noted to be elevated and reach a maximum on the fifth postpartum day with 12% of patients having a DBP exceeding 100 mmHg [51]. Certainly, in clinical practice, this physiology is accentuated in women with HDP. Women are counseled that BP will rise between days 3 and 5 postpartum, requiring clinical vigilance and appropriate medical management.

Choice of antihypertensive agent in the postpartum period is influenced by breastfeeding. Methyldopa, nifedipine, labetalol, and hydralazine are safe in breastfeeding with low neonatal exposure in breast milk [52]. Sufficient data exists for the safety of enalapril, captopril, and quinalapril for breastfeeding, and women with a strong indication for renin–angiotensin system blockade are switched to one of these agents postpartum [53]. There is insufficient evidence for the safety of ARBs; thus, these are avoided during lactation.

Diuretics are generally avoided while breastfeeding due to theoretical reduction in milk volume although milk concentrations of diuretics are low and considered safe. A short course of furosemide could be considered if there were maternal indications for prompt diuresis including severe peripheral edema or pulmonary edema [54].

References

[1]   Steegers EAP, Von Dadelszen P, Duvekot JJ, Pijnenborg RR. Pre-eclampsia, seminar. Lancet 2010;376(9741):631–644.
[2]   Wallis AB, Saftlas AF, Hsia J, Atrash HK. Secular trends in the rates of preeclampsia, eclampsia, and gestational hypertension, United States, 1987–2004. Am J Hypertens 2008;21(5):521–526.
[3]   Lo JO, Mission JF, Caughey AB. Hypertensive disease of pregnancy and maternal mortality. Curr Opin Obstet Gynecol 2013;25(2):124–132.
[4]   Magee LA, Pels A, Helewa M, Rey E, Von Dadelszen P. Diagnosis, evaluation, and management of the hypertensive disorders of pregnancy: executive summary. J Obstet Gynaecol Canada 2014;36(5):416–438.
[5]   American College of Obstetricians and Task Force on Hypertension in Pregnancy – Hypertension in pregnancy. Report of the American college of obstetricians and gynecologists' task force on hypertension in pregnancy. Obstet Gynecol 2013;122(5): 1122–1131.
[6]   ACOG – Clinical management guidelines for obstetrician – gynecologists. Obstet Gynecol 2019;133(76):168–186.
[7]   Reddy M, Rolnik DL, Harris K, et al. Challenging the definition of hypertension in pregnancy: a retrospective cohort study. Am J Obstet Gynecol 2020.
[8]   Martin JN, Thigpen BD, Moore RC, Rose CH, Cushman J, May W. Stroke and severe preeclampsia and eclampsia: a paradigm shift focusing on systolic blood pressure. Obstet Gynecol 2005;105(2):246–254.
[9]   ACOG – Clinical Management. Guidelines for obstetrician – gynecologists – gestational hypertension and preeclampsia. Obstet Gynecol 2019;133(76):168–186.
[10]   Barton JR, O'Brien JM, Bergauer NK, Jacques DL, Sibai BM. Mild gestational hypertension remote from term: progression and outcome. Am J Obstet Gynecol 2001;184(5):979–983.
[11]   Saudan P, Brown MA, Buddle ML, Jones M. Does gestational hypertension become pre-eclampsia?. Br J Obstet Gynaecol 1998 Nov;105(11):1177–1184.
[12]   Chobanian AV, Bakris GL, Black HR, et al. Seventh report of the joint national committee on prevention, detection, evaluation, and treatment of high blood pressure. Hypertension 2003;42(6):1206–1252.
[13]   ACOG Practice Bulletin No. 203. Chronic hypertension in pregnancy. Obstet Gynecol 2019 Jan;133(1):e26–e50.
[14]   Berks D, Steegers EAP, Molas M, Visser W. Resolution of hypertension and proteinuria. Obstet Gynecol 2009;114(6):1307–1314.
[15]   Brown MA, Mangos G, Davis G, Homer C. The natural history of white coat hypertension during pregnancy. BJOG An Int J Obstet Gynaecol 2005;112(5):601–606.
[16]   Seely EW, Ecker J. Chronic hypertension in pregnancy. Circulation 2014;129(11):1254–1261.

[17] De Haas S, Ghossein-Doha C, Van Kuijk SMJ, Van Drongelen J, Spaanderman MEA. Adaptación fisiológica del volumen del plasma materno durante el embarazo: Una revisi\xF3n sistemática y metaanálisis. Ultrasound Obstet Gynecol 2017;49(2):177–187.

[18] Lund CJ, Donovan JC. Blood volume during pregnancy. Significance of plasma and red cell volumes. Am J Obstet Gynecol 1967 Jun;98(3):394–403.

[19] Meah VL, Cockcroft JR, Backx K, Shave R, Stöhr EJ. Cardiac output and related haemodynamics during pregnancy: a series of meta-analyses. Heart 2016;102(7):518–526.

[20] Vongpatanasin W. Resistant hypertension: a review of diagnosis and management. JAMA – J Am Med Assoc 2014;311(21):2216–2224.

[21] Gilbert WV, Young AL, Danielsen B. Pregnancy outcomes in women with chronic hypertension: a population-based study. J Reprod Med 2007 Nov;52(11):1046–1051.

[22] ACOG. Clinical management guidelines for obstetrician. Gynecologists. Obstet Gynecol 2019;133(76):168–186.

[23] Bramham K, Parnell B, Nelson-Piercy C, Seed PT, Poston L, Chappell LC. Chronic hypertension and pregnancy outcomes: systematic review and meta-analysis. BMJ 2014;348(April):1–20.

[24] Butalia S, Audbiert FM, Cote FM, et al. Hypertension Canada's 2018 Guidelines for the Management of Hypertension in Pregnancy. Can J Cardiol 2018;34(5):526–531.

[25] Denolle T, Weber JL, Calvez C, et al. Diagnosis of White Coat Hypertension in Pregnant Women with Teletransmitted Home Blood Pressure. Hypertens Pregnancy 2008 Jan;27(3):305–313.

[26] Von Dadelszen P, Magee LA. Fall in mean arterial pressure and fetal growth restriction in pregnancy hypertension: an updated metaregression analysis. J Obstet Gynaecol Can 2002;24(12):941–945.

[27] Magee LA, Von Dadelszen P, Rey E, et al. Less-tight versus tight control of hypertension in pregnancy. N Engl J Med 2015;372(5):407–417.

[28] Brown MA, Magee LA, Kenny LC, et al. Hypertensive disorders of pregnancy: ISSHP classification, diagnosis, and management recommendations for international practice. Hypertension 2018;72(1):24–43.

[29] Liu S, Liston RM, Joseph KM, Heaman M, Sauve R, Kramer MS. Maternal mortality and severe morbidity associated with low-risk planned cesarean delivery versus planned vaginal delivery at term. CMAJ 2007;176(4):455–460.

[30] Decker WW, Godwin SA, Hess EP, Lenamond CC, Jagoda AS. Clinical policy: critical issues in the evaluation and management of adult patients with asymptomatic hypertension in the emergency department. Ann Emerg Med 2006;47(3):237–249.

[31] Duley L, Meher S, Jones L. Drugs for treatment of very high blood pressure during pregnancy. Cochrane Database Syst Rev 2013;7, 2013.

[32] Lowe SA, Bowyer L, Lust K, et al. The SOMANZ Guideline for the Management of Hypertensive Disorders of Pregnancy 2014.

[33] Cockburn J, Ounsted M, Moar VA, Redman CWG. Final report of study on hypertension during pregnancy: the effects of specific treatement on the growth and development of the children. Lancet 1982 Mar;319(8273):647–649.

[34] Schweitzer IL, Peters RL. Acute submassive hepatic necrosis due to methyldopa. A case demonstrating possible initiation of chronic liver disease. Gastroenterology 1974 Jun;66(6):1203–1211.

[35] Magee LA, Duley L. Oral beta-blockers for mild to moderate hypertension during pregnancy. Cochrane Database Syst Rev 2003;3.

[36] Butters L, Kennedy S, Rubin PC. Atenolol in essential hypertension during pregnancy. BMJ 1990 Sep;301(6752):587–589.

[37] Lydakis C, Lip GY, Beevers M, Beevers DG. Atenolol and fetal growth in pregnancies complicated by hypertension. Am J Hypertens 1999 Jun;12(6):541–547.

[38] Waterman EJ, Magee LA, Lim KI, Skoll A, Rurak D. and von Dadelszen P. Do commonly used oral antihypertensives alter fetal or neonatal heart rate characteristics? A systematic review. Hypertens Pregnancy 2004;23(2):155–169.

[39] Yakoob MY, Bateman BT, Ho E, et al. The risk of congenital malformations associated with exposure to β-blockers early in pregnancy: a meta-analysis. Hypertension 2013;62(2): 375–381.

[40] Aedla N, Fisher M, McKay G. Nifedipine in pregnancy. Pract Diabetes 2012;29(7):295–296.

[41] Magee LA, Schick B, Donnefeld AE, et al. The safety of calcium channel blockers in human pregnancy: a prospective, multicenter cohort study. Am J Obstet Gynecol 1996;174(3): 823–828.

[42] Puzey MS, Ackovic KL, Lindow SW, Gonin R. The effect of nifedipine on fetal umbilical artery Doppler waveforms in pregnancies complicated by hypertension. S Afr Med J 1991 Feb;79(4): 192–194.

[43] Brown MA, Buddle ML, Farrell T, Davis GK. Efficacy and safety of nifedipine tablets for the acute treatment of severe hypertension in pregnancy. Am J Obstet Gynecol 2002 Oct;187(4): 1046–1050.

[44] Zulfeen M, Tatapudi R, Sowjanya R. IV labetalol and oral nifedipine in acute control of severe hypertension in pregnancy-A randomized controlled trial. Eur J Obstet Gynecol Reprod Biol 2019 May;236:46–52.

[45] Widerlov E, Karlman I, Storsater J. Hydralazine-induced neonatal thrombocytopenia. N Engl J Med Nov 1980;303(21), United States:1235.

[46] Magee LA, Cham C, Waterman EJ, Ohlsson A, Von Dadelszen P. Hydralazine for treatment of severe hypertension in pregnancy: meta-analysis 2003:1–10.

[47] Pryde PG, Sedman AB, Nugent CE, Barr M. Angiotensin-converting enzyme inhibitor fetopathy. J Am Soc Nephrol 1993 Mar;3(9):1575–1582.

[48] Buttar HS. An overview of the influence of ACE inhibitors on fetal-placental circulation and perinatal development. Mol Cell Biochem 1997 Nov;176(1–2):61–71.

[49] Gubler MC. Renal tubular dysgenesis. Pediatr Nephrol 2014 Jan;29(1):51–59.

[50] Moretti ME, Caprara D, Drehuta I, et al. The fetal safety of angiotensin converting enzyme inhibitors and angiotensin ii receptor blockers. Obstet Gynecol Int 2012;2012.

[51] Bateman BT, Patrono E, Desai R, et al. Angiotensin-converting enzyme inhibitors and the risk of congenital malformations. Obstet Gynecol 2017 Jan;129(1):174–184.

[52] Walters BN, Thompson ME, Lee A, De Swiet M. Blood pressure in the puerperium. Clin Sci (Lond) 1986 Nov;71(5):589–594.

[53] A. A. of P. C. on Drug. Transfer of drugs and other chemicals into human milk.. Pediatrics 2001 Sep;108(3):776–789.

[54] White WB. Management of hypertension during lactation. Hypertens (Dallas, Tex 1979) 1984;6(3):297–300.

Laura Berall, Michelle A. Hladunewich
5 Kidney Disease in Pregnancy

5.1 Introduction

Women with chronic kidney disease (CKD) are at a higher risk of adverse maternal and fetal outcomes. Adverse maternal outcomes include worsening renal function, increased proteinuria, or a flare of underlying glomerular diseases. Women with CKD are also at a higher risk of hypertensive disorders of pregnancy, such as pre-eclampsia, and this can occur up to 10 times more frequently than in the general population [1–3]. Associated fetal risks include preterm birth and intrauterine growth restriction, which results in significant neonatal morbidity, and rarely neonatal death.

Early involvement of a nephrologist and a multidisciplinary team for prepregnancy counseling can assist women in identifying "a safe window of opportunity" for pregnancy and help mitigate the risk of a poor maternal and/or fetal outcome by optimizing a woman's prenatal condition. Further, women with genetic renal diseases should be offered genetic counseling to discuss risks of inheritance as well as options such as preimplantation genetics. When conception is not optimal or desired, effective contraception should be prescribed.

5.2 Renal Physiology in Normal Pregnancy and the Diagnosis of Kidney Disease

Multiple alternations to renal physiology occur in a normal pregnancy. There are anatomical changes, including increased kidney size and dilatation of the collecting system. Notable hemodynamic changes result in increased renal plasma flow, and hence, glomerular hyperfiltration. Finally, other expected changes include altered tubular function as well as changes in electrolyte balances [4–6].

Given these adaptations, a significant decline in serum creatinine concentration during the first trimester is anticipated. Creatinine will stabilize by the second trimester and return to baseline levels toward the end of the third trimester and into the postpartum period. This was demonstrated in a retrospective administrative database study which included more than 240,000 women without antecedent kidney disease [7]. The expected trend in creatinine is shown in Figure 5.1, wherein a "normal" serum creatinine or one that has not changed from baseline in fact represents renal insufficiency. This should be noted as a red flag, prompt closer monitoring, and trigger further evaluation. When assessing renal function, clinicians must be aware that equations to estimate glomerular filtration rate (GFR) are inaccurate in

https://doi.org/10.1515/9783110615258-005

pregnancy and tend to underestimate GFR [8, 9]. A 24 h urine for creatinine clearance can be considered, but this is cumbersome and often collected inappropriately without careful instructions.

In the nonpregnant state, a healthy adult should excrete less than 30 mg of albumin or less than 150 mg of protein in the urine per 24 h period. Due to the physiologic changes in pregnancy, including reduced tubular reabsorption, the degree of protein excretion in the urine may be somewhat higher than in the nonpregnant state [4]. Obstetric guidelines define an abnormal degree of proteinuria as a protein-to-creatinine ratio of ≥30 mg/mmol or ≥300 mg of protein per day on a 24 h urine collection [10]. Abnormal levels of proteinuria in pregnancy are rare, with studies suggesting that it may be on the order of 3–27% of pregnancies [11–13]. Any pregnant women with significantly abnormal levels of urinary protein excretion (>1 g/day) should be referred to a nephrologist for further investigation and management.

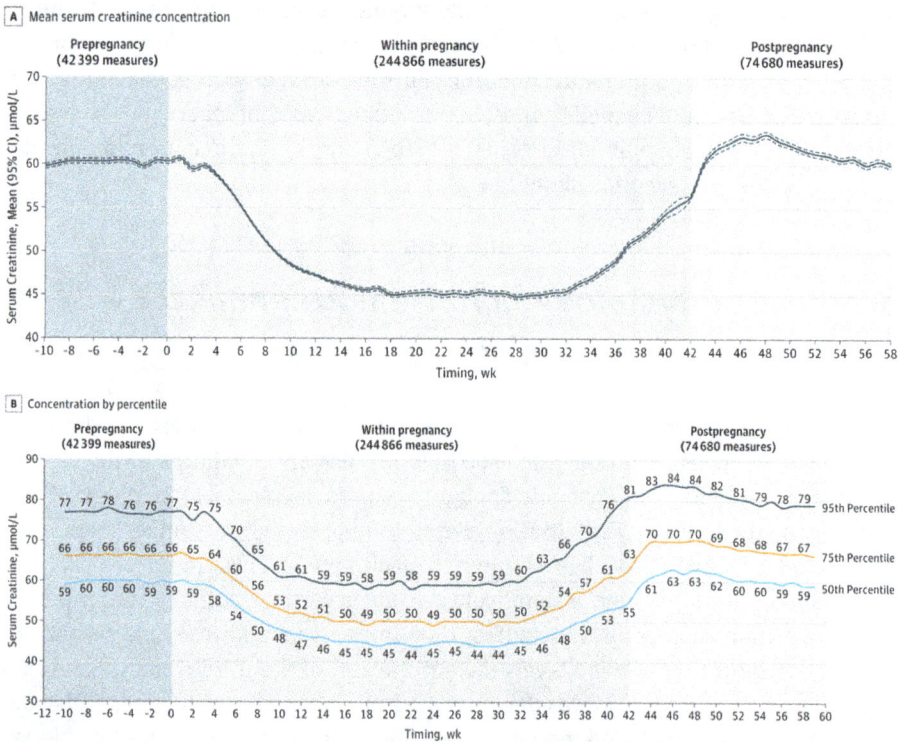

A, Dashed curves indicate upper and lower 95% CI bounds. B, Values adjacent to each curve indicate the percentile-specific corresponding serum creatinine values at each time point. To convert creatinine values to mg/dL, divide by 88.4.

Figure 5.1: Mean serum creatinine concentrations with 50th, 75th, and 95th percentile values among 243,534 women with singleton pregnancies and apparently healthy renal function. Figure reprinted with permission from [7].

5.3 Renal Biopsy in Pregnancy

Percutaneous native kidney biopsies can provide crucial diagnostic and prognostic information. While it is ideal to perform a renal biopsy prior to pregnancy, it is reasonable to request a biopsy early in a pregnancy if the diagnostic information will affect treatment selection. Establishing a diagnosis early in a disease course can allow for prompt initiation of appropriate therapy and can potentially avoid unnecessary treatments. This is particularly true for diagnosing acute versus CKD in a woman with no prepregnancy laboratory values, or in a woman presenting with new onset nephrotic syndrome.

As shown in a meta-analysis comparing 243 biopsies in pregnancy with 1,236 postpartum biopsies, there is a higher documented complication rate for biopsies conducted during pregnancy [14]. This study noted the risk of complications was 7% in biopsies performed during pregnancy compared to only 1% in postpartum biopsies ($P = 0.001$). Notably, complication rates were highest and most severe between 23 and 26 weeks of gestation. Otherwise, the complications mostly included loin pain and perirenal hematomas [14]. While renal biopsy is feasible in early gestation, pursuing a renal biopsy in later pregnancy can be challenging for several reasons, including patient positioning, as well as the risk of evolving hypertension and abnormal coagulation if the patient develops superimposed preeclampsia. As such, in later gestation the risks may begin to outweigh the benefits of a biopsy, and this should be clearly discussed with each woman prior to proceeding with the procedure.

5.4 Acute Kidney Injury in Pregnancy

Acute kidney injury (AKI) in pregnancy contributes to higher rates of both maternal and fetal morbidity and mortality. Fortunately, in both developing and developed countries, overall rates of AKI in pregnancy have decreased significantly over the last several decades. In India, for example, a recent study notes the rate of AKI to be 2.78% between 2014 and 2016 [15], improving significantly from earlier studies noting rates of approximately 10% [16]. These decreased rates are attributed to less peripartum sepsis and hemorrhage due to enhanced obstetrical care, despite increasing rates of gestational hypertension and preeclampsia. Similarly, there has been a slight increase in the rate of pregnancy-related AKI in the developed world in recent years, also attributed to increased rates of the hypertensive disorders of pregnancy. Specifically, Canadian data report an increased rate of pregnancy-related AKI from 1.66 per 10,000 deliveries between 2003 and 2004 to 2.68 per 10,000 deliveries from 2009 to 2010 [17]. Data from the United States show a similar trend with rates of AKI rising from 2.4 to 6.3 per 10,000 deliveries between 1999–2001 and 2010–2011, respectively [18]. Although increased rates may reflect increased vigilance in monitoring and reporting, the societal trend to delay childbirth results in the expanded use of reproductive assistance and more frequently associated comorbidities such as hypertension, diabetes, and obesity as maternal age advances. While in the developing world, the increased burden of obesity-associated comorbidities is further exacerbated by lack of access to care.

There are no specific criteria to define AKI in pregnancy. While specific criteria exist for the nonpregnant state, these have not been validated in a pregnant population. Additionally, as established above, equations to estimate GFR are not accurate [8, 9]. Further, the serum creatinine may in fact underestimate the level of AKI due to expected physiological changes of pregnancy. As such, careful clinical monitoring in women who do not demonstrate a renal accommodation to pregnancy is indicated [7].

Causes and frequencies of AKI in pregnancy vary somewhat by trimester. In the first trimester, AKI is often due to prerenal physiology secondary to volume depletion (e.g., severe hyperemesis gravidarum) or sepsis (e.g., septic abortion). Moving into the second and third trimesters, AKI from thrombotic microangiopathies become more prominent along with the hypertensive disorders of pregnancy. Although thrombotic thrombocytopenic purpura (TTP) can occur at any time during pregnancy, new onset disease or a relapse of TTP most commonly develops during the second or third trimester, as pregnancy is associated with a progressive deficiency of Von Willebrand factor cleaving protease (ADAMTS-13). Beyond 20 weeks of gestation, both preeclampsia and hemolysis, elevated liver enzymes, and low platelets (HELLP) syndrome may cause AKI. While AKI is a rare complication of preeclampsia (1%) [19], it is seen more frequently in the context syndrome of HELLP syndrome (7–15%) [20, 21]. Acute fatty liver of pregnancy (AFLP) is a rare condition that develops in the third trimester of pregnancy due to abnormal oxidation of fatty acids by fetal mitochondria [22, 23]. Fetal deficiency of long-chain 3-hydroxyl CoA dehydrogenase leads to excess fetal free fatty acids that cross the placenta, causing maternal hepatotoxicity and AKI due to acute tubular necrosis (ATN), fatty vacuolization of tubular cells, and occlusion of capillary lumens by fibrin-like material as noted on kidney biopsy [22, 24]. AKI, secondary to obstruction of the urinary tract, also most often occurs into the third trimester due to the gravid uterus. While atypical hemolytic uremic syndrome (aHUS), secondary to genetic mutations in complement regulatory proteins, tends to appear around the time of delivery with more than two-thirds of cases presenting postpartum, and more commonly in the second pregnancy [25]. In the approximately half of the patients with detected complement gene variants, severe disease including progression to end-stage renal disease (ESRD) is more likely to occur, making rapid diagnosis and treatment imperative [26]. Other rare obstetrical catastrophes (e.g., amniotic fluid embolism, massive hemorrhage, or placental abruption) can cause disseminated intravascular coagulation (DIC) and ischemic ATN, and, if severe enough can result in bilateral cortical necrosis, the most extreme form of hemodynamic kidney injury [27]. It is a pathologic diagnosis characterized by diffuse cortical necrosis on kidney biopsy with evidence of intravascular thrombosis. Pregnant women are uniquely at risk for this irreversible adverse event presumably due to the hypercoagulable state that accompanies pregnancy in the context of endothelial dysfunction. Finally, acute pyelonephritis or flares of underlying glomerulonephritis can cause AKI at any time during a pregnancy.

Establishing the underlying cause of an AKI in pregnancy can be challenging, particularly since many of the causes can manifest with similar clinical signs and symptoms. Specifically, it can be challenging to differentiate between preeclampsia, HELLP syndrome, aHUS, TTP, AFLP, and DIC, but an understanding on the pathophysiology can assist with the appropriate diagnosis. Table 5.1 compares and contrasts these conditions to assist in clinical differentiation.

Management of AKI in pregnancy is directed towards the specific underlying cause and includes supportive care, both for the mother and the fetus. In hypertensive disorders of pregnancy, such as severe preeclampsia, HELLP syndrome, and AFLP, timely fetal delivery is indicated. Plasmapheresis should be used in TTP and prompt therapy of aHUS with eculizumab can dramatically improve renal recovery. For proven glomerulonephritis, pregnancy-safe immunosuppressive therapy should be given as appropriate for the underlying glomerular condition. Maternal supportive care includes volume resuscitation and medical management of specific complications, for example, pregnancy-safe antibiotics for sepsis, treatment of acid–base disturbances with bicarbonate, transfusions for anemia, cautious use of diuretics in volume overload, and rarely, dialysis. Fetal supportive care involves close monitoring of fetal well-being, celestone for lung maturation (at <34 weeks' gestational age), and carefully timed delivery. Magnesium, given for either maternal and/or fetal neuroprotection, requires dose reductions as renally excreted, and women with severe AKI are at risk of magnesium toxicity (hyporeflexia and hypotension) and should be monitored closely.

Even when resolved, any episode of AKI is a risk factor for future adverse pregnancy outcomes. A recent study demonstrated that women who conceived within 18 months of an episode of AKI had a sevenfold higher rate of preeclampsia and a fourfold increase in having their infant require an admission to the neonatal intensive care unit (NICU). The risk was attenuated if they waited for at least 18 months after the episode of AKI to conceive [28].

Table 5.1: Clinical differentiation between major causes of acute kidney injury in pregnancy.

	Preeclampsia	HELLP	aHUS	TTP	AFLP	DIC
Cause	Abnormal placentation	Abnormal placentation	Abnormal complement function	ADAMTS 13 deficiency	Defects in fetal mitochondrial fatty acid beta-oxidation metabolism	Catastrophic events in pregnancy**
Timing of onset	>20 weeks' GA	>20 weeks' GA	Late gestation/ postpartum	2nd and 3rd trimester	Third trimester	Anytime
Notable symptoms	Headache, right upper quadrant pain, blurred vision, and swelling	Headache, right upper quadrant pain, blurred vision, and swelling	Nonspecific, but renal symptoms dominate	Nonspecific, but neurological symptoms dominate	Jaundice, nausea and vomiting, and abdominal pain	Nonspecific, bleeding/ oozing
Fever	–	–	–/+	+++	–	–/+
Hypertension (>140/90 mmHg)	+++	+++	++	+	+	–
Presence of abnormal proteinuria*	+++	+++	++	+	+	–/+
Hemolytic anemia	–	++	++	+++	+	+/++
Thrombocytopenia	–	++	++	+++	+	+/++
Clotting time						Prolonged
Hypoglycemia	–	–/+	–	–	+	–/+

Elevated liver enzymes	–	++	–/+	–/+	+++	–/+
ADAMTS 13 level	Normal	Normal	Normal	Low (<10%)	Normal	Normal
Complement levels	Normal	Normal	Decreased	Normal	Normal	Normal
Recovery	After delivery	After delivery	Not affected by delivery	Not affected by delivery	After delivery	After delivery (can depend on cause)

HELLP, hemolysis, elevated liver enzymes, low platelets; aHUS, atypical hemolytic uremic syndrome; TTP, thrombotic thrombocytopenic purpura; AFLP, acute fatty liver of pregnancy; GA, gestational age.

*Abnormal proteinuria is defined as a protein-to-creatinine ratio of ≥30 mg/mmol or ≥300 mg of protein per day on a 24 h urine collection.

**Catastrophic obstetrical events include severe sepsis, amniotic fluid embolism, pulmonary embolism, and placental abruption.

5.5 Pregnancy in Women with Chronic Kidney Disease

5.5.1 Prepregnancy Counseling and Optimization

Before confirming a woman with CKD is safe to proceed with a pregnancy, she should receive prepregnancy counseling and optimization. Ideally, she would work with her healthcare providers and nephrologist to ensure stabilization of her renal function, decrease proteinuria, control blood pressure, and finally to ensure ongoing emotional well-being. Underlying renal disease should be stable prior to conception, and there should be no recent episodes of AKI or flares of glomerular disease. Stable renal function, proteinuria less than 1 g/day, and well-controlled blood pressure are positive prognostic factors. All women with CKD should also be advised to initiate a prenatal vitamin with folic acid daily for at least 3 months prior to conception.

Prior to a pregnancy, it is important to review the risk for loss of kidney function, which is directly related to the degree of baseline renal insufficiency. In women with preserved kidney function, significant loss is unlikely, and pregnancy has not been noted to expedite progression to ESRD [3]. However, in women with more advanced kidney diseases at baseline, there is a higher chance of losing underlying renal function and progressing to a more severe stage of CKD or even dialysis. In an Italian cohort [2], 20% of women with stage 4 (GFR 15–29 mL/min/1.73 m^2) or stage 5 (GFR < 15 mL/min/1.73 m^2) non-dialysis CKD progressed to a more advanced stage of CKD or dialysis. Irrespective of the degree of renal dysfunction, inadequately treated concomitant hypertension may contribute to further renal damage even in women with only moderate renal insufficiency [29]. Further, when proteinuria exceeds 1 g/day in combination with significantly compromised GFR (<40 mL/min), accelerated postpartum loss of GFR has been noted [30].

Preconception, proteinuria should therefore also be treated aggressively, and ideally be less than 1 g/day preconception [3]. In diseases treated with immunosuppressive therapy, it is important to ensure that this target is achieved on pregnancy-safe immunosuppression. Examples of pregnancy-safe immunosuppression include glucocorticoids, azathioprine, and calcineurin inhibitors. Immunosuppressive medications often used for renal disease that should be stopped prior to conception include mycophenolic acid and cyclophosphamide. Specifically, for mycophenolic acid, it is advised that this is stopped at least 3 months prior to conception.

In the nonpregnant state, renin–angiotensin system (RAS) blockers are often used to treat proteinuria; however, RAS blockade cannot be used in pregnancy. Therefore, careful consideration about when to discontinue these medications must be undertaken. In renal diseases treated with immunosuppression, we often stop RAS blockade when planning a pregnancy to ensure immunosuppression can maintain proteinuria less than 1 g/day preconception. In renal diseases not treated with immunosuppression, such as diabetic nephropathy, the use of RAS blockers preconception has been shown to improve fetal outcomes [31, 32]. However, it is important to counsel your patient that these medications have teratogenicity in the second and third trimesters, and therefore must be stopped at the time of conception and by 8 weeks' gestation. Other conservative therapy that should be stopped prior to conception include statins, and diuretics (dose and type) need to be evaluated.

Women with chronic hypertension have higher rates of superimposed preeclampsia, caesarean section, preterm delivery at less than 37 weeks' gestation, low birth weight, NICU admission, and perinatal death [33, 34]. As such, obtaining tight blood pressure control prior to conception has been associated with improved fetal outcomes [35, 36]. This should ideally be achieved with pregnancy-safe medications including, but not limited to, nifedipine, methyldopa, labetalol, and hydralazine.

Finally, it is imperative to consider your patient's emotional well-being. Women with CKD must cope during a high-risk pregnancy as well as raise their children while having a chronic disease. This can trigger increased fear and anxiety [37, 38]. Early recognition and referral for support from social work and other mental health professionals when necessary is crucial.

5.5.2 Management of CKD in Pregnancy

Once women with CKD are pregnant, they must be closely followed by both a high-risk obstetrician and an experienced nephrologist. Maternal antenatal care is focused on monitoring for stability of renal function, worsening of proteinuria, as well as control of coincident conditions such as hypertension, lupus, or diabetes. Obstetrical care concentrates on the assessment of fetal well-being with serial obstetrical ultrasounds used to monitor fetal growth, placental morphology, and blood flow.

To help mitigate the risk of preeclampsia, women with CKD and/or chronic hypertension should initiate aspirin (150–162 mg daily) at 10–12 weeks' gestational age [39–43]. The beneficial effects of aspirin are maximized when taken at bedtime [44, 45] and when started before 16 weeks' gestation [40–42]. Aspirin is typically stopped between 35 and 36 weeks of gestation in preparation for delivery. Supplemental calcium, to target a total daily intake of 1,000 mg from diet and supplementary forms per day, may also help mitigate the risk of preeclampsia in high-risk women [46].

Pregnant women with CKD have higher rates of hypertension in pregnancy and should be treated to specific blood pressure targets of 120/80 to 140/90 mmHg with pregnancy-safe antihypertensive therapies [47, 48]. Home blood pressure monitoring with a calibrated device can help with titration of medication. Although no randomized controlled trials exist to establish optimal blood pressure targets among patients with CKD in the context of pregnancy, extrapolation from the Control of Hypertension in Pregnancy Study trial is reasonable [48]. While no significant difference in the risk of pregnancy loss or overall maternal complications was noted with less-tight (100 mmHg)) versus tight (85 mmHg) control of diastolic blood pressure, women with less-tight blood pressure control had a significantly higher frequency of severe maternal hypertension [48].

Diagnosing preeclampsia can be complex and challenging in women with CKD, given that worsening renal function, hypertension, and proteinuria can all be manifestations of worsening renal disease or superimposed preeclampsia. Thorough investigations should be undertaken to look for clinical or laboratory evidence of worsening renal disease or a flare (i.e., urine microscopy and serology). However, abnormal placental Doppler as well as a decreasing rate of interval fetal growth can hint toward superimposed preeclampsia, given that the pathogenesis of preeclampsia is related to abnormal placentation [49]. Recently, there is growing evidence that maternal circulating angiogenic markers, including plasma placental growth factor (PlGF), soluble Fms-like tyrosine kinase 1 (sFlt-1), and the ratio of sFlt-1/PlGF, can help differentiate CKD from preeclampsia [50, 51]. Further studies to guide the use of these markers in women with CKD are required. Due to these diagnostic challenges, the nephrologist and high-risk obstetrician should work closely together to determine the best next steps.

5.5.3 Postpartum Care

Women should be seen within 6 weeks of delivery to monitor for resolving preeclampsia or postpartum onset of preeclampsia. It is also important to follow serum creatinine in the postpartum period to determine if there was loss of renal function during the pregnancy. Adjustments to antihypertensive medications are frequently required. Additionally, if medications needed to be adjusted given altered pharmacokinetics in pregnancy, for example, calcineurin inhibitors, it is important to reassess these doses early in the postpartum period. Finally, in conjunction with the obstetrician and/or family physician, conversations should again be had around the value of contraception until she is ready to plan for her next pregnancy.

There is no contraindication to breastfeeding, and medications compatible with breastfeeding should be prescribed whenever possible. RAS blockade should be restarted early in the postpartum period to help maintain control of proteinuria and hypertension. This is a key management consideration for women with nonimmune-mediated proteinuric renal diseases such as diabetes or secondary focal segmental glomerulosclerosis, but can also be useful in immune-mediated conditions such as IgA nephropathy, to either supplement or to minimize exposure to immunosuppression. Enalapril, captopril, and quinapril are safe to be used in breastfeeding [52, 53].

5.6 Disease-Specific Comments

5.6.1 Lupus Nephritis in Pregnancy

It has been well demonstrated that active lupus nephritis at the time of conception and during a pregnancy is associated with worse pregnancy outcomes, with especially high rates of preterm birth [54–56]. Adverse pregnancy outcomes are less frequent when disease is stable and quiescent at time of conception and during pregnancy. This was demonstrated in the recent PROMISSE study, wherein 81% of pregnancies in women with inactive or stable active lupus were uncomplicated [57]. Experts therefore advise that women should have stable, quiescent lupus for at least 6 months prior to conception [47, 58, 59].

Prior to conception, all women should be tested for anti-SSA/Ro and anti-SSB/La antibodies as these can increase the risk of neonatal lupus and fetal heart block. These patients should undergo fetal echocardiography in the second trimester [60]. Hydroxychloroquine use in pregnancy can decrease the risk of congenital heart block by up to 50% [57, 61, 62]. Continuing hydroxychloroquine in pregnancy is safe [63, 64] and strongly advised as it has also been shown to also reduce the rate of maternal lupus flares [65, 66]. Additionally, hydroxychloroquine use during pregnancy reduces the probability of intrauterine growth restriction [56]. Finally, the presence of antiphospholipid antibodies have been associated with higher rates of preterm birth, hypertension, and fetal loss, and it is important to screen for these early [54, 56] so that appropriate treatment with either aspirin or low-molecular-weight heparin can be initiated.

When monitoring disease activity in pregnancy, it should be noted that complement levels often rise, and as such, a decrease in complements levels, even within the normal range, may be indicative of disease activity. After 24 weeks' gestation, it can be very difficult to distinguish between a lupus flare and preeclampsia. Clinical clues and laboratory investigations can help with the differentiation. Notably, in a lupus flare, complement levels may decrease while anti-double-stranded DNA antibody levels increase. As safe treatment options are limited, biopsy is rarely indicated.

5.6.2 Diabetic Nephropathy in Pregnancy

Prepregnancy optimization in women with diabetic nephropathy is a key component in managing the risks of pregnancy. Prior to attempting pregnancy, women with diabetes must have optimal diabetic control, as well as a recent retinal examination. As mentioned above, the use of RAS blockers preconception has been shown to minimize proteinuria, and therefore, improve maternal and fetal outcomes [31, 32].

Pregnancy outcomes are similar in women with type 1 and type 2 diabetes [67]. Women with pregestational diabetic nephropathy tend to have worse pregnancy outcomes than those without diabetic nephropathy [68]. In general, if a woman has well-preserved renal function prior to conception, pregnancy will likely not accelerate the progression of her renal disease [69]. However, a small study of women with diabetic nephropathy and moderate-to-severe renal impairment demonstrated a permanent decline in renal function postpartum in 45% of women [70]. There were also significant rates of hypertensive disorders of pregnancy, with 73% of these women developing worsening hypertension or preeclampsia [70]. With regard to other adverse pregnancy outcomes associated with diabetic nephropathy, studies have noted rates of preeclampsia to be as high as 64% [71] with rates of delivery at less than 37 weeks' gestation to be as high as 77% along with high rates of caesarean section (71%) [72]. Further, up to 45% of these mothers have a small for gestational age baby [71], and up to 49% of babies will need an admission to the NICU [71–73].

5.6.3 Hereditary Kidney Disease in Pregnancy

Women with a history of a hereditary kidney disease who wish to become pregnant should also be counseled by a genetics specialist who can help inform them about the disease heritability pattern, educate about available genetic screening, as well as the reproductive options, such as preimplantation genetics, which has been used successfully in both carriers of autosomal dominant and recessive polycystic kidney disease [74, 75]. In women with CKD, we advise single embryo transfer, as a multiple fetus pregnancy can further increase the risk of hypertensive disorders of pregnancy and preterm delivery. Limited data are available with regard to pregnancy outcomes in specific conditions with the exception of autosomal dominant polycystic kidney disease (ADPKD) and Alport's syndrome.

Women with ADPKD appear to have similar rates of fertility to women without ADPKD [76]. Additionally, a study of 235 women with ADPKD and 108 women without ADPKD found that normotensive women with ADPKD have similar pregnancy outcomes as their unaffected family members; however, ADKPKD women with preexisting hypertension had higher rates of maternal complications when compared to their unaffected family members (35% versus 19%; $P < 0.001$) [77]. A second study of 54 women with ADPKD compared to 92 women with simple cysts (control group) also found similar rates of fetal complications between the two groups with similar rates of spontaneous abortion and premature delivery. However again, the ADPKD group had higher risks of maternal complications, including hypertension, proteinuria, and preeclampsia [78].

Less information is available for counseling women with a diagnosis of Alport's syndrome on pregnancy outcomes. Most women who have minimal renal impairment and tight blood pressure control (<130/80 mmHg) prior to pregnancy have successful pregnancy outcomes, but progression to high-grade proteinuria during pregnancy and loss of renal function has also been noted. In a series of seven pregnancies in six women, wherein all women were taking anti-proteinuric therapy with RAS blockers prior to conception [79], only one of the six women had a completely normal pregnancy while the other five women, who had proteinuria prior to conception, all had worsening proteinuria with mild proteinuria progressing into nephrotic range during pregnancy in four pregnancies. There was also a high rate of preterm delivery. Further studies are needed in Alport's syndrome and other rare forms of hereditary renal diseases.

5.7 Pregnancy in End-Stage Kidney Disease

5.7.1 Pregnancy and Renal Transplant Recipients

In order to achieve the same risk of graft loss as women who did not have a pregnancy, the US registry data suggest that the optimal timing of conception posttransplant is after 3 years [80]. Acute graft dysfunction is relatively common in pregnancy; however, acute graft rejection during pregnancy is extremely rare [81]. In terms of immunosuppressive medications, it is advised to switch mycophenolic acid to azathioprine at least 3 months prior to conception to both assess graft stability and avoid teratogenicity. As well, the pharmacokinetics of calcineurin inhibitors is altered with hyperfiltration in pregnancy, and levels need to be closely monitored. Doses may need to be increased by up to 20–25% [82]. Given the common use of prednisone in women with renal transplant, there are higher rates of gestational diabetes, and early screening for gestational diabetes should be considered. Rates of preeclampsia in the renal transplant population are up to 30% higher than for the general population according to the US registry data [83, 84]. Preterm delivery, intrauterine growth restriction, and NICU admission are also more likely in women with a renal transplant than the general population. Overall maternal and fetal outcomes in patients with a renal transplant are similar to nontransplanted patients with CKD with similar levels of renal function [85]. Finally, urinary tract infections are common in women with renal transplants during pregnancy. Routine screening and prompt treatment of positive cultures is recommended.

5.7.2 Pregnancy in Women on Dialysis

While the rate of fertility in patients on dialysis is much lower than the general population, overall fertility rates are increasing and vary by dialysis modality and comorbidities [86]. Patients receiving more intensive nocturnal hemodialysis have been documented to have a higher pregnancy rate than those receiving conventional hemodialysis [87], while women receiving peritoneal dialysis have significantly lower pregnancy rates [88, 89]. As renally cleared, beta-hCG levels are not reliable in women with end-stage kidney disease [90], a diagnosis of pregnancy should be made with both a beta-hCG level and an ultrasound for fetal viability. Similarly, first-trimester screening for aneuploidy can be falsely positive, necessitating further screening studies (i.e., nuchal translucency and/or amniocentesis).

The primary dialysis team will closely monitor blood pressure, ultrafiltration, hemoglobin, iron stores, urea, bicarbonate, and electrolyte balance. Anemia is a frequent concern, and women should be treated with oral or parenteral iron, and erythropoietin stimulating agents as indicated to target a hemoglobin of greater than 100 g/L. In addition to fetal well-being and growth, the obstetrics team will follow cervical length, which can inform the clinician about cervical incompetence and risk of preterm birth as well as amniotic fluid volume, specifically polyhydramnios, which can be also associated with preterm labor and preterm premature rupture of membranes [91]. Both these complications occur in higher frequency in pregnant women on hemodialysis and may necessitate adjustments to the dialysis prescription [92].

Studies suggest that intensified dialysis improves overall pregnancy outcomes, and a dose response between dialysis intensity and pregnancy outcomes has been shown [92]. Women who received at least 36 h per week of dialysis had significantly longer gestational age and infant birth weight than women who were dialyzed 20 or less hours per week [93]. It is important to ensure this intense schedule is feasible for patients, and working closely with social work and the rest of the multidisciplinary team can help ensure adherence and emotional well-being.

In women who are progressing toward end-stage kidney disease, there is a paucity of evidence to support timing of dialysis initiation; however, elective initiation of hemodialysis should be considered when the estimated GFR is below 20 mL/min/1.73 m² or the maternal urea concentration is 17–20 mmol/L [47]. Initiating dialysis at these clinical parameters may mitigate the poor pregnancy outcomes associated with severe renal disease, though this has yet to be proven in the literature.

5.8 Conclusion

Physicians caring for women with CKD of childbearing age should maintain a comfortable environment for conversation about renally safe contraception as well as pregnancy planning. Early involvement of a nephrologist and a maternal–fetal medicine specialist in the prepregnancy counseling and optimization stages can help mitigate the increased maternal and fetal risks faced by this population, and multidisciplinary care is recommended at all stages of the pregnancy journey.

References

[1]   Nevis IF, Reitsma A, Dominic A et al. Pregnancy outcomes in women with chronic kidney disease: a systematic review. Clin J Am Soc Nephrol 2011;6(11):2587–2598.

[2]   Piccoli GB, Cabiddu G, Attini R et al. Risk of adverse pregnancy outcomes in women with CKD. J Am Soc Nephrol 2015;26:2011–2022.

[3]   Zhang JJ, Ma XX, Hao L et al. A systematic review and meta-analysis of outcomes of pregnancy in CKD and CKD outcomes in pregnancy. Clin J Am Soc Nephrol 2015;10(11): 1964–1978.

[4]   Odutayo A, Hladunewich M. Obstetric nephrology: renal hemodynamic and metabolic physiology in normal pregnancy. Clin J Am Soc Nephrol 2012;7(12):2073–2080.

[5]   Davison JM, Dunlop W. Renal hemodynamics and tubular function in normal human pregnancy. Kidney Int 1980;18(2):152–161.

[6]   Cornelis T, Odutayo A, Keunen J, Hladunewich M. The kidney in normal pregnancy and preeclampsia. Semin Nephrol 2011;31(1):4–14.

[7]   Harel Z, McArthur E, Hladunewich M et al. Serum creatinine levels before, during, and after pregnancy. JAMA 2019;321(2):205.

[8]   Ahmed SB, Bentley-Lewis R, Hollenberg NK et al. A comparison of prediction equations for estimating glomerular filtration rate in pregnancy. Hypertens Pregnancy 2009;28(3):243–255.

[9]   Smith M, Moran P, Ward M, Davison J. Assessment of glomerular filtration rate during pregnancy using the MDRD formula. BJOG 2007;115(1):109–112.

[10] Brown MA, Magee LA, Kenny LC et al. The hypertensive disorders of pregnancy: ISSHP classification, diagnosis & management recommendations for international practice. Pregnancy Hypertens 2018;13(May):291–310.

[11] Beunis M, Schweitzer K, Hooff MV, Weiden RVD. Midtrimester screening for microalbuminuria in healthy pregnant women. J Obstet Gynaecol 2004;24(8):863–865.

[12] Konstantin-Hansen KF, Hesseldahl H, Pedersen SM. Microalbuminuria as a predictor of preeclampsia. Acta Obstet Gynecol Scand 1992;71(5):343–346.

[13] Erman A, Neri A, Sharoni R et al. Enhanced urinary albumin excretion after 35 weeks of gestation and during labour in normal pregnancy. Scand J Clin Lab Invest 1992;52(5): 409–413.

[14] Piccoli G, Daidola G, Attini R et al. Kidney biopsy in pregnancy: evidence for counselling? A systematic narrative review. BJOG 2013;120(4):412–427.

[15] Prakash J, Ganiger V, Prakash S et al. Acute kidney injury in pregnancy with special reference to pregnancy-specific disorders: a hospital based study (2014–2016). J Nephrol 2018;31(1): 79–85.

[16] Prakash J, Kumar H, Sinha D et al. Acute renal failure in pregnancy in a developing country: twenty years of experience. Ren Fail 2006;28(4):309–313.

[17] Mehrabadi A, Liu S, Bartholomew S et al. Hypertensive disorders of pregnancy and the recent increase in obstetric acute renal failure in Canada: population based retrospective cohort study. BMJ 2014;349:g4731.

[18] Mehrabadi A, Dahhou M, Joseph KS, Kramer MS. Investigation of a Rise in Obstetric Acute Renal Failure in the United States, 1999–2011. Obstet Gynecol. 2016 May;127(5):899–906.

[19] Kuklina EV, Ayala C, Callaghan WM. Hypertensive disorders and severe obstetric morbidity in the United States. Obs Gynecol 2009;113(6):1299–1306.

[20] Sibai B, Ramadan M, Usta I et al. Maternal morbidity and mortality in 442 pregnancies with hemolysis, elevated liver enzymes, and low platelets (HELLP Syndrome). Am J Obs Gynecol 1993;169(4):1000–1006.

[21] Gul A, Aslan H, Cebeci A et al. Maternal and fetal outcomes in HELLP syndrome complicated with acute renal failure. Ren Fail 2004;26(5):557–562.

[22] Ibdah JA, Bennett MJ, Rinaldo P et al. A fetal fatty-acid oxidation disorder as a cause of liver disease in pregnant women. NEJM 1999;340(22):1723–1731.

[23] Wilcken B, Leung K, Hammond J et al. Pregnancy and fetal long-chain 3-hydroxyacyl coenzyme A dehydrogenase deficiency. Lancet 1993;341(8842):407–408.

[24] Slater D, Hague W. Renal morphological changes in idiopathic acute fatty liver of pregnancy. Histopathology 1984;8(4):567–581.

[25] Fakhouri F, Roumenina L, Provot F et al. Pregnancy-associated hemolytic uremic syndrome revisited in the era of complement gene mutations. J Am Soc Nephrol 2010;21(5):859–867.

[26] Bruel A, Kavanagh D, Noris M et al. Hemolytic uremic syndrome in pregnancy and postpartum. CJASN 2017;12(8):1237–1247.

[27] Frimat M, Decambron M, Lebas C et al. Renal cortical necrosis in postpartum hemorrhage: a case series. Am J Kidney Dis 2016;68(1):50–57.

[28] Tangren JS, Wan M, Adnan WAH, Powe CE et al. Risk of preeclampsia and pregnancy complications in women with a history of acute kidney injury. Hypertension 2018;72(2):451–459.

[29] Hou S, Grossman S, Madias N. Pregnancy in women with renal disease and moderate renal insufficiency. Am J Med 1985;78(2):185–194.

[30] Imbasciati E, Gregorini G, Cabiddu G et al. Pregnancy in CKD stages 3 to 5: fetal and maternal outcomes. Am J Kidney Dis 2007;49(6):753–762.

[31] Hod M, van Dijk DJ, Weintraub N et al. Diabetic nephropathy and pregnancy: the effect of ACE inhibitors prior to pregnancy on fetomaternal outcome. Nephrol Dial Transplant 1995;10(12): 2328–2333.

[32] Bar J, Chen R, Schoenfeld A et al. Pregnancy outcome in patients with insulin dependent diabetes mellitus and diabetic nephropathy treated with ACE inhibitors before pregnancy. J Pediatr Endocrinol Metab 1999;12(5):659–665.

[33] Bramham K, Parnell B, Nelson-Piercy C et al. Chronic hypertension and pregnancy outcomes: systematic review and meta-analysis. BMJ 2014;348:2301.

[34] Gilbert WM, Young AL, Danielsen B. Pregnancy outcomes in women with chronic hypertension: a population-based study. J Reprod Med 2007;52(11):1046–1051.

[35] Carr D, Koontz G, Gardella C et al. Diabetic Nephropathy in pregnancy: suboptimal hypertensive control associated with preterm delivery. Am J Hypertens 2006;19(5):513–519.

[36] Packham DK, North RA, Fairley KF et al. Primary glomerulonephritis and pregnancy. Q J Med 1989;71(266):537–553.

[37] Tong A, Jesudason S, Craig JC, Winkelmayer WC. Perspectives on pregnancy in women with chronic kidney disease: systematic review of qualitative studies. 2014;30(4):652–661.

[38] Tong A, Brown MA, Winkelmayer WC et al. Perspectives on pregnancy in women with CKD: a semistructured interview study. Am J Kidney Dis 2015;66(6):951–961.

[39] Rolnik DL, Wright D, Poon LC et al. Aspirin versus placebo in pregnancies at high risk for preterm preeclampsia. N Engl J Med 2017;377(7):613–622.

[40] Roberge S, Nicolaides K, Demers S et al. The role of aspirin dose on the prevention of preeclampsia and fetal growth restriction: systematic review and meta-analysis. Am J Obstet Gynecol 2017;216(2):110–120.e6.

[41] Roberge S, Nicolaides KH, Demers S et al. Prevention of perinatal death and adverse perinatal outcome using low-dose aspirin: a meta-analysis. Ultrasound Obstet Gynecol 2013;41(5):491–499.

[42] Bujold E, Roberge S, Lacasse Y et al. Prevention of preeclampsia and intrauterine growth restriction with aspirin started in early pregnancy. Obstet Gynecol 2010;116(2,Part 1)): 402–414.

[43] Henderson JT, Whitlock EP, O'Conner E et al. Low-dose Aspirin for the Prevention of Morbidity and Mortality from Preeclampsia: a Systematic Evidence Review for the U.S. Preventative Services Task Force. Rockville (MD): Agency for Healthcare Research and Quality (US), 2014.

[44] Bonten T, Saris A, van Oostrom M et al. Effect of aspirin intake at bedtime versus on awakening on circadian rhythm of platelet reactivity. Thromb Haemost 2014;112(12):1209–1218.

[45] Ayala DE, Ucieda R, Hermida RC. Chronotherapy with low-dose aspirin for prevention of complications in pregnancy. Chronobiol Int 2013;30(1–2):260–279.

[46] Hofmeyr G, Lawrie T, Atallah A, Torloni M. Calcium supplementation during pregnancy for preventing hypertensive disorders and related problems. Cochrane Database Syst Rev 2018;10:10.

[47] Wiles K, Chappell L, Clark K et al. Clinical practice guideline on pregnancy and renal disease. BMC Nephrol 2019;20(1):401.

[48] Magee LA, von Dadelszen P, Rey E et al. Less-tight versus tight control of hypertension in pregnancy. N Engl J Med 2015;372(5):407–417.

[49] Piccoli GB, Gaglioti P, Attini R et al. Pre-eclampsia or chronic kidney disease? The flow hypothesis. Nephrol Dial Transplant 2013;28(5):1199–1206.

[50] Rolfo A, Attini R, Tavassoli E et al. Is it possible to differentiate chronic kidney disease and preeclampsia by means of new and old biomarkers? A prospective study. Dis Markers 2015;2015:1–8.

[51] Bramham K, Seed PT, Lightstone L et al. Diagnostic and predictive biomarkers for pre-eclampsia in patients with established hypertension and chronic kidney disease. Kidney Int 2016;89(4):874–885.

[52] Beardmore KS, Morris JM, Gallery EDM. Excretion of antihypertensive medication into human breast milk: a systematic review. Hypertens Pregnancy 2002;21(1):85–95.

[53] Begg EJ, Robson RA, Gardiner SJ et al. Quinapril and its metabolite quinaprilat in human milk. Br J Clin Pharmacol 2001;51(5):478–481.

[54] Smyth A, Oliveira GHM, Lahr BD et al. A systematic review and meta-analysis of pregnancy outcomes in patients with systemic lupus erythematosus and lupus nephritis. Clin J Am Soc Nephrol 2010;5(11):2060–2068.

[55] Wei S, Lai K, Yang Z, Zeng K. Systemic lupus erythematosus and risk of preterm birth: a systematic review and meta-analysis of observational studies. Lupus 2017;26(6):563–571.

[56] Moroni G, Doria A, Giglio E et al. Fetal outcome and recommendations of pregnancies in lupus nephritis in the twenty-first century. A prospective multicenter study. J Autoimmun 2016;74:6–12.

[57] Buyon JP, Kim MY, Guerra MM et al. Predictors of pregnancy outcomes in patients with lupus: a cohort study. Ann Intern Med 2015;163(3):153–163.

[58] Lightstone L, Hladunewich M. Lupus nephritis and pregnancy: concerns and management. Semin Nephrol 2017;37(4):347–353.

[59] Gonzalez Suarez ML, Kattah A, Grande JP, Garovic V. Renal disorders in pregnancy: core curriculum 2019. Am J Kidney Dis 2019;73(1):119–130.

[60] Buyon JP, Hiebert R, Copel J et al. Autoimmune-associated congenital heart block: demographics, mortality, morbidity and recurrence rates obtained from a national neonatal lupus registry. J Am Coll Cardiol 1998;31(7):1658–1666.

[61] Izmirly PM, Costedoat-Chalumeau N, Pisoni CN et al. Maternal use of hydroxychloroquine is associated with a reduced risk of recurrent anti-SSA/Ro-antibody-associated cardiac manifestations of neonatal lupus. Circulation 2012;126(1):76–82.

[62] Izmirly PM, Kim MY, Llanos C et al. Evaluation of the risk of anti-SSA/Ro-SSB/La antibody-associated cardiac manifestations of neonatal lupus in fetuses of mothers with systemic lupus erythematosus exposed to hydroxychloroquine. Ann Rheum Dis 2010;69(10):1827–1830.

[63] Abarientos C, Sperber K, Shapiro DL et al. Hydroxychloroquine in systemic lupus erythematosus and rheumatoid arthritis and its safety in pregnancy. Expert Opin Drug Saf 2011;10(5):705–714.

[64] Motta M, Tincani A, Faden D et al. Follow-up of infants exposed to hydroxychloroquine given to mothers during pregnancy and lactation. J Perinatol 2005;25(2):86–89.

[65] Koh JH, Ko HS, Kwok S-K et al. Hydroxychloroquine and pregnancy on lupus flares in Korean patients with systemic lupus erythematosus. Lupus 2015;24(2):210–217.

[66] Clowse MEB, Magder L, Witter F, Petri M. Hydroxychloroquine in lupus pregnancy. Arthritis Rheum 2006;54(11):3640–3647.

[67] Damm JA, Ásbjörnsdóttir B, Callesen NF et al. Diabetic nephropathy and microalbuminuria in pregnant women with type 1 and type 2 diabetes. Diabetes Care 2013;36:3489–3494.

[68] Biesenbach G, Grafinger P, Zazgornik J, Stöger H. Perinatal complications and three-year follow up of infants of diabetic mothers with diabetic nephropathy stage IV. Ren Fail 2000;22 (5):573–580.

[69] Rossing K, Jacobsen P, Hommel E et al. Pregnancy and progression of diabetic nephropathy. Diabetologia 2002;45(1):36–41.

[70] Purdy LP, Hantsch CE, Molitch ME et al. Effect of pregnancy on renal function in patients with moderate-to-severe diabetic renal insufficiency. Diabetes Care 1996;19(10):1067–1074.

[71] Ekbom P, Damm P, Feldt-Rasmussen B et al. Pregnancy outcome in type 1 diabetic women with microalbuminuria. Diabetes Care 2001;24(10):1739–1744.

[72] Klemetti MM, Laivuori H, Tikkanen M et al. Obstetric and perinatal outcome in type 1 diabetes patients with diabetic nephropathy during 1988–2011. Diabetologia 2015;58(4):678–686.

[73] Nielsen LR, Damm P, Mathiesen ER. Improved pregnancy outcome in type 1 diabetic women with microalbuminuria or diabetic nephropathy. Diabetes Care 2009;32(1):38–44.

[74] Verlinsky Y, Rechitsky S, Verlinsky O et al. Preimplantation genetic diagnosis for polycystic kidney disease. Fertil Steril 2004;82(4):926–929.

[75] Murphy E, Droher M, DiMaio M, Dahl N. Preimplantation genetic diagnosis counseling in autosomal dominant polycystic kidney disease. Am J Kidney Dis 2018;72(6):866–872.

[76] Milutinovic J, Fialkow PJ, Agodoa LY et al. Fertility and pregnancy complications in women with autosomal dominant polycystic kidney disease. Obs Gynecol 1983;61(5):566–570.

[77] Chapman AB, Johnson AM, Gabow PA. Pregnancy outcome and its relationship to progression of renal failure in autosomal dominant polycystic kidney disease. J Am Soc Nephrol 1994;5(5): 1178–1185.

[78] Wu M, Wang D, Zand L et al. Pregnancy outcomes in autosomal dominant polycystic kidney disease: a case-control study. J Matern Fetal Neonatal Med 2016;29(5):807–812.

[79] Brunini F, Zaina B, Gianfreda D et al. Alport syndrome and pregnancy: a case series and literature review. Arch Gynecol Obstet 2018;297(6):1421–1431.

[80] Rose C, Gill J, Zalunardo N et al. Timing of pregnancy after kidney transplantation and risk of allograft failure. Am J Transplant 2016;16(8):2360–2367.

[81] Deshpande NA, James NT, Kucirka LM et al. Pregnancy outcomes in kidney transplant recipients: a systematic review and meta-analysis. Am J Transplant 2011;11(11):2388–2404.

[82] Kim H, Jeong JC, Yang J et al. The optimal therapy of calcineurin inhibitors for pregnancy in kidney transplantation. Clin Transplant 2015;29(2):142–148.

[83] Bramham K. Pregnancy in renal transplant recipients and donors. Semin Nephrol 2017;37(4): 370–377.

[84] Webster P, Lightstone L, Mckay DB, Josephson MA. Pregnancy in chronic kidney disease and kidney transplantation. Kidney Int 2017;91:1047–1056.

[85] Piccoli GB, Cabiddu G, Attini R et al. Outcomes of pregnancies after kidney transplantation. Transplantation 2017;101(10):2536–2544.

[86] Shah S, Christianson AL, Meganathan K et al. Racial differences and factors associated with pregnancy in ESKD patients on dialysis in the United States. J Am Soc Nephrol 2019;30(12): 2437–2448.

[87] Barua M, Hladunewich M, Keunen J et al. Successful pregnancies on nocturnal home hemodialysis. Clin J Am Soc Nephrol 2008;3(2):392–396.

[88] Shahir AK, Briggs N, Katsoulis J, Levidiotis V. An observational outcomes study from 1966–2008, examining pregnancy and neonatal outcomes from dialysed women using data from the ANZDATA Registry. Nephrology (Carlton) 2013;18(4):276–284.

[89] Okundaye I, Abrinko P, Hou S. Registry of pregnancy in dialysis patients. Am J Kidney Dis 1998;31(5):766–773.

[90] Haninger-Vacariu N, Herkner H, Lorenz M et al. Exclusion of pregnancy in dialysis patients: diagnostic performance of human chorionic gonadotropin. BMC Nephrol 2020;21(1):70.

[91] Hladunewich MA, Melamad N, Bramham K Pregnancy across the spectrum of chronic kidney disease. 2016.

[92] Piccoli G, Minelli F, Versino E et al. Pregnancy in dialysis patients in the new millennium: a systematic review and meta-regression analysis correlating dialysis schedules and pregnancy outcomes. Nephrol Dial Transpl 2016;31(11):1915–1934.

[93] Hladunewich MA, Hou S, Odutayo A et al. Intensive hemodialysis associates with improved pregnancy outcomes: a Canadian and United States cohort comparison. J Am Soc Nephrol 2014;25(5):1103–1109.

Kelsey McLaughlin, Melanie C. Audette, Sebastian R. Hobson,
John C. Kingdom

6 Preeclampsia

6.1 Introduction

Hypertensive disorders of pregnancy are a leading cause of maternal morbidity and mortality, accounting for 14% of maternal deaths worldwide [1]. Depending on the population risk profile, the incidence of preeclampsia varies between 2% and 5% of pregnancies [2]. The diagnosis of preeclampsia has much greater significance relative to other hypertensive disorders of pregnancy, as it is a systemic vasculopathy with the potential for acute clinical deterioration and multi-organ injury [3–5]. Established preeclampsia is associated with an increased risk of iatrogenic preterm birth, often by caesarean section [6]. Placental damage associated with preeclampsia mediates additional risks of severe perinatal outcomes, including placental abruption, fetal growth restriction (FGR), and stillbirth [6]. Preeclampsia is now acknowledged as a significant risk factor for future maternal cardiovascular disease; women with a history of severe preeclampsia are at a 73% increased risk of cardiovascular disease-related mortality and cerebrovascular-related morbidity [6].

Preeclampsia is clinically defined after 20 weeks' gestation by new onset or worsening preexisting hypertension accompanied by evidence of specific maternal organ injury and/or FGR. The majority of women (approximately 80%) who develop preeclampsia present with relatively mild disease near term, typically with proteinuria and minimal additional symptoms, and can be safely managed by expediting delivery, leading to favorable outcomes [4]. However, a subset of pregnant women with preeclampsia (approximately 20%) develops manifestations of severe disease, typically presenting in the late second or early third trimester. Early-onset disease is characterized by substantially greater degrees of maternal complications, including maternal seizures, hemolysis, elevated liver enzymes, low platelets (HELLP) syndrome, kidney and liver failure, and cardiorespiratory distress, while fetal complications include preterm delivery, low birth weight, hypoxia-induced neurological injury, and perinatal death.

The heterogeneous and incompletely understood pathways mediating preeclampsia largely account for the lack of standard screening algorithms to effectively identify pregnant women at high-risk for preeclampsia development. In the absence of a comprehensive and effective screening program, the scenario of an urgent preeclampsia presentation, which may rapidly deteriorate into a hypertensive emergency requiring hospitalization, stabilization, and preterm delivery, continues to challenge all health care systems. Treatments for such women with established

https://doi.org/10.1515/9783110615258-006

preeclampsia are largely focused on managing disease severity, specifically stabilizing hypertension and minimizing organ damage via delivery.

6.2 Preeclampsia Pathogenesis: Stage 1

The pathogenesis of preeclampsia is generally considered to follow a two-step pathway: initial placental dysfunction which in turn manifests in maternal systemic vascular dysfunction. Figure 6.1 demonstrates the relative contributions of maternal characteristics relative to placental contribution to the phenotype of the disease.

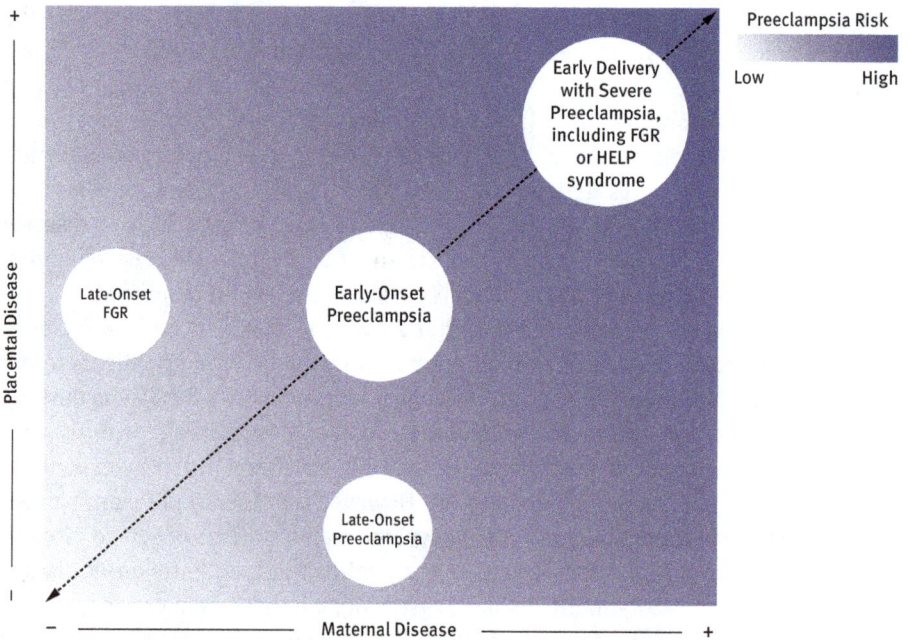

Figure 6.1: Contributions of maternal and placental disease to the development of distinct preeclampsia phenotypes. HELLP syndrome indicates hemolysis, elevated liver enzymes, low platelets; FGR indicates fetal growth restriction.

6.2.1 Abnormal Placentation

In normal pregnancy, the placenta develops and transforms the surrounding maternal tissue and structures to support fetal growth. The radial arteries of the uterus divide into two or more branches: the basal arteries, which perfuse the superficial myometrium and decidua, along with the spiral arteries, which perfuse the intervillous space [7]. Extravillous cytotrophoblast cells invade and transform the distal spiral arteries into high-flow, low-resistance vessels early in normal pregnancy, which ultimately direct large volumes of blood at low pressure into the intervillous space [7]. The transition to the early second trimester is characterized by the further establishment of intervillous blood flow. Placental derived proteins, such as the pro-angiogenic placental growth factor (PlGF) and anti-angiogenic soluble fms-like tyrosine kinase-1 (sFlt-1) proteins, are secreted by the syncytiotrophoblast layer covering the developing placental villi, reliably enter the maternal blood and circulation and promote placental vasculogenesis and maternal circulatory regulation.

Early-onset preeclampsia is hypothesized to largely originate from defective early placentation during the first trimester, with failure of the extravillous cytotrophoblast to transform the distal uterine spiral arteries. Diseased spiral arteries exhibit fibrinoid necrosis and thrombosis, which may occlude their lumens and lead to infarction of the overlying villous tissues [8]. Consequently, as the second trimester begins and fetal oxygen demands rise, the developing placental villi enter a progressive state of chronic ischemia [9]. In preeclampsia arising from shallow cytotrophoblast invasion, growth of the developing fetus is ultimately limited by disordered utero-placental blood flow [10, 11].

The perfused placental villi become chronically hypoxic which impairs the normal growth and specialization of the placental villi, impairing fetal growth, and leading to dysregulated secretion of angiogenic growth factors, which then cause abnormal maternal vascular function. The inherently unstable perfusion of the placenta via diseased spiral arteries generates oxidative stress in the developing placental villi, resulting in dysregulation of the heme oxygenase vasodilator pathway and endoplasmic reticulum stress within the syncytiotrophoblast [9, 12–14]. These changes subsequently suppress the synthesis of key proteins in the outer syncytiotrophoblast layer, which is in contact with maternal blood, especially nutrient transporter proteins and the pro-angiogenic PlGF protein [15–18].

In addition to the development of adequate blood flow across the placenta, appropriate maternal immune adaptations are required at the maternal-placental interface to tolerate and support normal pregnancy. Research indicates that women with preeclampsia exhibit both systemic and local (placental bed) immune abnormalities.

6.3 Preeclampsia Pathogenesis: Stage 2

While the majority of women who develop the early-onset, severe phenotype of preeclampsia typically exhibit evidence of abnormal placentation, preeclampsia ultimately presents as a maternal vascular disorder, manifested by hypertension, systemic endothelial dysfunction and multi-organ ischemic injury. An autopsy series of women who died of eclampsia described brain lesions characterized by perivascular edema and hemorrhage, periportal/portal necrosis and sinusoidal fibrin in hepatic analysis, and glomerular endotheliosis in renal analysis [19]. Vascular injury is the hypothesized mechanistic link between abnormal placentation and the maternal syndrome of preeclampsia, where the diseased placenta exerts powerful influence upon the maternal cardiovascular system.

6.3.1 Placental-Derived Angiogenic Proteins

It has long been hypothesized that the preeclamptic placenta releases soluble factors into the maternal system, mediating detrimental effects on the maternal systemic vasculature. It is now well documented that preeclampsia is a state of angiogenic imbalance between pro- and anti-angiogenic proteins synthesized by placental villi.

PlGF, a member of the vascular endothelial growth factor (VEGF) family, is a pro-angiogenic protein released by the placenta that mediates large reductions in peripheral vascular resistance, establishing a high-volume, low-resistance state that is highly protective against the development of hypertension in pregnancy [20]. PlGF levels rise substantially during the second trimester of pregnancy, before declining during the third trimester to term [21]. As normal pregnancy nears term, the circulating levels of sFlt-1 (the soluble form of VEGF receptor-1) increase, binding to and sequestering both PlGF and VEGF [21].

Low circulating levels of PlGF early in pregnancy are associated with the subsequent development of preeclampsia, specifically with the more severe early-onset preeclampsia phenotype, relative to normotensive pregnant women [21]. As pregnancy progresses, women who subsequently develop preeclampsia exhibit significantly increased levels of sFlt-1 prior to the clinical presentation of preeclampsia [21]. In high concentrations, sFlt-1 is capable of inducing a state of systemic maternal endothelial dysfunction in systemic arterioles via competitive inhibition of VEGF and PlGF, mediating the loss of nitric oxide-mediated endothelium-dependent vasodilation of the maternal circulatory system [22, 23]. The anti-angiogenic protein soluble endoglin has also been implicated in the pathogenesis of preeclampsia, with increased circulating levels in women with preeclampsia [23, 24].

6.3.2 Systemic Maternal Endothelial Dysfunction

Healthy pregnancy is characterized by significant increases in the synthesis and local release of nitric oxide in the systemic endothelial layer of the maternal circulation, mediating significant decreases in total peripheral resistance by 25% in the third trimester, relative to pre-pregnancy levels [25–31]. This dramatic change in total peripheral resistance is required to counterbalance large increases in cardiac output and blood volume that occur in early pregnancy [32].

Widespread systemic endothelial dysfunction mediates many of the clinical manifestations of preeclampsia. Pregnant women with preeclampsia exhibit significantly impaired endothelium-dependent vasodilation prior to the clinical diagnosis of preeclampsia, and these changes persist into the postpartum period [33, 34].

6.3.3 Maternal Hemodynamics and Hypertension

The maternal cardiovascular system undergoes significant adaptations throughout normal pregnancy to adapt to chronic volume overload, beginning as early as the first trimester to establish a high-volume, low-resistance hemodynamic state [30]. Maternal systemic vascular resistance decreases by approximately 25% by the third trimester to protect against the development of hypertension [30]. Normal pregnancy is characterized by a decrease in blood pressure in the first trimester, before rising to nonpregnant levels by term. The pregnant heart also begins to structurally adapt by increasing left ventricular thickness, muscle mass, and right heart diameters; normal pregnancy is associated with significant increases in heart rate, stroke volume, and cardiac output [30]. Maternal cardiovascular adaptations that occur during normal pregnancy are disrupted in women who develop preeclampsia; however, the nature of the hemodynamic abnormalities is not consistent across all types of preeclampsia and is dependent on the timing of clinical onset.

Although women who develop early- or late-onset preeclampsia each exhibit clinical hypertension and some evidence of organ injury, these disease subtypes exhibit contrasting hemodynamic and cardiovascular phenotypes. Relative to normotensive pregnant women, women with late-onset preeclampsia exhibit a hemodynamic profile characterized by increased stoke volume, cardiac output and heart rate, and decreased vascular resistance, as well as significant cardiovascular dysfunction, including global diastolic dysfunction and myocardial damage [35–38]. In contrast, women who develop early-onset preeclampsia exhibit a hemodynamic profile characterized by significantly increased systemic vascular resistance and decreased heart rate, stroke volume, and cardiac output [35–37]. Their cardiovascular impairment is more severe, including biventricular systolic dysfunction, and may lead to left ventricular hypertrophy [37]. There is a strong association between preeclampsia and peripartum cardiomyopathy, possibly due to a shared pathogenesis [39].

In addition to abnormal levels of circulating angiogenic proteins, agonistic autoantibodies to the angiotensin II type 1 receptor have also been implicated in the development of hypertension in preeclamptic women [40].

6.3.4 Glomerular Endotheliosis

The classic clinical presentation of preeclampsia new-onset hypertension is accompanied by proteinuria, indicating renal dysfunction characterized by glomerular endotheliosis. This specific renal injury is hypothesized to be caused by deprivation of VEGF signaling in the renal podocytes, resulting in podocyte fragmentation and loss of the podocytes' ability to retain circulating proteins such as albumin [41]. Podocyte fragments (or the protein podocin) can be detected in the urine of women at risk of severe preeclampsia in advance of disease presentation, and are thus indirect evidence of high circulating sFlt-1 levels [42, 43].

6.4 Risk Factors for Preeclampsia

Clinical risk factors associated with increased risk of preeclampsia development can be broadly classified into genetic predisposition, preexisting maternal health along with pregnancy history and characteristics. The Society of Obstetricians and Gynaecologists of Canada (SOGC) recommends consultation with an obstetrician if women have a history of preeclampsia or other factors that would increase the risk of developing preeclampsia, including multiple pregnancy, antiphospholipid antibody syndrome, significant proteinuria early in pregnancy, preexisting hypertension, diabetes mellitus, or renal disease [44].

6.4.1 Genetic Predisposition

Overall, the heritability of preeclampsia is estimated to be 55%, with 35% contribution from maternal factors and 20% contribution from fetal factors, impacted by paternal genes [45, 46]. Family history of preeclampsia, diabetes, coronary artery disease, or myocardial infarction before 60 years of age are significant risk factors for the development of preeclampsia, suggesting an underlying genetic component [4, 47–49]. Race is also a risk factor for preeclampsia, with increased risk amongst women of Afro-Caribbean racial origin and decreased risk amongst white women [50, 51]. Women with A or AB blood groups are at increased risk of preeclampsia, relative to O-type women [52, 53]. Severe preeclampsia is associated with higher risk of being carriers of either an inherited or acquired thrombophilia, including factor V Leiden [54].

6.4.2 Pre-Existing Maternal Health

Women with antiphospholipid antibody syndrome, preexisting hypertension, diabetes, dyslipidemia, pre-pregnancy obesity (BMI > 30), chronic kidney disease, advanced maternal age > 35 years, and systemic lupus erythematosus are at increased risk of developing preeclampsia [48–50]. Cigarette smoking is associated with a reduced risk of preeclampsia, possibly due to increased carbon monoxide exposure [55, 56].

6.4.3 Pregnancy History and Characteristics

Nulliparous women, as a group, contribute the bulk of disease burden mediated by preeclampsia; nulliparity is a significant risk factor for the development of preeclampsia, potentially due to the lack of fetal immune tolerance [49]. Whilst these women have no parous history, their prior reproductive performance, expressed as a history of infertility or miscarriages, is highly important. Early miscarriage prior to an ongoing pregnancy with the same partner confers a lower risk, whereas both the need for assisted reproductive technologies and a history of recurrent losses, or any loss >16 weeks, confers a higher risk [4, 49, 50, 57]. Longer inter-pregnancy interval, shorter period of cohabitation with a partner prior to conception, and conception with a new partner are also associated with an increased preeclampsia risk, possibly also attributable to immune memory [50]. While healthy multiparous women generally have a lower risk of the disease, they are at increased risk of preeclampsia if there is a history of preeclampsia, placental abruption, or stillbirth in prior pregnancies [49]. Women with multifetal pregnancies or who have utilized assisted reproductive technologies are also at increased risk of preeclampsia [49].

6.5 Clinical Definition of Preeclampsia

Preeclampsia (referring to the clinical state prior to the development of seizures, or eclampsia) was traditionally characterized by the development of new-onset hypertension after 20 weeks' gestation accompanied by proteinuria [58]. The scope of defining preeclampsia has since expanded to reflect the heterogeneous nature of this disease. Preeclampsia is now characterized by the American College of Obstetricians and Gynecologists (ACOG) as new-onset hypertension after 20 weeks' gestation (systolic blood pressure ≥140 mmHg or diastolic blood pressure ≥90 mmHg on more than two occasions at least 4 hours apart, or one measurement of systolic blood pressure ≥160 mmHg or diastolic blood pressure ≥110 mmHg) with additional evidence of end-organ injury, defined as proteinuria (urinary excretion of ≥0.3 g of protein in a 24 hour collection, protein/creatinine ratio of ≥0.3 mg/dL, or dipstick reading of >

2+), thrombocytopenia (platelet count <100,000 × 10^9/L), renal insufficiency (serum creatinine concentrations >1.1 mg/dL or a doubling of the serum creatinine concentration in the absence of overt renal disease), impaired liver function (elevated liver transaminases), abdominal pain, peripheral edema, pulmonary edema, new-onset headache (unresponsive to medication), or visual symptoms [59].

6.6 Diagnosis of Preeclampsia

Preeclampsia is commonly characterized based on the timing of disease presentation and severity of clinical symptoms; however, these characterizations can be ambiguous which may be difficult to diagnose. Often several factors are taken into consideration when making the diagnosis of preeclampsia which includes repeat blood pressure readings, patient's reported symptoms, physical exam findings, maternal blood/urine testing, and monitoring of fetal growth and wellbeing. Preeclampsia is typically distinguished as "early-onset" disease (clinical presentation prior to 34 weeks' gestation) or "late-onset" disease (clinical presentation after 34 weeks' gestation). The reason for this distinction is based on the severity of clinical presentation, as women presenting with early-onset disease tend to develop a more severe disease phenotype than women presenting with late-onset disease, and the subsequent clinical course of management. The time course of disease development is hypothesized related to the underlying pathogenesis of preeclampsia, as each subset confer its own unique disease risk [60]. It is hypothesized that women who present with early-onset disease typically exhibit a more severe phenotype that is predominately mediated by abnormal placentation. In contrast, the late-onset disease that is typically a less severe phenotype is thought to be mediated by maternal factors, such as preexisting cardiovascular dysfunction and systemic inflammation. Consistent with this approach, the SOGC refers to early-onset preeclampsia as "placental" preeclampsia, due to the large contribution of impaired placentation to disease development, while late-onset preeclampsia is referred to as "maternal" preeclampsia, due to the lowered maternal threshold to pregnancy or excessive placental demands [44].

The SOGC defines severe preeclampsia as preeclampsia with severe complications, including those involving the maternal central nervous system (eclampsia, blindness, retinal detachment, stroke), cardiorespiratory system (uncontrolled severe hypertension, pulmonary edema, myocardial infarction), hematological system (thrombocytopenia with platelet count <50 × 10^9/L, disseminated intravascular coagulation), renal system (acute kidney injury, dialysis initiation), hepatic dysfunction (severe hepatitis, sub-capsular hemorrhage, or rupture), or the placenta (abruption, FGR, stillbirth) [44]. The SOGC also recognizes feto-placental involvement, including FGR, placental abruption and stillbirth, as a diagnostic criteria for preeclampsia [44].

6.7 Preventative Strategies for Preeclampsia

6.7.1 Lifestyle Strategies for Preeclampsia Prevention

Physical activity in the pre-conception period is protective against the development of preeclampsia [48, 61, 62]. A joint clinical practice guideline from the SOGC and Canadian Society for Exercise Physiology recommends that all women without contraindication should be physically active throughout pregnancy, with at least 150 min of moderate-intensity physical activity per week [63]. Exercise in pregnancy is associated with significantly lower incidence of hypertensive disorders of pregnancy and gestational diabetes [64]. Once women are diagnosed with preeclampsia, exercise is contraindicated [63].

6.7.2 Therapies for Preeclampsia Prevention

Pregnant women, determined to be at increased risk of developing preeclampsia through the assessment of preexisting maternal health, pregnancy history, and current pregnancy characteristics, are recommended by SOGC, National Institute for Health and Care Excellence (NICE), and ACOG to receive take low-dose aspirin (SOGC: 75–162 mg/day, ACOG: 81 mg/day, NICE: 75–150 mg/day) for preeclampsia prevention [44, 59, 65]; low-dose aspirin should be initiated early in pregnancy if possible (SOGC: before 16 weeks' gestation; ACOG: between 12 and 28 weeks' gestation, optimally before 16 weeks' gestation, NICE: from 12 weeks' gestation) and continued until delivery. The ASPRE trial determined that low-dose aspirin (150 mg/day) initiated prior to 14 weeks' gestation in multi-modal screen-positive women reduced the risk of preterm preeclampsia by 62%, with no serious reported adverse events [66]. In addition, the ASPIRIN trial determined that lose-dose aspirin (81 mg/day) given widely to nulliparous women with singleton pregnancies from low-income and middle-income countries significantly reduced the risk of preterm birth, perinatal mortality, fetal loss, and the incidence of women who delivered <34 weeks' gestation with hypertensive disorders of pregnancy [67].

Calcium supplementation is an effective preventative therapy against the development of preeclampsia in women with low-calcium diets [68]. The SOGC recommends at least 1 g/day of calcium supplementation for women with dietary intake of calcium <600 mg/day [44]. The SOGC recommends the use of low-molecular-weight heparin for the prevention of recurrent severe or early-onset preeclampsia, preterm delivery and/or small for gestational age infants [44]. Use of a folate-containing multivitamin in the preconception and pregnancy period is also recommended for the prevention of preeclampsia [44].

Dietary antioxidant supplementation with vitamins C and E did not significantly reduce the risk of preeclampsia, severe preeclampsia, preterm birth, or small-for-gestational-age infants [69]. Similarly, vitamin D supplementation above the current recommended intake amount and magnesium supplementation in pregnant women did not impact the risk of preeclampsia, preterm birth, and low birthweight [70, 71]. Finally, the SOGC recommends against the use of prostaglandin precursors and supplementation with zinc for the prevention of preeclampsia [44].

6.8 Treatment Options for Established Preeclampsia

Once preeclampsia has been diagnosed, therapies are utilized to prevent the development a severe hypertensive crisis and seizures (eclampsia).

Antihypertensive therapies are recommended for pregnant women with severe hypertension to prevent progression of a hypertensive emergency and associated cardiovascular complications, including myocardial ischemia, renal dysfunction, and stroke [59]. The SOGC recommends blood pressure targets of systolic blood pressure <160 mmHg and diastolic blood pressure <110 mmHg for women with severe hypertension [44]. The CHIPS trial determined that lower diastolic blood pressure target (85 mmHg vs. 100 mmHg) in pregnant women was associated with reduced frequency of severe maternal hypertension, supporting the importance of proper blood pressure control [72]. For pregnant women with severe hypertension, the SOGC recommends initiation of antihypertensive therapy in the hospital setting, utilizing intravenous labetalol or hydralazine, or nifedipine short-acting capsules. A nitroglycerin infusion may be used in circumstances that include left ventricular failure [44]. Until maternal blood pressure is stable, continuous fetal heart rate monitoring is recommended to identify fetal hypoxia.

The SOGC also recommends antihypertensive therapy for women with non-severe hypertension, with blood pressure targets of systolic blood pressure between 130–155 mmHg and diastolic between 80 and 105 mmHg [44]. Given the lessened emergency of this cohort, the choice of oral antihypertensive therapy is more varied and is dominated by labetalol, short- or long-acting nifedipine, and methyldopa. Selection is currently empirical, and largely based on patient characteristics and physician familiarity [44, 73].

The use of angiotensin-converting enzyme inhibitors and angiotensin receptor blockers is contraindicated during pregnancy. In addition atenolol and prazosin are not recommended prior to delivery [44].

Magnesium sulfate therapy is the first-line therapy recommended for eclampsia prophylaxis in pregnant women with severe preeclampsia [44, 59]. Magnesium therapy was also associated with reduced risk of placental abruption and increased risk of caesarean delivery. Approximately 25% of women experienced side effects with magnesium sulfate therapy, primarily flushing [74]. There is currently no consensus to recommend the administration of magnesium sulfate for non-severe preeclampsia; the decision to administer magnesium sulfate to this population should be based on clinical judgement and institutional guidelines [59]. It is typically administered as a loading dose of 4 grams IV, followed by 1-2 g/hr for 24 hours.

6.8.1 Expectant Management Versus Delivery

Delivery of the placenta and fetus is the only effective approach to reverse the clinical syndrome of preeclampsia. The main challenge for clinicians when managing a woman with preeclampsia is determining when to use an expectant management approach versus intervene to initiate delivery, and the optimal timing for delivery. This decision should ultimately be made to balance maternal and fetal health by weighing the risks and benefits at each specific gestational age, thereby aiming to prevent or limit the risk of major maternal or fetal complications. Expectant management of women with preeclampsia consists of transferring to a regional perinatal center for in depth assessments, when required, and family-centered counseling, inpatient or outpatient monitoring, and treatment to effectively control blood pressure and avoid severe manifestations of preeclampsia. The SOGC recommends Doppler-based assessment of the utero-placental, umbilical, and fetal circulations to elucidate the role of the placenta in the development of preeclampsia, combined with serial monitoring of fetal growth. Acute tests of fetal well-being include the biophysical profile, fetal Doppler, and nonstress tests should also be utilized.

6.8.2 Term Preeclampsia (37+ weeks)

The SOGC and ACOG recommend delivery for women presenting with preeclampsia at or after 37 weeks' gestation without severe disease characteristics [44, 59]. In women with preeclampsia without severe characteristics before 37 weeks' gestation, ACOG recommends continued monitoring until term, at which point delivery is recommended [59].

6.8.3 Late Preterm Preeclampsia (34–37 weeks)

ACOG recommends urgent delivery of women presenting with severe characteristics of preeclampsia beyond 34 weeks' gestation, if the maternal or fetal condition begins to deteriorate during expectant management; conditions that would necessitate delivery include uncontrolled maternal blood pressure, stroke, myocardial infarction, HELLP syndrome, eclampsia, placental abruption, fetal death, anticipated fetal death, and persistent reversed end-diastolic flow of the umbilical artery [59]. The

SOGC recommends immediate delivery for all women with severe preeclampsia, regardless of gestational age, and immediate delivery for women with HELLP syndrome, following 35 weeks' gestation [44]. FGR in the absence of additional abnormal fetal findings is not considered an indication for delivery [59]. A clinical trial determined that planned delivery in women with preeclampsia who present between 34 and 35 + 6 weeks' gestation reduces maternal morbidity and severe hypertension and increased neonatal unit admissions without greater neonatal morbidity, relative to expectant management [75].

6.8.4 Preterm Preeclampsia (<34 weeks)

The clinical decision to employ an expectant management approach to pregnant women presenting with severe preeclampsia prior to 34 weeks' gestation is based on pregnancy prolongation in order to promote fetal development and reduce risk of morbidity and mortality associated with premature delivery, while balancing maternal health. This strategy should be utilized in settings with appropriate resources and when neonatal survival is expected [59]. If delivery is indicated in this population prior to 34 weeks' gestation, guidelines recommend administration of corticosteroids for fetal lung maturation and decrease neonatal adverse outcomes for women who are stable in the short term; delivery is recommended 48 h posttreatment [44, 59].

6.8.5 Mode of Delivery

Clinicians should determine the mode of delivery for women with preeclampsia, based on gestational age, possibility of maternal and fetal complications, and obstetric history [59]. SOGC recommends that vaginal delivery should be considered for all hypertensive women, unless caesarean delivery is required for standard obstetric indications [44]. Careful consideration should be given to the ability of the fetus to withstand labor induction [76]. If Doppler abnormalities of the umbilical and/or middle cerebral artery circulation are found, an oxytocin challenge test is wise prior to formal cervical ripening initiation to avoid acute fetal distress [44, 77]. Planned caesarean section should be considered in certain circumstances such as older nulliparous women at earlier gestations, especially before 34 weeks' gestation.

In women with severe HELLP syndrome, an intravenous dexamethasone rescue regimen may provide temporary relief from thrombocytopenia and abnormal liver function tests to permit a successful induction of labor with epidural analgesia [78]. Women with major fluid shifts, pulmonary edema or subclinical heart failure may best be delivered by planned caesarean section under epidural anesthesia, followed by fluid restriction and vasodilator therapies to improve cardiac output and lower peripheral vascular resistance. This is preferable to a prolonged attempt at induction, as oxytocin use may result in unwanted fluid accumulation and hyponatremia [79]. However, there is evidence to suggest that caesarean section may benefit hypertensive pregnant women remote from term with evidence of fetal compromise [44].

6.9 Postpartum Care

Despite removal of the placenta and fetus, preeclampsia can extend into the postpartum period, or previously normotensive women can develop de novo preeclampsia in the postpartum period. It has been reported that one quarter of eclamptic seizures occur more than 48 hours following delivery, with a third of HELLP cases occurring postpartum [59, 80]. In the immediate postpartum period, SOCG recommends continuing blood pressure monitoring up to 6 days following delivery, continuing antihypertensive therapy in women with antenatal preeclampsia, and maintaining a healthy blood pressure for women with co-morbidities [44]. The use of non-steroidal anti-inflammatory agents is controversial in the postpartum period, as they may contribute to worsening hypertension [44, 81, 82]. The provision of a calibrated ambulatory blood pressure monitoring device empowers women in their disease management, including drug dose adjustments at home in the early postpartum period [83]. Postpartum thromboprophylaxis should also be considered in women with preeclampsia, especially in older women delivered by caesarean section, women who have early onset disease characterized by hemoconcentration, women who receive blood products, or have a family history of venous thromboembolism events [44]. ACOG recommends that magnesium sulfate be considered the drug of choice for the prevention of eclampsia in the early (24–48 h) postpartum period [59]. Women should be counselled to seek medical advice in the postpartum period if they experience preeclampsia-like symptoms; the most common symptom for postpartum preeclampsia is headache [84].

Half of women who had a preeclamptic pregnancy remain hypertensive in the postpartum period, suggesting that this population of women may require referral to a blood pressure specialist, or a postpartum cardiovascular rehab program to manage persistent hypertension and future cardiovascular risk [83]. Preeclampsia is a significant risk factor for future maternal cardiovascular health; women with a history of severe preeclampsia are at significantly higher risk of cardiovascular disease-related morbidity and mortality, cerebrovascular-related morbidity and ischemic heart disease [6].

Figure 6.2 presents a template to guide investigations, monitoring and management from the pre-pregnancy stage through to delivery.

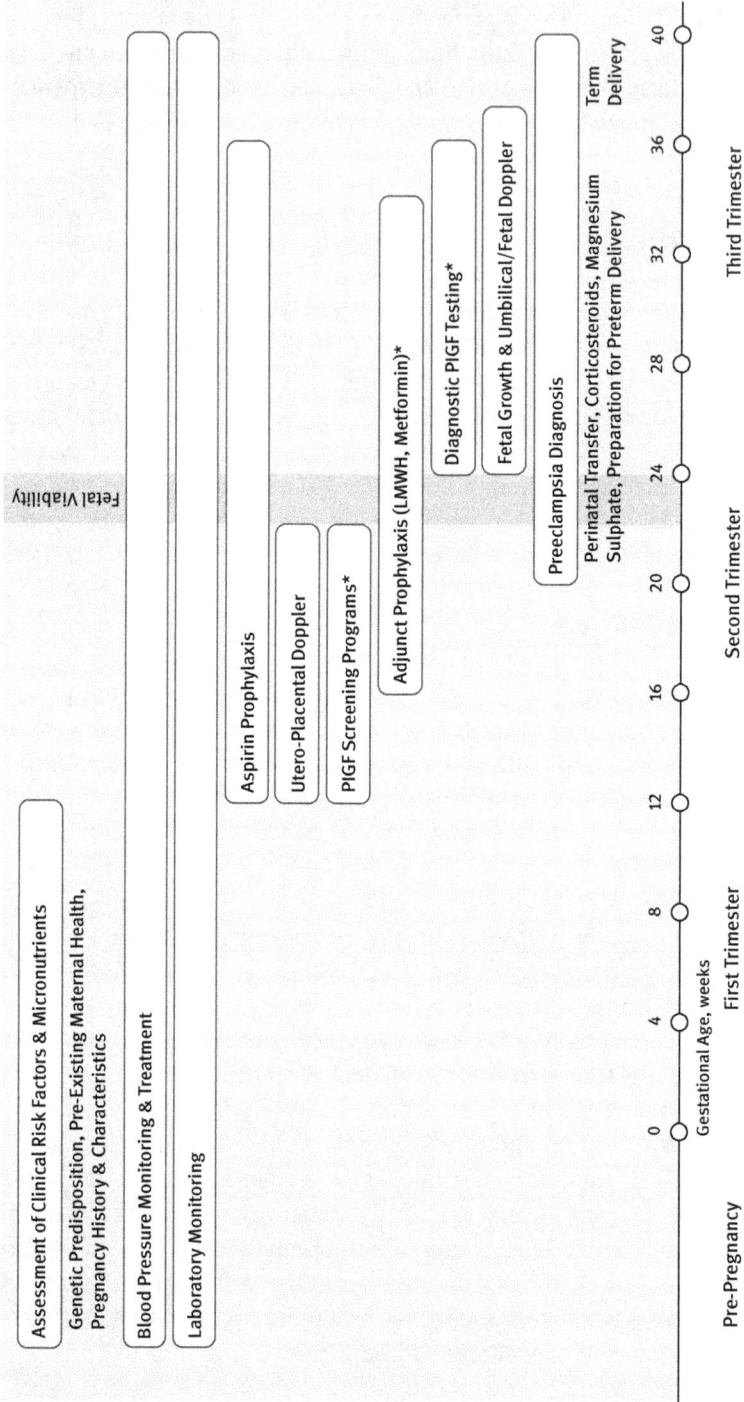

Figure 6.2: Overview of contemporary care of pregnant women at risk of preeclampsia in high-resource settings. Strategies under investigation and not yet integrated into standard clinical care are indicated (*). PlGF indicates placental growth factor.

6.10 Innovations in Preeclampsia

6.10.1 Prediction of Preeclampsia

Improving the prediction of preeclampsia across a wide range of risk populations in distinct geographical locations is a critical clinical initiative. Recent screening approaches have centered around evaluating circulating levels of placental-derived angiogenic proteins for the prediction of preeclampsia [85–87]. Maternal hemodynamics have also been investigated in a limited manner for the prediction of preeclampsia [20].

6.10.2 Diagnosis and Clinical Management of Preeclampsia

Recent evidence emphasizes the promise of angiogenic protein testing for the diagnosis of preeclampsia, aiding clinicians in the recognition and clinical intervention of women with the most severe placenta-mediated disease, and prevents unnecessary clinical intervention and iatrogenic premature delivery in low-risk pregnant women [88, 89].

6.10.3 Phenotypes of Preeclampsia

Scientific innovations have allowed the field to move past phenotyping preeclampsia based on timing of clinical presentation and severity alone [21, 35, 90–95]. Recent findings support the integration of consolidated assessment of maternal hemodynamics, clinical characteristics and circulating levels of angiogenic proteins into clinical care, to develop pathway-specific screening programs with tailored preventative strategies through phenotype pregnant women [60].

6.10.4 Therapeutic Strategies

There has been a significant focus on developing novel therapies for the prevention of preeclampsia with the progression of research elucidating the pathogenesis and phenotypes of preeclampsia. Novel therapeutic strategies include exogenous PlGF [96–98], heparin [95, 99–102], statins [103, 104], metformin [105], melatonin [106], and sFlt-1 apheresis [107, 108].

6.11 Conclusions

Preeclampsia is a complex hypertensive disorder of pregnancy, characterized by new-onset hypertension with subsequent maternal organ injury. Significant research in the past 10 years has identified distinct phenotypes of preeclampsia, mediated by multiple pathways with unique clinical presentations. It remains a challenge to prevent preeclampsia and provide tailored-treatment therapies for women presenting with preeclampsia. Integrating novel scientific findings and innovative clinical strategies to improve maternal and fetal health should be the aim of future work to help reduce this obstetrical disease burden.

References

[1]   Say L, Chou D, Gemmill A, et al. Global causes of maternal death: a WHO systematic analysis. Lancet Glob Health 2014;2:e323–33.
[2]   Roberts CL, Ford JB, Algert CS, et al. Population-based trends in pregnancy hypertension and pre-eclampsia: an international comparative study. BMJ Open 2011;1:e000101.
[3]   Bokslag A, Van Weissenbruch M, Mol BW, De Groot CJ. Preeclampsia; short and long-term consequences for mother and neonate. Early Hum Dev 2016;102:47–50.
[4]   North RA, McCowan LM, Dekker GA, et al. Clinical risk prediction for pre-eclampsia in nulliparous women: development of model in international prospective cohort. BMJ (Clinical Research Ed) 2011;342:d1875.
[5]   Melamed N, Ray JG, Hladunewich M, Cox B, Kingdom JC. Gestational hypertension and preeclampsia: are they the same disease?. J Obstet Gynaecol Can: JOGC = J D'obstet Gynecol Can: JOGC 2014;36:642–647.
[6]   Shen M, Smith GN, Rodger M, White RR, Walker MC, Wen SW. Comparison of risk factors and outcomes of gestational hypertension and pre-eclampsia 2017;12:e0175914.
[7]   Brosens I, Robertson WB, Dixon HG. The physiological response of the vessels of the placental bed to normal pregnancy. J Pathol Bacteriol 1967;93:569–579.
[8]   Robertson WB, Brosens I, Dixon HG. The pathological response of the vessels of the placental bed to hypertensive pregnancy. J Pathol Bacteriol 1967;93:581–592.
[9]   Phipps EA, Thadhani R, Benzing T, Karumanchi SA. Pre-eclampsia: pathogenesis, novel diagnostics and therapies. Nat Rev Nephrol 2019;15:275–289.
[10] Brosens IA, Robertson WB, Dixon HG. The role of the spiral arteries in the pathogenesis of preeclampsia. Obstet Gynecol Annu 1972;1:177–191.
[11] Lyall F, Robson SC, Bulmer JN. Spiral artery remodeling and trophoblast invasion in preeclampsia and fetal growth restriction: relationship to clinical outcome. Hypertension (Dallas, Tex: 1979) 2013;62:1046–1054.
[12] Ahmed A, Rahman M, Zhang X, et al. Induction of placental heme oxygenase-1 is protective against TNFalpha-induced cytotoxicity and promotes vessel relaxation. Mol Med (Cambridge, Mass) 2000;6:391–409.
[13] Zhao H, Wong RJ, Kalish FS, Nayak NR, Stevenson DK. Effect of heme oxygenase-1 deficiency on placental development. Placenta 2009;30:861–868.

[14] Lian IA, Loset M, Mundal SB, et al. Increased endoplasmic reticulum stress in decidual tissue from pregnancies complicated by fetal growth restriction with and without pre-eclampsia. Placenta 2011;32:823–829.

[15] Speake PF, Glazier JD, Ayuk PT, Reade M, Sibley CP, Sw D. L-Arginine transport across the basal plasma membrane of the syncytiotrophoblast of the human placenta from normal and preeclamptic pregnancies. J Clin Endocrinol Metab 2003;88:4287–4292.

[16] Myers JE, Kenny LC, McCowan, et al Angiogenic factors combined with clinical risk factors to predict preterm pre-eclampsia in nulliparous women: a predictive test accuracy study. BJOG: Int J Obstet Gynaecol 2013;120:1215–1223.

[17] Drewlo S, Levytska K, Sobel M, Baczyk D, Lye SJ, Kingdom JC. Heparin promotes soluble VEGF receptor expression in human placental villi to impair endothelial VEGF signaling. J Thromb Haemost 2011;9:2486–2497.

[18] Huppertz B, Kingdom J, Caniggia I, et al. Hypoxia favours necrotic versus apoptotic shedding of placental syncytiotrophoblast into the maternal circulation. Placenta 2003;24:181–190.

[19] Hecht JL, Ordi J, Carrilho C, et al. The pathology of eclampsia: an autopsy series. Pregnancy Hypertens 2017;36:259–268.

[20] Vasapollo B, Novelli GP, Valensise H. Total vascular resistance and left ventricular morphology as screening tools for complications in pregnancy. Hypertension (Dallas, Tex: 1979) 2008;51:1020–1026.

[21] Levine RJ, Maynard SE, Qian C, et al. Circulating angiogenic factors and the risk of preeclampsia. N Engl J Med 2004;350:672–683.

[22] Ahmad S, Ahmed A. Elevated placental soluble vascular endothelial growth factor receptor-1 inhibits angiogenesis in preeclampsia. Circ Res 2004;95:884–891.

[23] Maynard SE, Min JY, Merchan J, et al. Excess placental soluble fms-like tyrosine kinase 1 (sFlt1) may contribute to endothelial dysfunction, hypertension, and proteinuria in preeclampsia. J Clin Invest 2003;111:649–658.

[24] Levine RJ, Lam C, Qian C, et al. Soluble endoglin and other circulating antiangiogenic factors in preeclampsia. N Engl J Med 2006;355:992–1005.

[25] Williams DJ, Vallance PJ, Neild GH, Spencer JA, Imms FJ. Nitric oxide-mediated vasodilation in human pregnancy. Am J Physiol 1997;272:H748–52.

[26] Dorup I, Skajaa K, Sorensen KE. Normal pregnancy is associated with enhanced endothelium-dependent flow-mediated vasodilation. Am J Physiol 1999;276:H821–5.

[27] Anumba DO, Robson SC, Boys RJ, Ford GA. Nitric oxide activity in the peripheral vasculature during normotensive and preeclamptic pregnancy. Am J Physiol 1999;277:H848–54.

[28] Stewart FM, Freeman DJ, Ramsay JE, Greer IA, Caslake M, Ferrell WR. Longitudinal assessment of maternal endothelial function and markers of inflammation and placental function throughout pregnancy in lean and obese mothers. J Clin Endocrinol Metab 2007;92: 969–975.

[29] Takase B, Goto T, Hamabe A, et al. Flow-mediated dilation in brachial artery in the second half of pregnancy and prediction of pre-eclampsia. J Hum Hypertens 2003;17:697–704.

[30] Melchiorre K, Sharma R, Khalil A, Thilaganathan B. Maternal cardiovascular function in normal pregnancy: evidence of maladaptation to chronic volume overload. Hypertension (Dallas, Tex: 1979) 2016;67:754–762.

[31] Meah VL, Cockcroft JR, Backx K, Shave R, Stohr EJ. Cardiac output and related haemodynamics during pregnancy: a series of meta-analyses. Heart (British Cardiac Society) 2016;102:518–526.

[32] Lopes VBVA, Van Gansewinkel TAG, De Haas S, et al Physiological adaptation of endothelial function to pregnancy: systematic review and meta-analysis. Ultrasound Obstet Gynecol: Off J Int Soc Ultrasound Obstet Gynecol 2017;50(697–708).

[33] Weissgerber TL, Milic NM, Milin-Lazovic JS, Garovic VD. Impaired flow-mediated dilation before, during, and after preeclampsia: a systematic review and meta-analysis. Hypertension 2016;67:415–423.

[34] Yinon Y, Kingdom JC, Odutayo A, et al. Vascular dysfunction in women with a history of preeclampsia and intrauterine growth restriction: insights into future vascular risk. Circulation 2010;122:1846–1853.

[35] Valensise H, Vasapollo B, Gagliardi G, Novelli GP. Early and late preeclampsia: two different maternal hemodynamic states in the latent phase of the disease. Hypertension (Dallas, Tex: 1979) 2008;52:873–880.

[36] Melchiorre K, Sutherland G, Sharma R, Nanni M, Thilaganathan B. Mid-gestational maternal cardiovascular profile in preterm and term pre-eclampsia: a prospective study. BJOG: Int J Obstet Gynaecol 2013;120:496–504.

[37] Melchiorre K, Sutherland GR, Watt-Coote I, Liberati M, Thilaganathan B. Severe myocardial impairment and chamber dysfunction in preterm preeclampsia. Pregnancy Hypertens 2012;31:454–471.

[38] Melchiorre K, Sutherland GR, Baltabaeva A, Liberati M, Thilaganathan B. Maternal cardiac dysfunction and remodeling in women with preeclampsia at term. Hypertension (Dallas, Tex: 1979) 2011;57:85–93.

[39] Bello N, Rendon ISH, Arany Z. The relationship between pre-eclampsia and peripartum cardiomyopathy: a systematic review and meta-analysis. J Am Coll Cardiol;2013(62): 1715–1723.

[40] Wallukat G, Homuth V, Fischer T, et al. Patients with preeclampsia develop agonistic autoantibodies against the angiotensin AT1 receptor. J Clin Invest 1999;103:945–952.

[41] Eremina V, Sood M, Haigh J, et al. Glomerular-specific alterations of VEGF-A expression lead to distinct congenital and acquired renal diseases. J Clin Invest 2003;111:707–716.

[42] Powe CE, Levine RJ, Karumanchi SA. Preeclampsia, a disease of the maternal endothelium: the role of antiangiogenic factors and implications for later cardiovascular disease. Circulation 2011;123:2856–2869.

[43] Wang Y, Zhao S, Loyd S, Groome LJ. Increased urinary excretion of nephrin, podocalyxin, and betaig-h3 in women with preeclampsia. Am J Physiol Renal Physiol 2012;302:F1084–9.

[44] Magee LA, Pels A, Helewa M, Rey E, Von Dadelszen P. Diagnosis, evaluation, and management of the hypertensive disorders of pregnancy: executive summary. J Obstet Gynaecol Can: JOGC = J D'obstet Gynecol Can: JOGC 2014;36:575–576.

[45] Gray KJ, Saxena R, Karumanchi SA. Genetic predisposition to preeclampsia is conferred by fetal DNA variants near FLT1, a gene involved in the regulation of angiogenesis. Am J Obstet Gynecol 2018;218:211–218.

[46] Lie RT, Rasmussen S, Brunborg H, Gjessing HK, Lie-Nielsen E, Irgens LM. Fetal and maternal contributions to risk of pre-eclampsia: population based study. BMJ (Clinical Research Ed) 1998;316:1343–1347.

[47] Boyd HA, Tahir H, Wohlfahrt J, Melbye M. Associations of personal and family preeclampsia history with the risk of early-, intermediate- and late-onset preeclampsia. Am J Epidemiol 2013;178:1611–1619.

[48] Egeland GM, Klungsoyr K, Oyen N, Tell GS, Naess O, Skjaerven R. Preconception cardiovascular risk factor differences between gestational hypertension and preeclampsia: cohort norway study. Hypertension (Dallas, Tex: 1979) 2016;67:1173–1180.

[49] Bartsch E, Medcalf KE, Park AL, Ray JG. Clinical risk factors for pre-eclampsia determined in early pregnancy: systematic review and meta-analysis of large cohort studies. BMJ (Clinical Research Ed) 2016;353:i1753.

[50] Wright D, Syngelaki A, Akolekar R, Poon LC, Nicolaides KH. Competing risks model in screening for preeclampsia by maternal characteristics and medical history. Am J Obstet Gynecol 2015;213:62.e1–62.e10.

[51] Caughey AB, Stotland NE, Washington AE, Escobar GJ. Maternal ethnicity, paternal ethnicity, and parental ethnic discordance: predictors of preeclampsia. Obstet Gynecol 2005;106: 156–161.

[52] Phaloprakarn C, Tangjitgamol S. Maternal ABO blood group and adverse pregnancy outcomes. J Perinatol: Off J Calif Perinatal Assoc 2013;33:107–111.

[53] Lee BK, Zhang Z, Wikman A, Lindqvist PG, Reilly M. ABO and RhD blood groups and gestational hypertensive disorders: a population-based cohort study. BJOG: Int J Obstet Gynaecol 2012;119:1232–1237.

[54] Mello G, Parretti E, Marozio L, et al. Thrombophilia is significantly associated with severe preeclampsia: results of a large-scale, case-controlled study. Hypertension (Dallas, Tex: 1979) 2005;46:1270–1274.

[55] Wikstrom AK, Stephansson O, Cnattingius S. Tobacco use during pregnancy and preeclampsia risk: effects of cigarette smoking and snuff. Hypertension (Dallas, Tex: 1979) 2010;55:1254–1259.

[56] Mehendale R, Hibbard J, Fazleabas A, Leach R. Placental angiogenesis markers sFlt-1 and PlGF: response to cigarette smoke. Am J Obstet Gynecol 2007;197:363.e1–5.

[57] Shevell T, Malone FD, Vidaver J, et al. Assisted reproductive technology and pregnancy outcome. Obstet Gynecol 2005;106:1039–1045.

[58] Report of the National High Blood Pressure Education Program Working Group on High Blood Pressure in Pregnancy. *American journal of obstetrics and gynecology*. 2000;183:S1–s22.

[59] ACOG Practice Bulletin. No. 202: gestational Hypertension and Preeclampsia. Obstet Gynecol 2019;133:e1–e25.

[60] McLaughlin K, Zhang J, Lye SJ, Parker JD, Kingdom JC. Phenotypes of pregnant women who subsequently develop hypertension in pregnancy. J Am Heart Assoc 2018:7.

[61] Scholten RR, Hopman MT, Lotgering FK, Spaanderman ME. Aerobic exercise training in formerly preeclamptic women: effects on venous reserve. Hypertension (Dallas, Tex: 1979) 2015;66:1058–1065.

[62] Scholten RR, Spaanderman ME, Green DJ, Hopman MT, Thijssen DH. Retrograde shear rate in formerly preeclamptic and healthy women before and after exercise training: relationship with endothelial function. Am J Physiol Heart Circ Physiol 2014;307:H418–25.

[63] Mottola MF, Davenport MH, Ruchat SM, et al. No. 367-2019 Canadian Guideline for Physical Activity throughout Pregnancy. J Obstet Gynaecol Can: JOGC = J D'obstet Gynecol Can: JOGC 2018;40:1528–1537.

[64] Di Mascio D, Magro-Malosso ER, Saccone G, Marhefka GD, Berghella V. Exercise during pregnancy in normal-weight women and risk of preterm birth: a systematic review and meta-analysis of randomized controlled trials. Am J Obstet Gynecol 2016;215:561–571.

[65] Webster K, Fishburn S, Maresh M, Findlay SC, Chappell LC. Diagnosis and management of hypertension in pregnancy: summary of updated NICE guidance. BMJ (Clinical Research Ed) 2019;366:l5119.

[66] Rolnik DL, Wright D, Poon LC, et al. Aspirin versus Placebo in Pregnancies at High Risk for Preterm Preeclampsia. N Engl J Med 2017;377:613–622.

[67] Hoffman MK, Goudar SS, Kodkany BS, et al. Low-dose aspirin for the prevention of preterm delivery in nulliparous women with a singleton pregnancy (ASPIRIN): a randomised, double-blind, placebo-controlled trial. Lancet (London, England) 2020;395:285–293.

[68]   Hofmeyr GJ, Lawrie TA, Atallah AN, Torloni MR. Calcium supplementation during pregnancy for preventing hypertensive disorders and related problems. Cochrane Database Syst Rev 2018;10:Cd001059.

[69]   Rumbold A, Duley L, Crowther CA, Haslam RR. Antioxidants for preventing pre-eclampsia. Cochrane Database Syst Rev 2008:Cd004227.

[70]   De-Regil LM, Palacios C, Ansary A, Kulier R, Pena-Rosas JP. Vitamin D supplementation for women during pregnancy. Cochrane Database Syst Rev 2012:Cd008873.

[71]   Makrides M, Crosby DD, Bain E, Crowther CA. Magnesium supplementation in pregnancy. Cochrane Database Syst Rev 2014:Cd000937.

[72]   Magee LA, Von Dadelszen P, Rey E, et al. Less-tight versus tight control of hypertension in pregnancy. N Engl J Med 2015;372:407–417.

[73]   McLaughlin K, Scholten RR, Kingdom JC, Floras JS, Parker JD. Should maternal hemodynamics guide antihypertensive therapy in preeclampsia?. Hypertension (Dallas, Tex: 1979) 2018;71: 550–556.

[74]   Duley L, Gulmezoglu AM, Henderson-Smart DJ, Chou D. Magnesium sulphate and other anticonvulsants for women with pre-eclampsia. Cochrane Database Syst Rev 2010: Cd000025.

[75]   Chappell LC, Brocklehurst P, Green ME, et al. Planned early delivery or expectant management for late preterm pre-eclampsia (PHOENIX): a randomised controlled trial. Lancet (London, England) 2019;394:1181–1190.

[76]   Griffin M, Seed PT, Duckworth S, et al. Predicting delivery of a small-for-gestational-age infant and adverse perinatal outcome in women with suspected pre-eclampsia. Ultrasound Obstet Gynecol: Off J Int Soc Ultrasound Obstet Gynecol 2018;51:387–395.

[77]   El S, Jy T, Jc K, et al Intrapartum magnesium sulfate is associated with neuroprotection in growth-restricted fetuses. Am J Obstet Gynecol 2018;219:606.e1–606.e8.

[78]   Woudstra DM, Chandra S, Hofmeyr GJ, Dowswell T. Corticosteroids for HELLP (hemolysis, elevated liver enzymes, low platelets) syndrome in pregnancy. Cochrane Database Syst Rev 2010:Cd008148.

[79]   Tarnow-Mordi WO, Shaw JC, Liu D, Gardner DA, Flynn FV. Iatrogenic hyponatraemia of the newborn due to maternal fluid overload: a prospective study. Br Med J (Clinical Research Ed) 1981;283:639–642.

[80]   Chames MC, Livingston JC, Ivester TS, Barton JR, Sibai BM. Late postpartum eclampsia: a preventable disease?. Am J Obstet Gynecol 2002;186:1174–1177.

[81]   Makris A, Thornton C, Hennessy A. Postpartum hypertension and nonsteroidal analgesia. Am J Obstet Gynecol 2004;190:577–578.

[82]   Bramham K, Nelson-Piercy C, Brown MJ, Chappell LC. Postpartum management of hypertension. BMJ (Clinical Research Ed) 2013;346:f894.

[83]   Ditisheim A, Wuerzner G, Ponte B, et al. Prevalence of hypertensive phenotypes after preeclampsia: a prospective cohort study. Hypertension (Dallas, Tex: 1979) 2018;71:103–109.

[84]   Al-Safi Z, Imudia AN, Filetti LC, Hobson DT, Bahado-Singh RO, Awonuga AO. Delayed postpartum preeclampsia and eclampsia: demographics, clinical course, and complications. Obstet Gynecol 2011;118:1102–1107.

[85]   Agrawal S, Cerdeira AS, Redman C, Vatish M. Meta-analysis and systematic review to assess the role of soluble fms-like tyrosine kinase-1 and placenta growth factor ratio in prediction of preeclampsia: the sappphire study. Hypertension (Dallas, Tex: 1979) 2018;71:306–316.

[86]   Zeisler H, Llurba E, Chantraine F, et al. Predictive Value of the sFlt-1: PlGFRatio in Women with Suspected Preeclampsia. N Engl J Med 2016;374:13–22.

[87] Agrawal S, Shinar S, Cerdeira AS, Redman C, Vatish M. Predictive performance of PlGF (Placental Growth Factor) for screening preeclampsia in asymptomatic women: a systematic review and meta-analysis. Hypertension (Dallas, Tex: 1979) 2019;74:1124–1135.

[88] McLaughlin K, Snelgrove JW, Audette MC, et al. PlGF (Placental Growth Factor) testing in clinical practice: evidence from a canadian tertiary maternity referral center. Hypertension (Dallas, Tex: 1979) 2021:Hypertensionaha12117047.

[89] Duhig KE, Myers J, Seed PT, et al. Placental growth factor testing to assess women with suspected pre-eclampsia: a multicentre, pragmatic, stepped-wedge cluster-randomised controlled trial. Lancet (London, England);2019(393):1807–1818.

[90] Villa PM, Marttinen P, Gillberg J, et al. Cluster analysis to estimate the risk of preeclampsia in the high-risk Prediction and Prevention of Preeclampsia and Intrauterine Growth Restriction (PREDO) study. PloS One 2017;12:e0174399.

[91] Ogge G, Chaiworapongsa T, Romero R, et al. Placental lesions associated with maternal underperfusion are more frequent in early-onset than in late-onset preeclampsia. J Perinat Med 2011;39:641–652.

[92] Faupel-Badger JM, Fichorova RN, Allred EN, et al. Cluster analysis of placental inflammatory proteins can distinguish preeclampsia from preterm labor and premature membrane rupture in singleton deliveries less than 28 weeks of gestation. Am J Reprod Immunol (New York, NY: 1989) 2011;66:488–494.

[93] Leavey K, Bainbridge SA, Cox BJ. Large scale aggregate microarray analysis reveals three distinct molecular subclasses of human preeclampsia. PloS One 2015;10:e0116508.

[94] Leavey K, Benton SJ, Grynspan D, Kingdom JC, Bainbridge SA, Cox BJ. Unsupervised placental gene expression profiling identifies clinically relevant subclasses of human preeclampsia. Hypertension (Dallas, Tex: 1979) 2016;68:137–147.

[95] McLaughlin K, Scholten RR, Parker JD, Ferrazzi E, Kingdom JCP. Low molecular weight heparin for the prevention of severe preeclampsia: where next?. Br J Clin Pharmacol 2018;84: 673–678.

[96] Suzuki H, Ohkuchi A, Matsubara S, et al. Effect of recombinant placental growth factor 2 on hypertension induced by full-length mouse soluble fms-like tyrosine kinase 1 adenoviral vector in pregnant mice. Hypertension (Dallas, Tex: 1979) 2009;54:1129–1135.

[97] Spradley FT, Tan AY, Joo WS, et al. Placental growth factor administration abolishes placental ischemia-induced hypertension. Hypertension (Dallas, Tex: 1979) 2016;67:740–747.

[98] Makris A, Yeung KR, Lim SM, et al. Placental growth factor reduces blood pressure in a uteroplacental ischemia model of preeclampsia in nonhuman primates. Hypertension (Dallas, Tex: 1979) 2016;67:1263–1272.

[99] Rodger MA, Gris JC, Jip DV, et al. Low-molecular-weight heparin and recurrent placenta-mediated pregnancy complications: a meta-analysis of individual patient data from randomised controlled trials. Lancet (London, England) 2016;388:2629–2641.

[100] Wat JM, Audette MC, Kingdom JC. Molecular actions of heparin and their implications in preventing pre-eclampsia. J Thromb Haemost: JTH 2018.

[101] McLaughlin K, Baczyk D, Potts A, Hladunewich M, Parker JD, Kingdom JC. Low molecular weight heparin improves endothelial function in pregnant women at high risk of preeclampsia. Hypertension (Dallas, Tex: 1979) 2017;69:180–188.

[102] Mello G, Parretti E, Fatini C, et al. Low-molecular-weight heparin lowers the recurrence rate of preeclampsia and restores the physiological vascular changes in angiotensin-converting enzyme DD women. Hypertension (Dallas, Tex: 1979) 2005;45:86–91.

[103] Costantine MM, Cleary K, Hebert MF, et al. Safety and pharmacokinetics of pravastatin used for the prevention of preeclampsia in high-risk pregnant women: a pilot randomized controlled trial. Am J Obstet Gynecol 2016;214:720.e1–720.e17.

[104] Ahmed A, Williams DJ, Cheed V, et al. Pravastatin for early-onset pre-eclampsia: a randomised, blinded, placebo-controlled trial. BJOG: Int J Obstet Gynaecol 2019.

[105] Cluver CA, Hiscock R, Decloedt EH et al. Use of metformin to prolon ggestation in preterm pre-eclampsia: randomised, double blind, placebo controlled trial. BMJ 2021;374:n2103

[106] Hobson SR, Gurusinghe S, Lim R, et al. Melatonin improves endothelial function in vitro and prolongs pregnancy in women with early-onset preeclampsia. J Pineal Res 2018;65:e12508.

[107] Thadhani R, Kisner T, Hagmann H, et al. Pilot study of extracorporeal removal of soluble fms-like tyrosine kinase 1 in preeclampsia. Circulation 2011;124:940–950.

[108] Thadhani R, Hagmann H, Schaarschmidt W, et al. Removal of soluble fms-like tyrosine kinase-1 by dextran sulfate apheresis in preeclampsia. J Am Soc Nephrol: JASN 2016;27: 903–913.

Omri Zamstein, Eyal Sheiner

7 Late Consequences of Pregnancy-Associated Hypertensive Disorders

7.1 Introduction

Hypertensive disorders of pregnancy are one of the most common conditions known to affect pregnancy, with a prevalence of over 15% worldwide [1, 2]. This group of disorders is generally divided into either preexisting hypertension (present before 20th week of gestation or persists chronically postpartum) or gestational hypertension and preeclampsia that first appear late in gestation, with the latter distinguished from the former by the presence of end-organ dysfunction [3]. The various hypertensive disorders have different courses, where preeclampsia is considered the most clinically significant of them all, as it mandates careful management to prevent development of both maternal and fetal complications from disease progression [4]. While gestational hypertension and preeclampsia are both induced by abnormal development of the placenta [5, 6] and thus ultimately resolves after delivery, there is a growing body of evidence supporting the hypothesis that these pregnancy-associated complications could either stimulate or unmask nonadaptive maternal physiology. Established risk factors for cardiovascular morbidity such as endothelial dysfunction [7], insulin resistance, inflammatory activation, and dyslipidemia [9] could all be elicited by the process of abnormal placentation and can eventually contribute to elevated risk of various maternal comorbidities (Table 7.1), particularly cardiovascular disease (CVD), and carry implications for offspring's well-being as well.

7.2 Cardiovascular Disease

Well-established studies have found pregnancy-related hypertension to be strongly associated with future development of CVD. A 2008 systemic review that evaluated more than 116,000 women with preeclampsia found a 2-fold increased risk of cardiac, cerebrovascular, peripheral arterial disease, as well as total CVD mortality compared to women with uncomplicated pregnancies, even after controlling for other common cardiovascular risk factors. An even higher relative risk (RR) of 5.36 for future cardiac disease was noted in women with a history of more severe preeclampsia (95% CI 3.96–7.27; P < 0.0001), that is, preeclampsia that was complicated by preterm delivery or fetal demise [10]. Similar results were later determined in a meta-analysis by Wu et al. that included 258,000 women with preeclampsia. The authors found a 2-fold increased risk in coronary heart disease, stroke, and CVD-related mortality, and up to 4-fold increase in the risk for future heart failure. Notably, the risk became nonsignificant

https://doi.org/10.1515/9783110615258-007

Table 7.1: Key findings from articles assessing the relationship between pregnancy-associated hypertension and maternal morbidity, as compared to women with normotensive pregnancies.

Reference	Total participants included in analysis	Main outcomes assessed	RR/OR
Wu et al. [11]	1,986,285	Heart failure	4.19
	2,068,673	Coronary artery disease	2.5
	2,614,180	CVD-related mortality	2.21
	4,131,344	CVA	1.81
McDonald et al. [10]	2,375,751	CVA	2.03
		PVD	1.87
		CVD-related mortality	2.29
Brown et al. [12]	822,555	Hypertension	3.31
	1,426,488	CVA	1.77
	2,010,656	CVD	2.28
Kessous et al. [14]	96,370	Major cardiovascular events	2.4
		Renal-related hospitalizations	3.7
Callaway et al. [25]	3,639	Diabetes mellitus	1.76
Kristensen et al. [31]	1,072,330	Chronic renal disease	2.06
Vikse et al. [30]	570,433	End-stage renal disease	3.2–15.5

CVA, cerebrovascular accident; CVD, cardiovascular disease; PVD, peripheral vascular disease; OR, odds ratio.

10 years after the affected pregnancy, probably because of the inevitable effects of aging on the general population comprising the control group as well as the low number of events [11]. Another meta-analysis that included 32 articles in which elevated blood pressure was evaluated as an outcome reported that women who previously experienced preeclampsia were at increased risk of developing hypertension (RR = 3.13, 95% CI 2.51–3.89) [12]. A recent observational cohort study that included 58,671 parous women found that compared with women who were normotensive during pregnancy, those with gestational hypertension (2.9%) or preeclampsia (6.3%) in their first pregnancy developed chronic hypertension at a 2- to 3-fold higher rate. Although elevated rates of chronic hypertension were observed throughout a long follow-up of up to 50 years, the risk was highest in the first 5 years from birth. Type 2 diabetes mellitus and hypercholesterolemia, two other established risk factors for CVD, were also increased by 70% and 30%, respectively [13]. Dose–response relationship may exist, whereas women with early-onset, severe, or recurring preeclampsia

are at greater risk for adverse sequelae. In their observational study of over 96,370 parturients, Kessous et al. showed that the link between preeclampsia and CVD is becoming more substantial in the subgroup of patients with severe compared to mild disease (5.2% vs. 4.5%, respectively; p = 0.001) and recurrent episodes compared to a single episode of preeclampsia (6.0% vs. 4.4%, respectively; p = 0.001) [14]. Likewise, in a systemic review, Brouwers et al. observed that women with recurrent preeclampsia had a 3-fold increased risk of heart failure, 2- to 3-fold risk of hypertension and ischemic heart disease, and approximately 2-fold risk of CVA and overall CVD, when compared with women with only a single event of preeclampsia and subsequent uneventful pregnancies [15]. Early-onset preeclampsia is also predictive of worse cardiovascular outcomes, as evident from the child health and development studies cohort, where women with onset of preeclampsia by 34 weeks of gestation had 9.5-fold increased risk of subsequent CVD-related death. The corresponding risk for later-onset preeclampsia was lower at 2.08 (95% CI 1.26–3.44) [16]. With regard to hypertension, a prospective study of 131 women with early-onset preeclampsia found that almost 40% developed hypertension 9–16 years after pregnancy [17].

It is still not clear if the increased risk of late cardiovascular morbidity and mortality is attributed to predisposing factors that put women at risk for development of both conditions or whether preeclampsia itself induces vascular and metabolic changes that negatively influence future health [18]. According to one observation, women who develop preeclampsia already had unfavorable cardiovascular profile (in the form of elevated blood pressure) to begin with, thus indicating that preeclampsia only unmasks a subclinical tendency toward hypertension [19]. When Romundstad et al. studied a group of women who experienced preeclampsia and gestational hypertension, they noticed significant attenuation of post-pregnancy BMI (body mass index), blood pressure, and metabolic profile after adjustment for prepregnancy measurements, suggesting that CVD risk factors are actually present before the hypertensive pregnancy [20]. On the other hand, it could be that preeclampsia causally increases CVD risk. Research from animal models revealed that s-Flt1-induced preeclampsia (see chapter 6 for details) enhanced the expression of proteins that are associated with CVD [21]. Additional abnormalities such as impaired vascular function, dyslipidemia, and elevated insulin levels, all been observed in women with previous preeclampsia, may also play a contributory role in future maternal vascular disease [8, 22]. While the optimal screening and preventive strategy have not been established [23], a history of hypertensive pregnancy may help identify women who are at increased risk for cardiovascular disease. And indeed, the American Heart Association, the American Stroke Association, and the American College of Obstetrics and Gynecology acknowledge preeclampsia as a risk factor for future CVD and recommend screening for these conditions [24] and suggest closer follow-up and lifestyle interventions as part of a risk reduction strategy [3].

7.3 Diabetes Mellitus

Other than the cardiovascular risk, women with a history of preeclampsia appear to exhibit increased risk for developing Type 2 diabetes mellitus. According to one prospective study that included more than 3,600 women, those who experienced hypertensive disorders during pregnancy had a 2-fold increased risk of diabetes mellitus after more than 20 years, compared to uncomplicated pregnancy. While the elevated risk was partially explained by increased body weight, it remained significant even after adjusting for BMI and waist circumference [25]. Another study by Lykke et al. found that women with severe preeclampsia were at even higher risk by a 3.7-fold for developing Type 2 diabetes mellitus after a mean follow-up of 15 years [26]. Results from a Norwegian population-based prescription database similarly showed that although gestational diabetes mellitus was the strongest predictor of future diabetes, women with only preeclampsia had 3 times higher risk of receiving drugs used to treat diabetes during the first 5 years after birth (95% CI 2.4–3.6) [27]. While it is possible that unmeasured confounders contribute to the association between preeclampsia and diabetes mellitus, these observations further highlight the importance of comprehensive lifestyle modification in women who have had preeclampsia [28, 29].

7.4 Chronic Kidney Disease

A history of preeclampsia has been linked with increased risk of chronic and even end-stage kidney disease (ESKD) [14]. According to a national cohort-based study following more than 570,000 Norwegian women, although the total incidence of ESKD was low, preeclampsia was associated with a relative risk of ESKD ranging between 3.2 (when preeclampsia complicated the first pregnancy) and 15.5 (preeclampsia during two or three pregnancies) [30]. Another large cohort study consisting of over 1,000,000 participants found significant association between preeclampsia and later chronic kidney disease, where women with a history of preeclampsia had overall twice the risk of later chronic kidney disorder. The risk increased 4-fold for early preterm preeclampsia and was most prominent within 5 years of the affected pregnancy (hazard ratio 6.11; 95% CI 3.84–9.72). Interestingly, the observed association remained even after adjustment for potential mediators of chronic kidney disease such as hypertension [31]. Once again, it is still unclear whether the association between preeclampsia and kidney disease is explained merely by the common underlying factors of both conditions [32], or if preeclampsia leads or at least worsens subclinical kidney disease [33].

7.5 Additional Morbidities Related to Pregnancy-Associated Hypertension

There are several reports linking pregnancy-associated hypertension with various other maternal health conditions, including ophthalmic disease, hypothyroidism, malignancy, and dementia. Demonstrating the future microvascular consequence of preeclampsia, Beharier et al. found that a history of preeclampsia was associated with emergence of maternal ophthalmic morbidity, with declining prognosis as a function of disease severity (0.3% and 2.2% vs. 0.2% for women with mild preeclampsia and eclampsia versus women without preeclampsia, respectively) [34]. Furthermore, in the first study to evaluate the occurrence of age-related macular degeneration (AMD), a leading cause of blindness worldwide, Curtin et al. showed that women who experienced hypertension disorder during pregnancy were 80% more likely to develop choroidal neovascularization AMD ("wet" AMD) before the age of 70 years [35]. Although available evidence is inconsistent [36], a history of preeclampsia may also predispose to subclinical hypothyroidism by a nonimmune mechanism, as suggested by elevated thyroid-stimulating hormone without the presence of thyroid autoantibodies, compared with women who had a normotensive pregnancy [37]. Few observational studies additionally found support for a link between preeclampsia and altered cerebrovascular function, visual memory impairment, brain structural changes, and clinical cognitive impairment, all contributing to the developments of the common forms of dementia, that is, vascular dementia and Alzheimer's disease [38, 39].

7.6 Prognosis of Offspring of Hypertensive Pregnancies

Apart from the long-term maternal risks, inadequate placentation could also be meaningful for future offspring's health. A meta-analysis of over 1,500 children exposed to preeclampsia in utero found them to have mild but significant rise in blood pressure and BMI during childhood and young adulthood [40]. Another large population-based study of over 230,000 deliveries that assessed cardiovascular risk factors among singletons exposed to preeclampsia in utero with those unexposed reported significant linear relationship between the severity of preeclampsia and diagnosis of hypertension in the offspring. Children exposed to mild preeclampsia, severe preeclampsia, and eclampsia had significantly higher rates of cardiovascular morbidity compared with children born after normotensive pregnancies (0.33%, 0.51%, and 2.73% vs. 0.24%, respectively, p < 0.001). Similar trends were observed for hypertension specifically, with children exposed to mild preeclampsia, severe preeclampsia, and eclampsia having significantly greater rates of hypertension compared with children born after nonpreeclamptic pregnancies (0.11%, 0.14%, and 1.37% vs. 0.06%, respectively, p < 0.001) [41]. Two other cohort studies based on a heterogeneous population of almost quarter of a million children also related preeclampsia with the development of respiratory morbidity, specifically asthma [42], as well as gastrointestinal-related hospitalizations during childhood [43]. Limited number of studies have additionally found preeclampsia to be associated with autism spectrum disorder [44] and childhood neuropsychiatric morbidity [45], highlighting the possible consequences of inadequate transplacental nutrient transport on fetal neurological development.

7.7 Conclusion

In summary, there is a growing body of evidence indicating that, despite prior beliefs that "delivery was the cure," women who survive preeclampsia may have long-term sequelae from the syndrome and may benefit from ongoing monitoring and counseling of these risks.

References

[1]   Phipps EA, Thadhani R, Benzing T, Karumanchi SA. Pre-eclampsia: pathogenesis, novel diagnostics and therapies. Nat Rev Nephrol 2019;15(5):275–289.
[2]   Stuart JJ, Tanz LJ, Cook NR, et al. Hypertensive disorders of pregnancy and 10-year cardiovascular risk prediction. J Am Coll Cardiol 2018;72(11):1252–1263.
[3]   ACOG Practice Bulletin No. 202. Gestational hypertension and preeclampsia. Obstetrics and gynecology 2019;133(1):e1–e25.
[4]   Von Dadelszen P, Payne B, Li J, et al. Prediction of adverse maternal outcomes in pre-eclampsia: development and validation of the fullPIERS model. Lancet (London, England) 2011;377(9761):219–227.
[5]   Pijnenborg R, Vercruysse L, Hanssens M. The uterine spiral arteries in human pregnancy: facts and controversies. Placenta 2006;27(9–10):939–958.
[6]   Tomimatsu T, Mimura K, Matsuzaki S, Endo M, Kumasawa K, Kimura T. Preeclampsia: maternal systemic vascular disorder caused by generalized endothelial dysfunction due to placental antiangiogenic factors. Int J Mol Sci 2019;20(17).
[7]   Chambers JC, Fusi L, Malik IS, Haskard DO, De Swiet M, Kooner JS. Association of maternal endothelial dysfunction with preeclampsia. Jama 2001;285(12):1607–1612.
[8]   Hermes W, Ket JC, Van Pampus MG, et al. Biochemical cardiovascular risk factors after hypertensive pregnancy disorders: a systematic review and meta-analysis. Obstet Gynecol Surv 2012;67(12):793–809.
[9]   Van Rijn BB, Nijdam ME, Bruinse HW, et al. Cardiovascular disease risk factors in women with a history of early-onset preeclampsia. Obstet Gynecol 2013;121(5):1040–1048.
[10] McDonald SD, Malinowski A, Zhou Q, Yusuf S, Devereaux PJ. Cardiovascular sequelae of preeclampsia/eclampsia: a systematic review and meta-analyses. Am Heart J 2008;156(5): 918–930.

[11] Wu P, Haththotuwa R, Kwok CS, et al. Preeclampsia and future cardiovascular health: a systematic review and meta-analysis. Circ Cardiovasc Qual Outcomes 2017;10(2).

[12] Brown MC, Best KE, Pearce MS, Waugh J, Robson SC, Bell R. Cardiovascular disease risk in women with pre-eclampsia: systematic review and meta-analysis. Eur J Epidemiol 2013;28(1):1–19.

[13] Stuart JJ, Tanz LJ, Missmer SA, et al. Hypertensive disorders of pregnancy and maternal cardiovascular disease risk factor development: an observational cohort study. Ann Intern Med 2018;169(4):224–232.

[14] Kessous R, Shoham-Vardi I, Pariente G, Sergienko R, Sheiner E. Long-term maternal atherosclerotic morbidity in women with pre-eclampsia. Heart (British Cardiac Society) 2015;101(6):442–446.

[15] Brouwers L, Van Der Meiden-van Roest AJ, Savelkoul C, et al. Recurrence of pre-eclampsia and the risk of future hypertension and cardiovascular disease: a systematic review and meta-analysis. BJOG: Int J Obstet Gynaecol 2018;125(13):1642–1654.

[16] Mongraw-Chaffin ML, Cirillo PM, Cohn BA. Preeclampsia and cardiovascular disease death: prospective evidence from the child health and development studies cohort. Hypertension (Dallas, Tex: 1979) 2010;56(1):166–171.

[17] Bokslag A, Teunissen PW, Franssen C, et al. Effect of early-onset preeclampsia on cardiovascular risk in the fifth decade of life. Am J Obstet Gynecol 2017;216(5):523.e1–e7.

[18] Seely EW, Tsigas E, Rich-Edwards JW. Preeclampsia and future cardiovascular disease in women: how good are the data and how can we manage our patients?. Semin Perinatol 2015;39(4):276–283.

[19] Magnussen EB, Vatten LJ, Lund-Nilsen TI, Salvesen KA, Davey Smith G, Romundstad PR. Prepregnancy cardiovascular risk factors as predictors of pre-eclampsia: population based cohort study. BMJ (Clinical Research Ed) 2007;335(7627):978.

[20] Romundstad PR, Magnussen EB, Smith GD, Vatten LJ. Hypertension in pregnancy and later cardiovascular risk: common antecedents?. Circulation 2010;122(6):579–584.

[21] Bytautiene E, Bulayeva N, Bhat G, Li L, Rosenblatt KP, Saade GR. Long-term alterations in maternal plasma proteome after sFlt1-induced preeclampsia in mice. Am J Obstet Gynecol 2013;208(5):388.e1–e10.

[22] Yinon Y, Kingdom JC, Odutayo A, et al. Vascular dysfunction in women with a history of preeclampsia and intrauterine growth restriction: insights into future vascular risk. Circulation 2010;122(18):1846–1853.

[23] Bro Schmidt G, Christensen M, Breth Knudsen U. Preeclampsia and later cardiovascular disease – What do national guidelines recommend?. Pregnancy Hypertens 2017;10:14–17.

[24] Bushnell C, McCullough LD, Awad IA, et al. Guidelines for the prevention of stroke in women: a statement for healthcare professionals from the American Heart Association/American Stroke Association. Stroke 2014;45(5):1545–1588.

[25] Callaway LK, Lawlor DA, O'Callaghan M, Williams GM, Najman JM, McIntyre HD. Diabetes mellitus in the 21 years after a pregnancy that was complicated by hypertension: findings from a prospective cohort study. Am J Obstet Gynecol 2007;197(5):492.e1–7.

[26] Lykke JA, Langhoff-Roos J, Sibai BM, Funai EF, Triche EW, Paidas MJ. Hypertensive pregnancy disorders and subsequent cardiovascular morbidity and type 2 diabetes mellitus in the mother. Hypertension (Dallas, Tex: 1979) 2009;53(6):944–951.

[27] Engeland A, Bjorge T, Daltveit AK, et al. Risk of diabetes after gestational diabetes and preeclampsia. A registry-based study of 230,000 women in Norway. Eur J Epidemiol 2011;26(2):157–163.

[28] Wu P, Kwok CS, Haththotuwa R, et al. Pre-eclampsia is associated with a twofold increase in diabetes: a systematic review and meta-analysis. Diabetologia 2016;59(12):2518–2526.

[29] Sheiner E, Kapur A, Retnakaran R, et al. FIGO (International Federation of Gynecology and Obstetrics) Postpregnancy initiative: long-term maternal implications of pregnancy complications – follow-up considerations 2019;147(S1):1–31.

[30] Vikse BE, Irgens LM, Leivestad T, Skjaerven R, Iversen BM. Preeclampsia and the risk of end-stage renal disease. N Engl J Med 2008;359(8):800–809.

[31] Kristensen JH, Basit S, Wohlfahrt J, Damholt MB, Boyd HA. Pre-eclampsia and risk of later kidney disease: nationwide cohort study. BMJ (Clinical Research Ed) 2019;365:l1516.

[32] Sibai BM, Gordon T, Thom E, et al. Risk factors for preeclampsia in healthy nulliparous women: a prospective multicenter study. The National Institute of Child Health and Human Development Network of Maternal-Fetal Medicine Units. Am J Obstet Gynecol 1995;172(2 Pt 1): 642–648.

[33] Bar J, Kaplan B, Wittenberg C, et al. Microalbuminuria after pregnancy complicated by pre-eclampsia. Nephrol Dialysis Transplant: off Publ Eur Dialysis Transplant Assoc Eur Renal Assoc 1999;14(5):1129–1132.

[34] Beharier O, Davidson E, Sergienko R, et al. Preeclampsia and future risk for maternal ophthalmic complications. Am J Perinatol 2016;33(7):703–707.

[35] Curtin K, Theilen LH, Fraser A, Smith KR, Varner MW, Hageman GS. Hypertensive disorders of pregnancy increase the risk of developing neovascular age-related macular degeneration in later life. Hypertens Pregnancy 2019;38(3):141–148.

[36] Mannisto T, Karumanchi SA, Pouta A, et al. Preeclampsia, gestational hypertension and subsequent hypothyroidism. Pregnancy Hypertens 2013;3(1):21–27.

[37] Levine RJ, Vatten LJ, Horowitz GL, et al. Pre-eclampsia, soluble fms-like tyrosine kinase 1, and the risk of reduced thyroid function: nested case-control and population based study. BMJ (Clinical Research Ed) 2009;339:b4336.

[38] Miller KB, Miller VM, Barnes JN. Pregnancy history, hypertension, and cognitive impairment in postmenopausal women. Curr Hypertens Rep 2019;21(12):93.

[39] Basit S, Wohlfahrt J, Boyd HA. Pre-eclampsia and risk of dementia later in life: nationwide cohort study. BMJ (Clinical Research Ed) 2018;363:k4109.

[40] Andraweera PH, Lassi ZS. Cardiovascular risk factors in offspring of preeclamptic pregnancies-systematic review and meta-analysis. J Pediatr 2019;208(104–13.e6).

[41] Nahum Sacks K, Friger M, Shoham-Vardi I, et al. Prenatal exposure to preeclampsia as an independent risk factor for long-term cardiovascular morbidity of the offspring. Pregnancy Hypertens 2018;13:181–186.

[42] Nahum Sacks K, Friger M, Shoham-Vardi I, Sergienko R, Landau D, Sheiner E. In utero exposure to pre-eclampsia as an independent risk factor for long-term respiratory disease. Pediatr Pulmonol 2020.

[43] Leybovitz-Haleluya N, Wainstock T, Sheiner E. Maternal preeclampsia and the risk of pediatric gastrointestinal diseases of the offspring: a population-based cohort study. Pregnancy Hypertens 2019;17:144–147.

[44] Dachew BA, Mamun A, Maravilla JC, Alati R. Pre-eclampsia and the risk of autism-spectrum disorder in offspring: meta-analysis. Br J Psychiatry J Mental Sci 2018;212(3):142–147.

[45] Nahum Sacks K, Friger M, Shoham-Vardi I, et al. Long-term neuropsychiatric morbidity in children exposed prenatally to preeclampsia. Early Hum Dev 2019;130:96–100.

Harrison Banner, Jack M. Colman, Mathew Sermer

8 Cardiovascular Disease in Pregnancy

8.1 Introduction

The incidence of pregnancy complicated by cardiovascular disease is rising, primarily due to an increased number of women with congenital heart disease (CHD) reaching childbearing age. With the exception of patients with severe conditions, maternal death during pregnancy in women with heart disease is relatively rare [1–6]. However, pregnant women with heart disease do remain at risk for cardiac, obstetric, and fetal–neonatal complications. The most common maternal cardiac complications are congestive heart failure (CHF) and arrhythmia [1, 6–8]. Fetal risks include preterm birth and its associated sequelae, intrauterine growth restriction, pregnancy loss, and stillbirth.

For women with cardiac disease contemplating pregnancy, preconception evaluation and counseling by a cardiologist with expertise in the management of heart disease in pregnancy and a maternal–fetal medicine specialist are recommended to optimize outcomes. Baseline testing can be arranged, pregnancy-related risk stratification can be established, and interventions can be planned if necessary. Medications should be reviewed and, depending on teratogenic potential, can be discontinued, altered, or, if safe, continued. Discussion regarding the impact of pregnancy on heart disease as well as of heart disease on the potential pregnancy should be discussed. Recently, the discipline providing this type of specialized interdisciplinary care has been named Cardio-Obstetrics [9].

8.2 Cardiovascular Physiology and Adaptation to Pregnancy

Substantial maternal cardiovascular changes occur in pregnancy, beginning as soon as the early first trimester. Blood volume increases by approximately 40%, and there is a 30% decrease in peripheral vascular resistance and a 10–20% increase in heart rate by late pregnancy. These changes result in the 25–50% increase in cardiac output (CO) which occurs over the course of pregnancy. During labor and delivery, there is an additional 50% increase in CO due to catecholaminergic response to pain and anxiety and auto-transfusion caused by uterine contractions. Following delivery, relief of caval compression and autotransfusion from the empty uterus result in a further transient increase in CO. Most of the hemodynamic changes of pregnancy resolve by the second postpartum week, however a complete return to baseline may not occur until 6 months after delivery. In addition to these

https://doi.org/10.1515/9783110615258-008

hemodynamic stressors, pregnancy is a prothrombotic state, increasing the risk of thromboembolic complications in women with preexisting cardiovascular disease.

Normal hemodynamic adaptations to pregnancy may produce symptoms and signs which mimic cardiac decompensation. Normal physiologic pregnancy changes can lead to presyncope, palpitations, dyspnea, and exercise intolerance in women with a structurally normal heart. Normal physical examination findings in pregnancy can mimic heart disease, such as prominent jugular venous pulsations, displacement of the apical impulse, presence of a murmur or gallop sound and/or peripheral edema. This can make differentiating between normal physiologic changes and cardiac disease difficult. A complete history, physical exam, electrocardiogram, and transthoracic echocardiogram should be performed when heart disease is suspected. Serum B-type natriuretic peptide may be a useful adjunct, as normal levels have been noted to have a negative predictive value of 100% for identifying adverse cardiac events during pregnancy [10].

8.3 Risk Assessment

8.3.1 Maternal Risk

For women with preexisting heart disease, assessment of pregnancy risk includes a detailed cardiac, surgical, and obstetrical history, including a review of any operative notes for patients with previous cardiac interventions. Maternal functional status, using tools such as the New York Heart Association NYHA functional classification are predictive of pregnancy-related morbidity and mortality. A physical exam should include a detailed cardiorespiratory examination, as well as documentation of oxygen saturation. Baseline 12-lead electrocardiogram and transthoracic echocardiogram are necessary. Prepregnancy exercise testing can occasionally be helpful, as impaired chronotropic response on cardiopulmonary exercise testing correlates with adverse pregnancy outcomes [11].

Several risk assessment tools have been developed to predict maternal cardiac complications in pregnancy, including the cardiac disease in pregnancy (CARPREG) risk score [12], the modified WHO (mWHO) classification [13, 14], and the ZAHARA risk score [15]. Recently, the CARPREG II risk score was published [16], which incorporates information about the specific lesion, the patient's history of prior cardiac complications, the timing of their presentation to care, as well as current functional status, to predict the likelihood of an adverse cardiac event occurring in pregnancy (see Figure 8.1).

In addition to discussing the risk of an adverse cardiac event in pregnancy, women with a high-risk cardiac lesion need counseling regarding maternal life expectancy. A patient with limited physical capacity or a condition that may result in

PREDICTOR	POINTS
History of heart failure, stroke or arrhythmias	3
Baseline NYHA III-IV or cyanosis	3
Mechanical valve	3
Ventricular dysfunction	2
High risk left-sided valve disease/left ventricular outflow tract obstruction	2
Pulmonary hypertension	2
Coronary artery disease	2
High risk aortopathy	2
No Prior cardiac intervention	1
Late pregnancy assessment	1

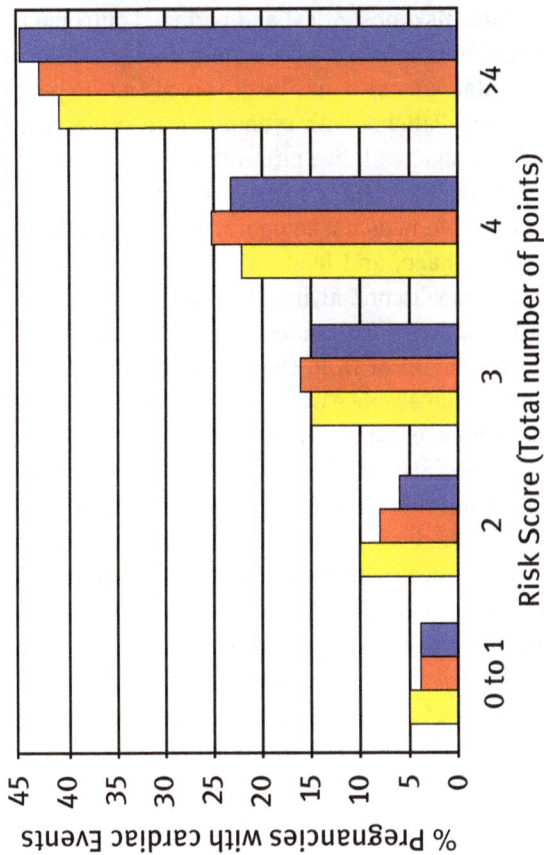

Figure 8.1: CARPREG II Risk Prediction Index: Incidence of Adverse Cardiac Events Stratified According to CARPREG II Risk Scores. Modified from Silversides et al, 2012 [reference 16]

premature death should be advised of her potential inability to look after her child. Additionally, women whose condition imparts a high likelihood of fetal complications must be apprised of these added risks.

There are a small number of specific cardiac conditions associated with high maternal morbidity and mortality. These conditions include severe pulmonary hypertension (PH), severe systemic ventricular dysfunction, poor exercise tolerance (NYHA functional class III–IV), ejection fraction < 40%, peripartum cardiomyopathy (PPCM) with residual ventricular dysfunction, severe left heart obstructive lesions including aortic stenosis (AS) and mitral stenosis (MS), and Marfan syndrome with an aortic root diameter > 44 mm [12, 14, 17]. Women with these conditions should be counseled carefully, noting that pregnancy carries significant risk, including mortality, and should perhaps be avoided or deferred until corrective surgery, if possible, can be performed.

8.3.2 Fetal/Neonatal Risk

In addition to maternal cardiac risk, obstetrical and perinatal outcome risks should be considered when discussing pregnancy with a patient with cardiovascular disease. Suboptimal fetal-neonatal outcomes may be driven, at least in part, by insufficient uteroplacental perfusion. Patients with cyanotic heart disease, for example, are at increased risk of miscarriage, with live birth rates of 43% overall, and 12% in women with oxygen saturations ≤85% [18]. Adverse obstetrical outcomes, including preterm delivery and its associated neonatal complications, intrauterine fetal growth restriction, postpartum hemorrhage, and fetal and neonatal death have all been shown to be increased in women with underlying CHD [17, 19–21].

Mothers with a genetic condition with autosomal dominant inheritance (such as Marfan syndrome, 22q11 deletion or Holt–Oram syndrome) have a 50% risk of recurrence in the offspring. In the absence of an identifiable anomaly with Mendelian inheritance, the fetal recurrence risk is generally in the range of 3–5%, compared with the background population risk of about 0.8% [22, 23]. Reported recurrence risks of individual lesions are quite variable, ranging from as low as 0.6% for mothers with transposition of the great arteries [8] to as high as 18% in the presence of maternal left ventricular outflow tract obstruction [24]. The type of CHD seen in offspring may differ from the lesion seen in the mother [25].

Screening fetal echocardiography is recommended for women with structural CHD and is best performed between 18 and 22 weeks gestation [26, 27], though recent advances in ultrasound technology mean that large anomalies can now be identified sooner than this [28]. Fetal echocardiography allows for early counseling and decision-making for parents and for advance preparation for delivery and appropriate care during the early neonatal period in the event that a fetal cardiac abnormality is detected.

8.4 Advanced Cardiac Imaging During Pregnancy

On occasion, more sophisticated cardiac imaging than that afforded by transthoracic echocardiography is required during pregnancy. Trans-esophageal echocardiography is considered to be safe during pregnancy, although the operator should be aware of the increased risk of vomiting and aspiration, such that airway protection is indicated in later pregnancy.

Coronary angiography should be performed if indicated in cases of suspected acute coronary syndrome to clarify the diagnosis and so that percutaneous angioplasty and stenting, if indicated, can proceed without delay. Estimated exposure to the unshielded maternal abdomen after conventional coronary angiography is ~1.5 mSv (equivalent to 75 chest X-rays) and after percutaneous coronary intervention is ~3 mSV (equivalent to 150 chest X-rays); however, with tissue attenuation, <20% of this radiation exposure reaches the fetus. Further minimization of fetal exposure to radiation in the catheterization laboratory can be achieved by using a radial artery approach, adequate shielding of the maternal abdomen, and minimizing fluoroscopic time.

Cardiac computed tomography can offer an alternative imaging modality for assessment of the coronary arteries; however, it is not recommended in pregnancy as radiation doses generally exceed those of conventional angiography [29]. Cardiovascular magnetic resonance (CMR) may provide useful information during pregnancy, particularly regarding arterial and/or venous structures which are suboptimally seen on echocardiography. Current recommendation is not to use gadolinium with CMR in pregnancy due to concerns regarding gadolinium effect on the developing fetus [30, 31]; however, MRI without gadolinium is considered quite safe from a fetal perspective [32].

8.5 General Principles for the Management of Patients with Cardiac Disease in Pregnancy

8.5.1 Antepartum Management

Women with cardiac disease at intermediate or high risk for complications should be managed in a high-risk pregnancy unit by a multidisciplinary team from maternal–fetal medicine, cardiology, anesthesia, and pediatrics. Initial consultation and risk stratification should be done early in pregnancy – preferably by the end of the first trimester. Initial investigations, including baseline echocardiography and other tests as appropriate should be arranged at that time. The cardio-obstetrics team should meet early in the pregnancy to develop and distribute a written management plan for the complex patient. For women in a "low risk" group, consultation can be arranged at a regional referral center whereas subsequent management can often be carried out at a community hospital.

Patients who are at high risk of developing cardiac complications in pregnancy should be seen by both maternal-fetal medicine and an obstetrical cardiologist at regular intervals, with ongoing monitoring for new cardiac symptoms, echocardiographic changes, or deterioration in functional status. In women with structural cardiac lesions and NYHA III or IV symptoms, activity limitation is advisable. Hospital admission by mid-second or third trimester is only rarely necessary. Gestational hypertension, hyperthyroidism, infection and anemia should be identified early and treated vigorously, as these conditions can escalate cardiac decompensation.

8.5.2 Management During Labor and Delivery

Vaginal delivery is generally recommended for most patients with cardiac disease [33] as it is associated with decreased risks of infectious morbidity, blood loss, and thrombotic complications compared to caesarean delivery [34]. Elective caesarean delivery for cardiac indications should be reserved for patients with severe PH, intractable heart failure, aortic dissection, Marfan syndrome with dilated aortic root, and failure to switch from warfarin to heparin prior to labor [14], though there is debate about whether caesarean delivery is protective in all of these cases. Preterm induction is rarely indicated, but once fetal lung maturity is assured, a planned induction is preferred in high-risk situations so that appropriate support will be readily available. For cardiac patients who do not experience spontaneous labor beforehand, a scheduled induction of labor between 39 and 40 weeks gestation has been suggested by recent guidelines [35].

The use of invasive hemodynamic peripartum monitoring, particularly central venous pressure catheters and pulmonary arterial lines, has decreased over time [19]. Intra-arterial monitoring can be used for patients in whom the interpretation of external monitoring is difficult, or in whom a sudden drop in systemic blood pressure would require an immediate response.

For patients requiring antepartum anticoagulation, UH is discontinued 12–24 h prior to induction, or reversed with protamine if spontaneous labor develops, and can usually be resumed 6–12 h postpartum. For patients on low-molecular-weight heparin (LMWH), a 24 h interval prior to delivery is recommended (see section 8.6.1 for more details). According to current guidelines [14], routine prophylactic antibiotic therapy is not indicated due to the rarity of infective endocarditis following vaginal birth or caesarean section [36, 37].

Epidural anesthesia with adequate volume preloading is the technique of choice to prevent abrupt pressure or volume changes in cardiac patients. In the presence of an intracardiac shunt, air and particulate filters should be placed in all intravenous lines to prevent embolism. Early placement of an epidural catheter for analgesia is advantageous in decreasing maternal pain and anxiety which has the effect of blunting the release of maternal circulating catecholamines, thereby attenuating the increases in CO during labor [38, 39].

For patients with active cardiac disease, assessment should be made prior to labor by the cardio-obstetric team regarding recommendations for a "cardiac vaginal delivery." For these patients, early epidural placement is recommended for the reasons outlined above. Labor is conducted in the left lateral decubitus position to minimize hemodynamic fluctuations associated with contractions in the supine position. Once full dilatation is reached, careful management of the two phases of the second stage of labor allows for a minimum of maternal effort to be expended during delivery. The first (or latent) phase of the second stage should be lengthened. During this period, passive descent of the fetal presenting part is allowed to occur by uterine activity alone without the need for active maternal expulsive effort. The second phase of the second stage of labor can then be shortened with an assisted vaginal delivery using either vacuum or forceps to minimize the need for maternal expulsive effort and the associated increase in CO and blood pressure. Assisted vaginal delivery is indicated in patients with significant risk of CHF or arrhythmia, as these patients are most likely to be affected by the hemodynamic stressors of prolonged active pushing. A significant proportion of patients can undergo spontaneous vaginal delivery without the need for instrumental assistance [19].

Patients with cardiac disease should be monitored postpartum as hemodynamics do not immediately return to baseline following delivery. Mortality risk for PH and Eisenmenger syndrome persists for several weeks following delivery [40, 41], and these patients should have close cardiac follow-up during the postpartum period. Adverse cardiac events in pregnancy predict poorer long-term outcomes for patients with heart disease; therefore, these patients warrant ongoing cardiac care after pregnancy [42].

8.6 Management of Artificial Heart Valves in Pregnancy

Bioprosthetic valves are associated with elevated risk of structural valve deterioration and dysfunction and increased need for replacement over time compared to mechanical valves. Most women with a bioprosthetic valve will tolerate pregnancy well if the valve is functioning well and they have normal systolic ventricular function. Patients with a previous Ross operation (pulmonary autograft aortic valve replacement), for example, are at low risk for cardiac complications during pregnancy [43, 44]. Pregnancy has not been clearly shown to accelerate degeneration of bioprosthetic valves [45, 46].

Although mechanical heart valves are more durable than bioprosthetic heart valves, they are associated with increased frequency of complications during pregnancy, primarily related to valve thrombosis and bleeding secondary to anticoagulation. Because of such complications, women with mechanical heart valves carry an elevated mortality risk during pregnancy compared to patients with bioprosthetic valves [47].

8.6.1 Anticoagulation for Mechanical Heart Valves

All women with mechanical valves are at increased risk of valve thrombosis in pregnancy; thus, maintaining therapeutic anticoagulation throughout pregnancy is crucial. Current recommendations from the European Society of Cardiology and the American College of Cardiology suggest vitamin K antagonists (VKA), such as warfarin, be used throughout pregnancy, under strict INR control, for optimal prevention of valve thrombosis [14, 48, 49]. Use of VKAs in the first trimester has been associated with "warfarin embryopathy" (limb defects, nasal hypoplasia, stippled epiphyses), while "warfarin fetopathy" (central nervous system and ocular anomalies, lowered IQ, fetal loss and stillbirth) has been associated with use of these medications later in pregnancy [50]. Since unfractionated heparin (UH) and low molecular weight heparin (LMWH) do not cross the placenta, substitution of one of these agents up to week 12 can be considered in order to decrease the risks of embryopathy, hemorrhage, and pregnancy loss, though patients should be counseled that this switch does increase their valve thrombosis risk in comparison to continued VKA therapy [51]. A further option is to maintain patients on UH or LMWH for the duration of pregnancy, which minimizes embryopathy and fetopathy risk and maximizes the likelihood of a livebirth at the expense of increased maternal risk of thromboembolic complications [52, 53]. As a result of the complicated balance of risks necessary to guide decision-making around choice of anticoagulant, we advocate that informed patient preference guide the decision after detailed counseling by the cardio-obstetrics team.

Recent anesthesia guidelines recommend that patients on LMWH in pregnancy should receive their last dose of anticoagulation on the morning prior to a planned induction of labor or caesarean section, to allow at least 24 hours between LMWH administration and placement of regional anesthesia [54, 55]. Patients who are on VKAs during pregnancy should be transitioned to either UH or LMWH 2 weeks prior to expected delivery, to minimize bleeding risk for both mother and neonate at the time of delivery, and to allow for safe placement of neuraxial anesthesia. For these patients, as well as those on daily therapeutic dose LMWH, the last dose of LMWH should be given 36 h prior to the planned delivery, when they can be transitioned to an IV infusion of UH. This should be stopped when the patient is in active labor or 4–6 h prior to the placement of an epidural catheter and then recommenced 4–6 h after delivery [54, 55]. Patients can then be transitioned back to VKA with bridging during the postpartum period [50]. For patients delivering by caesarean section at our center, this is done 2 weeks postpartum to decrease the risk of wound hematoma following caesarean delivery. Patients requiring emergency delivery while on a VKA can be given prothrombin complex and vitamin K to quickly reverse maternal VKA effect. Caesarean section is recommended in this circumstance since fetal VKA effect cannot quickly be reversed and risk of fetal intracranial hemorrhage in the event of vaginal delivery is not eliminated.

8.7 Evaluation and Management of Specific Structural Cardiac Lesions

8.7.1 Volume Overload Lesions: Left-to-Right Shunts

Patients with left-to-right shunts experience increased CO on the volume-loaded right ventricle (RV) in the presence of an atrial septal defect (ASD), or left ventricle (LV) in the context of a ventricular septal defect (VSD) or patent ductus arteriosus. This is mitigated by the physiologic decrease in peripheral vascular resistance during pregnancy and as a result, in the absence of PH, pregnancy and delivery are generally well tolerated [1, 50–56]. Paradoxical embolization is a rare complication in a patient with an open shunt, particularly when increase in pulmonary vascular resistance promotes transient right-to-left shunting at the atrial level.

Due to their complexity, atrioventricular septal defects may be less well tolerated in pregnancy than simpler shunts. These patients are at increased risk of postpartum persistence of NYHA class deterioration, arrhythmias, and worsening of preexisting atrioventricular valve regurgitation [57].

8.7.2 Volume Overload Lesions: Regurgitant Valves

Severe pulmonary regurgitation (PR) is common in patients who have had a previous tetralogy of Fallot (TOF) repair, particularly in those repaired with a transannular patch. Sequelae of severe PR include RV dilation and dysfunction. In one study of women with repaired and unrepaired TOF, cardiovascular events occurred in 14% of pregnancies and included supraventricular arrhythmia, CHF, PH, and pulmonary embolus. Cardiovascular complications were more likely in patients with severe PR with RV dilation, RV hypertension, and peripartum LV dysfunction [58]. Another study of pregnancies in women with corrected TOF found cardiac complications in 12% of pregnancies, consisting of CHF, arrhythmia, or both [59].

Aortic and mitral regurgitation can result from rheumatic, congenital, or degenerative causes in women of childbearing age. These lesions can be tolerated during pregnancy if mild; however, women with severe regurgitation, those who are symptomatic, and those with compromised LV function are at risk of heart failure [60, 61].

Tricuspid regurgitation may be functional, secondary to a dilated RV annulus, or due to congenital malformation of the tricuspid valve itself. Ebstein anomaly is one cause, in which apical displacement of the tricuspid valve leads to atrialization of the RV, tricuspid regurgitation, and a dilated RA. The result of this is a functionally small RV, probably also myopathic, which may not be able to accommodate the increased stroke volume of pregnancy, resulting in worsening tricuspid insufficiency, raised right atrial pressure, and right-to-left shunting across the atrial septum if there is an ASD or a PFO. Assessment of a woman with Ebstein anomaly requires careful consideration of the specific manifestations in the individual because the condition is so varied, from trivial to very severe with right-to-left shunt and cyanosis, and pregnancy risk varies accordingly [62].

8.7.3 Pressure Overload Lesions (Left Heart): Aortic Stenosis

AS is often due to a bicuspid aortic valve (BAV), which may also be associated with aortic coarctation and/or ascending aortopathy. Women with moderate or severe AS are at risk for pulmonary edema or arrhythmia during pregnancy, even if they are asymptomatic prior to conception [1, 56, 63, 64]. Those with symptomatic severe AS should delay pregnancy until after surgical correction [29, 65]. In asymptomatic women with severe AS, prepregnancy evaluation should establish that LV systolic function is normal. Exercise testing can be used to determine functional capacity, blood pressure response to exertion, and to rule out arrhythmia [14]. Patients with severe AS can destabilize secondary to postpartum hemorrhage, uncontrolled epidural anesthesia, or during Valsalva maneuvers associated with maternal expulsive efforts during the second stage of labor. As a result of their fixed outflow tract obstruction, these patients may not be able to meet the increased demand in situations where systemic blood pressure is decreased leading to coronary hypoperfusion and ischemic coronary events. Despite these risks, there are several studies reporting either no or low maternal mortality in appropriately selected patients with AS in pregnancy [63, 64, 66, 67].

For patients requiring surgical intervention for symptomatic AS during pregnancy, percutaneous balloon valvuloplasty is preferable to open cardiac surgery because the latter carries substantial fetal mortality risk [63, 68–71].

8.7.4 Pressure Overload Lesions (Left Heart): Mitral Stenosis

Congenital mitral stenosis (MS) is rare. Most cases of MS affecting pregnancy result from complications of rheumatic fever. The hypervolemia and tachycardia associated with pregnancy exacerbate the impact of mitral valve obstruction. Elevated left atrial pressure as a result of MS increases the likelihood of both pulmonary edema and atrial fibrillation (AF) [72]. Even patients with mild to moderate MS who are asymptomatic prior to pregnancy may develop AF and heart failure during the antepartum and peripartum periods, contributing to substantial maternal morbidity, fetal complications related to preterm birth and growth restriction [61, 73, 74].

For patients with MS in pregnancy, beta-blockade with β1-selective beta blockers β-blockers, and activity restriction, if needed, are the mainstays of medical treatment [9] because bradycardia allows increased time for LV filling and lower LA pressure. Percutaneous mitral valvuloplasty should be considered during pregnancy in suitable symptomatic patients who are refractory to medical therapy [75–77].

8.7.5 Pressure Overload Lesions (Left Heart): Coarctation of the Aorta

Individuals with surgically corrected coarctation generally tolerate pregnancy well, though there is elevated risk of hypertensive disorders and miscarriage [1, 56, 78, 79]. In uncorrected coarctation, satisfactory control of upper body hypertension may lead to hypotension below the coarctation site, compromising fetal growth. For patients with unrepaired coarctation there is an increased risk of serious complications including dissection. Following coarctation repair, the risk of dissection and rupture is reduced but not eliminated, particularly in the setting of systemic hypertension [78, 80]. Pregnant women with repaired coarctation are at increased risk for pregnancy-induced hypertension, likely as a result of abnormal aortic compliance [1, 56, 78].

8.7.6 Pressure Overload Lesions (Left Heart): Aortopathy

Marfan syndrome, BAV, vascular-type Ehlers–Danlos syndrome (EDS), Turner syndrome, Loeys–Dietz syndrome, and other inherited aortopathies are associated with increased risks in pregnancy. In addition to a heritable condition, risk factors for aortic dilatation include hypertension and advanced maternal age. Maternal morbidity and mortality are primarily related to the risk of dissection. The majority of deaths occur in women not previously known to have an aortopathy [14]. For patients with known aortic root or ascending aortic dilatation in pregnancy, current guidelines recommend strict blood pressure control as well as monthly or bimonthly echocardiographic measurement of the ascending aorta during pregnancy to detect expansion early. As well, serial follow-up with MRI (without gadolinium) is recommended for monitoring of known aortic arch, descending aorta, or abdominal aortic dilatation [81].

In Marfan syndrome, maternal morbidity and mortality are primarily due to aortic dissection resulting from medial aortopathy. Risk is elevated in pregnancy due to both hemodynamic stress and hormonal effects on the aorta. The overall risk of aortic dissection in pregnancy for women with Marfan syndrome is around 3% [82]. Risk of dissection is increased in pregnant patients with aortic root size greater than 45 mm compared to those with normal aortic root size and no history of prior dissection [73, 83]. The overall dissection rate in Marfan syndrome has been reported to be 3%, although this risk is still 1% in the population of patients with a root <40 mm [82, 84].

Surgical correction of a dilated aortic root is offered to Marfan patients when the root diameter is greater than 50 mm [85]. Surgical correction can be offered at 45 mm to patients embarking on pregnancy though this may not fully normalize the risk of dissection thereafter [86, 87].

Less is known about risk factors for dissection in pregnant women with a dilated aorta in the context of a BAV. BAV is common, occurring in 1–2% of the general population. Half of the patients with BAV have an associated aortopathy [85]. Although aortic dissection in the context of BAV is reported, it is less common than in the setting of other aortopathies [87, 88] and is uncommon in the pregnant population [89]. Recent guidelines suggest that pregnancy be avoided in patients with BAV and ascending aorta ≥50 mm, though the risk of dissection for BAV patients is substantially lower at a given root diameter than it is for patients with Marfan disease [87].

Women with vascular EDS (formerly called type IV EDS) carry elevated maternal mortality related to the risk of uterine rupture, bowel rupture, and dissection of major arteries and veins including the aorta [90]. The risk of arterial dissection was shown to be 9.2% in one reported cohort [91], while another study found the maternal mortality rate to be 6.6% [90]. For these reasons, many experts strongly caution women with vascular EDS wishing to undergo pregnancy about the risk of mortality [14, 87, 92].

In Turner syndrome, elevated dissection risk has been identified when the indexed aortic size exceeds 2.5 cm/m^2 outside of pregnancy [93]. For this reason, experts would strongly counsel these patients against pregnancy when the aortic size exceeds 2.5 cm/m^2, or 2.0 cm/m^2 if there is evidence of BAV, elongated transverse aorta, coarctation of the aorta, or hypertension [94], due to substantial risk of cardiovascular mortality.

8.7.7 Pressure Overload Lesions (Right Heart): Pulmonary Stenosis

Unlike AS, pulmonary stenosis (PS) is not often associated with significant cardiovascular complications during pregnancy [1, 56, 67, 95, 96], though one study did report rates of hypertension, thromboembolism, and premature delivery in 15%, 4%, and 17% of pregnancies, respectively [95]. Balloon valvuloplasty during pregnancy is often feasible if women with severe PS decompensate.

8.7.8 Pressure Overload Lesions (Right Heart): Pulmonary Hypertension

Pulmonary hypertension (PH) can occur secondary to several different causes resulting in an elevation in mean pulmonary arterial pressure. Maternal outcome differs based on the underlying etiology of PH; however, mortality can reach 16–30% for some, particularly those with pulmonary arterial hypertension (PAH) [97]. For patients with PH, cardiovascular complications are most likely to occur at term and during the first month postpartum [4, 40, 98].

Eisenmenger syndrome occurs when a patient with congenital systemic-to-pulmonary communication with left-to-right shunt develops increased pulmonary vascular resistance causing bidirectional or reversed (right-to-left) shunt. It is often associated with cyanosis. Patients with Eisenmenger syndrome have a maternal mortality risk as high as 30% with deaths secondary to factors including right heart failure, pulmonary hypertensive crisis, and pulmonary thrombosis.

Survival for patients with pulmonary arterial hypertension during pregnancy has improved somewhat over the last few decades [40]. This may be attributed, at least in part, to an increase in the use of selective pulmonary vasodilator therapy in the more recent era. Mortality rates for patients with PH vary considerably based on underlying etiology, with an overall maternal death rate of 3.3% reported in one recent cohort, but a rate of 43% among those with idiopathic pulmonary arterial hypertension [97]. Other significant morbidities associated with PH include heart failure, premature delivery, low birth weight, and fetal–neonatal mortality [40].

Patients with severe PH considering a pregnancy should be made aware of the significant maternal mortality risk and fetal risk involved [99]. For patients with shunts, pregnancy-related systemic vasodilatation may increase the magnitude of right-to-left shunting, leading to further hypoxemia and downstream effects on both maternal and fetal health. Decreased pulmonary blood flow due to right-to-left shunting can also increase the risk of pulmonary tree hypoperfusion and increased thrombosis in the pulmonary vasculature. Patients with severe PH are particularly sensitive to volume depletion and hypotension; pulmonary perfusion and CO will fall to a greater extent than in absence of PH, and, in patients with a shunt, augmentation of right-to-left shunting will result in worsening cyanosis.

Fetal complications with PH include spontaneous abortion, intrauterine growth restriction, and preterm labor. The high perinatal mortality rate of 28% in patients with severe PH is largely related to prematurity [4]. For additional information on pulmonary hypertension in pregnancy, please refer to Chapter 13.

8.8 Arrhythmia

The risk of arrhythmia is elevated in pregnancy in general due to a number of factors, including an altered hormonal milieu, enhanced sympathetic tone and cardiac chamber dilation [100]. Premature atrial or ventricular beats are common and generally benign in normal pregnancy.

8.8.1 Atrial Arrhythmias

Atrial tachyarrhythmias such as paroxysmal supraventricular tachycardia (SVT) or AF may present for the first time or become more frequent in pregnancy. AF in particular has been associated with increased mortality risk [101], although mortality is still quite uncommon. For some women with recurrent arrhythmia, catheter ablation prior to pregnancy may decrease the risk of serious adverse events. Adverse fetal and neonatal sequelae have been reported due to recurrent arrhythmia during pregnancy [102].

For women who present with acute SVT, vagal maneuvers and adenosine can be used. In the hemodynamically unstable patient, electrical cardioversion is safe in pregnancy [103].

In women with recurrent symptomatic SVT, beta-blockers or verapamil are often used as first-line prophylactic therapy. Patients with Wolff–Parkinson–White syndrome may be treated with prophylactic flecainide or propafenone.

Tachyarrhythmias such as atrial flutter or AF are more common in patients with structural heart disease. Sustained atrial flutter or fibrillation can be associated with hemodynamic instability and should therefore be treated promptly. If adenosine does not successfully convert, then ibutilide or flecainide may be used for the hemodynamically stable patient, and cardioversion if the patient is unstable [14].

8.8.2 Ventricular Arrhythmias

Ventricular tachycardia is less common than atrial tachycardia. New-onset ventricular tachycardia in the last 6 weeks of pregnancy or early in the postpartum period should prompt consideration of underlying structural heart disease, as well as PPCM or long QT syndrome as a potential underlying diagnosis [104]. Idiopathic RV outflow tract tachycardia is the most common type of VT and may be treated with prophylactic beta-blockade, verapamil, or other antiarrhythmics including sotalol or flecainide if necessary. Catheter ablation or the insertion of an implantable cardioverter defibrillator (ICD) can be done in pregnancy if medical treatment fails [14].

8.9 Cardiomyopathy and Heart Failure

Pregnancy-associated cardiomyopathy comprises both acquired and inherited disease, including PPCM, hypertrophic cardiomyopathy (HCM), dilated cardiomyopathy (DCM), Takotsubo cardiomyopathy, and storage diseases. Any of these can cause maternal complications in pregnancy, particularly when the left ventricular systolic function is severely impaired.

PPCM presents toward the end of pregnancy or in the weeks to months following delivery with symptoms of heart failure secondary to LV systolic dysfunction. Other causes of heart failure must be excluded. In addition to heart failure, patients may present with ventricular arrhythmia or cardiac arrest. The EF is typically <45%. Poor prognostic signs on echocardiography include initial LVEF <30%, marked LV dilatation, and RV involvement [105]. For patients whose EF has not recovered to >50–55%, subsequent pregnancy should be cautioned against. Patients who do recover their heart function have gone on to have successful subsequent pregnancies, though they should be counseled regarding risk of recurrence of PPCM and monitored carefully [106].

HCM is a genetically determined disease of the heart muscle which manifests with left ventricular hypertrophy leading to any of LV outflow obstruction, diastolic dysfunction, myocardial ischemia, or mitral regurgitation. These patients generally tolerate pregnancy well, though they may experience worsening symptoms of heart failure due to increasing cardiac demand in pregnancy and are at elevated risk of preterm birth [107, 108]. A small subset of patients with HCM are at risk of sudden cardiac death, progressive heart failure, and both supraventricular and ventricular arrhythmias. Patients with a history of arrhythmia or heart failure should be maintained on beta-blocker therapy. Cardioversion is safe in pregnancy for poorly tolerated AF [109], and an ICD may be considered for patients considered to be at high risk of lethal arrhythmia [14].

DCM may be caused by prior viral infection, drugs, and cardiac ischemia leading to LV dilatation and dysfunction. Half of the cases are idiopathic and may be hereditary [110]. Pregnancy is tolerated poorly by women with DCM who have moderate or severe LV systolic dysfunction (EF < 40%), evidence of mitral regurgitation, and those with compromised functional status manifested as NYHA class III/IV [111]. As a result of the potential for irreversible deterioration in ventricular function, maternal mortality, and fetal loss in patients with known DCM, pregnancy should be carefully considered and planned. Many of these patients are on medications including angiotensin-converting enzyme (ACE) inhibitors, angiotensin receptor blockers, and mineralocorticoid receptor antagonists, which should be stopped prior to pregnancy due to their teratogenic potential, and the maternal risks of their withdrawal need to be taken into account. These patients should be optimized on beta-blockers if possible [14].

Patients presenting with heart failure in pregnancy, or the puerperium, should be managed by an interdisciplinary team including cardiology. Typical therapy for acute heart failure during pregnancy includes ensuring adequate oxygenation, diuretics for pulmonary edema, and afterload reduction with hydralazine and isosorbide dinitrates. For the unstable patient, inotropic support and/or vasopressors may be necessary. If not available locally, patients may need to be transferred to a center with the availability of mechanical support and transplant services for patients with severe left ventricular systolic dysfunction.

Postpartum, ACE inhibitors can be used for afterload reduction. For patients with PPCM, some centers advocate bromocriptine use postpartum to improve LV recovery and clinical outcome, though this remains controversial [112].

8.10 Conclusion

The majority of women with cardiac disease can be expected to do well during pregnancy with appropriate risk stratification and medical optimization. A preconception cardiac evaluation is highly recommended so that medications can be reviewed and revised if need be, pregnancy-related risk stratification can be established and necessary interventions can be planned prior to pregnancy. Pregnancies deemed to be at intermediate or high risk should be managed and delivered in a tertiary care Cardio-Obstetric center by an experienced team including cardiologists, maternal–fetal medicine specialists, and anesthetists with expertise in pregnancy and heart disease. Antepartum multidisciplinary conferences are very helpful for complex cases to coordinate management, and care plans should be distributed. Postpartum monitoring and follow-up are an important aspect of care.

References

[1]   Siu SC, Sermer M, Colman JM, et al. Prospective multicenter study of pregnancy outcomes in women with heart disease. Circulation 2001;104(5):515–521.
[2]   Chan WS, Anand S, Ginsberg JS. Anticoagulation of pregnant women with mechanical heart valves: A systematic review of the literature. Arch Intern Med 2000;160(2):191–196.
[3]   Elkayam U, Tummala PP, Rao K, et al. Maternal and fetal outcomes of subsequent pregnancies in women with peripartum cardiomyopathy. N Engl J Med 2001;344(21): 1567–1571.
[4]   Weiss BM, Zemp L, Seifert B, Hess OM. Outcome of pulmonary vascular disease in pregnancy: A systematic overview from 1978 through 1996. J Am Coll Cardiol 1998;31(7): 1650–1657.
[5]   Pyeritz R. Maternal and fetal complications of pregnancy in the Marfan syndrome. Am J Med 1981;71:784–790.

[6]   Avila WS, Rossi EG, Ramires JA, et al. Pregnancy in patients with heart disease: Experience with 1,000 cases. Clin Cardiol 2003;26(3):135–142.

[7]   Khairy P, Ouyang DW, Fernandes SM, Lee-Parritz A, Economy KE, Landzberg MJ. Pregnancy outcomes in women with congenital heart disease. Circulation 2006;113(4):517–524.

[8]   Drenthen W, Pieper PG, Roos-Hesselink JW, et al. Outcome of pregnancy in women with congenital heart disease: A literature review. J Am Coll Cardiol 2007;49(24):2303–2311.

[9]   Mehta LSWC, Bradley E, Burton T, et al on behalf of the American Heart Association Council on Clinical Cardiology. Cardiovascular considerations in caring for pregnant patients A scientific statement from the American Heart Association. Circulation 2020;141:e1–e20.

[10] Tanous D, Siu SC, Mason J, et al B-type natriuretic peptide in pregnant women with heart disease. J Am Coll Cardiol 2010;56(15):1247–1253.

[11] Lui GK, Silversides CK, Khairy P, et al. Heart rate response during exercise and pregnancy outcome in women with congenital heart disease. Circulation 2011;123(3):242–248.

[12] Siu SCSM, Colman JM, Alvarez AN, et al. Prospective multicenter study of pregnancy outcomes in women with heart disease. Circulation 2001;104(5):515–521.

[13] Thorne SMA, Nelson-Piercy C. Risks of contraception and pregnancy in heart disease. Heart 2006;92:1520–1525.

[14] Regitz-Zagrosek VR-HJ, Bauersachs J, Blomstrom-Lundqvist C, et al. ESC Guidelines for the management of cardiovascular diseases during pregancy. Eur Heart J 2018;2018(39):3165–3241.

[15] Drenthen WBE, Balci A, Moons P, et al for the ZAHARA Investigators. Predictors of pregnancy complications in women with congenital heart disease. Eur Heart J 2010;31(17):2124–2132.

[16] Silversides CGJ, Mason J, Sermer M, et al. Pregnancy outcomes in women with heart disease The CARPREG II study. J Am College Cardiol 2018;71(21):2419–2430.

[17] Khairy POD, Fernandes SM, Lee-Parritz A, Economy KE, Landzberg MJ. Pregnancy outcomes in women with congenital heart disease. Circulation 2006;113(4):517–524.

[18] Presbitero PSJ, Stone S, Aruta E, Spiegelhalter D, Rabajoli F. Pregnancy in cyanotic congenital heart disease. Outcome of mother and fetus. Circulation 1994;89(6):2673–2676.

[19] Robertson JESC, Mah ML, Kulikowski J, et al. A contemporary approach to the obstetric management of women with heart disease. J Obstet Gynaecol Can 2012;34(9):812–819.

[20] Balci A-S-SK, Van Der Bijl AG, et al. for the ZAHARA-II Investigators. Prospective validation and assesment of cardiovascular and offspring risk models for pregnant women with congenital heart disease. Heart 2014;100:1373–1381.

[21] Siu SC, Colman JM, Sorensen S, et al. Adverse neonatal and cardiac outcomes are more common in pregnant women with cardiac disease. Circulation 2002;105(18):2179–2184.

[22] Nora JJ. From generational studies to a multilevel genetic-environmental interaction. J Am Coll Cardiol 1994;23(6):1468–1471.

[23] Uebing A, Steer PJ, Yentis SM, Gatzoulis MA. Pregnancy and congenital heart disease. Bmj 2006.

[24] Nora JJ, Nora AH. Maternal transmission of congenital heart diseases: New recurrence risk figures and the questions of cytoplasmic inheritance and vulnerability to teratogens. Am J Cardiol 1987;59(5):459–463.

[25] Whittemore R, Wells JA, Castellsague X. A second-generation study of 427 probands with congenital heart defects and their 837 children. J Am Coll Cardiol 1994;23(6):1459–1467.

[26] Rychik J, Ayres N, Cuneo B, et al. American Society of Echocardiography guidelines and standards for performance of the fetal echocardiogram. J Am Soc Echocardiogr 2004;17(7): 803–810.

[27] Thangaroopan MWR, Silversides C, Mason J, et al. Incremental diagnostic yield of pediatric cardiac assessment after fetal echocardiography in the offspring of women with congenital heart disease: Prospective study. Pediatrics 2008;121(3):e660–e5.

[28] Yu DSL, Zhang N. Performance of first-trimester fetal echocardiography in diagnosing fetal heart defects: Meta-analysis and systematic review. J Ultrasound Med 2020;39(3):471–480.

[29] Regitz-Zagrosek V, Blomstrom Lundqvist C, Borghi C, et al. ESC Guidelines on the management of cardiovascular diseases during pregnancy: The task force on the management of cardiovascular diseases during pregnancy of the european society of cardiology (ESC). Eur Heart J 2011;32(24):3147–3197.

[30] De Wilde JP, Rivers AW, Price DL. A review of the current use of magnetic resonance imaging in pregnancy and safety implications for the fetus. Prog Biophys Mol Biol 2005;87 (2–3):335–353.

[31] Kanal E, Barkovich AJ, Bell C, et al. ACR guidance document for safe MR practices: 2007. AJR Am J Roentgenol 2007;188(6):1447–1474.

[32] Ray JGVM, Bharatha A, Montanera WJ, Park AL. Association between MRI exposure during pregnancy and fetal and childhood outcomes. JAMA 2016;316(9):952–961.

[33] Ruys TPER-HJ, Pijuan-Domenech A, Vasario E, et al. Is a planned caesarean section in women with cardiac disease beneficial?. Heart 2015;101:530–536.

[34] Liu SLR, Joseph KS, Heaman M, Sauve R, Kramer MS. Maternal health study group of the Canadian perinatal surveillance system. Maternal mortality and severe morbidity associated with low-risk planned cesarean delivery versus planned vaginal delivery at term. Can Med Assoc J 2007;176:455–460.

[35] ACOG Practice Bulletin No. 212. Pregnancy and heart disease. Obstet Gynecol 2019;133(5): e320–e56.

[36] Kuijpers JMKD, Groenink M, Peels KCH, et al. Incidence, risk factors, and predictors of infective endocarditis in adult congenital heart disease: Focus on the use of prosthetic material. Eur Heart J 2017;38:2048–2056.

[37] Kebed KYBK, Al Adham RI, Baddour LM, et al. Pregnancy and postpartum infective endocarditis: A systematic review. Mayo Clin Proc 2014;89:1143–1152.

[38] Robson SHS, Boys R, Dunlop W, Bryson M. Changes in cardiac output during epidural anaesthesia for caesarean section. Anaesthesia 1989;44:475–479.

[39] Arendt KWLK. Obstetric anesthesia management of the patient with cardiac disease. Int J Obstet Anest 2019;37:73–85.

[40] Bedard EDK, Gatzoulis MA. Has there been any progress made on pregnancy outcomes among women with pulmonary arterial hypertension?. Eur Heart J 2009;30(3):256–265.

[41] Weiss BMZL, Seifert B, Hess OM. Outcome of pulmonary vascular disease in pregnancy: A systematic overview from 1978 through 1996. J Am Coll Cardiol 1998;31(7):1650–1657.

[42] Balint OHSS, Mason J, Grewal J, et al. Cardiac outcomes after pregnancy in women with congenital heart disease. Heart 2010;96:1656–1661.

[43] Yap SC, Drenthen W, Pieper PG, et al. Outcome of pregnancy in women after pulmonary autograft valve replacement for congenital aortic valve disease. J Heart Valve Dis 2007;16(4): 398–403.

[44] Dore A, Somerville J. Pregnancy in patients with pulmonary autograft valve replacement. Eur Heart J 1997;18(10):1659–1662.

[45] North RA, Sadler L, Stewart AW, McCowan LM, Kerr AR, White HD. Long-term survival and valve-related complications in young women with cardiac valve replacements. Circulation 1999;99(20):2669–2676.

[46] Salazar E, Espinola N, Roman L, Casanova JM. Effect of pregnancy on the duration of bovine pericardial bioprostheses. Am Heart J 1999;137(4 Pt 1):714–720.

[47] Van Hagen IMR-HJ, Ruys TP, Merz WM, et al. Pregnancy in women with a mechanical heart valve: Data of the European Society of Cardiology Registry of Pregnancy and Cardiac Disease (ROPAC). Circulation 2015;132:132–142.

[48] Nishimura RAOC, Bonow RO, Carabello BA, et al. AHA/ACC guideline for the management of patients with valvular heart disease: A report of the American College of Cardiology/ American Heart Association Task Force on Practice Guidlines. J Am Coll Cardiol 2014;63(22): e57–185.

[49] Nishimura RAOC, Bonow RO, Carabello BA, et al. AHA/ACC focused update of the 2014 AHA/ ACC guideline for the management of patients with valvular heart disease. J Am Coll Cardiol 2017;70(2):252–289.

[50] D'Souza RSC, McLintock C. Optimal anticoagulation for pregnant women with mechanical heart valves. Semin Thromb Hemost 2016;42(7):798–804.

[51] Xu ZFJ, Luo X, Zhang WB, et al. Anticoagulation regimens during pregnancy in patients with mechanical heart valves: A systematic review and meta-analysis. Can J Cardiol 2016;32: 1248e1–e9.

[52] D'Souza ROJ, Shah PS, Silversides CK, et al. Anticoagulation for pregnant women with mechanical heart valves: A systematic review and meta-analysis. Eur Heart J 2017;38: 1509–1516.

[53] Yinon YSS, Warshafsky C, Maxwell C, et al Use of low molecular weight heparin in pregnant women with mechanical heart valves. Am J Cardiol 2009;104:1259–1263.

[54] Horlocker TTVE, Kopp SL, Gogarten W, Leffert LR, Benzon HT. Regional anesthesia in the patient receiving antithrombotic or thrombolytic therapy: American Society of Regional Anesthesia and Pain Medicine evidence-based guidelines (fourth edition). Reg Anesth Pain Med 2018;43:263–309.

[55] Leffert LBA, Carvalho B, Arendt K, et al Society of Obstetric Anesthesia and Perinatology VTE Taskforce. The society for obstetric anesthesia and perinatology consensus statement on the anesthetic management of pregnant and postpartum women receiving thromboprophylaxis or higher dose anticoagulants. Anesth Analg 2018;126:928–944.

[56] Siu SC, Sermer M, Harrison DA, et al. Risk and predictors for pregnancy-related complications in women with heart disease. Circulation 1997;96(9):2789–2794.

[57] Drenthen W, Pieper PG, Van Der Tuuk K, et al. Cardiac complications relating to pregnancy and recurrence of disease in the offspring of women with atrioventricular septal defects. Eur Heart J 2005;26(23):2581–2587.

[58] Veldtman GR, Connolly HM, Grogan M, Ammash NM, Warnes CA. Outcomes of pregnancy in women with tetralogy of Fallot. J Am Coll Cardiol 2004;44(1):174–180.

[59] Meijer JM, Pieper PG, Drenthen W, et al. Pregnancy, fertility, and recurrence risk in corrected tetralogy of Fallot. Heart 2005;91(6):801–805.

[60] Lesniak-Sobelga ATW, KostKiewicz M, Podolec P, Pasowicz M. Clinical and echocardiographic assessment of pregnant women with valvular heart diseases-maternal and fetal outcome. Int J Cardiol 2004;94:15–23.

[61] Van Hagen TS, Taha N, Youssef G, et al (ROPAC Investigators and EORP Team). Pregnancy outcomes in women with rheumatic mitral valve disease: results from the Registry of Pregnancy and Cardiac Disease. Circulation 2018;137:806–816.

[62] Connolly H, Warnes C. Ebstein's anomaly: outcome of pregnancy. J Am Coll Cardiol 1994;23: 1194–1198.

[63] Lao T, Sermer M, MaGee L, Farine D, Colman J. Congenital aortic stenosis and pregnancy–a reappraisal. Am J Obstet Gynecol 1993;169:540–545.

[64] Silversides CK, Colman JM, Sermer M, Farine D, Siu SC. Early and intermediate-term outcomes of pregnancy with congenital aortic stenosis. Am J Cardiol 2003;91(11):1386–1389.

[65] Bonow RO, Carabello BA, Kanu C, et al. ACC/AHA 2006 guidelines for the management of patients with valvular heart disease: a report of the American College of Cardiology/ American Heart Association Task Force on Practice Guidelines (writing committee to revise

the 1998 Guidelines for the Management of Patients With Valvular Heart Disease): developed in collaboration with the Society of Cardiovascular Anesthesiologists: endorsed by the Society for Cardiovascular Angiography and Interventions and the Society of Thoracic Surgeons. Circulation 2006;114(5):e84–231.

[66] Yap SC, Drenthen W, Pieper PG, et al. Risk of complications during pregnancy in women with congenital aortic stenosis. Int J Cardiol 2007.

[67] Hameed A, Karaalp IS, Tummala PP, et al. The effect of valvular heart disease on maternal and fetal outcome of pregnancy. J Am Coll Cardiol 2001;37(3):893–899.

[68] Myerson SG, Mitchell AR, Ormerod OJ, Banning AP. What is the role of balloon dilatation for severe aortic stenosis during pregnancy?. J Heart Valve Dis 2005;14(2):147–150.

[69] Bhargava B, Agarwal R, Yadav R, Bahl VK, Manchanda SC. Percutaneous balloon aortic valvuloplasty during pregnancy: use of the Inoue balloon and the physiologic antegrade approach. Cathet Cardiovasc Diagn 1998;45(4):422–425.

[70] Banning AP, Pearson JF, Hall RJ. Role of balloon dilatation of the aortic valve in pregnant patients with severe aortic stenosis. Br Heart J 1993;70(6):544–545.

[71] Arnoni RT, Arnoni AS, Bonini RC, et al. Risk factors associated with cardiac surgery during pregnancy. Ann Thorac Surg 2003;76(5):1605–1608.

[72] Elkayam U, Bitar F. Valvular heart disease and pregnancy part I: native valves. J Am Coll Cardiol 2005;46(2):223–230.

[73] Silversides CKCJ, Sermer M, Siu SC. Cardiac risk in pregnant women with rheumatic mitral stenosis. Am J Cardiol 2003;91:1382–1385.

[74] Ducas RAJD, D'Souza R, Silversides CK, Tsang W. Pregnancy outcomes in women with significant valve disease: a systematic review and meta-analysis. Heart 2020;106:512–519.

[75] Desai DK, Adanlawo M, Naidoo DP, Moodley J, Kleinschmidt I. Mitral stenosis in pregnancy: a four-year experience at King Edward VIII Hospital, Durban, South Africa. Bjog 2000;107(8): 953–958.

[76] Mangione JA, Lourenco RM, Dos Santos ES, et al Long-term follow-up of pregnant women after percutaneous mitral valvuloplasty. Catheter Cardiovasc Interv 2000;50(4):413–417.

[77] De Souza JA, Martinez EE Jr., Ambrose JA, et al. Percutaneous balloon mitral valvuloplasty in comparison with open mitral valve commissurotomy for mitral stenosis during pregnancy. J Am Coll Cardiol 2001;37(3):900–903.

[78] Beauchesne LM, Connolly HM, Ammash NM, Warnes CA. Coarctation of the aorta: outcome of pregnancy. J Am Coll Cardiol 2001;38(6):1728–1733.

[79] Vriend JW, Drenthen W, Pieper PG, et al. Outcome of pregnancy in patients after repair of aortic coarctation. Eur Heart J 2005;26(20):2173–2178.

[80] Plunkett MD, Bond LM, Geiss DM. Staged repair of acute type I aortic dissection and coarctation in pregnancy. Ann Thorac Surg 2000;69(6):1945–1947.

[81] Hiratzka LFBG, Beckman JA, Bersin RM, et al. ACCF/AHA/AATS/ACR/ASA/SCA/SCAI/SIR/STS/ SVM Guidelines for the diagnosis and management of patients with thoracic aortic disease. Circulation 2010;2010(121):e266–e369.

[82] Smith KGB. Pregnancy-related acute aortic dissection in Marfan syndrome: a review of the literature. Congen Heart Dis 2017;12:251–260.

[83] Meijboom LJ, Vos FE, Timmermans J, Boers GH, Zwinderman AH, Mulder BJ. Pregnancy and aortic root growth in the Marfan syndrome: a prospective study. Eur Heart J 2005;26(9): 914–920.

[84] Goland S, Elkayam U. Cardiovascular problems in pregnant women with marfan syndrome. Circulation 2009;119(4):619–623.

[85] Boodhwani MAG, Leipsic J, Lindsay T, McMurtry S, Therrien J, Siu SC. Canadian Cardiovascular Society position statement on the management of thoracic aortic disease. Can J Cardiol 2014;30:577–589.

[86] McDermott CD, Sermer M, Siu SC, David TE, Colman JM. Aortic dissection complicating pregnancy following prophylactic aortic root replacement in a woman with Marfan syndrome. Int J Cardiol 2007;120(3):427–430.

[87] Wanga SSC, Dore A, De Waard V, Mulder B. Pregnancy and thoracic aortic disease: managing the risks. Can J Cardiol 2016;32:78–85.

[88] McKellar SHMR, Michelena HI, Connolly HM, Sundt TM. Frequency of cardiovascular events in women with a congenitally bicuspid aortic valve in a single community and effect of pregnancy on events. Am J Cardiol 2011;107:96–99.

[89] Immer FF, Bansi AG, Immer-Bansi AS, et al. Aortic dissection in pregnancy: analysis of risk factors and outcome. Ann Thorac Surg 2003;76(1):309–314.

[90] Murray MLPM, Peterson S, Byers PH. Pregnancy-related deaths and complications in women with vascular Ehlers-Danlos syndrome. Genet Med 2014;16:874–880.

[91] Pepin MSU, Superti-Furga A, Byers PH. Clinical and genetic features of Ehlers-Danlos syndrome type IV, the vascular type. N Engl J Med 2000;342:673–680.

[92] Bons LRR-HJ. Aortic disease and pregnancy. Curr Opin Cardiol 2016;31(6):611–617.

[93] Matura LA, Ho VB, Rosing DR, Bondy CA. Aortic dilatation and dissection in Turner syndrome. Circulation 2007;116(15):1663–1670.

[94] Gravholt CHAN, Conway GS, Dekkers OM, et al International Turner Syndrome Consensus Group. Clinical practice guidelines for the care of girls and women with Turner syndrome: proceedings from the 2016 Cincinnati International Turner Syndrome Meeting. Eur J Endocrinol 2017;177(3):G1.

[95] Drenthen W, Pieper PG, Roos-Hesselink JW, et al. Non-cardiac complications during pregnancy in women with isolated congenital pulmonary valvar stenosis. Heart 2006;92(12):1838–1843.

[96] Hameed AB, Goodwin TM, Elkayam U. Effect of pulmonary stenosis on pregnancy outcomes–a case-control study. Am Heart J 2007;154(5):852–854.

[97] Sliwa KV, Budts W, Swan L, et al Pulmonary hypertension and pregnancy outcomes: data from the registry of pregnancy and cardiac disease (ROPAC) of the European Society of Cardiology. Eur J Heart Failure 2016;18:1119–1128.

[98] Bedard E, Dimopoulos K, Gatzoulis MA. Has there been any progress made on pregnancy outcomes among women with pulmonary arterial hypertension?. Eur Heart J 2009;30(3): 256–265.

[99] Kiely D, Elliot C, Webster V, Stewart P. Pregnancy and pulmonary hypertension: new approaches to the management of a life-threatening condition. In: Steer P, Gatzoulis M, Baker P, editors. Heart Disease and Pregnancy. London: RCOG Press; 2006, 79–95.

[100] Mak S, Harris L. Arrhythmia in pregnancy. In: Wilansky S, Willerson J, editors. Heart Disease in Women, 1st. Philadelphia: Churchill Livingstone; 2002, 497–514.

[101] Vaidya VRAS, Patel N, Badheka AO, et al. Burden of arrhythia in pregnancy. Circulation 2017;135:619–621.

[102] Silversides CK, Harris L, Haberer K, Sermer M, Colman JM, Siu SC. Recurrence rates of arrhythmias during pregnancy in women with previous tachyarrhythmia and impact on fetal and neonatal outcomes. Am J Cardiol 2006;97(8):1206–1212.

[103] Al-Khatib SMSW, Ackerman MJ, Bryant WJ, et al. AHA/ACC/HRS guideline for management of patients with ventricular arrhythmias and the prevention of sudden cardiac death. Circulation 2017;138(13):e272–e391.

[104] Sliwa KMA, Hilfiker-Kleiner D, Petrie MC, et al. Clinical characteristics of patients from the worldwide registry on peripartum cardiomyopathy (PPCM): EURObservational Research

Programme in conjunction with the Heart Failure Association of the European Society of Cardiology Study Group on PPCM. Eur J Heart Fail 2017;19:1131–1141.

[105] Ponikowski PVA, Anker SD, Bueno H, et al. ESC guidelines for the diagnosis and treatment of acute and chronic heart failure. Eur Heart J 2016;2016(37):2129–2200.

[106] Hilfiker-Kleiner DHA, Masuko D, Nonhoff J, et al. Outcome of subsequent pregnancies in patients with a history of peripartum cardiomyopathy. Eur J Heart Fail 2017;19:1723–1728.

[107] Van Tintelen JPPP, Van Spaendonck-Zwarts KY, Van Den Berg MP. Pregnancy, cardiomyopathies, and genetics. Cardiovasc Res 2014;101:571–578.

[108] Schinkel AFL. Pregnancy in women with hypertrophic cardiomyopathy. Cardiol Rev 2014;22: 217–222.

[109] Kirchhof PBS, Kotecha D, Ahlsson A, et al. ESC guidelines for the management of atrial fibrillation developed in collaboration with FACTS. Eur Heart J 2016;37:2893–2962.

[110] Ware JSLJ, Mazaika E, Yasso CM, et al. Shared genetic predisposition in peripartum and dilated cardiomyopathies. N Engl J Med 2016;374:233–244.

[111] Grewal JSS, Ross HJ, Mason J, et al. Pregnancy outcomes in women with dilated cardiomyopathy. J Am Coll Cardiol 2009;55:45–52.

[112] Desplantie OT-GM, Avram R, Marquis-Gravel G, Ducharme A, Jolicoeur EM. The medical treatment of new-onset peripartum cardiomyopathy: a systematic review of prospective studies. Can J Cardiol 2015;31:1421–1426.

Emilie Laflamme, Rachel M. Wald

9 Cardiac Arrest in Pregnancy

9.1 Introduction and Epidemiology

Cardiac arrest in pregnancy represents a unique clinical scenario which has simultaneous and critical impact on two patients, a woman and her fetus. While
maternal mortality has decreased globally over the past 25 years [1, 2], recent decades have seen an increase in numbers of maternal deaths related to pregnancy
in North America [3, 4]. As a result of late maternal age in women with concomitant cardiovascular comorbidities [5–9], the incidence of maternal cardiac arrest
in pregnancy is rising in the developed world [10]. Specifically, the incidence of
cardiac arrest during pregnancy is approximately 8–8.5/100,000 deliveries in
North America and approximately 6.3–7.6/100,000 deliveries in Europe [10–13].
A recent Canadian study demonstrated a 10% increase in the incidence of severe
maternal morbidities (17.2 cases/1,000 deliveries in 2004–2005 to 18.9 cases/1,000
deliveries in 2014–2015) correlating with a proportional increase in number of pregnancies in women older than 40 years of age [7]. Although an infrequent occurrence,
maternal cardiac arrest will pose a challenge to even the most highly trained and specialized of medical teams. In this chapter, we review the most frequent causes of maternal cardiac arrest with a particular focus on distinct aspects of management
related to pregnancy.

9.2 Etiology of Cardiac Arrest in Pregnancy

Maternal cardiac arrest has been attributed to numerous obstetric and non-obstetric
etiologies, as shown in Table 9.1 [11–14]. A retrospective study which included data
from several centers in the United States reviewed the reported etiologies for more
than 4,000 episodes of cardiac arrest occurring during hospitalization for delivery. The most frequent causes were hemorrhage (38%), heart failure (13%), amniotic
fluid embolism (13%), and sepsis (11%) [11]. Another study, focused exclusively on
cardiovascular causes of maternal cardiac arrest, revealed that arrhythmia accounted
for more than half of cases (54%), followed by cardiomyopathy (13%), aortic dissection (8%), congenital heart disease (3%) and valvular heart disease (4%) [15].

https://doi.org/10.1515/9783110615258-009

Table 9.1: Non-obstetric and obstetric causes of maternal cardiac arrest [11–14].

Non-obstetric	Obstetric
Cardiovascular (11–33%)	Hemorrhagic (18–60%)
Arrhythmia	Uterine atony
Myocardial infarction	Placenta accreta
Heart failure	Placenta abruptio
Congenital heart disease	Placenta previa
Aortic dissection	Uterine rupture
Tamponade	Disseminated intravascular coagulation
Stroke (ischemic/hemorrhagic)	Transfusion reaction
Pulmonary (7–24%)	Anesthesia related (3–13%)
Pulmonary embolism	High neuraxial block
Asthma	Aspiration
Hypoxemia	Toxicity of local anesthetic
	Hypotension
	Respiratory depression
Trauma/suicide (2–3%)	Amniotic fluid embolism (13–16%)
Hypertensive disorders (7–18%)	
Pheochromocytoma	Eclampsia/HELLP
Infection/sepsis (3–11%)	
Drug related (3–9%)	
Anaphylaxis	Toxicity from tocolytic therapy
Illicit drug use	Hypermagnesemia
Opioids	
Insulin	

HELLP: Hemolysis, Elevated Liver enzymes, and Low Platelet level.

9.3 Management of Cardiac Arrest in Pregnancy

While many of the management recommendations apply broadly to pregnant and non-pregnant women alike, there are several features of advanced life support which are specific to the parturient (see Figure 9.1). When cardiac arrest occurs in a hospital setting, expeditious notification and activation of the appropriate team is of critical importance. In institutions where resources allow, a designated maternal code blue team should be assigned [16]. This team would ideally include representation from multiple specialties (internal medicine [i.e., critical care], obstetrics, pediatrics [i.e., neonatology]) and should span multiple disciplines (including physicians, nurses, and respiratory therapists). Because a response team will invariably include a relatively large number of individuals with varying medical expertise, effective

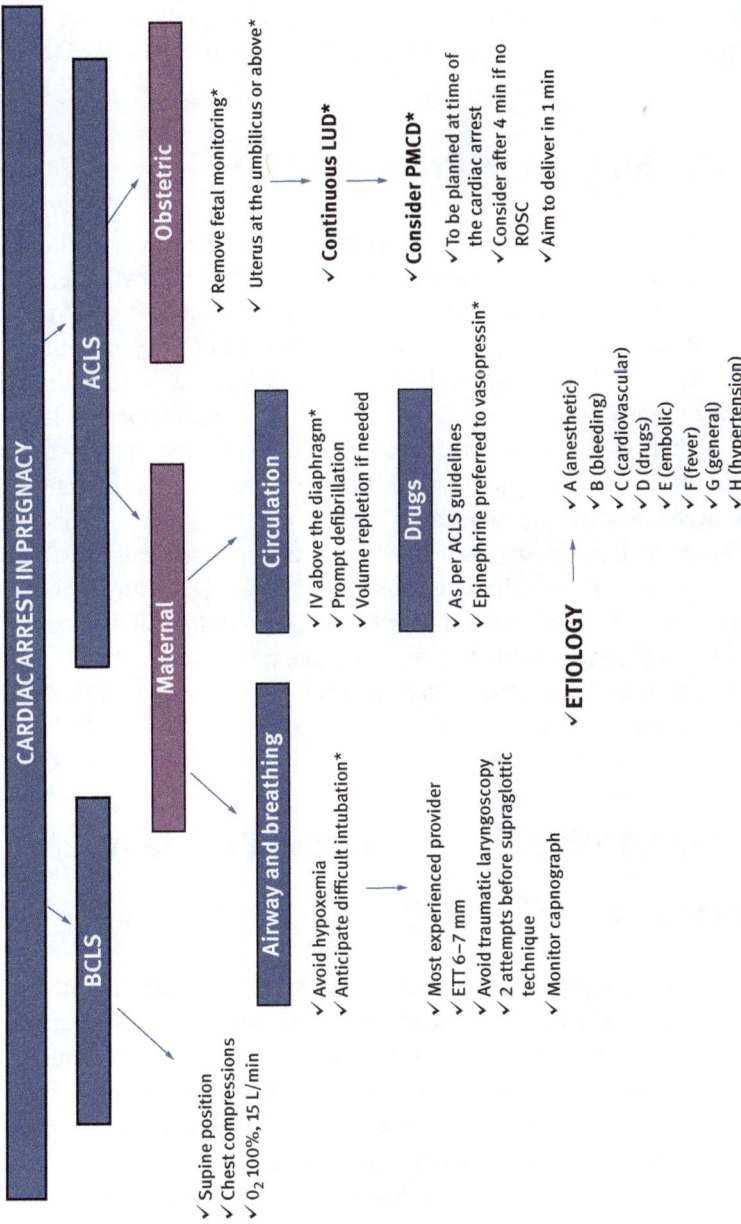

Figure 9.1: Algorithm for cardiac arrest in pregnancy. Adapted from Jeejeebhoy et al. [16].
The asterisks (*) highlight special considerations in maternal resuscitation.
ACLS, advanced cardiac life support; BCLS, basic cardiac life support; ETT, endotracheal tube; IV,
intravenous; L, liters; LUD, left uterine displacement; mm, millimeters; min, minute; PMCD,
perimortem caesarian section delivery; ROSC, return of spontaneous circulation.

communication is of utmost importance. A single team member should therefore assume the position of leader throughout the duration of the resuscitation [16].

9.4 Basic Life Support in Pregnancy

As in the non-pregnant patient, chest compressions in a pregnant woman should be initiated promptly with a target thoracic depression of 5 cm at a rhythm of 100 beats per minute [16, 17]. Because the efficacy of chest compressions in a tilt position has not been studied, it is recommended that the resuscitation continue in the supine position, with a backboard placed if the patient is found on a soft surface [16, 18]. It had been previously suggested that the site for compressions be landmarked slightly higher on the thorax of the pregnant woman, however this is no longer advised due to the lack of supporting evidence [16]. When indicated, defibrillation should be accomplished without delay. The same energy should be delivered irrespective of the stage in pregnancy as it is expected that minimal energy will be delivered to the fetus [16, 18, 19]. Adhesive pads should be applied with anterolateral positioning while avoiding placement over breast tissue [16]. Fetal monitoring is not only considered unnecessary during resuscitation, but monitors should also be removed if present to facilitate perimortem caesarian section delivery (PMCD), if necessary (described below).

9.5 Advanced Cardiac Life Support in Pregnancy

9.5.1 Airway and Breathing

Pregnant women are uniquely susceptible to progressive hypoxemia and respiratory deterioration as a result of several factors such as increased oxygen consumption and reduced lung capacity [20, 21]. Delivery of 100% oxygen at a rate of 15 L/min or greater should be administered and two-handed bag-mask ventilation should ideally be performed. Although it is important to avoid undue interruption in chest compressions, the pregnant state may necessitate earlier attention to airway management and a higher likelihood of difficult intubation should be anticipated. Edema within the upper airway and increased risk of aspiration may further complicate airway management. Repeated traumatic laryngoscopy can result in bleeding and promote localized edema and it is therefore crucial that an experienced operator be involved whenever possible [22–25].

9.5.2 Circulation

The first important step toward effective hemodynamic management is optimization of venous access. Although femoral access could be of benefit in some emergency situations in the non-pregnant individual, it is likely a suboptimal location for intravenous placement during pregnancy given vascular compression from the enlarging uterus. Therefore, it is preferable that venous lines be located above the diaphragm [16]. Following initiation of initial life support maneuvers, prompt determination of gestational age is necessary to direct further management. Measurement of symphysis fundal height allows for estimation of gestational age if more precise dating information is unavailable at the time of resuscitation. Generally, for a singleton pregnancy, the fundal height in centimeters corresponds to the number of weeks between 16 and 36 weeks of gestation (i.e., 20 weeks of gestation corresponds to fundal height located at the level of the umbilicus and 36 weeks of gestation to a fundal height located at the xyphoid process) [26, 27].

Importantly, aortocaval compression is more likely to occur after 20 weeks of gestation and may disadvantage the resuscitation efforts [16, 27, 28]. Although there are limited data on direct measures to mitigate the effects of aortocaval compression during resuscitation, maternal left uterine displacement (LUD) is generally recommended [16, 18]. Of note, it has been previously demonstrated that LUD during caesarian section results in reduced hypotension and ephedrine requirements as compared with maternal tilt position [29, 30]. The application of LUD is indicated throughout the resuscitation effort and is best accomplished from the right side of the patient with the uterus lifted upward and leftward [16]. Finally, the use of medication, when indicated, should follow the same algorithm as outlined for advanced cardiac life support in the non-pregnant patient [17]. Importantly, the US Food and Drug Administration categories of fetal risk are not applicable to medication selection during a resuscitation scenario [16]. Although it is known that the volume of distribution and drug metabolism are altered during pregnancy [31], there are no data to support modification of the dosage of any medication.

9.6 Perimortem Caesarian Section Delivery

PMCD is a critical procedure which allows for relief of aortocaval compression and therefore should be considered in every individual in whom return of spontaneous circulation does not occur despite 4 min of active resuscitation [16]. The rationale of PMCD is restoration of optimal hemodynamics for ongoing resuscitation following relief of aortocaval compression as well as limiting risk of anoxic brain injury to the fetus. As time is of the essence during PMCD, preparation should ideally occur at the time of diagnosis of maternal cardiac arrest and should be completed at the site of the arrest; transportation of the patient for PMCD is not indicated, and in fact has been associated with decreased efficacy of resuscitation and reduced survival of the pregnant person [10, 32]. Aside from a scalpel, no additional instrumentation is recommended, and it is advised that time should not be devoted to achievement of aseptic technique [16]. Based on recognized physiologic changes of pregnancy and data from case series, Katz et al. proposed that PMCD should occur 4 minute (min) after cardiac arrest with the aim of delivery of the fetus within 1 min [33]. Return of spontaneous circulation and improvement in maternal hemodynamics have been well-documented after PMCD [33–37]. Although a 4 min window of time for initiation of PMCD has long been advocated, published reports suggest that this is only achieved in the minority of patients [14, 34, 38, 39] and very few deliveries (approximately 10%) are completed within 1 min [39]. However, a recent series from the United Kingdom revealed that most PMCD will occur within 5 min of onset of cardiac arrest and may reflect contemporary training as compared with more historic reports [10]. Of note, maternal survival is associated with shorter mean times from cardiac arrest to PMCD [10, 13, 14]. Intact survival of woman and baby decrease significantly with longer time to PMCD and has been reported to be only 50% at 25 min in one series [39].

9.7 Mechanical Support and Intensive Care Management

Only few published case reports describe the successful use of extracorporeal membrane oxygenation (ECMO) during a cardiac arrest in a pregnant patient [40–42]. There are several challenges imposed by the physiology of pregnancy which need to be considered when initiating ECMO, notably maintenance of high maternal cardiac output and achievement of the optimal balance between anticoagulation and hemostasis [40]. Currently, there are no published recommendations pertaining to the use of ECMO in the resuscitation efforts of a pregnant woman and decision-making should be individualized on a case-by-case basis.

Following successful resuscitation, the patient should be admitted to the intensive care unit for ongoing investigations and management. If the woman remains pregnant, attention should be given to minimizing aortocaval compression, such as left lateral decubitus positioning. The cause of the cardiac arrest should be maintaining and treatment should be tailored accordingly. Therapeutic hypothermia is the standard of care following cardiac arrest for patients who remain unable to respond to verbal commands immediately after resuscitation given favorable impact on neurological outcomes [43, 44]. However, scarce data are available regarding the application of therapeutic hypothermia in pregnant women. Two case reports suggest favorable outcomes for woman and babies [45, 46] and one report describes fetal demise following prolonged resuscitation efforts [47]. We submit that pregnancy is not an absolute contraindication for therapeutic hypothermia and its use should be individualized. In contrast to active resuscitation, fetal monitoring is mandatory during therapeutic hypothermia, particularly as the impact on the fetus remains unclear. As hypothermia is associated with heightened risk of bleeding and infection, close monitoring of the woman is also necessary.

9.8 Outcomes and Training Perspectives

Maternal survival to hospital discharge following maternal cardiac arrest varies widely in the literature with estimates ranging between 17% and 71% [10–12, 14, 34, 48, 49]. As would be expected, lower survival rates are associated with out-of-hospital cardiac arrest [13, 50, 51]. Neonatal survival to hospital discharge varies from 63% to 86% and has been reported to be higher when PMCD is performed within 5 min of maternal cardiac arrest [10, 12, 14, 49]. Outcomes following resuscitation are linked to timelines of response and level of expertise of the arrest team. To date, knowledge about management of cardiac arrest in pregnancy is generally thought to be suboptimal [52–54]. For instance, two previous reports have documented that effective LUD is rarely achieved during the resuscitation efforts [10, 13]. Teaching and maintenance of competence, ideally with clinical simulations, can ensure that health care professionals have the tools that they require to effectively manage the complexities and intricacies of the rare occurrence of cardiac arrest in pregnancy [55–57].

References

[1]   WHO, UNICEF, UNFPA WBG and the UNPD. WHO | Trends in maternal mortality: 1990 to 2015. *Who*. 2016.
[2]   Alkema L, Chou D, Hogan D, et al. Global, regional, and national levels and trends in maternal mortality between 1990 and 2015, with scenario-based projections to 2030: A systematic analysis by the un Maternal Mortality Estimation Inter-Agency Group. Lancet 2016;387 (10017):462–474.
[3]   WHO, UNICEF, UNFPA, World Bank Group, United Nations population division. Trends in maternal mortality: 2000 to 2017. *Geneva.*:https://data.worldbank.org/indicator/SH.STA. MMRT.
[4]   Cook JL, Majd M, Blake J, et al. Measuring maternal mortality and morbidity in Canada. J Obstet Gynaecol Canada 2017;39(11):1028–1037.
[5]   Davis NL, Hoyert DL, Goodman DA, Hirai AH, Callaghan WM. Contribution of maternal age and pregnancy checkbox on maternal mortality ratios in the United States, 1978–2012. Am J Obstet Gynecol 2017;217(3):352.e1–352.e7.
[6]   Matthews TJ, Hamilton BE. First births to older women continue to rise. NCHS Data Brief 2014;152:1–8.

[7]   Aoyama K, Pinto R, Ray JG, et al. Association of maternal age with severe maternal morbidity and mortality in Canada. JAMA Netw Open 2019;2(8):e199875.

[8]   Londero AP, Rossetti E, Pittini C, Cagnacci A, Driul L. Maternal age and the risk of adverse pregnancy outcomes: a retrospective cohort study. BMC Pregnancy Childbirth 2019;19(1): 1–10.

[9]   Metcalfe A, Wick J, Ronksley P. Racial disparities in comorbidity and severe maternal morbidity/mortality in the United States: an analysis of temporal trends. Acta Obstet Gynecol Scand 2018;97(1):89–96.

[10] Beckett VA, Knight M, Sharpe P. The CAPS study: incidence, management and outcomes of cardiac arrest in pregnancy in the UK: a prospective, descriptive study. BJOG An Int J Obstet Gynaecol 2017;124(9):1374–1381.

[11] Mhyre JM, Tsen LC, Einav S, Kuklina EV, Leffert LR, Bateman BT. Cardiac arrest during hospitalization for delivery in the United States, 1998–2011. Anesthesiology 2014;120(4): 810–818.

[12] Balki M, Liu S, León JA, Baghirzada L. Epidemiology of cardiac arrest during hospitalization for delivery in Canada: a nationwide study. Anesth Analg 2017;124(3):890–897.

[13] Schaap TP, Overtoom E, Van Den Akker T, Zwart JJ, Van Roosmalen J, Bloemenkamp KWM. Maternal cardiac arrest in the Netherlands: a nationwide surveillance study. Eur J Obstet Gynecol Reprod Biol 2019;237:145–150.

[14] Einav S, Kaufman N, Sela HY. Maternal cardiac arrest and perimortem caesarean delivery: evidence or expert-based?. Resuscitation 2012;83(10):1191–1200.

[15] Krexi D, Sheppard MN. Cardiovascular causes of maternal sudden death. Sudden arrhythmic death syndrome is leading cause in UK. Eur J Obstet Gynecol Reprod Biol 2017;217:177.

[16] Jeejeebhoy FM, Zelop CM, Lipman S, et al. Cardiac arrest in pregnancy: a scientific statement from the American heart association. Circulation 2015;132(18):1747–1773.

[17] Panchal AR, Berg KM, Kudenchuk PJ, et al. American heart association focused update on advanced cardiovascular life support use of antiarrhythmic drugs during and immediately after cardiac arrest: an update to the american heart association guidelines for cardiopulmonary resuscitation and Em. Circulation 2018;138(23):e740–e749.

[18] Jeejeebhoy FM, Zelop CM, Windrim R, Carvalho JCA, Dorian P, Morrison LJ. Management of cardiac arrest in pregnancy: a systematic review. Resuscitation 2011;82(7):801–809.

[19] Nanson J, Elcock D, Williams M, Deakin CD. Do physiological changes in pregnancy change defibrillation energy requirements?. Br J Anaesth 2001;87(2):237–239.

[20] Pernoll M, Metcalfe J, Schienker T, Welch J, Matsumoto J. Oxygen consumption at rest and during exercise in pregnancy. Respiro Physiol 1975;25(3): 285–293.

[21] Baldwin GR, Moorthi DS, Whelton, MacDonnell JAKF. New lung functions and pregnancy. Am J Obstet Gynecol 1977;127(3):235–239.

[22] McDonnell NJ, Paech MJ, Clavisi OM, Scott KL. Difficult and failed intubation in obstetric anaesthesia: an observational study of airway management and complications associated with general anaesthesia for caesarean section. Int J Obstet Anesth 2008;17(4):292–297.

[23] Quinn AC, Milne D, Columb M, Gorton H, Knight M. Failed tracheal intubation in obstetric anaesthesia: 2 yr national case-control study in the UK. Br J Anaesth 2013;110(1):74–80.

[24] Mhyre JM, Healy D. The unanticipated difficult intubation in obstetrics. Anesth Analg 2011;112 (3):648–652.

[25] Balki M, Cooke ME, Dunington S, Salman A, Goldszmidt E. Unanticipated difficult airway in obstetric patients. Development of a new algorithm for formative assessment in high-fidelity simulation. Anesthesiology 2012;117(4): 883–897.

[26] Stallard T, Burns B. Emergency delivery and perimortem C-section. Emerg Med Clin North Am 2003;21(3): 679–693.

[27] Mackway-Jones K. Towards evidence based emergency medicine: best BETs from the Manchester Royal Infirmary. Emerg Med J 2008;25(11):764–765.

[28] Ueland K, Novy M, Peterson E, Mercalfe J. Maternal cardiovascular dynamics. IV. The influence of gestational age on the maternal cardiovascular response to posture and exercise. Am J Obstet Gynecol 1969;104(6): 856–864.

[29] Kundra P, Khanna S, Habeebullah S, Ravishankar M. Manual displacement of the uterus during Caesarean section. Anaesthesia 2007;62(5):460–465.

[30] Cluver C, Novikova N, Hofmeyr GJ, Hall DR. Maternal position during caesarean section for preventing maternal and neonatal complications. Cochrane Database Syst Rev 2013;2013:3.

[31] Feghall M, Venkataramanan R, Carltls S. Pharmacokinetics of drugs in pregnancy. Semin Perinatol 2015;39(7): 512–519.

[32] Lipman SS, Wong JY, Arafeh J, Cohen SE, Carvalho B. Transport decreases the quality of cardiopulmonary resuscitation during simulated maternal cardiac arrest. Anesth Analg 2013;116(1):162–167.

[33] Katz VL, Dotters DJ, Droegemueller W. Perimortem cesarean delivery. Obstet Gynecol 1986;68 (4): 571–576.

[34] Dijkman A, Huisman CMA, Smit M, et al. Cardiac arrest in pregnancy: increasing use of perimortem caesarean section due to emergency skills training?. BJOG An Int J Obstet Gynaecol 2010;117(3):282–287.

[35] McDonnell NJ. Cardiopulmonary arrest in pregnancy: two case reports of successful outcomes in association with perimortem Caesarean delivery. Br J Anaesth 2009;103(3):406–409.

[36] Stehr SN, Liebich I, Kamin G, Koch T, Litz RJ. Closing the gap between decision and delivery-Amniotic fluid embolism with severe cardiopulmonary and haemostatic complications with a good outcome. Resuscitation 2007;74(2):377–381.

[37] O'Connor RL, Sevarino FB. Cardiopulmonary arrest in the pregnant patient: a report of a successful resuscitation. J Clin Anesth 1994;6(1):66–68.

[38] Katz V, Balderston K, Defreest M, Nageotte M, Parer J. Perimortem cesarean delivery: were our assumptions correct?. Am J Obstet Gynecol 2005;192(6):1916–1920.

[39] Benson MD, Padovano A, Bourjeily G, Zhou Y. Maternal collapse: challenging the four-minute rule. EBioMedicine 2016;6:253–257.

[40] Biderman P, Carmi U, Setton E, Fainblut M, Bachar O, Einav S. Maternal salvage with extracorporeal life support: lessons learned in a single center. Anesth Analg 2017;125(4): 1275–1280.

[41] Depondt C, Arnaudovski D, Voulgaropoulos A, et al. Venoarterial extracorporeal membrane oxygenation as supportive therapy after cardiac arrest after amniotic fluid embolism. A A Pract 2019;13(2):1.

[42] Moore SA, Dietl CA, Coleman DM. Extracorporeal life support during pregnancy. J Thorac Cardiovasc Surg 2016;151(4):1154–1160.

[43] Bernard SA, Gray TW, Buist MD, et al. Treatment of comatose survivors of out-of-hospital cardiac arrest with induced hypothermia. N Eng J Med 2002;346(8):557–563.

[44] Holzer M, Sterz F, Darby JM, et al. Mild therapeutic hypothermia to improve the neurologic outcome after cardiac arrest. N Engl J Med 2002;346(8):549–556.

[45] Rittenberger JC, Kelly E, Jang D, Greer K, Heffner A. Successful outcome utilizing hypothermia after cardiac arrest in pregnancy: a case report. Crit Care Med 2008;36(4):1354–1356.

[46] Chauhan A, Musunuru H, Donnino M, McCurdy MT, Chauhan V, Walsh M. The use of therapeutic hypothermia after cardiac arrest in a pregnant patient. Ann Emerg Med 2012;60 (6):786–789.

[47] Wible EF, Kass JS, Lopez GA. A report of fetal demise during therapeutic hypothermia after cardiac arrest. Neurocrit Care 2010;13(2):239–242.

[48] Zelop CM, Einav S, Mhyre JM, et al. Characteristics and outcomes of maternal cardiac arrest: a descriptive analysis of Get with the guidelines data. Resuscitation 2018;132(August):17–20.

[49] Baghirzada L, Balki M. Maternal cardiac arrest in a tertiary care centre during 1989–2011: a case series. Can J Anesth 2013;60(11):1077–1084.

[50] Lipowicz AA, Cheskes S, Gray SH, et al. Incidence, outcomes and guideline compliance of out-of-hospital maternal cardiac arrest resuscitations: a population-based cohort study. Resuscitation 2018;132(September):127–132.

[51] Maurin O, Lemoine S, Jost D, et al. Maternal out-of-hospital cardiac arrest: a retrospective observational study. Resuscitation 2019;135(November 2018):205–211.

[52] Cohen SE, Andes LC, Carvalho B. Assessment of knowledge regarding cardiopulmonary resuscitation of pregnant women. Int J Obstet Anesth 2008;17(1):20–25.

[53] Einav S, Matot I, Berkenstadt H, Bromiker R, Weiniger CF. A survey of labour ward clinicians' knowledge of maternal cardiac arrest and resuscitation. Int J Obstet Anesth 2008;17(3): 238–242.

[54] Lipman SS, Daniels KI, Carvalho B, et al. Deficits in the provision of cardiopulmonary resuscitation during simulated obstetric crises. Am J Obstet Gynecol 2010;203(2):179. e1–179.e5.

[55] Lee A, Sheen JJ, Richards S. Intrapartum maternal cardiac arrest: a simulation case for multidisciplinary providers. MedEdPORTAL J Teach Learn Resour 2018;14:10768.

[56] Gogle J. Using simulation-based learning to prepare for a potential cardiac emergency on the labor unit. Nurs Womens Health 2017;21(1):20–27.

[57] Adams J, Cepeda Brito JR, Baker L, et al. Management of maternal cardiac arrest in the third trimester of pregnancy: a simulation-based pilot study. Crit Care Res Pract 2016;2016(590).

Stephanie C. Lapinsky, Stephen E. Lapinsky

10 Critical Care in Pregnancy

10.1 Introduction

Management of a critically ill pregnant patient is a relatively unusual situation with which few physicians gain expertise. It is stressful to obstetricians, obstetric medicine physicians, and insensivists alike. The usual clinical management approach may be altered by the physiologic changes induced by pregnancy, by the relatively uncommon pregnancy-specific conditions, and also by perceived limitations on therapy produced by the presence of a fetus.

10.2 Physiologic Changes in Pregnancy

Physiology changes during pregnancy, and several adaptations are relevant to the management of critical illness (see Table 10.1). The upper airways develop edema and hyperemia and this may increase the difficulty of endotracheal intubation and alter the planned approach. Changes in lung volumes occur as the uterus enlarges, most signifi-cantly a 10–25% decrease in functional residual capacity (FRC) [1]. Total lung capacity decreases only minimally due to widening of the thorax to compensate. Forced expira-tory volume in 1 s is unchanged in the pregnant state. Although lung compliance is not altered, the chest wall and total respiratory compliance do decrease [2].

Ventilation increases in pregnancy, stimulated by rising progesterone levels, which increases the sensitivity of the respiratory center to carbon dioxide. Minute ventilation rises with increasing gestation (largely mediated by an increased tidal volume), reaching 20–40% above baseline by term [3]. The median respiratory rate at 12 weeks of gestation is 15/min (3rd–97th percentile: 9–22/min), and does not change with gestation [4]. This hyperventilation produces a lowered maternal CO_2 (28–32 mmHg) which facilitates transfer of CO_2 from the fetal to maternal circulation. A mild respiratory alkalosis occurs, with metabolic compensation occurring through bicarbonate excretion ($PaCO_2$ 28–32 mmHg; HCO_3^- 18–21 mEq/L). Oxygen consump-tion (and CO_2 production) increases to levels of up to 20–30% above baseline by term, due to maternal metabolic processes and the demands of the fetus. Arterial PO_2 remains unchanged throughout pregnancy but mild hypoxemia can occur near term, particularly in the supine position, as a result of airway closure with the diminishing FRC producing an increased alveolar-arterial oxygen tension difference.

Physiological changes also occur in the cardiovascular system to allow adequate oxygen delivery to the placenta and fetus. Volume expansion occurs, mediated by sodium retention from increased aldosterone production. Maternal blood volume and

https://doi.org/10.1515/9783110615258-010

Table 10.1: Physiologic changes in pregnancy.

Parameter	Change
Respiratory	
Functional residual capacity	Decreased 10–25%
Minute ventilation	Increased 20–40%
Tidal volume	Increases 30–35%
Respiratory rate	No change
Arterial partial pressure of oxygen	No change
Arterial partial pressure of carbon dioxide	Reduced to 28–32 mmHg
Serum bicarbonate	Reduced to 18–21 mEq/L
Cardiac	
Blood volume	Increase 40%
Heart rate	Increased 10–30%
Pulmonary capillary wedge pressure	No change
Cardiac output	Increased 30–50%
Systemic vascular resistance	Decreased 20–30%
Pulmonary vascular resistance	Decreased 20–30%

cardiac output increase during pregnancy, peaking by about 28 weeks, with levels reaching 30–50% above baseline [5]. This increase in cardiac output is accompanied by a 20–30% reduction in systemic vascular resistance and pulmonary vascular resistance. Cardiac output is further augmented in labor and the immediate postpartum period by the auto-transfusion of 300–500 mL of blood from the uterus to the central circulation [6]. Vena caval and aortic obstruction by the gravid uterus can occur in the supine position, reducing cardiac output which can be ameliorated by positioning in the left lateral decubitus position [7].

Oxygen delivery to the fetus is dependent on maternal oxygen content (hemoglobin concentration × oxygen saturation) and uterine blood flow. Fetal oxygenation is therefore affected by both maternal oxygen saturation and factors which cause uterine artery vasoconstriction [5]. Uterine arterial blood flow is reduced by maternal hypotension, alkalosis (e.g., hyperventilation), as well as endogenous or exogenous catecholamines. Uterine blood flow is also reduced transiently by uterine contractions. Umbilical venous blood returning to the fetus from the placenta has a relatively low oxygen tension, but a high oxygen content due to the left shift of the oxygen dissociation curve of fetal hemoglobin.

10.3 Critical Illness in Pregnancy

Admission of the pregnant or postpartum woman to the intensive care unit is uncommon, representing about 2% of all ICU admissions [8], and up to 5% of maternities may require a higher level of care [9]. It can be difficult to identify women who are at risk of dying, and conventional ICU risk prediction models are not very useful [10]. Risk prediction models are affected by the altered maternal physiology (and therefore vital signs) and by pregnancy-specific conditions which have varying prognoses.

Several studies have documented the limitations of conventional, non-obstetric risk prediction models, such as APACHE II and SAPS II. Although they have a high level of discrimination, they are poorly calibrated and tend to overestimate mortality [10]. A systematic review of risk prediction models for maternal mortality identified 38 studies using 12 prediction models [10]. Five of these models had been developed specifically for an obstetric population. Two models had good discrimination and calibration with both low risk of bias and low concern of applicability: the CIPHER score and the maternal severity index (MSI). The CIPHER model was developed from a cohort of pregnant ICU patients from high-, middle-, and low-income countries and utilizes 10 risk parameters [11], but so far has not been externally validated. The MSI was based on WHO criteria for the identification of maternal near-miss and has been externally validated in multi-national cohorts [12]. Other scores include the obstetric early warning score, developed by the Intensive Care National Audit and Research Centre (ICNARC) in the United Kingdom in 2013, which was reported to have excellent operating characteristics, but validation was done internally [13]. More recently, ICNARC has developed two new multivariable logistic regression models; one for the outcome of acute hospital mortality (8 risk factors) and one for a composite outcome of death or prolonged ICU stay (17 risk factors) [14]. These models have been validated internally utilizing a temporally different ICNARC cohort. Their risk model for hospital mortality utilizes eight commonly available variables, namely PaO_2/FO_2 ratio, pH, systolic blood pressure, lactate, sodium, preexisting medical conditions, and direct/indirect (i.e., obstetric/non-obstetric) maternal admission. It demonstrated excellent operating characteristics with an area under the receiver operating characteristics curve (AUROC) of 0.96 (95% CI 0.91–1.0).

A concern with many of these prediction models is that information derived solely from patients already admitted to the ICU may not be generalizable to the assessment of patients deteriorating on the ward. Furthermore, the rate of admission of obstetric patients to the ICU is very variable, even in a similar healthcare environment. There is also significant variability in the type of obstetric patient admitted to the ICU. These factors will have a large impact on the study derivation cohort. These types of prediction models are generally not used for clinical decision making in the individual patient, but could act as an aid in communication with patients and their families, and in comparing critical care units from a quality perspective.

10.4 Critical Care Management: ICU Drug Therapy in Pregnancy

10.4.1 Catecholamines

Catecholamines commonly used in the ICU such as dobutamine, dopamine, norepinephrine, and epinephrine may reduce uterine blood flow, either due to arterial vasoconstriction or by shunting blood away from the uterus (e.g., vasodilators such as dobutamine). However, maternal hypotension is potentially harmful to the fetus and rapid correction is important. Both ephedrine boluses and phenylephrine by bolus or infusion have been shown to be safe and effective for transient hypotension induced by neuraxial anesthesia [62, 63]. Nonpharmacologic maneuvers such as volume replacement and left lateral positioning or manual displacement of the uterus are essential to the management of hypotension in the pregnant patient. However, if vasopressor infusion therapy is required to support maternal hemodynamics, this therapy should not be withheld because of concerns for potential adverse effects on the fetus. An approach similar to that used in the nonpregnant patient is usually appropriate. Electronic fetal heart-rate monitoring may be useful to assess whether these hemodynamic interventions are beneficial to the fetus.

10.4.2 Sedation, Analgesia, and Neuromuscular Blockade

The current approach for sedation in the ICU patient is to minimize the use of pharmacotherapy, and this is clearly advantageous to the fetus. Little data exist on which drugs are optimal for prolonged sedation, analgesia, or neuromuscular blockade in the critically ill pregnant woman. Benzodiazepine use in early pregnancy has been associated with a small risk of congenital malformations, mainly cleft lip and palate [15]. However, studies of use of benzodiapines for anxiety in pregnant women show no significant concerns [16]. Midazolam crosses the placenta to a lesser degree than diazepam, which can accumulate in the fetus at levels greater than in the mother. Propofol has been used as an induction agent for caesarean section, but there is limited data on the prolonged use for ICU sedation. A single case report describes the development of non-anion gap acidosis in two pregnant women receiving propofol infusion for prolonged neurosurgical procedures [17]. Congenital malformations have not been demonstrated with use of narcotic analgesics such as morphine, meperidine, and fentanyl. Nondepolarizing neuromuscular blocking agents including pancuronium, vecuronium, and atracurium do cross the placenta to a varying degree [18], but transfer is unlikely to have clinical effects on the fetus in the short term. However, if delivery occurs while the mother is on sedative or paralyzing agents, it is essential that this information is communicated to those responsible for managing the neonate. The need for ventilatory support for the fetus and possible neonatal abstinence syndrome should be anticipated.

10.5 Ventilatory Support

10.5.1 Noninvasive Ventilation

Noninvasive ventilation (NIV) avoids the potential adverse effects of endotracheal intubation in the pregnant patient, such as airway trauma, the risk of nosocomial pneumonia, and the complications associated with sedation. NIV is ideally suited to short-term ventilatory support which is often the case in many obstetric complications which reverse rapidly [19]. A major concern with mask ventilation in pregnancy is the risk of aspiration due to the increased intraabdominal pressure, delayed gastric emptying, and reduced lower esophageal sphincter tone which occur in pregnancy. NIV is appropriate for the pregnant woman who is protecting her airway, and with an expectation of a relatively brief requirement for mechanical ventilatory support.

10.5.2 Airway Management

Due to the physiological changes to the upper airway and significantly reduced safe apnea time, failed intubation is more common in the obstetric population than in other populations undergoing anesthetic intubations. The diminished FRC and increased oxygen consumption reduces oxygen reserve and produces rapid desaturation during apnea or hypoventilation [20]. Preoxygenation with 100% oxygen may help, but hyperventilation and respiratory alkalosis must be avoided due to its adverse effects on uterine blood flow. Upper airway hyperemia and edema may reduce visualization and necessitate use of a smaller endotracheal tube. The diameter of the oropharynx narrows and the Mallampati class may increase during labor and delivery [21]. Nasal intubation should be avoided as the risk of bleeding is increased. In view of the delayed gastric emptying and the elevated intraabdominal pressure occurring in pregnancy, these patient should always be considered to have a full stomach and appropriate precautions should be taken.

10.5.3 Mechanical Ventilation

There is limited data specific to pregnancy to guide prolonged mechanical ventilation of pregnant patients. Hyperventilation should be avoided as maternal respiratory alkalosis reduces uterine blood flow and may also adversely affect fetal cerebral blood flow [22, 23]. Current ventilator approaches in the nonpregnant patient should be followed such as avoiding excessive lung stretch by limiting tidal volume and pressure, although permissive hypercapnia has not been assessed in pregnancy. The usual pressure limits (e.g., plateau pressure of 35 cm H_2O) may not be applicable in the near-term patient, where chest wall compliance is reduced. It is likely that transpulmonary pressures are not elevated at a plateau pressure of 35 cm H_2O, and slightly higher ventilatory pressures may be accepted in pregnant women near term.

Although pregnancy produces a mild respiratory alkalosis, maternal hypercapnia up to 60 mmHg (in the presence of adequate oxygenation) does not appear to be detrimental to the fetus [24, 25]. Maternal respiratory acidosis may produce fetal hypercapnia and acidosis, but this does not have the same ominous implications as fetal acidosis due to fetal hypoxia causing lactic acidosis [26]. However, this acidosis will cause a right shift of the fetal oxygen–hemoglobin dissociation curve which may negate the beneficial oxygen carrying characteristics of fetal hemoglobin. If marked respiratory acidosis results from permissive hypercapnia, bicarbonate therapy may improve maternal and fetal acidemia.

Many references suggest that maternal arterial oxygenation should be maintained greater than 70 mmHg (or saturation >95%) [27], but this recommendation is not based on evidence. Maternal oxygen saturation is only one of the factors affecting fetal oxygen supply to the fetus, uterine blood flow playing a major role. Optimizing maternal oxygenation is a reasonable clinical approach, but harm from mild maternal hypoxemia has not been clearly established and hyperoxia is also harmful [28, 29]. Supplemental oxygen therapy should be provided for maternal hypoxia and not routinely for nonreassuring fetal status [30].

It may seem reasonable to think that delivery of the pregnant patient with respiratory failure will improve the mother's respiratory status. A number of small case series addressing this issue have not found a consistent significant benefit to the mother, and delivery carries a risk of harm [31]. Delivery should not be carried out purely in the hope of improving "maternal condition." If the fetus is considered viable and appears to be at risk due to severe maternal hypoxia, delivery may benefit the fetus. These decisions are usually made in consultation with the obstetrician, neonatologist, and intensivist. Obstetric indications should always determine the mode of delivery.

10.6 Pregnancy-Specific Conditions Requiring ICU Care

The following section will outline several conditions which may necessitate critical care in pregnancy. Many conditions are discussed elsewhere in the book.

10.6.1 Acute Fatty Liver of Pregnancy

Acute fatty liver of pregnancy (AFLP) is a rare and potentially fatal complication of pregnancy, which typically manifests in the late third trimester, but can occur from as early as 30 weeks of gestation up until the puerperium. Earlier diagnosis and improvements in the management of AFLP have resulted in significantly improved maternal and fetal outcomes, with maternal and fetal mortality estimated at approximately 7% and 15%, respectively [32]. Pathophysiology is unclear, but this condition is associated with a fetal autosomal recessive inborn error of fatty acid metabolism (L-CHAD deficiency) which leads to the accumulation and deposition of fetal fatty acids in the maternal liver, resulting in diffuse microvesicular fatty infiltration [33]. Typical laboratory findings include elevated transaminases, 5–10 times the upper limit of normal and higher than typically seen in HELLP but less than would be expected in other causes of acute hepatitis. Leukocytosis and hypoglycemia are common, and coagulation studies can be abnormal with evidence of microangiopathic hemolytic anemia. Fulminant hepatic failure can occur and result in encephalopathy, renal failure, pancreatitis, hemorrhage, disseminated intravascular coagulation (DIC), seizures, coma, or death.

Definitive treatment involves obstetrical delivery, along with supportive care often requiring admission to ICU. Supportive therapy follows the same principles as other causes of fulminant hepatic failure including correction of coagulation abnormalities and hypoglycemia. Management of hepatic encephalopathy requires attention to airway protection, dietary protein restriction, bowel sterilization, and oral or rectal lactulose administration. Complications such as hemorrhage, pancreatitis, renal failure, diabetes insipidus, and infection should be sought and treated. Transient worsening of hepatic function may occur following delivery with improvement usually beginning within 2–3 days. A small subset of patients continue to show worsening hepatic function following delivery, and need for liver transplantation has been described [32].

10.6.2 Amniotic Fluid Embolism

Amniotic fluid embolism (AFE) is a rare complication of pregnancy, occurring in 1/8,000 to 1/80,000 live births [34]. It carries a mortality rate of 10% to 86% and has been estimated to account for up to 10% of maternal deaths [35]. It usually occurs during labor and delivery but it may also occur with uterine manipulations, uterine trauma, terminations, or in the early postpartum period, and presents with sudden onset dyspnea, hypoxemia, and cardiovascular collapse. Occasionally, the presenting symptom is fetal distress, seizures, or postpartum hemorrhage secondary to DIC [34, 36]. The mechanism involves amniotic fluid entering the vascular circulation through endocervical veins or uterine tears. Cellular contents and humoral factors in the amniotic fluid produce acute pulmonary hypertension and biventricular dysfunction, with resulting hemodynamic collapse resembling anaphylaxis, potentially related to sensitivity to amniotic fluid contents [37, 38]. The diagnosis is clinical and no specific test has been validated, although many have been reported. C1-esterase inhibitor levels have potential diagnostic value as extremely low levels have been demonstrated in patients with AFE [39].

Treatment involves cardiovascular resuscitation and support, including mechanical ventilation and inotropic therapy. Extracorporeal life-support may also play a role in managing oxygenation and hemodynamics [40]. Following the hypothesis that the process involves an anaphylactoid reaction to amniotic fluid contents, a role for corticosteroids has been suggested [35]. Survivors of the initial process may develop DIC and acute respiratory distress syndrome (ARDS). Neurologic damage caused by the initial hypotension and hypoxemia is common.

10.6.3 Obstetric Hemorrhage

Obstetric hemorrhage requires supportive management in keeping with any massive hemorrhage. This includes rapid volume replacement, supplemental oxygen administration, red cell transfusion, and management of any dilutional coagulopathy with FFP, platelets, and fibrinogen transfusion [41]. This may be best carried out using an institutional massive transfusion protocol. Complications of obstetric hemorrhage include acute kidney injury, myocardial ischemia, and DIC [42].

In addition to blood product resuscitation, various pharmacologic agents are used to control uterine bleeding. Tranexamic acid, an antifibrinolytic agent, can be safely used in pregnancy and should be administered in a dose of 1 g intravenously within 3 h of onset of hemorrhage, with a repeat dose if bleeding does not settle within 30 min [43]. High-dose intravenous oxytocin infusion is commonly used, up to 100 mU/min (e.g., 40 U in 1,000 mL normal saline at 150 mL/h). At these high doses, oxytocin can produce an antidiuretic effect and resulting hyponatremia. A prostaglandin F_{2a} analogue (carboprost tromethamine, Hemabate) given intramuscularly or intramyometrially in a dose of 0.25 mg (repeated every 15–90 min to maximum 2 mg) is effective in treating atony and controlling hemorrhage. Side effects include bronchoconstriction (therefore contraindicated in severe asthma), vomiting, diarrhea, and increased intrapulmonary shunt [44–46]. Methylergonovine (0.2 mg IM) may also be useful in the presence of uterine atony but is contraindicated in women with hypertension.

Additional options in the management of severe postpartum hemorrhage include interventional and surgical management. Intrauterine balloon devices may be placed to tamponade bleeding, with high success rates [47]. Consideration should be given to antibiotic prophylaxis while the balloon is in place and analgesia is essential. If the above methods fail to control bleeding, radiologic embolization of the internal iliac or uterine artery, or surgical exploration with arterial ligation may be necessary [48]. Laparotomy and hysterectomy may become necessary as a life-saving procedure.

10.6.4 Tocolytic Pulmonary Edema

β-Adrenergic agonists can be administered to inhibit uterine contractions in pre-term labor, although this practice is less frequent due to evidence regarding a lack of fetal benefit. A complication of this β-agonist therapy in pregnancy is the development of acute pulmonary edema, the mechanisms of which are not clear [49]. Treatment involves discontinuing the β-agonist and supportive treatment with diuresis, oxygen therapy, and occasionally mechanical ventilation. If the pulmonary edema does not resolve within 24 h, an alternative diagnosis should be sought.

10.7 Conditions Not Specific to Pregnancy

10.7.1 Acute Respiratory Distress Syndrome in Pregnancy

ARDS is the clinical expression of diverse processes causing lung injury, and is characterized by hypoxemia and bilateral pulmonary infiltrates (non-cardiogenic pulmonary edema) in the absence of left heart failure. The pregnant patient may develop ARDS from pregnancy-associated complications (e.g., AFE and preeclampsia) as well as other conditions (e.g., sepsis, pneumonia, and aspiration) [50]. The pregnant patient appears to develop ARDS more frequently than the nonpregnant patient, likely due to their increased blood volume, the reduced albumin level occurring in pregnancy, increased capillary leak, and a degree of upregulation of components of the acute inflammatory response [51].

Little data are available to direct management of ARDS in pregnancy, and a similar approach to the nonpregnant patient is used. Adequate maternal oxygenation is important for fetal well-being, and is addressed with supplemental oxygen administration and mechanical ventilation with positive end-expiratory pressure (discussed above). Survival from ARDS during pregnancy is as good as or better than that in the general population, likely because of these patients' young age, lack of comorbidity, and the reversibility of many of the predisposing conditions. Delivery is often considered and may improve the maternal condition in some, but not all cases, and should usually be reserved for situations where the fetus is likely also to benefit.

10.7.2 Thyroid Storm

Thyroid storm during pregnancy is uncommon, but occurs at a higher rate in hyperthyroid pregnant women than in the nonpregnant hyperthyroid population. It can lead to adverse maternal and fetal outcomes including abruption, preeclampsia, maternal heart failure, intrauterine fetal demise, and maternal death [52]. It occurs most commonly in women with known hyperthyroidism who are exposed to a stressor (e.g., labor and delivery, surgery including cesarean section, or severe infection), or in the context of a gestational trophoblastic neoplasm (GTN), in which the high levels of βHCG stimulate the thyroid gland [56, 57]. Presentation is with hyperthermia, tachycardia, and agitation or other central nervous system findings [53]. Close monitoring and supportive measures are essential, including the careful administration of IV fluids (noting that heart failure may occur), antipyretics and oxygen.

Pharmacologic treatment follows similar guidelines as in the nonpregnant individual with acute symptom control with beta-blockade, a thionamide (propylthiouracil preferred during the first trimester, or methimazole preferred after first trimester), a concentrated iodide, and corticosteroids [54, 55]. Unless deemed necessary, delivery should be delayed until after the patient has been stabilized, however, in the case of GTN-associated thyrotoxicosis, evacuation of the uterus is also an essential step in definitive management [55, 56]. Anesthesia for evacuation can precipitate thyroid storm, so preoperative beta-blockers should be administered. Plamsapheresis has been used for rapid control of thyroid hormone excess, particularly when usual pharmacological therapy is not tolerated [57].

10.7.3 Trauma

Trauma is a leading cause of non-obstetric maternal death [58]. Due to the anatomic and physiologic changes which occur during pregnancy, the manifestations and severity of traumatic injury may be altered as compared to a nonpregnant trauma patient. Penetrating abdominal injuries predominantly affect the uterus in late pregnancy, while the intraabdominal viscera are compressed and relatively protected. However, due to this compression of organs, even minor upper abdominal injury can result in significant visceral injury [59]. Due to the high uterine blood flow in late pregnancy, severe hemorrhage can occur as a result of uterine injury. Uterine injury may also precipitate placental abruption or rarely uterine rupture. Uterine rupture presents with maternal shock, abdominal pain, and palpable fetal parts abdominally. Pelvic fractures can result in severe retroperitoneal hemorrhage due to the marked dilation of pelvic veins.

Maternal trauma is also associated with fetal risks including fetal loss, due to direct fetal or placental injury, or due to maternal shock or hypoxia. Placental abruption is the most common cause of fetal demise in blunt trauma, and may present with vaginal bleeding or fluid leakage, abdominal cramps or uterine tenderness, and fetal distress or maternal hypovolemic shock [60]. DIC is also commonly associated with placental abruption due to release of thromboplastin into the maternal circulation. Transplacental fetomaternal hemorrhage may occur and can result in fetal exsanguination and maternal Rh sensitization. Blunt maternal trauma may cause direct fetal injury, usually involving fetal head injury associated with maternal pelvic fractures. Maternal burns to greater than 30% of the body surface area is associated with high fetal mortality.

Evaluation of the pregnant trauma patient requires a detailed abdominal examination, bearing in mind the altered position of organs and the reduced peritoneal sensitivity that occurs in pregnancy [61]. Initial investigations should include blood type including Rh status and a Kleihauer–Betke test, which identifies and quantifies fetal cells in the maternal blood film, and can estimate the volume of fetal hemorrhage. Fetal evaluation includes heart rate assessment by auscultation or Doppler probe. When the fetus is known or estimated to be at a viable gestation, obstetric consultation and continuous fetal cardiotocography are important. Ultrasound is useful both for evaluation of the fetus for injury and biophysical profile, and to assess for maternal intraabdominal injuries. Ultrasound-guided paracentesis or diagnostic peritoneal lavage (by open technique, above the uterus) may aid in detecting bowel perforation or intraperitoneal hemorrhage.

A multidisciplinary approach is essential in the care of the severely injured pregnant patient involving the emergency physician, trauma surgeon, obstetrician, intensivist, and neonatologist. Initial efforts should follow usual resuscitation principles and be directed at stabilizing the mother, as correction of maternal hemodynamics is beneficial to the fetus. Uterine blood flow will be markedly reduced when maternal circulation is compromised and the fetus is extremely vulnerable to hypotension and hypoxemia. Maternal blood pressure and heart rate may not be reliable predictors of the degree of hemorrhage, and fluid replacement may need to be given more rapidly than in nonpregnant women because of the physiologic increase in plasma volume [61]. Left lateral positioning is an important consideration in the hypotensive patient to prevent supine hypotensive syndrome. All Rh-negative mothers with abdominal trauma should receive Rh immune globulin even with a negative Kleihauer-Betke test, and additional doses of Rh immune globulin may be necessary in the presence of significant fetomaternal hemorrhage.

Management of maternal injuries takes precedence over fetal distress. Caesarean section may be an option if the fetus is considered viable, in the stable mother with severe injury, and also in the unsalvageable mother. The limits of viability are largely dependent on the level of neonatal care available. Resuscitative caesarean section may be considered in the unsalvageable mother with a potentially viable fetus.

References

[1]   Elkus R, Popovich J. Respiratory physiology in pregnancy. Clin Chest Med 1992;13:555–565.
[2]   Marx GF, Murthy PK, Orkin LR. Static compliance before and after vaginal delivery. Br J Anaesth 1970;42:1100–1104.

[3]   Rees GB, Pipkin FB, Symonds EM, Patrick JM. A longitudinal study of respiratory c changes in normal human pregnancy with cross-sectional data on subjects with pregnancy- induced hypertension. Am J Obstet Gynecol 1990;162:826–830.

[4]   Green LJ, Mackillop LH, Salvi D et al. Gestation-specific vital sign reference ranges in pregnancy. Obstet Gynecol 2020;135(3):653–664.

[5]   Mabie WC, DiSessa TG, Crocker LG et al. A longitudinal study of cardiac output in normal human pregnancy. Am J Obstet Gynecol 1994;170:849–856.

[6]   Robson SC, Dunlop W, Boys RJ, Hunter S. Cardiac output during labour. BMJ 1987;295: 1169–1171.

[7]   Kinsella SM, Lohmann G. Supine hypotensive syndrome. Obstet Gynecol 1994;83:774–788.

[8]   Pollock W, Rose L, Dennis CL. Pregnant and postpartum admissions to the intensive care unit: A systematic review. Intensive Care Med 2010;36:1465–1474.

[9]   Royal College of Anaesthetists: Care of the Critically Ill Woman in Childbirth: Enhanced Maternal Care. 2018. Available at: https://www.rcoa.ac.uk/sites/default/files/documents/ 2019-09/EMC-Guidelines2018.pdf. Accessed January 16, 2020

[10] Aoyama K, D'Souza R, Pinto R et al. Risk prediction models for maternal mortality: A systematic review and meta-analysis. PLoS One 2018;13:e0208563.

[11] Payne BA, Ryan H, Bone J et al.;. CIPHER Group: Development and internal validation of the multivariable CIPHER (Collaborative Integrated Pregnancy High-dependency Estimate of Risk) clinical risk prediction model. Crit Care 2018;22:278.

[12] Souza JP, Cecatti JG, Haddad SM et al.;. Brazilian Network for Surveillance of Severe Maternal Morbidity Group; Brazilian Network for Surveillance of Severe Maternal Morbidity: The WHO maternal near-miss approach and the maternal severity index model (MSI): Tools for assessing the management of severe maternal morbidity. PLoS One 2012;7:e44129.

[13] Carle C, Alexander P, Columb M et al. Design and internal validation of an obstetric early warning score: Secondary analysis of the intensive care national audit and research centre case mix programme database. Anaesthesia 2013;68:354–367.

[14] Simpson NB, Shankar-Hari M, Rowan KM et al. Maternal Risk Modeling in Critical Care – Development of a Multivariable Risk Prediction Model for Death and Prolonged Intensive Care. Crit Care Med 2020;48:663–672.

[15] Dolovich LR, Addis A, Vaillancourt JM, Power JD, Koren G, Einarson TR. Benzodiazepine use in pregnancy and major malformations or oral cleft: Meta-analysis of cohort and case-control studies. BMJ 1998;317:839–843.

[16] Vigod SN, Dennis CL. Benzodiazepines and the Z-Drugs in Pregnancy-Reasonably Reassuring for Neurodevelopment But Should We Really Be Using Them?. JAMA Netw Open 2019;2(4): e191430.

[17] Hilton G, Andrzejowski JC. Prolonged propofol infusions in pregnant neurosurgical patients. J Neurosurg Anesthesiol 2007;19:67–68.

[18] Guay J, Grenier Y, Varin F. Clinical pharmacokinetics of neuromuscular relaxants in pregnancy. Clin Pharmacokinet 1998;34:483.

[19] Al-Ansari MA, Hameed AA,
      Al-Jawder SE et al. Use of noninvasive positive pressure ventilation in pregnancy: Case series. Ann Thoracic Medicine 2007;2:23–25.

[20] Archer GW, Marx GF. Arterial oxygen tension during apnoea in parturient women. Br J Anaesth 1974;46:358–360.

[21] Kodali BS, Chandrasekhar S, Bulich LN, Topulos GP, Datta S. Airway changes during labor and delivery. Anesthesiology 2008;108:357–362.

[22] Buss DD, Bisgard GE, Rawlings CA, Rankin JH. Uteroplacental blood flow during alkalosis in the sheep. Am J Physiol 1975;228:1497–1500.

[23] Tomimatsu T, Kakigano A, Mimura K et al. Maternal carbon dioxide level during labor and its possible effect on fetal cerebral oxygenation: Mini review. J Obstet Gynaecol Res 2013;39: 1–6.

[24] Fraser D, Jensen D, Wolfe LA, Hahn PM, Davies GAL. Fetal heart rate response to maternal hypocapnia and hypercapnia in late gestation. J Obstet Gynaecol Can 2008;30:312–316.

[25] Elsayegh D, Shapiro JM. Management of the obstetric patient with status asthmaticus. J Intensive Care Med 2008;23:396–402.

[26] Low JA, Panagiotopoulos C, Derrick EJ. Newborn complications after intrapartum asphyxia with metabolic acidosis in the term fetus. Am J Obstet Gynecol 1994;170:1081–1087.

[27] Cole DE, Taylor TL, McCullough DM et al. Acute respiratory distress syndrome in pregnancy. Cr7it Care Med 2005;33:S269–78.

[28] Aoyama K, Seaward PG, Lapinsky SE. Fetal outcome in the critically ill pregnant woman. Crit Care 2014;18:307.

[29] Raghuraman N, Temming LA, Stout MJ, Macones GA, Cahill AG, Tuuli MG. Intrauterine hyperoxemia and risk of neonatal morbidity. Obstet Gynecol 2017;129:676–682.

[30] Hamel MS, Anderson BL, Rouse DJ. Oxygen for intrauterine resuscitation: Of unproved benefit and potentially harmful. Am J Obstet Gynecol 2014;211:124–127.

[31] Lapinsky SE, Rojas-Suarez JA, Crozier TM et al. Mechanical ventilation in critically-ill pregnant women: A case series. Int J Obstet Anesth 2015;24(4):323–328.

[32] Nelson DB, Byrne JJ, Cunningham FG. Acute Fatty Liver of Pregnancy. Obstet Gynecol 2021Mar1;137(3):535–546.

[33] Ibdah JA, Bennett MJ, Rinaldo P et al. A fetal fatty-acid oxidation disorder as a cause of liver disease in pregnant women. N Engl J Med 1999;340:1723–1731.

[34] Rudra A, Chatterjee S, Sengupta S, Nandi B, Mitra J. Amniotic fluid embolism. Indian J Crit Care Med 2009;13(3):129–135. doi: 10.4103/0972-5229.58537.

[35] Clark SL, Hankins GD, Dudley DA et al. Amniotic fluid embolism: Analysis of the national registry. Am J Obstet Gynecol 1995;172:1158–1167.

[36] Kaur K, Bhardwaj M, Kumar P, Singhal S, Singh T, Hooda S. Amniotic fluid embolism. J Anaesthesiol Clin Pharmacol 2016;32(2):153–159. doi: 10.4103/0970-9185.173356.

[37] Clark SL, Cotton DB, Gonik B et al. Central hemodynamic alterations in amniotic fluid embolism. Am J Obstet Gynecol 1988;158:1124–1126.

[38] Conde-Agudelo A, Romero R. Amniotic fluid embolism: An evidence-based review. Am J Obstet Gynecol 2009;201(5):445e441–e413.

[39] Tamura N1, Kimura S, Farhana M et al. C1 esterase inhibitor activity in amniotic fluid embolism. Crit Care Med 2014;42:1392–1396.

[40] Viau-Lapointe J, Filewod N. Extracorporeal therapies for amniotic fluid embolism. Obstet Gynecol 2019;134:989–994.

[41] Segal S, Shemesh IY, Blumenthal R. Treatment of obstetric hemorrhage with recombinant activated factor VII (rFVIIa). Arch Gynecol Obstet 2003;268:266–267.

[42] Karpati PC, Rossignol M, Pirot M, Cholley B, Vicaut E, Henry P et al. High incidence of myocardial ischemia during postpartum hemorrhage. Anesthesiology 2004;100(1):30–36.

[43] WOMAN Trial Collaborators. Effect of early tranexamic acid administration on mortality, hysterectomy, and other morbidities in women with post-partum haemorrhage (WOMAN): An international, randomised, double-blind, placebo-controlled trial. Lancet 2017;389: 2105–2116.

[44] Shevell T, Malone FD. Management of obstetric hemorrhage. Semin Perinatol 2003;27: 86–104.

[45] Hayashi RH, Castillo MS, Noah ML. Management of severe postpartum hemorrhage with a prostaglandin F_{2a} analogue. Obstet Gynecol 1984;63:806–814.

[46] Gallos ID et al. Uterotonic agents for preventing postpartum haemorrhage: A network meta-analysis. Cochrane Database Syst Rev 2018Dec19;12(12):CD011689.

[47] Georgiou C. Balloon tamponade in the management of postpartum haemorrhage: A review. BJOG 2009;116:748.

[48] Hansch E, Chitkara U, McAlpine J et al. Pelvic arterial embolization for control of obstetric hemorrhage: A five-year experience. Am J Obstet Gynecol 1999;180:1454–1460.

[49] Pisani RJ, Rosenow EC. 3rd. Pulmonary edema associated with tocolytic therapy. Ann Intern Med 1989;110:714–718.

[50] Bandi VD, Munnur U, Matthay MA. Acute lung injury and acute respiratory distress syndrome in pregnancy. Crit Care Clin 2004;20:577–607.

[51] Lapinsky SE. Pregnancy joins the hit list. Crit Care Med 2012;40(5):1679–1680.

[52] Krajewski DA, Burman KD. Thyroid disorders in pregnancy. Endocrinol Metab Clin North Am 2011;40(4):739–763. doi: 10.1016/j.ecl.2011.08.004PMID: 22108278.

[53] Burch HB, Wartofsky L Life-threatening thyrotoxicosis. Thyroid storm Endocrinol Metab Clin North Am 1993Jun 222 263–277PMID: 8325286.

[54] Molitch ME. Endocrine emergencies in pregnancy. Baillieres Clin Endocrinol Metab 1992Jan;6(1):167–191. doi: 10.1016/s0950-351x(05)80337-4PMID: 1739393.

[55] Thyroid Disease in Pregnancy. ACOG Practice Bulletin, Number 223. Obstet Gynecol 2020Jun;135(6):e261–e274. doi: 10.1097/AOG.0000000000003893. PMID: 32443080.

[56] Pereira JV, Lim T. Hyperthyroidism in gestational trophoblastic disease – a literature review. Thyroid Res 2021;14(1):1. doi: 10.1186/s13044-021-00092-3. PMID: 33446242; PMCID: PMC7807451.

[57] Adali E, Yildizhan R, Kolusari A, Kurdoglu M, Turan N. The use of plasmapheresis for rapid hormonal control in severe hyperthyroidism caused by a partial molar pregnancy. Arch Gynecol Obstet 2009;279:569–571.

[58] El-Kady D, Gilbert WM, Anderson J, Danielsen B, Towner D, Smith LH. Trauma during pregnancy: An analysis of maternal and fetal outcomes in a large population. Am J Obstet Gynecol 2004;190(6):1661–1668.

[59] Pearlman MD, Tintinalli JE, Lorenz RP. A prospective controlled study of outcome after trauma during pregnancy. Am J Obstet Gynecol 1990;162:665–671.

[60] Drost TF, Rosemurgy AS, Sherman HF et al. Major trauma in pregnant women: Maternal/fetal outcome. J Trauma 1990;30:574–578.

[61] Pearlman MD, Tintinalli JE, Lorenz RP. Blunt trauma during pregnancy. N Engl J Med 1990;323: 1609–1613.

[62] Fitzgerald JP, Fedoruk KA, Jadin SM, Carvalho B, Halpern SH. Prevention of hypotension after spinal anaesthesia for caesarean section: A systematic review and network meta-analysis of randomised controlled trials. Anaesthesia 2020 Jan;75:109–121.

[63] Mohta M, Aggarwal M, Sethi AK, Harisinghani P, Guleria K. Randomized double-blind comparison of ephedrine and phenylephrine for management of post-spinal hypotension in potential fetal compromise. Int J Obstet Anesth 2016;27:32–40.

Dina Refaat, Mohamed Momtaz

11 Amniotic Fluid Embolism

11.1 Introduction

Let us be careful not to make it (the diagnosis of amniotic fluid embolism) a waste-basket for all cases of unexplained death in labor. [1]

N. J. Eastman, 1 1948
Editor of Williams Obstetrics (1950–1966)

11.1.1 History

Amniotic fluid embolism (AFE) is a rare catastrophic obstetric emergency, which can be a significant cause of maternal mortality [2, 3]. The first physician who described a case that matches the description of AFE was Matthew Baillie in 1789, as he reported a case of a multiparous female, with uterine rupture near the round ligament, who died suddenly before delivery. He explained the possibility of amniotic fluid entry into the maternal system through an anatomic connection between mother and fetus [4].

Subsequently, Ricardo Meyer reported this condition in 1926 as he described the presence of fetal cellular debris in maternal circulation [5]. In spite of its early discovery, it was not until 1941 when AFE was recognized as a syndrome by Steiner and Lushbaugh. They performed an autopsy series on 42 women who died during delivery of sudden shock. The autopsies of eight of the included mortalities showed fetal mucin and squamous cells in the pulmonary vasculature [6].

In 1949, Shotton and Taylor published a case report of pulmonary embolism caused by amniotic fluid [7]. They described the clinical presentation as sudden onset of profound shock, dyspnea, cyanosis, and pulmonary edema. The onset was closely related to labor, uterine contractions, or shortly after delivery, which resulted in stillbirth as well as maternal mortality within minutes to hours. The authors emphasized the importance of maternal autopsy in reaching a definitive diagnosis, depending on illustrating the presence of amniotic fluid, containing fetal particulates, in pulmonary, as well as uterine and cerebral vessels.

AFE was not listed as a separate cause of maternal mortality until 1957 when it was defined as obstetric shock. Since then, more and more cases have been documented, probably as a result of an increased awareness.

https://doi.org/10.1515/9783110615258-011

11.1.2 Definition

The International Network of Obstetric Survey Systems is a collaboration of over 15 countries conducting prospective population-based studies of uncommon and severe complications in pregnancy and childbirth using comparable surveillance systems [8]. They defined AFE as an acute cardiorespiratory collapse within 6 h after labor, or ruptured membranes, with no other identifiable cause, followed by acute coagulopathy in those women who survive the initial event.

Clark and colleagues [9] proposed a structured definition of AFE for research purposes. This definition is based on the presence of four diagnostic criteria, all of which must be present:

1. Sudden onset of cardiorespiratory arrest or both hypotension (systolic blood pressure <90 mmHg) and respiratory compromise (dyspnea, cyanosis, or peripheral capillary oxygen saturation <90%).
2. Documentation of overt disseminated intravascular coagulation (DIC) after appearance of these initial signs or symptoms, using the scoring system of the Scientific and Standardization Committee on DIC of the International Society on Thrombosis and Hemostasis, modified for pregnancy. Coagulopathy must be detected before loss of sufficient blood loss, since massive hemorrhage itself can lead to dilutional or shock-related consumptive coagulopathy.
3. Clinical onset during labor or within 30 min of delivery of placenta.
4. No fever (≥38 °C) during labor.

The UK Obstetric Surveillance System [10] suggested another definition, which is: In the absence of any other clear cause, *either* acute maternal collapse with one or more of the following features: acute fetal compromise, cardiac arrest, cardiac rhythm problems, coagulopathy hypotension, maternal hemorrhage, premonitory symptoms (i.e., restlessness, numbness, agitation, tingling), seizure, shortness of breath, excluding women with maternal hemorrhage as the first presenting feature in whom there was no evidence of early coagulopathy *or* cardiorespiratory compromise or women in whom the diagnosis was made at postmortem examination with the finding of fetal squames or hair in the lungs.

11.1.3 Incidence

It is difficult to estimate the correct incidence of AFE but it is said to be in the range from 1 in 8,000 to 1 in 80,000 pregnancies [11, 12]. The reported incidences ranged from 1.9 cases per 100,000 maternities (UK) to 6.1 per 100,000 maternities (Australia), which can vary considerably, depending on the period, region of study, and the definition [3, 13].

11.2 Risk Factors

There are no specific risk factors that were proved to cause AFE. However, historically, both Steiner and Lushbaugh described certain factors to be more linked to cases of AFE as; multiparity, increased maternal age, and hyper stimulated labor. Others have suggested that saline amnioinfusion, complicated labor, the use of oxytocin, advanced gestational age of the fetus, and vaginal prostaglandins can be considered as additional factors that increase the occurrence of AFE [6].

Clark et al. found no recognizable maternal risk factor related to the incidence of AFE, although the vast majority of patients with AFE experienced it during labor or immediately after delivery [14].

11.3 Pathophysiology

There are two main theories that were suggested to explain the AFE:

The first one is based historically on the hypothesis of the occlusion of the pulmonary arteries by amniotic fluid or fetal debris [3, 15]. But owing to the advancement in pulmonary artery catheterization by 1980, more arterial histologic specimens from living patients were obtained [3]. This subsequently led to several reports of pathologic findings, which were previously thought to be diagnostic of AFE, were also found in pregnant women who did not actually have AFE. These reports doubted the previously diagnosed AFE cases, as they were exclusively dependent on pathologic findings.

The second and more commonly accepted theory is that when AFE enters the circulation, it causes an initiation of a series of complex reactions involving an abnormal activation of pro-inflammatory mediators in the host leading to an immunologic response [3, 13, 15]. This reaction mimics the systemic inflammatory response syndrome. Amniotic fluid contains various procoagulant factors including platelet-activating factor, leukotrienes, bradykinin, cytokines, thromboxane, and arachidonic acid, which can explain why DIC is observed in 80% or more of women diagnosed with AFE [3, 10, 16]. In association with these responses, severe circulatory changes cause maternal collapse and death in patients with AFE. Consequently, during the first minutes, an abrupt rise in pulmonary vascular resistance as a result of an inflammatory/anaphylactoid vasoconstriction leads to a right ventricular dysfunction and dilatation, leading to left shift of the interventricular septum and lowering of the left ventricular filling pressures, resulting in hypotension and cardiovascular collapse [17]. This severe pulmonary vasoconstriction produces an oxygen shunt, with ventilation–perfusion mismatching and severe hypoxia. Additionally, left ventricular failure may occur as a result of myocardial injury secondary to either inflammatory mediators or myocardial ischemia [18]. Complement activation is thought to have a role in the pathophysiology of AFE. Hypothetically, all patients diagnosed with AFE develop some degree of acute respiratory distress syndrome. Many case series evaluating serum complement levels in patients with AFE have reported marked drop in the levels of C3 and C4 compared to a control group of normal parturient females [16]. Decreased levels of C3 are thought to be consistent with complement activation.

Owing to the marked similarity between amniotic fluid embolism and anaphylaxis, Clarke et al. have suggested a synonym of the syndrome as "anaphylactoid syndrome of pregnancy" [14].

11.4 Clinical Presentations

The classical presentation of AFE includes a triad of sudden hypoxia and hypotension, followed in many cases by coagulopathy, all occurring in relation to labor and delivery [14].

Cases of AFE typically pass by series of events:

1. Initially, a period of anxiety, change in mental status, agitation, and a sensation of doom may precede the event [19].
2. Then, patients may progress to cardiac arrest, with pulseless electrical activity, asystole, ventricular fibrillation, or pulseless ventricular tachycardia. In cases occurring prior to delivery, electronic fetal monitoring will demonstrate decelerations, loss of variability, and terminal bradycardia as oxygenated blood is shifted away from the uterus, and catecholamine induced hypertonic uterus causes more decline in uterine perfusion [3, 9].

11.5 Diagnosis

International criteria for diagnosis of AFE are:

United Kingdom and Australia:
Clinical diagnosis of AFE (acute hypotension or cardiac arrest, acute hypoxia, or coagulopathy in the absence of any other potential explanation for signs and symptoms observed) or pathologic diagnosis of fetal squames or hair in lungs [20, 21].

Japan:
1. Symptoms appeared during pregnancy or within 12 h of delivery.
2. Intensive medical intervention was conducted to treat one of the following symptoms/diseases: (a) cardiac arrest, (b) severe bleeding of unknown origin within 2 h of delivery (>1,500 mL), (c) DIC, or (d) respiratory failure.
3. If findings or symptoms obtained could not be explained by other diseases, consumptive coagulopathy/DIC due to evident etiologies such as abnormal

placentation, trauma during labor, and severe preeclampsia/eclampsia should be excluded [22].

11.6 Differential Diagnosis

There is a long list of conditions that may result in either acute cardiac or respiratory or hematological failure in pregnancy, which includes myocardial infarction, pulmonary embolism, air embolism, anesthetic complications, anaphylaxis, and eclampsia and in some cases sepsis [23].

11.6.1 Myocardial Infarction

When considering this diagnosis, there are a number of risk factors such as advanced maternal age, diabetes, chronic hypertension, smoking, obesity, dyslipidemia, and a previous history of coronary artery disease that are usually present in the patient's history. Urgent quantification of cardiac troponins and a 12 lead electrocardiograph should be obtained. Echocardiography may be helpful in diagnosing cardiac shock (resulting from myocardial ischemia) as well as ruling out conditions such as a peripartum dilated cardiomyopathy [24].

11.6.2 Pulmonary Embolism

It is also a complication that is closely linked to pregnancy. Computed tomography angiography or a ventilation perfusion scan may be useful in eliminating this possibility. However, if the condition is associated with severe hemorrhage, it is highly unlikely to be associated with thromboembolism [23].

11.6.3 Anesthetic Complications

- *High spinal anesthesia* may cause apnea but is unlikely to cause a marked drop in cardiac output or hemorrhagic manifestations [25].
- *Unintended intravascular injection of local anesthetics* may result in convulsions as well as cardiovascular collapse. The timing between injection and onset of symptoms is essential to establish this diagnosis [26].

11.6.4 Air Embolism

It may also cause acute cardiorespiratory compromise. It may be venous or arterial [23].

11.6.5 Eclampsia

It is a very common possibility in a patient in the second half of pregnancy with new-onset seizures, although eclampsia does not usually present with cardiorespiratory arrest and acute profound coagulopathy [23].

11.6.6 Transfusion Reactions

Complications of blood transfusion may simulate the clinical presentation of AFE as incompatible blood transfusion may result in coagulopathy, and acute pulmonary edema can be related to the condition "transfusion related acute lung injury" [23].

11.6.7 Anaphylactic Shock

It is a potential cause especially when the patient presents with urticarial rash, and laryngospasm or bronchospasm immediately following the administration of medication known to cause anaphylaxis. In cases of AFE, bronchospasm has been reported in about 15%. To differentiate between the two conditions, anaphylaxis is not usually accompanied by coagulopathy, and cardiac dysfunction is not usually profound as hypotension associated with anaphylaxis is mainly due to vasodilation and increased vascular permeability [23].

11.7 Management

As AFE diagnosis is based on exclusion of a long list of possible causes, physicians caring for pregnant females with an acute clinical event or cardiorespiratory failure should attempt to quickly shorten this list to clinically relevant diagnoses that require specific treatment strategies. It is crucial to know that the exact diagnosis is not required to start treatment, as the suggested treatment for AFE is basically supportive measures [23].

The principal steps for successful management of AFE include early diagnosis, aggressive cardiovascular support, treatment of hypoxia, management of hemorrhage and coagulopathy, and delivery of the fetus [10].

In 2015, the society of maternal neonatal medicine guidelines and the consensus statement from the Society for Obstetric Anesthesia and Perinatology [23, 27] pointed out the importance of *immediate delivery of the fetus*. They suggested a delivery in less than 5 min from maternal circulatory collapse (perimortom cesarean delivery) [24]; this would lower the fetal morbidity and improve maternal outcomes by alleviating the aorto-caval compression by the gravid uterus [28].

Although a number of new therapeutic modalities have been suggested for cardiovascular collapse secondary to AFE as extracorporeal membrane oxygenation [29–31], cardiopulmonary bypass [17], intra-aortic balloon pump [31], pulmonary artery thromboembolectomy [32], hemofiltration [33], and plasma exchange transfusions [34], still there is no evidence to support the beneficial outcomes of these procedures.

One of the most common presentations of AFE is severe bleeding. In this condition, aggressive transfusion protocols should be commenced. Transfusion should be initiated with O negative RBC without delay [35].

Prevention and treatment of *coagulopathy* requires early and ongoing administration of fresh frozen plasma (FFP), platelets, and cryoprecipitate. The optimal RBC to FFP ratio is not known, but given the associated coagulopathy with AFE, a 1:1–1.5 ratio may be preferable [35, 36]. Uncontrolled hemorrhage may require hysterectomy as a life-saving procedure [15].

Hemorrhage may also result from amniotic fluid-induced thrombocytopenia [3], that is why platelet transfusions should be started immediately. Fibrinogen is also an essential element for hemostasis and is the first coagulation factor to decrease in obstetric hemorrhage. Its levels can be used as a predictor of severity of obstetric hemorrhage; *hypofibrinogenemia* have been found in cases of AFE [36, 37]. The most appropriate replacement would be cryoprecipitate and/or human plasma-derived fibrinogen concentrates. For early diagnosis of hypofibrinogenemia, rotational thromboelastometry has been recently introduced (ROTEM, Tem International, Munich, Germany). It is a visco-elastometric method used to explore plasma coagulation. It is used to fasten the diagnosis if compared with standard hemostasis testing (such as prothrombin time or activated thrombin time. It provides the results as a bedside test within approximately 10 min, compared to 1 h for traditional testing. This aids in an early diagnosis of AFE, prediction of subsequent severe PPH, initiating good venous access, extra manpower, and the early administration of fibrinogen concentrate, tranexamic acid, and prostaglandins when PPH started [38, 39].

As antifibrinolytics agents have proved to be effective in control of non-AFE obstetric hemorrhage, their use has been described in cases of hemorrhage secondary to AFE [40]. On the contrary, a recent review of the use of recombinant factor VIIa in cases with AFE demonstrated poorer outcomes and increased mortality, consequently, it is currently not recommended for routine use [41].

On the other hand, some cases might present with *coagulopathy*, which is not an uncommon complication. Antithrombin concentrates have previously been proposed, and may lead to improved outcomes in patients with AFE-associated coagulopathy [42]. Heparin has also been proposed in these cases; however, owing to the great risk of massive hemorrhage in cases of AFE, heparin is currently not a recommended treatment [36].

If *uterine atony* occurs in a case of AFE, standard pharmacologic interventions should be commenced including oxytocin, carboprost tromethamine, methylergonovine, and misoprostol, and surgical interventions including Bakri balloon tamponade, uterine artery ligation/embolization, B-lynch suture, or hysterectomy as required [43].

Based on the *anaphylactic impact* of the AFE, plasma exchange has been used as a method to eliminate chemical mediators and cytokines responsible for the anaphylactoid response [44]. High-dose corticosteroid treatment may be used for presumed inflammatory-mediated anaphylactoid response [17]. Another novel treatment is the use of synthetic C1 esterase inhibitors (C1NH) [45]. C1NHs inhibit C1 esterase, Factor XIIa, and complement activation; low levels of C1NH may play a role in development of AFE. Kanayama and Tamura [36] found that women with AFE had decreased serum levels of C1NH, which responded to treatment with FFP, which contains C1NH.

11.8 Complications

Mortality and case fatality mortality ratios ranged from 0.4 per 100,000 live births in the Netherlands from 1993 to 2005 to 1.3 per 100,000 live births in the United States in 1997–2001 and 1.1 in Australia excluding Victoria in 1994–2005. Case-fatality rates ranged from 11% to 43% [13].

Owing to the marked improvement in resuscitation methods, the maternal mortality rates have dramatically decreased in developed countries over the past 30 years. Despite the decline in the maternal mortality rates, still the maternal and fetal morbidity are quite high [10].

11.8.1 Maternal Complications

The majority of patients with AFE (85%) showed mental status changes and encephalopathy with temporary or permanent neurologic complications [14]. Neurological complications included cerebral injury, which was noted in 6% of women with AFE in the UK, and cerebral infarction, occurred in 20% of women with AFE in New South Wales. Although seizures were very common in Clark's analysis of the national registry (30%) [46], in more recent studies the rate of recorded seizure-like activity was only 2.22%, which is still higher than the seizure rate for total obstetric population (0.03%) [47].

Cardiopulmonary arrest rates were reported by Clark et al. to be 87% [14], while in more recent study, the cardiac arrest and other cardiac complications rates were 22.22%. Obstetric shock was observed in 15.56% cases. Regarding Coagulopathy, including DIC, occurred in 66% of patients in a recent study from Gilber and Danielsen [46].

11.8.2 Fetal Complications

Reports from published literature showed poor neonatal outcomes, such as UK registry where only 78% of neonates survived [11], also Clark et al. demonstrated a similar (79%) survival rate with only 50% of the fetuses that survived being neurologically intact [14]. However, reports from a more recent study showed an improvement in the survival to be nearly 97.77% [47].

This markedly improved fetal survival rates could be attributed not only to improved healthcare but also to the inclusion of milder cases of AFE in our database when compared to reporting the outcomes of most severe cases in the published case series. The diagnosis of a "mild" or "atypical" case has been proposed in several case reports and is based on milder symptomatology such as transient headache, increased uterine bleeding during a vaginal delivery or a caesarean section, evidence of coagulopathy and presence of increased numbers of fetal blood cells in the maternal circulation [48–50].

Improvements in medical care have subsequently improved neonatal outcomes, which were reflected in a recent report by the National Centre for Health Statistics (NCHS). The NCHS reports that over the more recent period, 1990–2001, the infant mortality rate declined 26% (from 9.2 to 6.8 per 1,000) for an average decrease of 3% per year [51]. The rates of NICU admission were significantly increased in neonates born to mothers with AFE, with nearly 49% of neonates admitted.

A recent study reported a significant decrease in maternal and infant morbidity and mortality. This could be due to the reporting of "milder" cases and improvements in perinatal healthcare [47]. With recent advances in intensive care, better outcomes are expected in the future, while more studies are still needed to discover the pathophysiology and risk factors behind the AFE.

References

[1]   Eastman NJ. Editorial comment. Obstet Gynecol Surv 1948;3:35–36.
[2]   Kramer MS, Rouleau J, Liu S, Bartholomew S, Joseph KS. Maternal health study group of the canadian perinatal surveillance system. amniotic fluid embolism: incidence, risk factors, and impact on perinatal outcome. BJOG 2012 Jun;119(7):874–879.
[3]   Clark SL. Amniotic fluid embolism. Obstet Gynecol 2014;123:337–348.
[4]   Attwood HD. Matthew Baillie – a possible early description of amniotic fluid embolism. Aust N Z J Obstet Gynaecol 1979;19:176–177.
[5]   Meyer JR. Embolia pulmonary amino caseosa. Bras Med 1926;2:301–303.
[6]   Steiner PE, Lushbaugh CC. Landmark article, Oct. 1941: Maternal pulmonary embolism by amniotic fluid as a cause of obstetric shock and unexpected deaths in obstetrics. By Paul E. Steiner and C. C. Lushbaugh. JAMA 1986 Apr 25;255(16):2187–2203.
[7]   Shotton DM, Taylor CW. Pulmonary embolism by amniotic fluid; a report of a fatal case, together with a review of the literature. J Obstet Gynaecol Br Emp 1949 Feb;56(1):46–53.
[8]   Knight M. Inoss. The International Network of Obstetric Survey Systems (INOSS): Benefits of multicountry studies of severe and uncommon maternal morbidities. Acta Obstet Gynecol Scand 2014;93(2):127–131.
[9]   Clark SL, Romero R, Dildy GA, et al. Proposed diagnostic criteria for the case definition of amniotic fluid embolism in research studies. Am J Obstet Gynecol 2016 Oct;215(4):408–412.
[10]   Knight M, Tuffnell D, Brocklehurst P, Spark P, Kurinczuk JJ. UK obstetric surveillance system. Incidence and risk factors for amniotic-fluid embolism. Obstet Gynecol 2010 May;115(5): 910–917.
[11]   Tuffnell DJ. United kingdom amniotic fluid embolism register. BJOG 2005 Dec;112(12):1625–1629.
[12]   Morgan M. Amniotic fluid embolism. Anaesthesia 1979 Jan;34(1):20–32.
[13]   Ito F, Akasaka J, Koike N, Uekuri C, Shigemitsu A, Kobayashi H. Incidence, diagnosis and pathophysiology of amniotic fluid embolism. J Obstet Gynaecol 2014 Oct;34(7):580–584.
[14]   Clark SL, Hankins GD, Dudley DA, Dildy GA, Porter TF. Amniotic fluid embolism: Analysis of the national registry. Am J Obstet Gynecol 1995 Apr;172(4 Pt 1):1158–1167, discussion 1167–9.
[15]   Tamura N, Farhana M, Oda T, Itoh H, Kanayama N. Amniotic fluid embolism: Pathophysiology from the perspective of pathology. J Obstet Gynaecol Res 2017 Apr;43(4):627–632.
[16]   Benson MD. Current concepts of immunology and diagnosis in amniotic fluid embolism. Clin Dev Immunol 2012;2012:946576.
[17]   Stanten RD, Iverson LI, Daugharty TM, Lovett SM, Terry C, Blumenstock E. Amniotic fluid embolism causing catastrophic pulmonary vasoconstriction: Diagnosis by transesophageal echocardiogram and treatment by cardiopulmonary bypass. Obstet Gynecol 2003 Sep;102(3): 496–498.
[18]   James CF, Feinglass NG, Menke DM, Grinton SF, Papadimos TJ. Massive amniotic fluid embolism: Diagnosis aided by emergency transesophageal echocardiography. Int J Obstet Anesth 2004 Oct;13(4):279–283.
[19]   Clark SL. New concepts of amniotic fluid embolism: A review. Obstet Gynecol Surv 1990;45: 360–368.
[20]   Fitzpatrick KE, Tuffnell D, Kurinczuk JJ, Knight M. Incidence, risk factors, management and outcomes of amniotic-fluid embolism: A population-based cohort and nested case-control study. BJOG 2016 Jan;123(1):100–109.
[21]   McDonnell N, Knight M, Peek MJ, et al. The Australasian Maternity Outcomes Surveillance System (AMOSS). Amniotic fluid embolism: An Australian-New Zealand population-based study. BMC Pregnancy Childbirth 2015 Dec;24(15):352.

[22] Hasegawa J, Sekizawa A, Tanaka H, et al. Maternal death exploratory committee in Japan; Japan association of obstetricians and gynecologists. Current status of pregnancy-related maternal mortality in Japan: A report from the maternal death exploratory committee in Japan. BMJ Open 2016 Mar 21;6(3):e010304.

[23] Society for Maternal-Fetal Medicine (SMFM). Electronic address: Pubs@smfm.org, Pacheco LD, Saade G, Hankins GD, Clark SL. Amniotic fluid embolism: Diagnosis and management. Am J Obstet Gynecol 2016 Aug;215(2):B16–24.

[24] Stafford I, Sheffield J. Amniotic fluid embolism. Obstet Gynecol Clin North Am 2007;34: 545–553, xii.

[25] Marwick PC, Levin AI, Coetzee AR. Recurrence of cardiotoxicity after lipid rescue from bupivacaine-induced cardiac arrest. Anesth Analg 2009;108:1344–1346.

[26] Mazoit JX, Le Guen R, Beloeil H, Benhamou D. Binding of long-lasting local anesthetics to lipid emulsions. Anesthesiology 2009 Feb;110(2):380–386.

[27] Lipman S, Cohen S, Einav S, et al; Society for obstetric anesthesia and perinatology. The society for obstetric anesthesia and perinatology consensus statement on the management of cardiac arrest in pregnancy. Anesth Analg 2014 May;118(5):1003–1016.

[28] McDonnell N, Knight M, Peek MJ, et al. The Australasian Maternity Outcomes Surveillance System (AMOSS). Amniotic fluid embolism: An Australian-New Zealand population-based study. BMC Pregnancy Childbirth 2015 Dec;24(15):352.

[29] Sharma NS, Wille KM, Bellot SC, Diaz-Guzman E. Modern use of extracorporeal life support in pregnancy and postpartum. ASAIO J 2015 Jan-Feb;61(1):110–114.

[30] Ho CH, Chen KB, Liu SK, Liu YF, Cheng HC, Wu RS. Early application of extracorporeal membrane oxygenation in a patient with amniotic fluid embolism. Acta Anaesthesiol Taiwan 2009 Jun;47(2):99–102.

[31] Hsieh YY, Chang CC, Li PC, Tsai HD, Tsai CH. Successful application of extracorporeal membrane oxygenation and intra-aortic balloon counterpulsation as lifesaving therapy for a patient with amniotic fluid embolism. Am J Obstet Gynecol 2000 Aug;183(2):496–497.

[32] Esposito RA, Grossi EA, Coppa G, et al. Successful treatment of postpartum shock caused by amniotic fluid embolism with cardiopulmonary bypass and pulmonary artery thromboembolectomy. Am J Obstet Gynecol 1990 Aug;163(2):572–574.

[33] Weksler N, Ovadia L, Stav A, Ribac L, Iuchtman M. Continuous arteriovenous hemofiltration in the treatment of amniotic fluid embolism. Int J Obstet Anesth 1994 Apr;3(2):92–96.

[34] Dodgson J, Martin J, Boswell J, Goodall HB, Smith R. Probable amniotic fluid embolism precipitated by amniocentesis and treated by exchange transfusion. Br Med J (Clin Res Ed) 1987 May 23;294(6583):1322–1323.

[35] Burtelow M, Riley E, Druzin M, Fontaine M, Viele M, Goodnough LT. How we treat: Management of life-threatening primary postpartum hemorrhage with a standardized massive transfusion protocol. Transfusion 2007 Sep;47(9):1564–1572.

[36] Kanayama N, Tamura N. Amniotic fluid embolism: Pathophysiology and new strategies for management. J Obstet Gynaecol Res 2014;40:1507–1517.

[37] Collis RE, Collins PW. Haemostatic management of obstetric haemorrhage. Anaesthesia 2015 Jan;70(Suppl 1):78–86, e27–8.

[38] Brzan Simenc G, Ambrozic J, Prokselj K, et al. Ocular ultrasonography for diagnosing increased intracranial pressure in patients with severe preeclampsia. Int J Obstet Anesth 2018 Nov;36:49–55.

[39] Rosa N, Lanza M, Borrelli M, et al. Low intraocular pressure resulting from ciliary body detachment in patients with myotonic dystrophy. Ophthalmology 2011 Feb;118(2):260–264.

[40] Novikova N, Hofmeyr GJ, Cluver C. Tranexamic acid for preventing postpartum haemorrhage. Cochrane Database Syst Rev 2015 Jun;16(6):CD007872.

[41] Leighton BL, Wall MH, Lockhart EM, Phillips LE, Zatta AJ. Use of recombinant factor VIIa in patients with amniotic fluid embolism: a systematic review of case reports. Anesthesiology 2011 Dec;115(6):1201–1208.

[42] Kobayashi H. Amniotic fluid embolism: anaphylactic reactions with idiosyncratic adverse response. Obstet Gynecol Surv 2015 Aug;70(8):511–517.

[43] Goldszmidt E, Davies S. Two cases of hemorrhage secondary to amniotic fluid embolus managed with uterine artery embolization. Can J Anaesth 2003 Nov;50(9):917–921.

[44] Ogihara T, Morimoto K, Kaneko Y. Continuous hemodiafiltration for potential amniotic fluid embolism: dramatic responses observed during a 10-year period report of three cases. Ther Apher Dial 2012 Apr;16(2):195–197.

[45] Kramer MS, Abenhaim H, Dahhou M, Rouleau J, Berg C. Incidence, risk factors, and consequences of amniotic fluid embolism. Paediatr Perinat Epidemiol 2013 Sep;27(5): 436–441.

[46] Gilbert WM, Danielsen B. Amniotic fluid embolism: decreased mortality in a population-based study. Obstet Gynecol 1999 Jun;93(6):973–977.

[47] Spiliopoulos M, Puri I, Jain NJ, Kruse L, Mastrogiannis D, Dandolu V. Amniotic fluid embolism-risk factors, maternal and neonatal outcomes. J Matern Fetal Neonatal Med 2009 May;22(5): 439–444.

[48] Benson MD, Oi H. A mild case of amniotic fluid embolism?. J Matern Fetal Neonatal Med 2007 Mar;20(3):261–262.

[49] Ducloy-Bouthors AS, Wantellet A, Tournoys A, Depret S, Krivosic-Horber R. [Amniotic fluid embolism suspected in a case of seizure and mild uterine haemorrhage with activation of coagulation and fibrinolysis]. Ann Fr Anesth Reanim 2004 Mar;23(2):149–152.

[50] Awad IT, Shorten GD. Amniotic fluid embolism and isolated coagulopathy: atypical presentation of amniotic fluid embolism. Eur J Anaesthesiol 2001 Jun;18(6):410–413.

[51] Kochanek KD, Martin JA. Supplemental analyses of recent trends in infant mortality. Int J Health Serv 2005;35(1):101–115.

Sam Schulman, Aleksander Makatsariya

12 Venous Thromboembolism in Pregnancy

12.1 Introduction

The incidence of maternal death has stabilized at approximately 16 per 100,000 pregnancies during the past decade in the United States [1]. During the years 2011–2016, pulmonary embolism was the cause for 9.0% of the pregnancy-related deaths. United States is leading the statistics for maternal mortality in the developed world (see Table 12.1) [2]. In a systematic review of 20 studies, the incidence of venous thromboembolism (VTE) was 1.2 per 1,000 pregnancies with a case fatality rate of 0.68% [3]. Although the incidence of VTE in pregnancy is quite similar to the overall incidence of VTE in the population in the United States, it must be kept in mind that the risk of VTE rises exponentially with age. Thus, compared to nonpregnant women of the same age the risk is increased 4- to 5-fold. The highest incidence of VTE is in the third trimester and postpartum, the exception being thrombosis related to artificial reproductive technologies (ART) that tends to occur early.

Table 12.1: Examples of maternal mortality in different countries in 2015 [2].

Country	Maternal deaths, N	Maternal mortality ratio*
USA	1,063	26.4
Ukraine	116	24.0
Russia	340	18.7
United Kingdom	75	9.2
France	61	7.8
Sweden	5	4.4
Finland	3	3.8

*Per 100,000 live births.

12.2 Risk Factors for Venous Thromboembolism

Multiple factors have been reported to increase the risk for thrombosis in pregnancy. These can be classified as physiologic changes in pregnancy, pathology in pregnancy, and fetus-related and patient-related risk factors.

https://doi.org/10.1515/9783110615258-012

12.2.1 Physiological Changes in Pregnancy

As part of the host defense against potentially fatal bleeding at delivery, a number of changes occur in the hemostatic system with the common goal to enhance clot formation and to counteract rapid resolution of thrombi (fibrinolysis) (see Table 12.2) [4]. The resulting increase in thrombin generation is demonstrated by the rise in levels of thrombin–antithrombin complex and prothrombin fragment 1 + 2. Likewise, the typical increase in D-dimer level during pregnancy is a reflection of the tendency to clot formation. The exception in this procoagulant development is a decrease in platelet count, which is common, particularly in late pregnancy. This is partly due to hemodilution.

Table 12.2: Changes in the hemostatic system during pregnancy.

Primary hemostasis	
Von Willebrand factor	↑
Platelet count	↓
β-Thromboglobulin, thromboxane A2 derivatives	↑
Secondary hemostasis	
Factor VII, VIII, X, XII, fibrinogen	↑
Natural anticoagulants	
Acquired activated protein C resistance	↑
Protein S	↓
Coagulation activation products	
Prothrombin fragment 1 + 2	↑
Thrombin–antithrombin complex	↑
D-dimer	↑
Fibrinolytic system	
Plasminogen activator inhibitor type 1 and 2	↑
Tissue plasminogen activator	↓

Thromboelastography is a method that can visualize both clot formation and fibrinolysis in one test. During pregnancy, there is shortening of the R-value (time until start of clot formation), increased angle (rate of clot growth), increase of the maximum amplitude (clot strength), and decrease of the percent lysis after 30 min [5].

The growing uterus will exert pressure on the posteriorly located blood vessels. This effect is accentuated by the right common iliac artery crossing over the left common iliac vein with the lumbar vertebrae in the background. Thus, deep vein thrombosis (DVT) during pregnancy is in 90% of the cases located in the iliofemoral segment(s) of the left leg.

The above-described changes occur in all pregnancies and will add to the thrombogenic effect of any of the risk factors described below (Table 12.3). A wealth of data was derived from analysis of the Health Improvement Network database in the United Kingdom with 376,154 pregnancies [6] and from Danish national healthcare databases with 1.3 million pregnancies [7].

12.2.2 Pathology in Pregnancy

Preeclampsia and stillbirth confer probably the highest risks for VTE of the different pregnancy-related pathological conditions. However, if the earliest stage of pregnancy is taken into account, ART complicated by ovarian hyperstimulation syndrome increases the risk of VTE up to 100-fold [6, 8]. Other risk-prone conditions are preterm birth, intrauterine growth restriction, hyperemesis with hospitalization, caesarian section, and major obstetric hemorrhage (see Table 12.3).

12.2.3 Fetus-Related Risks

Some of the factors accounted for as pregnancy-related (above) could also be classified as fetus-related, for example, stillbirth and intrauterine growth restriction or low birth weight. In addition, multiple pregnancy might confer an increased risk for VTE, although the results are not consistent.

12.2.4 Patient-Related Risk Factors

This group can be split into maternal characteristics and maternal comorbidities. Of the former, advanced maternal age is not disputed, whereas for obesity the results vary and smoking seems to be more of a risk factor in puerperium than during pregnancy. Among comorbidities, infections requiring hospitalization, inflammatory bowel disease, and systemic lupus erythematosus seem to confer a high risk for VTE, but for cancer, this does not appear to be the case (see Table 12.3). A positive history for VTE is obviously a risk factor for recurrence during pregnancy or puerperium but the risk differs depending on the circumstances around the index event, presence of thrombophilic defects, and positive family history. In general, a positive history of VTE increases the antepartum risk for recurrence from 0.6 per 1,000 to 11 per 1,000, 36 per 1,000, and 64 per 1,000 in case the index VTE was provoked by temporary nonhormonal risk factor, unprovoked, or provoked by hormonal risk factor, respectively. The postpartum risk is even higher and since it is confined to a much shorter period (6 weeks) than the pregnancy, prophylaxis is justified in a wider population in puerperium than antepartum.

For asymptomatic women with identified thrombophilic defects the risk is relatively low for VTE in pregnancy in case of heterozygous form of factor V Leiden or prothrombin mutation with <1% risk even in the postpartum period. Conversely, women with homozygous form of factor V Leiden or prothrombin mutation, double heterozygotes, and those with antithrombin deficiency have a >10-fold increase in risk for VTE already during the antepartum period [9]. In a patient with a thrombophilic defect but without previous personal history of VTE, the presence of a positive family history increases the risk for VTE in pregnancy from 2- to 5-fold, whereas a personal history of VTE increases the risk 10- to 100-fold, depending on the underlying thrombophilia [10].

Table 12.3: Risk factors for pregnancy-associated venous thromboembolism and their importance.

Risk factor	Increase in VTE risk (95% CI) during pregnancy	Increase in VTE risk (95% CI) in puerperium
Assisted reproductive technologies	3.0 (2.1–4.3) [38]	
Ovarian hyperstimulation syndrome	100 (62–161) [8]	
Preeclampsia	5.1 (1.2–21.7) [39]	5.0 (3.1–7.8) [7]
Hyperemesis	2.5 (1.4–4.5) [7]	
Hospitalization	12.2 (8.7–17) [7]	5.9 (4.0–8.8) [7]
Multiple pregnancy	2.8 (1.9–4.2) [7]0.83 (0.26–2.61) [6]	1.3 (0.6–2.6) [7] 1.39 (0.65–2.93) [6]
Stillbirth		6.24 (2.77–14.1) [6]
Intrauterine growth restriction/fetal death		1.9 (0.9–4.4) [7]
Birth weight <2,500 g	2.98 (1.80–4.93) [40]	
Preterm birth		2.69 (1.99–3.65) [6]
Obstetric hemorrhage		2.89 (1.53–5.43) [6] 1.4 (1.0–2.1) [7]
Acute caesarian section		3.0 (2.3–4.0) [7]
Elective caesarian section		2.1 (1.4–3.1) [7]
Maternal age 35–44 years	1.42 (1.01–1.93) [6]	1.51 (1.15–1.98) [6]
Obesity	BMI ≥ 30 1.50 (0.99–2.28) [6] BMI > 35 0.7 (0.3–0.8) [7]	BMI ≥ 30 3.75 (2.76–5.08) [6] BMI > 35 3.5 (1.8–6.7) [7]
Current smoking	1.15 (0.83–1.58) [6] 0.9 (0.7–1.2) [7]	1.31 (1.01–1.71) [6] 1.2 (0.9–1.6) [7]

Table 12.3 (continued)

Risk factor	Increase in VTE risk (95% CI) during pregnancy	Increase in VTE risk (95% CI) in puerperium
Infection requiring antibiotics	1.8 (1.5–2.3) [7]	1.4 (1.0–1.9) [7]
Infection requiring hospitalization	4.3 (2.7–7.1) [7]	5.0 (2.4–10.6) [7]
Urinary tract infection	1.88 (1.28–2.77) [6]	1.15 (0.77–1.71) [6]
Respiratory tract infection	1.70 (0.97–2.99) [6]	1.65 (1.02–2.66) [6]
Preexisting diabetes	3.08 (1.42–6.39) [6]	0.88 (0.33–2.38) [6]
Inflammatory bowel disease	3.46 (1.11–10.7) [6]	4.56 (1.88–11.0) [6]
Sickle cell disease	6.7 (4.4–10.1) [11]	
Cancer	1.97 (0.87–4.44) [6]	1.21 (0.49–2.96) [6]
Systemic lupus		6.69 (0.95–47.0) [6]
Varicose veins	2.69 (1.53–4.60) [6]	3.83 (2.51–5.82) [6]
Previous VTE – see text	24.8 (17.1–36) [11]	

12.3 Diagnosis of VTE in Pregnancy

12.3.1 Deep Vein Thrombosis

The diagnostic method of choice for suspected DVT is compression duplex ultrasonography, which must include the iliac veins. For a negative ultrasound together with low level of DVT suspicion, no further investigation is needed [11]. When, however, a DVT is clinically suspected and no other diagnosis is more likely, there are three options: (1) check the D-dimer and if it is also negative (in addition to the ultrasound), DVT can be excluded [12], but the problem is that D-dimer rises progressively in normal pregnancy, (2) perform serial ultrasonography (day 3 and day 7), which implies the necessity of bringing the patient back twice, or (3) perform magnetic resonance venography [10], which may not be available everywhere [13]. D-dimer testing in pregnancy is not recommended by the Royal College of Obstetricians and Gynaecologists (RCOG) [14] or by the American Thoracic Society/Society of Thoracic Radiology [15]. A recent systematic review of 8 studies on serial compression ultrasound in 635 women with initial negative ultrasound revealed that 6 patients became positive during the serial testing (0.94%). During 3 months follow-up after the serial ultrasonography, three patients (0.47%) were eventually diagnosed with VTE. Thus, the yield of serial testing is quite low.

12.3.2 Pulmonary Embolism

A pregnant patient with symptoms of pulmonary embolism should, in case of concomitant symptoms or signs typical of DVT, first have a compression ultrasound. If that is positive, it is not necessary to perform imaging diagnostics for pulmonary embolism, since the management in the vast majority of cases will not change. In the absence of symptoms from the leg, the choice is between ventilation/perfusion (V/Q) lung scanning and computed tomography of the pulmonary arteries (CTPA). Each one of those has advantages and disadvantages (see Table 12.4). There is, in various guidelines, either no preference for either of the methods or a weak recommendation (suggestion) for V/Q scanning [13, 16]. Single-photon emission computed tomography (V/Q SPECT) has, however, improved the diagnostic accuracy compared to standard V/Q scanning. For patients with an initial chest X-ray showing an abnormal picture, CTPA is preferable, since it can distinguish between pneumonia, pulmonary edema, aortic dissection, and other pathologies.

Table 12.4: Advantages and disadvantages with V/Q scanning and CTPA for diagnosis of VTE in pregnancy.

	V/Q scanning	CTPA
Availability	Somewhat limited	Almost everywhere
Safety	Better for the mother	Better for the fetus
Cancer risk*	Childhood cancer	Breast cancer
Other risks	None	Fetal hypothyroidism*
Detection of other pathology	Limited	Better

*The absolute risk is very small

12.3.3 Clinical Prediction

In nonpregnant patients, various clinical decision rules are used to reduce the need for diagnostic imaging. In pregnant women, the LEFt score has been validated and shown to be of some value in the prediction of DVT (see Table 12.5) but it still needs to be evaluated in a prospective management study [17]. Two studies incorporating the LEFt score and D-dimer are currently recruiting patients (NCT01708239 and NCT02507180).

Table 12.5: Components of the LEFt score and results in validation study [17].

Criteria	Points
Left leg	1
Edema – ≥2 cm swelling	1
First trimester	1

Total score in validation study	N	Confirmed DVTn (%)
0	30	1 (3)
1	35	3 (9)
2	20	2 (10)
3	3	4 (75)

12.4 Prophylaxis

Prophylaxis with low-molecular-weight heparin (LMWH) or unfractionated heparin (UFH) reduces the risk for VTE in pregnancy by approximately 75% [13] and possibly as much as 88% in patients with a previous VTE [18]. Prophylaxis against VTE should preferably be given with LMWH and the typical once daily dose of enoxaparin 40 mg [19] or dalteparin 5,000 units [18] or tinzaparin 4,500 units is sufficient for most patients. For women with a body weight <50 kg, the dose should be reduced to enoxaparin 20 mg or dalteparin 2,500 units and for obese women, with the qualifying limit varying in different studies from 80 to 120 kg, the dose is increased to enoxaparin 60 mg or dalteparin 7,500 units.

A higher dose is recommended by some guidelines for certain high-risk patients. These include patients with (1) long-term anticoagulation with a vitamin K antagonist prior to the current pregnancy, (2) two or more prior episodes of VTE, and (3) high-risk thrombophilia with a previous VTE [20, 21].

The efficacy of LMWH prophylaxis in pregnancy is numerically better, although not statistically significant, than with UFH according to a systematic review of four randomized trials – risk ratio (RR) 0.47 (95% confidence interval [95% CI], 0.09–2.49) for symptomatic VTE [22]. There are fewer adverse events that result in cessation of prophylaxis with LMWH than with UFH (RR 0.07; 95% CI 0.01–0.54) and fewer fetal losses (RR 0.47; 95% CI 0.23–0.95) [22]. Furthermore, LMWH does not require twice-daily injections, carries a lower risk for heparin-induced thrombocytopenia and has a lower risk for osteoporosis during long-term use than UFH.

The most common conditions for which prophylaxis is discussed in the guidelines are reviewed in Table 12.7, including a section specifically for different hereditary thrombophilic defects in Table 12.7 [11, 13, 20, 21, 23]. The RCOG Guideline goes into particular detail with a vast number of risk factors that are included in a risk assessment tool, although this has not been validated yet [14].

Table 12.6: Recommendations regarding VTE chemoprophylaxis in clinical practice guidelines – excluding patients with thrombophilia.

	ACCP [23]	ACOG [20]	ASH [13]	RCOG [11]	SOGC [21]
Antepartum					
ART	No		No	(Yes)*	(Yes)*
ART + OHSS	Yes, 3 months		Yes	Yes, 3 months	Yes, 8–12 weeks
Prior cerebral vein thrombosis					Yes
Prior VTE, provoked, nonhormonal	No	No	No	No	
Prior VTE, provoked, hormonal	Yes	Yes	Yes	Yes	Yes
Prior VTE, unprovoked	Yes	Yes	Yes	Yes	Yes
>1 prior VTE		Yes		Yes	
Obstetric APS	Yes + ASA			Yes	
Inherited thrombophilia + pregnancy complications	No				
Miscarriages, neg APLA	No				
During admission for hyperemesis				Yes	
Puerperium					
Cesarean, no other risk factors	No			No	
Cesarean and ≥1 other risk factor	Yes, in hospital			Yes, 10 days	
Obesity, BMI > 40				Yes, 10 days	
Prior VTE	Yes, 6 weeks	Yes	Yes	Yes, 6 weeks	Yes
APS				Yes	Yes

ACCP, American College of Chest Physicians; ACOG, American College of Obstetricians and Gynecologists; ASH, American Society of Hematology; RCOG, Royal College of Obstetricians and Gynaecologists; SOGC, Society of Obstetricians and Gynaecologists of Canada; ART, assisted reproductive technology; OHSS, ovarian hyperstimulation syndrome; VTE, venous thromboembolism; APS, antiphospholipid syndrome; APLA, antiphospholipid antibodies; ASA, acetylsalicylic acid; BMI, body mass index.
*Only if together with one other (SOGC) [21] or three other risk factors (RCOG) [11]

Table 12.7: Recommendations regarding VTE chemoprophylaxis in clinical practice guidelines – excluding patients with thrombophilia.

Thrombophilia	ACCP [23]	ACOG [20]	ASH [13]	RCOG [11]	SOGC [21]
Antepartum – asymptomatic					
Heterozygous FVL or PGM	No	No	No	Not	No
Homozygous PGM	Yes	Yes	*Yes*	Yes	Yes
Homozygous FVL	Yes	Yes	Yes	Yes	Yes
Compound heterozygous FVL-PGM	No	Yes	Yes	Yes	Yes
Protein C or protein S deficiency	No	No	No	Yes	No
Antithrombin deficiency	No	Yes	*Yes*	Yes	Yes
Antepartum – prior VTE					
Heterozygous FVL or PGM	(Yes)*	Optional	(Yes)*	Yes	Yes
Homozygous PGM	(Yes)*	Yes	(Yes)*	Yes	Yes
Homozygous FVL	(Yes)*	Yes	(Yes)*	Yes	Yes
Compound heterozygous FVL-PGM	(Yes)*	Yes	(Yes)*	Yes	Yes
Protein C or protein S deficiency	(Yes)*	Optional	(Yes)*	Yes	Yes
Antithrombin deficiency	(Yes)*	Yes	(Yes)*	Yes	Yes
Puerperium – asymptomatic					5
Heterozygous FVL or PGM	*Yes*	Optional	No	Not	No‡
Homozygous PGM	Yes	Yes	Yes	Yes	Yes
Homozygous FVL	Yes	Yes	Yes	Yes	Yes
Compound heterozygous FVL-PGM	*Yes*	Yes	Yes	Yes	Yes
Protein C or protein S deficiency	*Yes*	Optional	*Yes*	Yes	No‡
Antithrombin deficiency	*Yes*	Yes	*Yes*	Yes	Yes
Puerperium – prior VTE					
Heterozygous FVL or PGM	(Yes)*	Yes	Yes	Yes	Yes
Homozygous PGM	(Yes)*	Yes	Yes	Yes	Yes
Homozygous FVL	(Yes)*	Yes	Yes	Yes	Yes
Compound heterozygous FVL-PGM	(Yes)*	Yes	Yes	Yes	Yes

Table 12.7 (continued)

Thrombophilia	ACCP [23]	ACOG [20]	ASH [13]	RCOG [11]	SOGC [21]
Protein C or protein S deficiency	(Yes)*	Yes	Yes	Yes	Yes
Antithrombin deficiency	(Yes)*	Yes	Yes	Yes	Yes

†Also recommended for patients with compound heterozygous FVL + PGM and for AT deficiency.
Recommendation in italics – pertains only to patients with a family history of VTE
*Not explicitly stated but understood from the context.
†Prophylaxis recommended for 10 days postpartum if one other risk factor; from 28 weeks of pregnancy if two other risk factors; for entire pregnancy if three other risk factors.
‡Recommended only when combined with at least one other risk factor.

12.5 Treatment

12.5.1 Initiation of Treatment

The RCOG guideline recommends that anticoagulant treatment is started as soon as there is clinical suspicion of DVT or PE and that it then is discontinued if objective testing leads to exclusion of the diagnosis [14]. Indeed, there is no measurable harm from one or two doses of potentially unnecessary LMWH. All guidelines give clear preference for LMWH over UFH and the main reason is the risk for fracture secondary to osteoporosis, which in a study of 184 pregnant women amounted to 2.2% [24]. There also a higher risk for heparin-induced thrombocytopenia, at least in nonpregnant patients, with UFH. Still, it is suggested that a platelet count is obtained when starting LMWH and 1 week later [21]. If the patient has received heparin within the last 100 days, the repeat platelet count should be done already 24 h after restarting LMWH/UFH [23]. LMWH can be given subcutaneously once or twice daily. The systematic review that showed lack of significant difference in outcomes between these two regimens included only studies in nonpregnant patients [25]. It can be argued that due to changes in pharmacokinetics with shorter half-life of LMWH in pregnancy, a twice daily regimen could be required, but two observational studies did not show any numerical difference between the regimens, and a third study with only a once daily regimen supported the overall low outcome event rate (see Table 12.8) [26–28]. It has been suggested that for women at high risk of bleeding, UFH could be the preferred treatment in view of its shorter half-life and with full reversibility by protamine [16]. Vitamin K antagonists should not be used during pregnancy in women with VTE.

For massive PE with hypotension (systolic blood pressure < 90 mmHg), there is no contraindication to thrombolysis, which can be life-saving. If this cannot be given immediately, an intravenous infusion with UFH should be started. This can quickly be reversed or reduced if thoracotomy or thrombolysis is chosen as the next step. For patients with DVT, thrombolysis should only be considered for patients in whom the

Table 12.8: Outcomes with LMWH treatment given once or twice daily for VTE in pregnancy.

Author, reference	Recurrent VTE n/N (%)		Major bleeding n/N (%)	
	Once daily	Twice daily	Once daily	Twice daily
Knight [26]	1/66 (1.5)	1/68 (1.5)	0/66 (0)	0/68 (0)
Voke [27]	0/83 (0)	0/39 (0)	0/83 (0)	0/39 (0)
Lepercq [28]	1/49 (2.0)	Not used	1/49 (2.0)	Not used

limb is threatened (*phlegmasia cerulea dolens* or *phlegmasia alba dolens*). In the largest randomized controlled trial comparing catheter-directed, pharmacomechanical clot removal versus standard anticoagulation, there was no benefit overall of the invasive method, although in the subset with iliofemoral location of the thrombus there was a significant reduction of the post-thrombotic syndrome [29]. This study was in nonpregnant patients, and a concern for pregnant women is the increased fetal radiation exposure and potential organ malformation due to the prolonged fluoroscopy.

The Canadian guideline suggests that pregnant patients diagnosed with VTE should be hospitalized or followed closely as outpatients for the first 2 weeks [21]. The Australian–New Zeeland guideline suggests a few days of observation as inpatients for women with PE [16], whereas the guideline from ASH suggests initial treatment as outpatients for those with low-risk VTE [13].

12.5.2 Maintenance Therapy

The question whether treatment with LMWH during pregnancy should be monitored with anti-factor Xa levels has often been raised. The background is that with the recommended, weight-based regimen of LMWH, even if given twice daily, many women will have progressively lower anti-Xa levels during the pregnancy [30]. There is only one small study that compared, monitored, and dose-adjusted LMWH to achieve peak anti-Xa levels between 0.5 and 1.0 IU/mL ($n = 11$) versus non-monitored, non-adjusted LMWH ($n = 15$) in a consecutive cohort design [31]. There was no recurrent VTE and no hemorrhage during pregnancy in either group. In addition, there is no validated therapeutic range for anti-Xa in the pregnant population and the inter-laboratory reproducibility of the test is low. Thus, current guidelines do not recommend routine monitoring [13, 14]. In specific cases such as morbidly obese (to check that levels are not far too low), renal impairment (to check that levels are not excessive), as well as in the very different population with mechanical heart valves, monitoring may still be justified.

After diagnosis, LMWH should be given at full treatment dose for at least 3 months and subsequently it may be reduced to a prophylactic dose, which should be maintained until 6 weeks postpartum [14, 21]. The Australian–New Zeeland guideline recommends 6 months of therapeutic dose for those with proximal DVT or with PE [16].

For patients with DVT, there is a high risk of post-thrombotic syndrome, which includes chronic swelling, pain, heaviness, varicose veins, hyperpigmentation, eczema, and, in a small proportion of patients, ultimately venous ulcers. The risk of developing this syndrome seems to be similar in pregnant patients as in nonpregnant. A 16-year follow-up study after DVT in pregnancy demonstrated deep venous reflux in 36% and leg swelling in 52% [32]. In a case–control study, women with DVT during pregnancy developed post-thrombotic syndrome in 42% compared to similar symptoms in 10% of those with uncomplicated pregnancy [33]. Although a meta-analysis of studies of moderate quality showed that the use of compression stockings reduces the risk of post-thrombotic syndrome from 46% to 26% in nonpregnant patients with DVT [34], a subsequent large, randomized, double-blind study could not demonstrate any benefit of graduated compression stockings to prevent this syndrome [35]. The recommendations in the guidelines vary from no suggestions [13], via a suggestion that the stockings can provide relief of DVT symptoms, that is, pain and swelling [14, 21], to a Level 1 recommendation that all women with a confirmed DVT need to wear a knee-high compression stocking for up to 2 years [16].

12.5.3 Around Time of Delivery

It is preferable to plan the time of delivery so that the last therapeutic dose LMWH is at least 24 h before induction or caesarian section [13]. In case labor starts before planned delivery, any further injections with LMWH must be held and neuraxial anesthesia cannot be given until 24 h after a therapeutic dose. For women with a VTE occurring close to or at term, the best option is to admit the patient the day before planned delivery and switch to intravenous UHF, which then is stopped 6 h before the start of induction, at which time also regional anesthesia can be provided [14]. At 6 h after delivery, the infusion with UFH is restarted at about half therapeutic dose and after another 6 h the infusion rate is doubled. A detailed protocol for this is provided in the Australian–New Zeeland guideline [16]. This type of regimen is also suitable for women at a high risk of bleeding [14].

Anticoagulation for the usual 6 weeks postpartum, or longer to complete at least 3 months of therapy can be given with LMWH, UFH, or a vitamin K antagonist, neither of which will generate any anticoagulant effect in the baby of the breastfeeding woman [13]. The options can be discussed at the last visit before delivery and then confirmed after delivery. After a normal delivery the VKA can be started the same evening, since it takes about 5 days to reach therapeutic international normalized ratio (INR). If, however, there is an increased risk for postpartum hemorrhage VKA should not be started until about 5 days later [14]. In a case-control study of 46 women initiated on warfarin, postpartum therapeutic INR was reached after a median of 7 days compared to 4 days in nonpregnant women despite similar doses given days 1–3 in both groups [36]. The maintenance weekly dose of warfarin also turned out to be higher in the postpartum women, 45 mg versus 24 mg.

12.6 Investigation for Thrombophilia

Tests for thrombophilic defects, except for mutations (factor V Leiden, prothrombin gene) should be avoided during pregnancy and puerperium due to risk of false results caused by high estrogen levels. Whether the investigation for acquired and inherited, thrombophilia should at all be done in women that suffered a VTE during pregnancy is not discussed in several of the guidelines. An American guideline recommends that it should be done [20], whereas the Canadian guideline suggests that routine testing in such patients should not be done unless there are family members with deficiency of one of the natural inhibitors or if the patient had thrombosis in an unusual site [21]. It also suggests testing for the antiphospholipid syndrome if the result may influence the anticoagulant treatment regimen. A similar strategy is suggested by the British guideline.

12.7 Conclusions

VTE is an important contributor to maternal morbidity and mortality. The pathogenesis is multifactorial in pregnancy with changes in many components of the hemostatic system, in blood flow and also local pressure on blood vessels, thus fulfilling the triad of Virchow [37]. Many additional risk factors during pregnancy may play a role for increased thrombus formation. Prophylaxis against VTE in pregnancy is recommended in some, but not all conditions with increased risk. The harm from bleeding, the inconvenience and cost of anticoagulant treatment has to be counterbalanced. For suspected VTE in pregnancy it is paramount to reach an accurate diagnosis without further delay, which in almost all cases requires imaging diagnostic methods. For treatment of VTE in pregnancy, LMWH is clearly favored. It should be continued at therapeutic dose for at least 3 months and until 6 weeks postpartum. Optimal management of VTE in pregnancy requires thorough patient education to achieve good adherence to the treatment and to understand the risk and appropriate actions in case of adverse events.

References

[1]   Pregnancy mortality surveillance system. (Accessed December 12, 2019, at cdc.gov/
       reproductivehealth/maternal-mortality/pregnancy-mortality-surveillance-system.htm?CDC

[2]   GBD 2015 Maternal Mortality Collaborators. Global, regional, and national levels of maternal
       mortality, 1990–2015: A systematic analysis for the global burden of disease study 2015.
       Lancet 2016;388:1775–1812.

[3]   Kourlaba G, Relakis J, Kontodimas S, Holm MV, Maniadakis N. A systematic review and meta-
       analysis of the epidemiology and burden of venous thromboembolism among pregnant
       women. Int J Gynaecol Obstet 2016;132:4–10.

[4]   Prisco D, Ciuti G, Falciani M. Hemostatic changes in normal pregnancy. Haematologica Rep
       2005;1:1–5.

[5]   Karlsson O, Sporrong T, Hillarp A, Jeppsson A, Hellgren M. Prospective longitudinal study of
       thromboelastography and standard hemostatic laboratory tests in healthy women during
       normal pregnancy. Anesth Analg 2012;115:890–898.

[6]   Sultan AA, Tata LJ, West J, et al. Risk factors for first venous thromboembolism around
       pregnancy: A population-based cohort study from the United Kingdom. Blood 2013;121:
       3953–3961.

[7]   Virkus RA, Lokkegaard E, Lidegaard O, et al. Risk factors for venous thromboembolism in
       1.3 million pregnancies: A nationwide prospective cohort. PLoS One 2014;9:e96495.

[8]   Rova K, Passmark H, Lindqvist PG. Venous thromboembolism in relation to in vitro
       fertilization: An approach to determining the incidence and increase in risk in successful
       cycles. Fertil Steril 2012;97:95–100.

[9]   Rodger M. Pregnancy and venous thromboembolism: 'TIPPS' for risk stratification.
       Hematology Am Soc Hematol Educ Program 2014;2014:387–392.

[10]   Rybstein MD, DeSancho MT. Risk factors for and clinical management of venous
       thromboembolism during pregnancy. Clin Adv Hematol Oncol 2019;17:396–404.

[11]   Royal College of Obstetricians and Gynaecologists. Reducing the Risk of Venous
       Thromboembolism during Pregnancy and Puerperium. Green-top Guideline No. 37b. London;
       2015, 1–40.

[12]   Nijkeuter M, Ginsberg JS, Huisman MV. Diagnosis of deep vein thrombosis and pulmonary
       embolism in pregnancy: A systematic review. J Thromb Haemost 2006;4:496–500.

[13]   Bates SM, Rajasekhar A, Middeldorp S, et al. American society of hematology 2018
       guidelines for management of venous thromboembolism: Venous thromboembolism in the
       context of pregnancy. Blood Adv 2018;2:3317–3359.

[14]   Royal College of Obstetricians and Gynaecologists. Thromboembolic Disease in Pregnancy
       and the Puerperium: Acute Management. Green-top Guideline No. 37a. London; 2015, 1–32.

[15]   Leung AN, Bull TM, Jaeschke R, et al. An official American Thoracic Society/Society of
       Thoracic Radiology clinical practice guideline: Evaluation of suspected pulmonary embolism
       in pregnancy. Am J Respir Crit Care Med 2011;184:1200–1208.

[16]   McLintock C, Brighton T, Chunilal S, et al. Recommendations for the diagnosis and treatment
       of deep venous thrombosis and pulmonary embolism in pregnancy and the postpartum
       period. Aust N Z J Obstet Gynaecol 2012;52:14–22.

[17]   Le Moigne E, Genty C, Meunier J, et al. Validation of the LEFt score, a newly proposed
       diagnostic tool for deep vein thrombosis in pregnant women. Thromb Res 2014;134:664–667.

[18]   Lindqvist PG, Bremme K, Hellgren M. Efficacy of obstetric thromboprophylaxis and long-term
       risk of recurrence of venous thromboembolism. Acta Obstet Gynecol Scand 2011;90:
       648–653.

[19] Cox S, Eslick R, McLintock C. Effectiveness and safety of thromboprophylaxis with enoxaparin for prevention of pregnancy-associated venous thromboembolism. J Thromb Haemost 2019;17:1160–1170.

[20] James A. Practice bulletin no. 123: Thromboembolism in pregnancy. Obstet Gynecol 2019;118: 718–729.

[21] Chan WS, Rey E, Kent NE, et al. Venous thromboembolism and antithrombotic therapy in pregnancy. J Obstet Gynaecol Can 2014;36:527–553.

[22] Bain E, Wilson A, Tooher R, Gates S, Davis LJ, Middleton P. Prophylaxis for venous thromboembolic disease in pregnancy and the early postnatal period. Cochrane Database Syst Rev 2014:CD001689.

[23] Bates SM, Greer IA, Middeldorp S, Veenstra DL, Prabulos AM, Vandvik PO. VTE, thrombophilia, antithrombotic therapy, and pregnancy: Antithrombotic therapy and prevention of thrombosis, 9th ed: American College of Chest Physicians Evidence-Based Clinical Practice Guidelines. Chest 2012;141:e691S–736S.

[24] Dahlman TC. Osteoporotic fractures and the recurrence of thromboembolism during pregnancy and the puerperium in 184 women undergoing thromboprophylaxis with heparin. Am J Obstet Gynecol 1993;168:1265–1270.

[25] Bhutia S, Wong PF. Once versus twice daily low molecular weight heparin for the initial treatment of venous thromboembolism. Cochrane Database Syst Rev 2013:CD003074.

[26] Knight M. Antenatal pulmonary embolism: Risk factors, management and outcomes. Bjog 2008;115:453–461.

[27] Voke J, Keidan J, Pavord S, Spencer NH, Hunt BJ. The management of antenatal venous thromboembolism in the UK and Ireland: A prospective multicentre observational survey. Br J Haematol 2007;139:545–558.

[28] Lepercq J, Conard J, Borel-Derlon A, et al. Venous thromboembolism during pregnancy: A retrospective study of enoxaparin safety in 624 pregnancies. Bjog 2001;108:1134–1140.

[29] Vedantham S, Goldhaber SZ, Julian JA, et al. Pharmacomechanical catheter-directed thrombolysis for deep-vein thrombosis. N Engl J Med 2017;377:2240–2252.

[30] Barbour LA, Oja JL, Schultz LK. A prospective trial that demonstrates that dalteparin requirements increase in pregnancy to maintain therapeutic levels of anticoagulation. Am J Obstet Gynecol 2004;191:1024–1029.

[31] McDonnell BP, Glennon K, McTiernan A, et al. Adjustment of therapeutic LMWH to achieve specific target anti-FXa activity does not affect outcomes in pregnant patients with venous thromboembolism. J Thromb Thrombolysis 2017;43:105–111.

[32] Rosfors S, Noren A, Hjertberg R, Persson L, Lillthors K, Torngren S. A 16-year haemodynamic follow-up of women with pregnancy-related medically treated iliofemoral deep venous thrombosis. Eur J Vasc Endovasc Surg 2001;22:448–455.

[33] Wik HS, Jacobsen AF, Sandvik L, Sandset PM. Prevalence and predictors for post-thrombotic syndrome 3 to 16 years after pregnancy-related venous thrombosis: a population-based, cross-sectional, case-control study. J Thromb Haemost 2012;10:840–847.

[34] Musani MH, Matta F, Yaekoub AY, Liang J, Hull RD, Stein PD. Venous compression for prevention of postthrombotic syndrome: a meta-analysis. Am J Med 2010;123:735–740.

[35] Kahn SR, Shapiro S, Wells PS, et al. Compression stockings to prevent post-thrombotic syndrome: a randomised placebo-controlled trial. Lancet 2014;383:880–888.

[36] Brooks C, Rutherford JM, Gould J, Ramsay MM, James DK. Warfarin dosage in postpartum women: a case-control study. Br J Obstet Gynaecol 2002;109:187–190.

[37] Virchow R. Ein Vortrag Über Die Thrombose Vom Jahre. Frankfurt: Von Medinger Sohn & Co; 1856.

[38] Hansen AT, Kesmodel US, Juul S, Hvas AM. Increased venous thrombosis incidence in pregnancies after in vitro fertilization. Hum Reprod 2014;29:611–617.

[39] Chan LY, Tam WH, Lau TK. Venous thromboembolism in pregnant Chinese women. Obstet Gynecol 2001;98:471–475.

[40] Blondon M, Quon BS, Harrington LB, Bounameaux H, Smith NL. Association between newborn birth weight and the risk of postpartum maternal venous thromboembolism: a population-based case-control study. Circulation 2015;131:1471–1476, discussion 6.

Shaun Yo, John Granton

13 Pulmonary Hypertension in Pregnancy

13.1 Introduction

Pulmonary hypertension (PH) is characterized by an elevation in pulmonary arterial pressure (PAP). The contemporary definition of PH is a mean PAP (mPAP) above 20 mmHg, two standard deviations above the population mean of 14 mmHg [1]. The WHO classification of PH informs the therapeutic approach by categorizing the etiologies of PH into five groups, based on entities that have similar pathophysiological, clinical, and hemodynamic features.

Clinical classification of PH:
1 Pulmonary arterial hypertension (PAH)
   1.1 Idiopathic PAH
   1.2 Heritable PAH
   1.3 Drug and toxin-induced PAH
   1.4 PAH associated with
      1.4.1 Connective tissue diseases
      1.4.2 HIV infection
      1.4.3 Portal hypertension
      1.4.4 Congenital heart disease
      1.4.5 Schistosomiasis
   1.5 PAH long-term responders to calcium channel blockers
   1.6 PAH with overt features of venous/capillaries (PVOD/PCH) involvement
   1.7 Persistent PH of the newborn syndrome
2 PH due to left heart disease
3 PH due to lung diseases and/or hypoxemia
4 PH due to pulmonary artery obstructions (e.g., thromboembolism)
5 PH with unclear and/or multifactorial mechanisms.

In this chapter, we will focus on group 1 – PAH, as it constitutes the salient patient group in relation to the discussion about pregnancy.

Group 1 PAH consists of a group of clinical conditions characterized by proliferative remodeling of the distal pulmonary arteries leading to progressive obstruction and obliteration [2]. This causes an increase in pulmonary vascular resistance (PVR), which is responsible for the elevation in PAP. The result is an increase in right ventricular (RV) afterload that leads to progressive RV dysfunction [3]. This manifests as symptoms of exertional dyspnea, chest pain, peripheral edema, abdominal distension, pre-syncope, and syncope. Untreated, RV failure and premature death ensues [4].

https://doi.org/10.1515/9783110615258-013

13.2 Epidemiology of PAH

As a group, PAH is uncommon, with an estimated prevalence of 10–25 per million population and incidence of 2–8 per million per year, based on registry data from the USA and Europe [5]. About half of these patients have idiopathic PAH (IPAH) or heritable PAH (HPAH). Of the associated PAH (APAH) conditions, connective tissue diseases (CTD) form the majority.

Traditionally, PAH was thought to be a disease predominantly of younger women. The first US NIH registry in 1987 demonstrated a mean age of 36 years and a female-to-male ratio of 1.7:1 [6]. The contemporary PAH patient population is older, with a mean age at diagnosis of between 50 and 65 years [5]. Nevertheless, there remains a significant female preponderance, with a ratio of up to 3.6:1 [7], and women of childbearing age continue to overrepresent the PAH patient population.

The prognosis of PAH has improved markedly since the availability of PAH-targeted therapy. Compared to the median survival of 2.8 years from diagnosis in the original NIH registry cohort three decades ago [8], the median survival is 9 years in the current era of advanced therapies [9].

However, for many, PAH remains a severe and incurable condition; patients with a high-risk status have an expected 1-year mortality of over 20% [4]. Given the progressive nature of the disease and the risk of abrupt deterioration, regular methodical risk assessment with a multiparametric approach is recommended by guidelines [4].

13.3 The Risk of Pregnancy in Patients with PAH

In the era before PAH-targeted therapy, pregnancy was associated with extremely high maternal and fetal risks, with maternal death in the range of 30–56% [10]. While outcomes have improved in the modern era with the availability of PAH-targeted treatments and advancements in high-risk pregnancy care, the risk of maternal mortality or need for urgent lung transplant remains substantial at 16–25%. The risk is greatest postpartum, when the majority of maternal deaths occur [11–14]. There is also an increased risk of adverse fetal/neonatal outcomes, with reports of fetal/neonatal mortality of up to 13%. Most fetal deaths are secondary to antepartum maternal death, whereas outcomes for live-born infants are much more favorable [11–15].

Given the unacceptably high maternal and fetal risks, guidelines continue to issue a strong recommendation for avoidance of pregnancy in patients with PAH, and that therapeutic abortion is offered to patients who get pregnant [16]. Nevertheless, women with PAH do become pregnant, intentionally or inadvertently; and occasionally, PAH manifests de novo during pregnancy. Therefore, it is imperative that clinicians treating patients with PAH have a sound understanding of the risks pertaining to pregnancy, and know how best to care for patients through this high risk period, should the decision be made to continue the pregnancy.

13.4 Physiological Effects of Pregnancy

Plasma volume expansion is a fundamental physiological change during pregnancy. This begins early in the first trimester, rises steeply in the second trimester, and by the end of the third trimester is around 50% above prepregnancy values [17]. This exceeds the 20–30% increase in red cell mass, resulting in a physiological dilutional anemia with normal hemoglobin levels as low as 105 g/L in the second and third trimesters [18, 19].

There is a sharp rise in cardiac output (CO) in the first trimester, followed by a more gradual increase to peak values of 30–50% above the pre-pregnancy baseline [20]. This is mediated by an early increase in stroke volume of up to 35% by the end of the second trimester, in conjunction with a progressive increase in heart rate of 10–20 bpm throughout the pregnancy [19, 21]. Oxygen consumption increases by 20% [22]. Although left ventricular (LV) and right ventricular (RV) ejection fractions remain unchanged, there is an increase in LV and RV end-diastolic volumes. LV and RV mass increase by 40–50% [23]. Systemic vascular resistance (SVR) decreases by up to 40%, mediated by the vasodilatory effects of progesterone and estrogen, in addition to the development of the high-flow, low-resistance uteroplacental circulation [19, 21].

The net effect of changes in CO and SVR is a slight decrease in systemic bloodpressure with a trough at 22–24 weeks of gestation, reaching a nadir of 7 and 5 mmHg lower than pre-pregnancy values in systolic and diastolic blood pressure, respectively [24]. In the pulmonary circulation, hormone-mediated vasodilation and recruitment of previously nonperfused pulmonary vessels lead to a decrease in PVR. This allows the pulmonary circulation to accommodate the increased CO with grossly unchanged pulmonary arterial pressures [19].

Abrupt and dramatic changes in the cardiovascular system occur during labor and delivery that affect preload and afterload. Pronounced respiratory efforts and Valsalva maneuvers cause significant intrathoracic pressure swings, which, in turn, lead to large fluctuations in central venous and arterial pressures [19]. There is an increase in blood volume from autotransfusion of 300–500 mL of blood into the systemic circulation after each uterine contraction. Intermittent inferior vena caval compression and release further contributes to volume shifts [21].

CO increases 60–80% above pre-labor levels, from a combination of increases in preload, heart rate, and circulating catecholamines [21]. However, blood loss can cause rapid and substantial drops in preload.

In the postpartum period, there is a rapid drop in estrogen and progesterone levels, followed by a gradual normalization of hormone levels and blood volume over 6 weeks [19].

13.5 The Perils of PAH and Pregnancy

Patients with PAH have markedly impaired compensatory mechanisms to adapt to the hemodynamic changes of pregnancy. Due to vasoconstriction, obstruction, and obliteration of the diseased pulmonary vascular bed, there is limited capacity to dilate and recruit pulmonary vasculature, and therefore an attenuation, or absence, of the normal physiological decrease in PVR [19].

The inability to modulate PVR to accommodate an increase in pulmonary blood flow leads to higher pulmonary pressures and an increase in RV afterload and RV work. Together with the increased preload, from an increase in plasma volume, the RV may become further distended, leading to an increase in RV wall stress. This increase in wall stress may, in turn, lead to RV ischemia and decreased RV contractility. Tricuspid regurgitation may also be aggravated – further increasing venous pressure that contributes to worsening peripheral edema and hepatic congestion. CO is compromised from a combination of reduced pulmonary blood flow and ventricular/atrial interdependence, where the dilated pressurized RA and RV leads to shift of the interatrial and interventricular septum, impairing LV filling. Systemic hypotension ensues, further impairing myocardial perfusion and exacerbating RV ischemia, thus setting up a perilous spiral into cardiogenic shock [19, 25, 26]. Impaired oxygen delivery is further compounded by increased peripheral oxygen consumption [22].

The risk of deterioration and death from RV failure is most pronounced at gestational weeks 20–24, during labor and delivery, and in the postpartum period [11, 12]. These represent the time points during which large and rapid changes in hemodynamics and volume status occur. Venous thromboembolism is an added risk and may contribute to RV failure and circulatory collapse in the peripartum period [19].

The effects of the sex hormones, in particular, estrogens, on the pulmonary circulation are complex and have yet to be fully elucidated. On the one hand, estrogens may have favorable vasodilatory and antiproliferative effects [27]. However, there are also concerns that proproliferative effects of estrogens [28] may worsen pulmonary vascular remodeling in pregnant PAH patients. There is a significant body of evidence of the salutary effects of estrogens on LV function and adaptations to LV injury [19]. However, there is a paucity of literature on the effects of sex hormones on the RV, particularly in the setting of pregnancy. The abrupt decrease in sex hormone levels, postpartum, is hypothesized to contribute to the high risk of cardiac decompensation during this period; however, this requires further investigation.

13.6 General Principles and Supportive Therapy in Pregnancy

Given the undue maternal and fetal risks, guidelines recommend that therapeutic abortion be offered to pregnant women with PAH, irrespective of markers of prognosis. Termination should be performed in the first trimester if possible, and at an experienced center [15, 19]. This is especially important for patients who demonstrate early deterioration, as it may be the crucial determinant of maternal survival [29]. There is lack of consensus on the mode of induced abortion in PAH patients; however, there are reports of generally favorable outcomes in early pregnancy, with both medical and surgical approaches [11, 13, 29, 30].

Women who decide to continue pregnancy should be managed at an expert center with a multidisciplinary team experienced in the care of pregnant PAH patients. The team should consist of a PH specialist, a cardiologist, an obstetrician, an anesthetist experienced in managing high-risk pregnancies, and a neonatologist [15, 19, 30].

A baseline multiparametric assessment of pregnancy risk should be performed. This should include a clinical evaluation of functional class and volume status, 6-minute walk testing, measurement of brain natriuretic peptide, and echocardiography. This systematic assessment of PH status should be performed at regular intervals. Patients should be followed closely. As a norm, reviews should occur monthly during the first trimester, fortnightly in the second trimester, and weekly in the third trimester. Naturally, patients at heightened risk will require more frequent assessment [19].

Volume status should be assiduously optimized with fluid and sodium restriction and use of diuretics (see Figure 13.1). Reducing RV overdistension is key to avoiding cardiac decompensation [25] and optimizing cardiac function. Furosemide is the preferred diuretic; spironolactone has anti-androgenic effects and is pregnancy category D [15]. Patients should be advised to lie in the lateral position to avoid IVC compression. Arrhythmias should be aggressively corrected. Significant anemia should be corrected to optimize oxygen delivery as much as possible [19]. Iron replacement should be considered for patients who are deficient [25].

Data on the need for anticoagulation for IPAH is conflicting, and for patients with associated forms of PAH it is not recommended [4]. However, in pregnancy, the use of heparin should be considered for prophylaxis of venous thromboembolism [19].

In normal health, blood flows from the resting circulating volume to the right heart and through the lung where it is oxygenated (Figure 13.1 A). During pregnancy, the vascular reservoir increases owing to expansion of plasma volume. There is an increase in end-diastolic cardiac volume and CO. Recruitment and vasodilation of the pulmonary vasculature allows for adaptation in the increase in flow through the pulmonary vascular bed (Figure 13.1 B). In PH, the vascular reserve of the pulmonary vasculature is attenuated. As such, there is a restriction in pulmonary blood flow and CO.

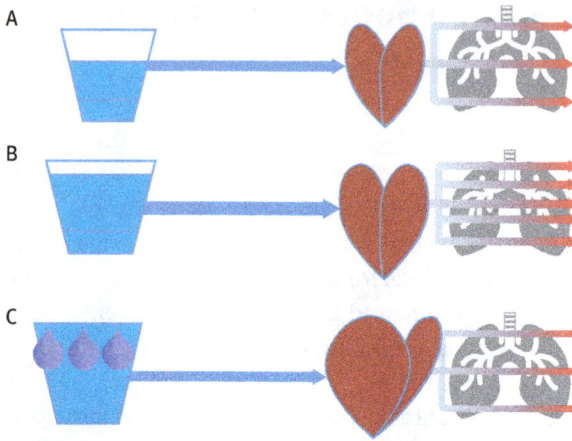

Figure 13.1: Influence of the loss of pulmonary vascular reserve on cardiac function in pregnancy.

This results in a reduction in venous return, leading to an increase in venous pressures and RV dilation. RV dilation leads to an increase in RV wall tension (increased cardiac work, oxygen consumption, and, if severe, RV ischemia). Additionally, the leftward shift of the interventricular septum leads to impairment in LV filling and contributes to a reduction in CO (Figure 13.1 C).

13.7 PAH-Targeted Medications in Pregnancy

Patients with PAH who choose to continue pregnancy will likely require PAH-targeted therapy adjusted to optimize hemodynamics and RV function prior to delivery, and tailored to prevent fetal toxicity. Currently available PAH therapies target three different pathways involved in the pathophysiology of the disease, that is, the prostacyclin, nitric oxide (NO), and endothelin pathways [16]. While the evidence supports the efficacy and safety of these therapeutics for the treatment of PAH, data on their use in pregnancy are scarce. The literature is largely comprised of retrospective reports of expert center experiences [13, 29, 30], small case series [22, 33], and a systematic review of these published cases, which showed a significantly lower maternal mortality compared to the era before PAH-targeted treatment [10, 12]. However, this should clearly be taken with a number of caveats, not in the least, reporting and publication biases. More recently, a multinational prospective registry reported outcomes of 26 pregnancies. Favorable outcomes were observed for women with well-controlled PAH on targeted therapy [11].

Prostacyclin and the prostacyclin analogs, epoprostenol, treprostinil, and iloprost, are potent vasodilators that also have antiproliferative properties [16]. These are administered parenterally, via the intravenous, subcutaneous, or inhaled route, and are pregnancy category B (epoprostenol and treprostinil) or C (iloprost). The usual indication for these agents is in patients of NYHA functional class III or IV, with a high-risk status based on multiparametric risk stratification, or patients who have had an inadequate response to oral therapies and are failing to meet treatment milestones [4, 16]. In pregnant PAH patients, there should be a low threshold for the initiation of parenteral prostanoids to optimize hemodynamics and RV function. Observational data suggest that these agents are safe in pregnancy and may potentially influence maternal outcomes [11, 12, 14, 22, 29, 30, 33]. There is lack of data to support the use of the oral prostacyclin IP receptor agonist, selexipag, in pregnancy.

The phosphodiesterase type 5 inhibitors (PDE-5i), sildenafil and tadalafil, act on the NO / cyclic GMP (cGMP) pathway to exert vasodilatory and antiproliferative effects [16]. These oral agents are considered safe in pregnancy (pregnancy category B). Data on their use in pregnancy is limited to published experience from expert centers and case series, often in combination with prostanoids [11, 13, 14, 30, 33, 34]. Although there is paucity of data on Tadalafil in the pregnant population, it is thought to have comparable safety and efficacy with the advantage of once-daily versus thrice-daily dosing.

Riociguat is a soluble guanylate cyclase inhibitor that acts upstream of PDE-5i in the common NO/cGMP pathway. It is pregnancy category X and should not be used in pregnancy [19].

The endothelin receptor antagonists (ERA), bosentan, ambrisentan, and macitentan are known to be teratogenic (pregnancy category X) and should not be used in pregnancy [19, 35].

Calcium channel blockers (CCB), amlodipine, nifedipine, and diltiazem, are used at high doses in selected IPAH patients who demonstrate an acute vasodilator response to inhaled nitric oxide or IV epoprostenol at the time of RHC, defined as $\geqslant 10$ mmHg reduction in mPAP to reach an absolute mPAP $\leqslant 40$ mmHg, with an increased or unchanged CO. However, only a subset of acute vasodilator responders has a sustained adequate clinical and hemodynamic response to CCB monotherapy after one year [36]. This group of long-term responders to CCB, which represents < 10% of IPAH patients, has a distinctively favorable clinical course, with essentially 100% survival at seven years and near-normal hemodynamics and functional status [1, 36]. Data on pregnancy in a very limited number of long-term responders to CCB who had near-normal hemodynamics showed that all had successful uncomplicated pregnancies [11, 29]. Patients who do not strictly meet the definition of an acute vasodilator response should not be treated with CCB due to the potential risk of hypotension and circulatory collapse.

13.8 Approach to PAH-targeted Treatment

There is no universal consensus on the approach to PAH-targeted therapy during pregnancy, including the timing of treatment initiation or escalation, and the choice of drugs. Varied approaches among expert centers reflect local experience and practical considerations. Additionally, treatment has to be individualized to take into account the severity of PAH, comorbidities, social and cultural aspects, and the patient's preferences. A number of important tenets form the cornerstone of contemporary PAH treatment. While these concepts were validated in the nonpregnant population, we believe that they should also shape the treatment approach for pregnant PAH patients.

Risk stratification has emerged as a fundamental paradigm in the PAH treatment strategy (see Figure 13.2). A global assessment incorporating clinical, functional, echocardiographic, and hemodynamic parameters is used to categorize patients into low-, intermediate- or high-risk according to expected 1-year mortality [4, 16]. Risk should be assessed at baseline and systematically on treatment, with the therapeutic goal of achieving a low-risk status. In case of inadequate treatment response, prompt escalation of PAH-targeted treatment is recommended [4]. A number of risk prediction models are in use, each with important prognostic implications validated by data from large PH registries [37–39].

There is a growing body of evidence in favor of combination therapy for PAH, and the landmark AMBITION study published in 2015 established upfront combination therapy as the standard of care [4, 16, 40]. While evidence is lacking in the pregnant PAH population, it is generally felt that a combination approach offers additive benefits on PAH control, compared to monotherapy. The usual combination in this setting is a PDE-5i and parenteral prostanoid, with the exception of the small minority, who are long-term responders to CCB [19]. Our recommendation is to maximize treatments early in the course of pregnancy, in advance of worsening in RV function, including aggressive up titration of parenteral therapies, and when appropriate, complete a full invasive hemodynamic review. In some women with known PAH, who are committed to considering pregnancy, we have adopted an aggressive approach using acceptable combination therapies that can be used safely in pregnancy to determine if we can achieve an acceptable risk profile.

During pregnancy, we use echocardiography to follow RV end-diastolic volume and RV function, in addition to markers such as Brain Naturetic Peptide (BNP), to guide treatment decisions and provide an ongoing risk assessment. The interprofessional team regularly assesses the mother's and baby's progress and make revisions to the care plan, accordingly.

Determinants of prognosis* (estimated 1-year mortality)	Low risk <5%	Intermediate risk 5–10%	High risk >10%
Clinical signs of right heart failure	Absent	Absent	Present
Progression of symptoms	No	Slow	Rapid
Syncope	No	Occasional syncope[b]	Repeated syncope[c]
WHO functional class	I, II	III	IV
6MWD	>440 m	165–440 m	<165 m
Cardiopulmonary exercise testing	Peak VO_2 >15 ml/min/kg (>65% pred.) VE/VCO_2 slope <36	Peak VO_2 11–15 ml/min/kg (35–65% pred.) VE/VCO_2 slope 36–44.9	Peak VO_2 <11 ml/min/kg (<35% pred.) VE/VCO_2 slope ≥ 45
NT-proBNP plasma levels	BNP <50 ng/l NT-proBNP <300 ng/l	BNP 50–300 ng/l NT-proBNP 300–1400 ng/l	BNP >300 ng/l NT-proBNP >1400 ng/l
Imaging (echocardiography, CMR imaging)	RA area <18 cm² No pericardial effusion	RA area 18–26 cm² No or minimal, pericardial effusion	RA area >26 cm² pericardial effusion
Haemodynamics	RAP <8 mmHg CI ≥ 2.5 l/min/m² SvO_2 > 65%	RAP 8–14 mmHg CI 2.0–2.4 l/min/m² SvO_2 60–65%	RAP >14 mmHg CI <2.0 l/min/m² SvO_2 <60%

Figure 13.2: PAH Determinates of Risk (General Population). 6-Minute Walk Distance (6MWD), Oxygen Consumption (VO2), Minute Ventilation (VE), N-Terminal Brain Natriuretic Peptide (NT-BNP), Brain Natriuretic Peptide (BNP), Right Atrium (RA), Right Atrial Pressure (RAP), Cardiac Index (CI), Mixed Venous Saturation (SvO2). Reproduced with permission from [4].

13.9 Peripartum Management

The optimal timing of elective delivery is uncertain and involves an evaluation of the maternal risk of continuing pregnancy and neonatal risk from preterm birth. For women who are stable, planned delivery around weeks 34–36 should be considered [19].

During the peripartum period, guidelines recommend monitoring in a high acuity setting, with continuous electrocardiogram, oxygen saturation, intra-arterial blood pressure, and central venous pressure [15]. There should be vigilant monitoring and correction of acute adverse conditions including hypoxemia, hypercapnia, acidemia, and hypothermia, as these can promote pulmonary vasoconstriction and further increase RV afterload [19, 25]. Swan–Ganz catheterization is not recommended as a routine because of the risk of complications, but may be considered in selected patients with severe RV failure to guide therapy [19].

Elective cesarean section is the preferred mode of delivery among many expert centers [19]. Vaginal delivery is associated with deleterious hemodynamic effects and imposes significant demands on the cardiovascular system. Normal vaginal delivery is associated with up to a 34% increase in CO. Frequent use of the Valsalva maneuver when pushing causes swings in intrathoracic pressure and fluctuations in venous return [30]. Combined with labor-induced vasovagal responses, this can lead to rapid and critical decreases in RV preload, which may precipitate cardiopulmonary collapse. Pain is associated with increased sympathetic activity and catecholamine release. This may contribute to hemodynamic instability from tachycardia and increases in pulmonary vascular tone. After delivery, autotransfusion from the contracting uterus and relief of IVC compression by the gravid uterus may lead to acute volume overload and RV overdistension. Lastly, agents and/or procedures to induce labor may precipitate deterioration [19].

In contrast, elective cesarean section avoids labor and its aforementioned detrimental hemodynamic consequences. It allows for meticulous multidisciplinary preparation, including planning of anesthesia, optimization of hemodynamics, and contingency planning [19]. Individualized management plans covering different eventualities are recommended. This includes premature onset of labor and emergency cesarean section for either the mother or baby. A tailored multi-professional approach is associated with improved outcomes [30].

Regional anesthesia is preferred. Epidural anesthesia with incremental doses has traditionally been the advocated approach [19]. Careful fractionated dosing is important to avoid precipitous drops in SVR, which can be complicated by hypotension, reduction of coronary perfusion, and RV failure [31]. Spinal anesthesia with a bolus technique should be avoided because of the risk of a rapid rise in block height, which may cause sympathetic block and hypotension [19, 31]. Low-dose combined spinal-epidural anesthesia is increasingly favored for its merits in providing a denser perineal sensory block, with minimal additive risk of hypotension [19, 29, 32].

General anesthesia is associated with significant risk in patients with PH [19, 31]. Observational data suggests increased mortality in parturients who receive general anesthesia compared to regional anesthesia [12]. Sedatives and general anesthetic agents may depress cardiac function, cause non-selective vasodilation, and lead to systemic hypotension and hemodynamic collapse [25, 26]. Laryngoscopy and endotracheal intubation increases PA pressures, and positive-pressure ventilation increases PVR [31]. If intubation and mechanical ventilation are unavoidable, administration of catecholamines prior to induction of anesthesia should be considered to mitigate hypotension and loss of RV contractility. Airway pressures should be kept as low as possible while avoiding hypercapnia, due to its deleterious effects on pulmonary hemodynamics [26]. For high risk pregnancies, we also consult our Ectracorporeal Membrane Oxygenation (ECMO) service to provide back up in the labor and delivery suite, in the event of cardiovascular collapse.

The early postpartum is a high-risk period for patients with PAH, with heart failure, sudden death, and thromboembolism being the leading causes of death [10, 12]. Close monitoring in ICU for several days after childbirth is recommended and prophylactic anticoagulation is crucial [19]. After placental delivery, it is crucial that oxytocin is infused slowly, as large boluses can cause significant hemodynamic perturbation [33]. We routinely keep patients in the ICU for 2–3 days following delivery, to be monitored and treated with vasopressors to support systemic blood pressure as needed and ensure the provision of aggressive diuresis (2–3 liters net negative per day), during the post-partum phase until they are euvolemic.

13.10 Conclusions

There have been major advances in the care of patients with PAH over the past several decades, with the advent of multiple classes of PAH-directed medications. However, PAH remains a severe, incurable disease with a high burden of morbidity and a high rate of premature death. Pregnancy continues to be associated with an unacceptably high risk of maternal mortality among women with PAH, and avoidance of pregnancy or early therapeutic abortion should be strongly recommended. Nonetheless, some women with PAH may decide to continue their pregnancy, in spite of the risks. These patients should be managed at experienced centers with close monitoring. There is suggestion from recent data from a limited sample that select patients with very well-controlled PAH may have favorable pregnancy outcomes. However, such an assessment of the safety of pregnancy should be based on an individualized assessment made by a highly experienced team, in conjunction with the patient and family.

References

[1]   Simonneau G, Montani D, Celermajer DS, et al. Haemodynamic definitions and updated clinical classification of pulmonary hypertension. Eur Respir J [Internet] 2019;53(1). Available from: http://dx.doi.org/10.1183/13993003.01913-2018.

[2]   Humbert M, Guignabert C, Bonnet S, et al. Pathology and pathobiology of pulmonary hypertension: State of the art and research perspectives. Eur Respir J [Internet] 2019;53(1). Available from: http://dx.doi.org/10.1183/13993003.01887-2018.

[3]   Vonk Noordegraaf A, Chin KM, Haddad F, et al. Pathophysiology of the right ventricle and of the pulmonary circulation in pulmonary hypertension: An update. Eur Respir J [Internet] 2019;53(1). Available from: http://dx.doi.org/10.1183/13993003.01900-2018.

[4]   Galiè Nazzareno, Humbert Marc, Jean-Luc Vachiery, et al. ESC/ERS Guidelines for the diagnosis and treatment of pulmonary hypertension. European Respiratory Journal 2015;46: 903–975. DOI: 10.1183/13993003.01032-2015.

[5]   McGoon MD, Benza RL, Escribano-Subias P, et al. Pulmonary arterial hypertension: Epidemiology and registries. J Am Coll Cardiol 2013;62(25SUPPL.).

[6]   Rich S, Dantzker DR, Ayres SM, et al. Primary pulmonary hypertension. Ann Intern Med 1987;107:216–223.

[7]   Frost AE, Badesch DB, Barst RJ, et al. The changing picture of patients with pulmonary arterial hypertension in the United States: How REVEAL differs from historic and non-US contemporary registries. Chest [Internet] 2011;139(1):128–137. Available from: http://dx.doi.org/10.1378/chest.10-0075.

[8]   D'Alonzo GE, Barst RJ, Ayres SM, et al. Survival in patients with primary pulmonary hypertension: Results from a national prospective registry. Ann Intern Med 1991;115(5): 343–349.

[9]   Benza RL, Miller DP, Barst RJ, Badesch DB, Frost AE, McGoon MD. An evaluation of long-term survival from time of diagnosis in pulmonary arterial hypertension from the reveal registry. Chest [Internet] 2012;142(2):448–456. Available from: http://dx.doi.org/10.1378/chest.11-1460.

[10]   Weiss BM, Zemp L, Seifert B, Hess OM. Outcome of pulmonary vascular disease in pregnancy: A systematic overview from 1978 through 1996. J Am Coll Cardiol [Internet] 1998;31(7):1650–1657. Available from: http://dx.doi.org/10.1016/S0735-1097(98)00162-4.

[11]   Jaïs X, Olsson KM, Barbera JA, et al. Pregnancy outcomes in pulmonary arterial hypertension in the modern management era. Eur Respir J 2012;40(4):881–885.

[12]   Bédard E, Dimopoulos K, Gatzoulis MA. Has there been any progress made on pregnancy outcomes among women with pulmonary arterial hypertension?. Eur Heart J 2009;30(3): 256–265.

[13]   Duarte AG, Thomas S, Safdar Z, et al. Management of pulmonary arterial hypertension during pregnancy: A retrospective, multicenter experience. Chest [Internet] 2013;143(5):1330–1336. Available from: http://dx.doi.org/10.1378/chest.12-0528.

[14]   Rosengarten D, Blieden LC, Kramer MR. Pregnancy outcomes in pulmonary arterial hypertension in the modern management era. Eur Respir J 2012;40(5):1304–1305.

[15]   Regitz-Zagrosek V, Roos-Hesselink JW, Bauersachs J, et al. 2018 ESC Guidelines for the management of cardiovascular diseases during pregnancy. Vol. 39. Eur Heart J 2018: 3165–3241.

[16]   Galiè N, Humbert M, Vachiery JL, et al. 2015 ESC/ERS Guidelines for the diagnosis and treatment of pulmonary hypertension. Eur Heart J 2016;37(1):67–119.

[17]   Aguree S, Gernand AD. Plasma volume expansion across healthy pregnancy: a systematic review and meta-analysis of longitudinal studies. BMC Pregnancy Childbirth 2019;19(1):1–11.

[18] Milman N, Bergholt T, Byg KE, Eriksen L, Hvas AM. Reference intervals for haematological variables during normal pregnancy and postpartum in 434 healthy Danish women. Eur J Haematol 2007;79(1):39–46.

[19] Hemnes AR, Kiely DG, Cockrill BA, et al. Statement on pregnancy in pulmonary hypertension from the pulmonary vascular research institute. Pulm Circ 2015;5(3):435–465.

[20] Van Oppen ACC, Stigter RH, Bruinse HW. 1996 Cardiac output in pregnancy.pdf. Obstet Gynecol 1996;87:310–318.

[21] Sanghavi M, Rutherford JD. Cardiovascular physiology of pregnancy. Circulation 2014;130(12):1003–1008.

[22] Bendayan D, Hod M, Oron G, et al. Pregnancy Outcome in Patients With Pulmonary Arterial Hypertension Receiving Prostacyclin Therapy. Obstet Gynecol 2005;106:1206–1210.

[23] Ducas RA, Elliott JE, Melnyk SF, et al. Cardiovascular magnetic resonance in pregnancy: insights from the cardiac hemodynamic imaging and remodeling in pregnancy (CHIRP) study. J Cardiovasc Magn Reson 2014;16(1):1–9.

[24] Grindheim G, Estensen ME, Langesaeter E, Rosseland LA, Toska K. Changes in blood pressure during healthy pregnancy: a longitudinal cohort study. J Hypertens 2012;30(2):342–350.

[25] Harjola VP, Mebazaa A, Čelutkiene J, et al. Contemporary management of acute right ventricular failure: a statement from the heart failure association and the working group on pulmonary circulation and right ventricular function of the European society of cardiology. Eur J Heart Fail 2016;18(3):226–241.

[26] Hoeper MM, Granton J. Intensive care unit management of patients with severe pulmonary hypertension and right heart failure. Am J Respir Crit Care Med 2011;184(10):1114–1124.

[27] Lahm T, Albrecht M, Fisher AJ, et al. 17β-Estradiol attenuates hypoxic pulmonary hypertension via estrogen receptor-mediated effects. Am J Respir Crit Care Med 2012;185(9):965–980.

[28] White K, Dempsie Y, Nilsen M, Wright AF, Loughlin L, MacLean MR. The serotonin transporter, gender, and 17β oestradiol in the development of pulmonary arterial hypertension. Cardiovasc Res 2011;90(2):373–382.

[29] Bonnin M, Mercier F, Sitbon O, et al. Severe Pulmonary Hypertension during Pregnancy. Surv Anesthesiol 2006;50(1):26–27.

[30] Kiely DG, Condliffe R, Webster V, et al. Improved survival in pregnancy and pulmonary hypertension using a multiprofessional approach. BJOG An Int J Obstet Gynaecol 2010;117(5): 565–574.

[31] Gille J, Seyfarth HJ, Gerlach S, Malcharek M, Czeslick E, Sablotzki A. Perioperative anesthesiological management of patients with pulmonary hypertension. Anesthesiol Res Pract 2012;2012.

[32] Duggan AB, Katz SG. Combined spinal and epidural anaesthesia for caesarean section in a parturient with severe primary pulmonary hypertension. Anaesth Intensive Care 2003;31(5): 565–569.

[33] Goland S, Tsai F, Habib M, Janmohamed M, Goodwin TM, Elkayam U. Favorable outcome of pregnancy with an elective use of epoprostenol and sildenafil in women with severe pulmonary hypertension. Cardiology 2010;115(3):205–208.

[34] Curry RA, Fletcher C, Gelson E, et al. Pulmonary hypertension and pregnancy-a review of 12 pregnancies in nine women. BJOG An Int J Obstet Gynaecol 2012;119(6):752–761.

[35] Treinen KA, Louden C, Dennis MJ, Wier PJ. Developmental toxicity and toxicokinetics of two endothelin receptor antagonists in rats and rabbits. Teratology 1999 Jan;59(1):51–59.

[36] Sitbon O, Humbert M, Jaïs X, et al. Long-term response to calcium channel blockers in idiopathic pulmonary arterial hypertension. Circulation 2005;111(23):3105–3111.

[37] Kylhammar D, Kjellström B, Hjalmarsson C, et al. A comprehensive risk stratification at early follow-up determines prognosis in pulmonary arterial hypertension. Eur Heart J 2018;39(47): 4175–4181.

[38] Benza RL, Miller DP, Foreman AJ, et al. Prognostic implications of serial risk score assessments in patients with pulmonary arterial hypertension: a registry to evaluate early and long-term pulmonary arterial hypertension disease management (REVEAL) analysis. J Hear Lung Transplant [Internet] 2015;34(3):356–361. Available from: http://dx.doi.org/ 10.1016/j.healun.2014.09.016.

[39] Boucly A, Weatherald J, Savale L, et al. Risk assessment, prognosis and guideline implementation in pulmonary arterial hypertension. Eur Respir J [Internet] 2017;50(2):1–10. Available from: http://dx.doi.org/10.1183/13993003.00889-2017.

[40] Galie N, Barbera JA, Frost AE, et al. Initial use of ambrisentan plus tadalafil in pulmonary arterial hypertension. N Engl J Med 2015;373(9):834–844.

Alina Blazer, Meyer Balter
14 Asthma in Pregnancy

14.1 Introduction

Asthma is a chronic inflammatory disorder characterized by airway hyperresponsiveness and variable airflow obstruction. It is the most common chronic medical condition affecting pregnancy and its prevalence in the population is only increasing [1, 2], with current estimates suggesting asthma affects 2–13% of pregnancies worldwide [2, 3]. Pregnancy can affect asthma control and, conversely, maternal asthma is associated with increased risk of adverse perinatal outcomes. Thus, optimizing asthma management prior to and during pregnancy is of critical importance to protecting the health of both mother and baby.

14.2 Changes in Respiratory Function During Pregnancy

Numerous physiological changes accompany pregnancy to meet the metabolic demands of the fetus and the mother (see Figure 14.1). Respiratory changes include an increase in minute ventilation that occurs by an increase in tidal volume without a change in respiratory rate, leading to a compensated respiratory alkalosis [4]. The enlarging gravid uterus affects chest wall compliance, causing a decrease of 10–25% in the functional residual capacity (FRC) as the pregnancy progresses [4, 5]. Expiratory reserve volume and residual volume also decline slightly; however, total lung capacity remains within the normal range [4, 5]. Forced vital capacity (FVC) remains stable or can exhibit a modest increase after 14–16 weeks gestation [6]. Pregnancy has no impact on the forced expiratory volume (FEV1) in 1 second, FEV1/FVC ratio, or peak expiratory flow [6, 7]. Thus, any abnormality or decline in spirometry should alert the health care practitioner to an underlying respiratory concern.

14.3 Effects of Pregnancy on Asthma

Multiple studies of pregnant women with asthma have demonstrated that asthma severity tends to improve in one-third of patients, stays the same in one-third, and worsens in one-third [8, 9]. While the course in an individual patient may be difficult to predict, two prospective studies reported that women with severe asthma are more likely to deteriorate than those with mild disease [9, 10]. In fact, more than

https://doi.org/10.1515/9783110615258-014

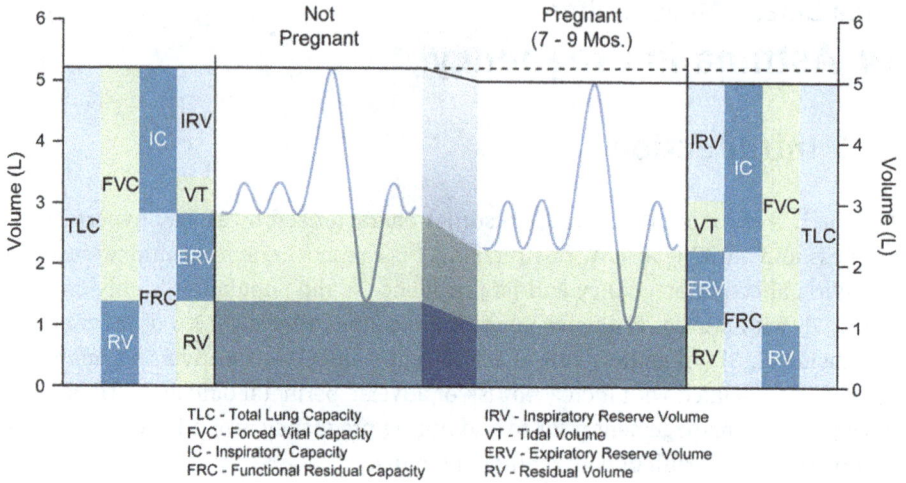

TLC - Total Lung Capacity
FVC - Forced Vital Capacity
IC - Inspiratory Capacity
FRC - Functional Residual Capacity

IRV - Inspiratory Reserve Volume
VT - Tidal Volume
ERV - Expiratory Reserve Volume
RV - Residual Volume

Figure 14.1: Comparison of lung volumes between pregnant and nonpregnant states. Reproduced with permission from [4].

half of women with severe asthma were found to experience exacerbations during pregnancy compared to 8–13% with mild disease [9, 10]. It follows that hospitalizations for asthma have also been shown to increase during pregnancy, with women of low socioeconomic status being at particularly increased risk [11]. Exacerbations most commonly occur between 24 and 36 weeks [10, 12] with respiratory viral infections cited as the most frequent trigger (34%), followed by poor adherence to inhaled corticosteroid therapy (29%) [10]. Other risk factors for worsened asthma control during pregnancy include obesity [13], ongoing smoking and uncontrolled comorbidities including rhinitis, gastrointestinal reflux disease (GERD), and depression [3, 12].

14.3.1 Mechanisms for the Effect of Pregnancy on Maternal Asthma

Physiological factors, including maternal hormonal fluctuations and alterations in immune function, have also been proposed to play a role in asthma control, in either beneficial or detrimental ways. Increased serum-free cortisol in pregnancy has been suggested to have anti-inflammatory effects [14], and elevated progesterone may contribute to improvement in asthma symptoms via its effect on smooth muscle relaxation and increased minute ventilation – both of these could improve asthma control [15]. Conversely, progesterone has also been implicated in worsening asthma status via progesterone-induced B2-adrenergic receptor downregulation and decreased bronchodilator responsiveness, as has been shown in nonpregnant females with asthma, following exogenous progesterone administration [16].

Pregnancy is a state that requires physiologic downregulation of the maternal immune system to tolerate the growing fetus, leading to suppression of cell-mediated immunity and the development of a predominantly Th2 cytokine environment [14]. Allergic asthma is a Th2-mediated inflammatory condition, leading researchers to suggest that the Th2-predominant environment of pregnancy may contribute to worsening asthma in some women [14]. Furthermore, modification of cell-mediated immunity may influence maternal response to infection and inflammation. Overall, the interplay of these multiple factors in a given individual may explain the variable prognoses of asthma during pregnancy.

14.4 Effects of Asthma on Pregnancy: Maternal and Fetal Outcomes

Numerous prospective and historical studies over the past decades have identified asthma as a risk factor for adverse perinatal outcomes such as preeclampsia, need for Caesarian section, perinatal mortality, preterm birth, and low birth weight [17, 18]. Although the exact mechanisms underlying these increased risks remain unclear, the most supported hypothesis is that poor asthma control contributes to chronic maternal hypoxia and inflammation, which, subsequently, negatively impacts placental function, fetal oxygen delivery, and growth [10, 19, 20].

The most comprehensive data on perinatal outcomes comes from a large meta-analysis that included 40 studies and over 1.5 million subjects, and showed maternal asthma was associated with an increased risk of low birthweight infants [relative risk (RR) 1.46, 95% confidence interval (CI) 1.22–1.75], intrauterine growth restriction (RR 1.22, 95% CI 1.14–1.31), preterm delivery (RR 1.41, 95% CI 1.22–1.61) and preeclampsia (RR 1.54, 95% CI 1.32–1.81) [17]. In addition to these risks, a large retrospective cohort study demonstrated an increased risk of congenital malformations associated with severe asthma exacerbations in the first trimester (adjusted odds ratio 1.64, 95% CI 1.02–2.64) [21]. Notably, the RR of preterm delivery and preterm labor were reduced to nonsignificant levels by active asthma management (RR 1.07, 95% CI 0.91–1.26 for preterm delivery; RR 0.96, 95% CI 0.73–1.26 for preterm labor) [17] and the risks of congenital malformations were not seen in mild-to-moderate exacerbations [21], suggesting that adequate asthma control is paramount to reducing negative perinatal outcomes.

In a complementary meta-analysis investigating adverse maternal outcomes, Wang *et al.* found that asthma was associated with a significantly increased risk of cesarean section (RR 1.31, 95% CI 1.22–1.39), gestational diabetes (RR 1.39, 95% CI 1.17–1.66), postpartum hemorrhage (RR 1.29, 95% CI 1.18–1.41), and premature rupture of membranes (RR 1.21, 95%CI 1.07–1.37) [18]. Similarly, higher asthma severity significantly increased the risk of cesarean section and gestational diabetes compared to mild asthma, whereas bronchodilator use was associated with a significantly lowered risk of gestational diabetes [18], providing consistent evidence for ensuring optimization of asthma symptoms in pregnancy.

Finally, a population cohort study investigating children born to women with acute asthma exacerbations during pregnancy showed they have an elevated risk of developing asthma (odds ratio 1.23, 95% CI 1.13–1.33) and pneumonia (odds ratio 1.12, 95% CI 1.03–1.22) during the first 5 years of life [22].

Taken together, these studies confirm that poor asthma control and increased asthma severity are associated with adverse outcomes in pregnancy, for both mother and baby. However, it is also important to remember that most pregnant women with mild and well-controlled asthma will experience no or minimal increased risks.

14.5 Treatment of Asthma in Pregnancy: General Principles

International guidelines are available that outline the goals of successful asthma management and recommendations for treatment of asthma during pregnancy. These goals include maintaining maternal quality of life and normal fetal growth by minimizing asthma symptoms and preventing exacerbations, using therapies with minimal or no adverse effects [23, 24]. Achievement of these aims requires patient engagement, regular monitoring of clinical symptoms, and correct administration of pharmacotherapies.

14.6 Nonpharmacological Management

Education is the cornerstone of asthma management, and pregnant patients with asthma should receive detailed counseling regarding trigger avoidance, medication adherence, and proper use of inhalers and devices [25].

Frequency and intensity of antenatal maternal monitoring should be based on individual patient risk factors, including the severity of asthma and adequacy of prepregnancy control. At a minimum, monthly monitoring of clinical symptoms is generally recommended [23, 24]. Monitoring can be accomplished via a multidisciplinary approach to coordinating asthma care, involving nurses, midwives, pharmacists, respiratory therapists, asthma educators, and primary care physicians [25–27].

Pregnancy is not a contraindication to pulmonary function testing. Spirometry and peak expiratory flow measurements should be performed at routine intervals antenatally to monitor lung function, with the exception being in patients suffering from cervical incompetence [28]. Pregnancy is, however, a relative contraindication to methacholine challenge testing. Methacholine was considered a pregnancy class C medication under the former FDA drug classification system, meaning that reproductive studies have not been performed and it is unknown whether methacholine is associated with fetal abnormalities. It is also unknown if it is excreted in breast milk [29].

Smoking cessation is an important issue for pregnant women, in general, and especially those with asthma. A significant proportion (20–30%) of asthmatic women continues to smoke during pregnancy, with studies suggesting they are more likely to experience severe symptoms and suffer from acute exacerbations [30]. In addition, they are at increased risk for worse perinatal outcomes from the combined effects of smoking, maternal asthma, and exacerbations [30]. Behavioral therapy and patient education should be recommended as first-line therapy for smoking cessation. A Cochrane systemic review of eight trials of nicotine replacement therapy (NRT) used with behavioral support in pregnancy showed borderline improvement in smoking cessation rates, with insufficient evidence to conclude positive or negative effects on birth outcomes [31]. Few trials have investigated the role of pharmacologic smoking cessation therapies in pregnancy, such as bupropion and varenicline. A single, small randomized controlled trial assessed the use of bupropion, with modest improvement in quit rates [32]. Limited data exist on varenicline in pregnancy, and it is not generally used. Current recommendations suggest offering NRT to pregnant patients if behavioral counseling alone fails, using the lowest effective dose required [33]. Bupropion could be considered with careful consideration if the benefits outweigh risks of ongoing maternal smoking.

14.7 Pharmacological Management

A stepwise approach to pharmacologic asthma treatment, similar to the non-pregnant population, is recommended during pregnancy, but with a few important considerations.

14.7.1 Beta-Agonists

Short-acting beta-agonists (SABAs) (e.g., salbutamol) are the reliever therapy of choice in current asthma guidelines, though minimizing use through optimizing asthma control is the goal. SABAs are regarded as safe, with no evidence of any associations with congenital anomalies, low birth weight, or increased rates of poor maternal or perinatal outcomes [8, 34]. SABA-only treatment for asthma management in adults is no longer recommended in the most recent Global Initiative for Asthma Control recommendations [24] and thus should be used in conjunction with a maintenance controller therapy. Long-acting beta-agonists (LABAs) (e.g., formoterol and salmeterol) are used as maintenance therapy in patients with moderate to severe asthma, in combination with inhaled corticosteroids (ICS). The use of LABAs during pregnancy has not been associated with an increased incidence of fetal abnormalities, with the majority of safety data available for salmeterol and formoterol [34–36]. In patients with persistent asthma symptoms not controlled by ICS alone, ICS/LABA combinations can be considered as additional therapy, with studies describing LABA addition more effective than increased ICS for reducing asthma exacerbation rates and SABA use [37].

14.7.2 Inhaled Corticosteroids

Inhaled corticosteroids (e.g., budesonide and fluticasone propionate) are considered the mainstay of controller therapy in asthma, in order to minimize symptoms and prevent acute exacerbations. While ICS remain under-prescribed to asthmatic pregnant patients [38], numerous studies evaluating their effectiveness have definitively shown they reduce the risk of exacerbations [39]. Furthermore, cessation of ICS in pregnancy has been shown to be an important contributing factor to the development of asthma exacerbations [12]. Low to moderate doses of ICS are not associated with increased incidence of congenital malformations or decreased fetal growth [21, 40]. While some studies have suggested a possible increased risk of congenital malformation in the higher dose range, it is impossible to account for confounding by asthma severity [40]. Budesonide is usually the drug of choice, as it has been studied in an analysis of over 6,000 pregnant asthmatics, but fluticasone propionate seems equally safe [35].

14.7.3 Other Asthma Medications

Leukotriene receptor antagonists (e.g., montelukast) are generally considered safe in pregnancy with no evidence of major congenital malformations in prospective human studies [41]. Theophylline can be continued in pregnancy but requires monitoring of serum concentrations (target level between 5 and 12 mcg/mL) to avoid toxicity [23]. Pregnancy outcomes of patients treated with the anti-IgE monoclonal antibody Omalizumab (Xolair) have been followed in the EXPECT Xolair Pregnancy Registry, and show no evidence of increased perinatal risks compared to the general asthma population [42]. New initiation is relatively contraindicated in pregnancy due to the risk of anaphylaxis; however, patients controlled on anti-IgE therapy prepregnancy can be continued with an informed discussion as to the risks and benefits. Newer biologic agents, including the anti-IL-5 monoclonal antibodies Benralizumab (Fasenra), Mepolizumab (Nucala), and Reslizumab (Cinqair), have had reassuring animal data but no human gestational studies are available yet.

14.7.4 Health Behaviors

Despite clear guidelines for the management of asthma during pregnancy, there is strong evidence that management remains suboptimal in many patients [43–45]. Nonadherence to asthma medications is a significant problem in pregnancy, with studies finding that up to one-third of patients discontinue regular preventative asthma therapy without consulting their healthcare professionals [45]. Another large longitudinal cohort study similarly demonstrated that pregnant women reduce their use of inhaled corticosteroids by 23%, SABA by 13%, and rescue oral corticosteroids by 54% [43]. Importantly, use of asthma medications below levels recommended by international guidelines is associated with more severe asthma during pregnancy [44]. Reasons for nonadherence have been explored and included lack of proactive support and information, and concerns regarding safety of the medications [46]. Further studies have shown that even physicians are reluctant to prescribe corticosteroids to pregnant women [47]. Overall, such concerns regarding harmful effects have not been borne out in studies. In fact, a systematic review of 33 published studies did not find any conclusive links between preventive asthma medications and adverse pregnancy outcomes [34]. Conversely, well-controlled maternal asthma has been shown to decrease the risks of congenital malformations and delivery complications. Thus, it is critical to emphasize to both patients and health care practitioners that the advantages of actively treating asthma and preventing exacerbations markedly outweigh any potential risk of maintenance and reliever therapy [24].

14.8 Treatment of Acute Exacerbations

Management of acute asthma exacerbations in pregnant women should mirror the treatment in nonpregnant patients. To avoid fetal hypoxia and adverse maternal outcomes, acute exacerbations should be aggressively treated with short-acting bronchodilators, supplemental oxygen, and early use of systemic corticosteroids [24].

As in nonpregnant patients, the practitioner should first identify the severity of the exacerbation as well as risk factors for clinical deterioration. Mild exacerbations can likely be managed as an outpatient with close follow-up, whereas moderate and severe exacerbations warrant inpatient monitoring, with a shared management model between obstetrical and asthma specialists [26]. Patients with a severe exacerbation in the advanced stages of pregnancy should undergo maternal-fetal monitoring with a biophysical profile [48]. Bedside peak expiratory flow measurements should be obtained and compared with usual or predicted values. Arterial blood gas measurements should be drawn, remembering that there is a baseline compensated respiratory alkalosis in pregnancy, and a normal arterial CO2 of 40 mmHg may indicate relative hypercapnia and impending respiratory failure.

Bronchodilators, including both SABA (e.g., salbutamol) and anticholinergic agents (i.e., ipratropium bromide), are the mainstays of therapy and can be delivered frequently in unstable presentations, such as 4–8 puffs every 20 min for 1 hour (h) and then reduced to hourly intervals. Maternal hypoxia should be promptly corrected with supplemental oxygen to a target oxygen saturation of 95% or greater in order to avoid fetal distress. Systemic corticosteroids should be administered early in the exacerbation at the usual recommended doses (i.e., prednisone 40–50 mg/day or equivalent for at least 5–7 days) [24]. While there are risks related to systemic corticosteroid use, including a small increased risk of cleft palate (0.1–0.3%) if given in the first trimester, the risks associated with uncontrolled asthma are deemed greater [49]. Systemic corticosteroid use beyond the first trimester has not been shown to be associated with adverse fetal effects.

Adjunctive therapies such as intravenous epinephrine should be avoided in pregnancy due to teratogenic effects and risk of placental vessel vasoconstriction [50]. Intravenous magnesium sulfate given at 2 g over 30 min is occasionally recommended in severe asthma exacerbations as a bronchodilator, and can be used in pregnant patients as well, although its efficacy remains unclear. In patients who fail to respond to maximal therapy, invasive ventilation and admission to the intensive care unit should be considered.

14.9 Labor and Delivery

Acute exacerbations during labor and delivery are uncommon but a proportion of patients do continue to demonstrate asthma symptoms [51, 52]. In a prospective observational study of over 1,700 pregnant asthmatic women, approximately 13% of patients with mild asthma and 46% with severe asthma exhibited asthma symptoms during labor [9]. Such symptoms can be well controlled with short-acting bronchodilators [51], and international guidelines support the use of ongoing controller therapy with additional reliever medication as needed in the peripartum period [24]. Importantly, high-dose beta-agonists can induce neonatal hypoglycemia, particularly in preterm infants; thus, if high-dose SABAs were used in the 48 h preceding delivery, blood glucose levels should be monitored in the neonate for the first 24 h of life [24]. Finally, medications such as oxytocin and prostaglandins E1 and E2 can safely be used for obstetrical purposes; however, prostaglandin F2α has been shown to cause bronchospasm and should not be used [23, 53].

14.10 Asthma Postpartum and Breastfeeding Implications

The postpartum period is generally not associated with an increased risk of asthma exacerbations [10, 51]. If a patient has experienced a change in asthma severity during pregnancy, they typically reverts back to prepregnancy severity within a few months postpartum. Limited data is available on the safety of asthma medications in breastfeeding; however, they are generally considered safe and should be continued.

14.11 Conclusion

Asthma is a common medical condition affecting pregnancy and can have a significant impact on maternal and fetal outcomes. The most effective strategy to prevent exacerbations and subsequent complications is optimization of asthma control via patient education, trigger avoidance, adherence to controller therapy, and regular monitoring by both obstetricians and asthma specialists. Asthma medications in pregnancy are generally considered safe, and exacerbations should be treated aggressively with similar management as in nonpregnant patients. Overall, patient and clinician engagement in ensuring optimal asthma control can improve clinical outcomes for both mother and child.

References

[1]   Kwon HL, Triche EW, Belanger K, Bracken MB. The epidemiology of asthma during pregnancy: prevalence, diagnosis, and symptoms. Immunol Allergy Clin North Am 2006;26(1):29–62. doi: 10.1016/j.iac.2005.11.002.

[2]   Jølving LR, Nielsen J, Kesmodel US, Nielsen RG, Beck-Nielsen SS, Nørgård BM. Prevalence of maternal chronic diseases during pregnancy – a nationwide population based study from 1989 to 2013. Acta Obstet Gynecol Scand 2016;95(11):1295–1304. doi: 10.1111/aogs.13007.

[3]   Bonham CA, Patterson KC, Strek ME. Asthma outcomes and management during pregnancy. Chest 2018;153(2):515–527. doi: 10.1016/j.chest.2017.08.029.

[4]   Hegewald MJ, Crapo RO. Respiratory Physiology in Pregnancy. Clin Chest Med 32 (2011) 1–13.

[5]   Milne JA. The respiratory response to pregnancy. Postgrad Med J 1979;55(643):318–324. doi: 10.1136/pgmj.55.643.318.

[6]   Contreras G, Gutiérrez M, Beroíza T et al. Ventilatory drive and respiratory muscle function in pregnancy. Am Rev Respir Dis 1991;144(4): 837–841. doi: 10.1164/ajrccm/144.4.837.

[7]   Grindheim G, Toska K, Estensen M-E, Rosseland LA. Changes in pulmonary function during pregnancy: a longitudinal cohort study. BJOG Int J Obstet Gynaecol 2012;119(1):94–101. doi: 10.1111/j.1471-0528.2011.03158.x.

[8] Milne JA, Mills RJ, Howie AD, Pack AI. Large airways function during normal pregnancy. BJOG Int J Obstet Gynaecol 1977;84(6):448–451. doi: 10.1111/j.1471-0528.1977.tb12621.x.

[9] Schatz M, Harden K, Forsythe A et al. The course of asthma during pregnancy, post partum, and with successive pregnancies: a prospective analysis. J Allergy Clin Immunol 1988;81(3): 509–517. doi: 10.1016/0091-6749(88)90187-X.

[10] Schatz M, Dombrowski MP, Wise R et al. Asthma morbidity during pregnancy can be predicted by severity classification. J Allergy Clin Immunol 2003;112(2): 283–288. doi: 10.1067/mai.2003.1516.

[11] Murphy VE, Gibson P, Talbot PI, Clifton VL. Severe asthma exacerbations during pregnancy. 2005;106(5):9.

[12] To T, Feldman LY, Zhu J, Gershon AS. Asthma health services utilisation before, during and after pregnancy: a population-based cohort study. Eur Respir J 2018;51(4):1800209. doi: 10.1183/13993003.00209-2018.

[13] Murphy VE. Asthma exacerbations during pregnancy: incidence and association with adverse pregnancy outcomes. Thorax 2006;61(2):169–176. doi: 10.1136/thx.2005.049718.

[14] Hendler I, Schatz M, Momirova V et al. Association of obesity with pulmonary and nonpulmonary complications of pregnancy in asthmatic women: Obstet Gynecol. 2006;108 (1):77–82. doi: 10.1097/01.AOG.0000223180.53113.0f.

[15] Murphy VE. Asthma during pregnancy: mechanisms and treatment implications. Eur Respir J 2005;25(4):731–750. doi: 10.1183/09031936.05.00085704.

[16] LoMauro A, Aliverti A. Respiratory physiology of pregnancy: physiology masterclass. Breathe 2015;11(4):297–301. doi: 10.1183/20734735.008615.

[17] Soong Tan K, McFarlane LC, Lipworth BJ. Paradoxical down-regulation and desensitization of β2-adrenoceptors by exogenous progesterone in female asthmatics. Chest 1997;111(4): 847–851. doi: 10.1378/chest.111.4.847.

[18] Murphy V, Namazy J, Powell H et al. A meta-analysis of adverse perinatal outcomes in women with asthma: adverse perinatal outcomes in women with asthma. BJOG Int J Obstet Gynaecol 2011;118(11): 1314–1323. doi: 10.1111/j.1471-0528.2011.03055.x.

[19] Wang G, Murphy VE, Namazy J et al. The risk of maternal and placental complications in pregnant women with asthma: a systematic review and meta-analysis. J Matern Fetal Neonatal Med 2014;27(9): 934–942. doi: 10.3109/14767058.2013.847080.

[20] Clifton VL, Giles WB, Smith R et al. Alterations of placental vascular function in asthmatic pregnancies. Am J Respir Crit Care Med 2001;164(4): 546–553. doi: 10.1164/ ajrccm.164.4.2009119.

[21] Murphy VE, Gibson PG, Giles WB et al. Maternal asthma is associated with reduced female fetal growth. Am J Respir Crit Care Med 2003;168(11): 1317–1323. doi: 10.1164/rccm.200303-3740C.

[22] Blais L, Kettani F-Z, Forget A, Beauchesne M-F, Lemiere C. Asthma exacerbations during the first trimester of pregnancy and congenital malformations: revisiting the association in a large representative cohort. Thorax 2015;70(7):647–652. doi: 10.1136/thoraxjnl-2014-206634.

[23] Abdullah K, Zhu J, Gershon A, Dell S, To T. Effect of asthma exacerbation during pregnancy in women with asthma: a population-based cohort study. Eur Respir J November 2019;1901335. doi: 10.1183/13993003.01335-2019.

[24] Busse WW, Cloutier M, Dombrowski M, et al. NATIONAL ASTHMA EDUCATION AND PREVENTION PROGRAM ASTHMA AND PREGNANCY WORKING GROUP.: 13.

[25] Global Initiative for Asthma. Global Strategy for Asthma Management and Prevention, 2019. pdf. 2019. www.ginasthma.org.

[26] Murphy VE, Gibson PG, Talbot PI, Kessell CG, Clifton VL. Asthma self-management skills and the use of asthma education during pregnancy. Eur Respir J 2005;26(3):435–441. doi: 10.1183/09031936.05.00135604.

[27] Lim AS, Stewart K, Abramson MJ, Walker SP, Smith CL, George J. Multidisciplinary Approach to Management of Maternal Asthma (MAMMA). Chest 2014;145(5):1046–1054. doi: 10.1378/chest.13-2276.

[28] Murphy V. Managing asthma in pregnancy. 2015;258–267.

[29] Coates AL, Graham BL, McFadden RG, McParland C. Spirometry in primary care. 2013;20(1):10.

[30] Guidelines for Methacholine and Exercise Challenge Testing – 1999. This official statement of the American thoracic society was adopted by the ATS Board of Directors, July 1999. Am J Respir Crit Care Med 2000;161(1):309–329. doi: 10.1164/ajrccm.161.1.ats11-99.

[31] Murphy VE, Clifton VL, Gibson PG. The effect of cigarette smoking on asthma control during exacerbations in pregnant women. Thorax 2010;65(8):739–744. doi: 10.1136/thx.2009.124941.

[32] Coleman T, Chamberlain C, Davey M-A, Cooper SE, Leonardi-Bee J. Pharmacological interventions for promoting smoking cessation during pregnancy. Cochrane Pregnancy and Childbirth Group, ed. Cochrane Database Syst Rev December 2015. doi: 10.1002/14651858.CD010078.pub2.

[33] Chan B, Einarson A, Koren G. Effectiveness of bupropion for smoking cessation during pregnancy. J Addict Dis 2005;24(2):19–23. doi: 10.1300/J069v24n02_02.

[34] Cressman AM, Pupco A, Kim E, Koren G, Bozzo P. Smoking cessation therapy during pregnancy. Can Fam Physician 2012;58(5):525.

[35] Lim A, Stewart K, König K, George J. Systematic review of the safety of regular preventive asthma medications during pregnancy. Ann Pharmacother 2011;45(7–8):931–945. doi: 10.1345/aph.1P764.

[36] Cossette B, Beauchesne M-F, Forget A et al. Relative perinatal safety of salmeterol vs formoterol and fluticasone vs budesonide use during pregnancy. Ann Allergy Asthma Immunol 2014;112(5): 459–464. doi: 10.1016/j.anai.2014.02.010.

[37] Eltonsy S, Forget A, Beauchesne M-F, Blais L. Risk of congenital malformations for asthmatic pregnant women using a long-acting β2-agonist and inhaled corticosteroid combination versus higher-dose inhaled corticosteroid monotherapy. J Allergy Clin Immunol 2015;135(1): 123–130. e2. doi: 10.1016/j.jaci.2014.07.051.

[38] Ulrik C, Lomholt Gregersen T. Safety of bronchodilators and corticosteroids for asthma during pregnancy: what we know and what we need to do better. J Asthma Allergy November 2013;117. doi: 10.2147/JAA.S52592.

[39] Robijn AL, Jensen ME, McLaughlin K, Gibson PG, Murphy VE. Inhaled corticosteroid use during pregnancy among women with asthma: a systematic review and meta-analysis. Clin Exp Allergy 2019;49(11):1403–1417. doi: 10.1111/cea.13474.

[40] Wendel P, Ramin SM, Barnett-Hamm C, Rowe TE, Cunningham EG. Asthma treatment in pregnancy" A randomized controlled study. AmJ Obstet Gynecol 1996;175(1):5.

[41] Blais L, Beauchesne M-F, Lemière C, Elftouh N. High doses of inhaled corticosteroids during the first trimester of pregnancy and congenital malformations. J Allergy Clin Immunol 2009;124(6):1229–1234. e4. doi: 10.1016/j.jaci.2009.09.025.

[42] Sarkar M, Koren G, Kalra S et al. Montelukast use during pregnancy: a multicentre, prospective, comparative study of infant outcomes. Eur J Clin Pharmacol 2009;65(12): 1259–1264. doi: 10.1007/s00228-009-0713-9.

[43] Namazy J, Cabana MD, Scheuerle AE et al. The Xolair Pregnancy Registry (EXPECT): the safety of Omalizumab use during pregnancy. J Allergy Clin Immunol 2015;135(2): 407–412. doi: 10.1016/j.jaci.2014.08.025.

[44] Enriquez R, Wu P, Griffin MR et al. Cessation of asthma medication in early pregnancy. Am J Obstet Gynecol 2006;195(1): 149–153. doi: 10.1016/j.ajog.2006.01.065.

[45] Belanger K, Hellenbrand ME, Holford TR, Bracken M Effect of pregnancy on maternal asthma symptoms and medication use: Obstet Gynecol. 2010;115(3):559–567. doi: 10.1097/ AOG.0b013e3181d06945.

[46] Sawicki E, Stewart K, Wong S, Paul E, Leung L, George J. Management of asthma by pregnant women attending an Australian maternity hospital: asthma management during pregnancy. Aust N Z J Obstet Gynaecol 2012;52(2):183–188. doi: 10.1111/j.1479-828X.2011.01385.x.

[47] Lim AS, Stewart K, Abramson MJ, Ryan K, George J. Asthma during pregnancy: the experiences, concerns and views of pregnant women with asthma. J Asthma 2012;49(5): 474–479. doi: 10.3109/02770903.2012.678024.

[48] Cydulka RK, Emerman CL, Schreiber D, Molander KH, Woodruff PG, Camargo CA. Acute asthma among pregnant women presenting to the emergency department. Am J Respir Crit Care Med 1999;160(3):887–892. doi: 10.1164/ajrccm.160.3.9812138.

[49] Schatz M. Asthma in pregnancy. N Engl J Med 2009;8.

[50] Park-Wyllie L, Mazzotta P, Pastuszak A et al. Birth defects after maternal exposure to corticosteroids: prospective cohort study and meta-analysis of epidemiological studies. Teratology 2000;62(6):385–392.

[51] Maselli DJ, Adams SG, Peters JI, Levine SM. Management of asthma during pregnancy. Ther Adv Respir Dis 2014;7(2):87–100.

[52] Stenius-Aarniala B, Piirila P, Teramo K. Asthma and pregnancy: a prospective study of 198 pregnancies. Thorax 1988;43(1):12–18. doi: 10.1136/thx.43.1.12.

[53] Stenius-Aarniala BS, Hedman J, Teramo KA. Acute asthma during pregnancy. Thorax 1996; 51(4):411–414. doi: 10.1136/thx.51.4.411.

[54] Arakawa H, Lötvall J, Kawikova I, Löfdahl C-G, Skoogh B-E. Leukotriene D4- and prostaglandin F2α-induced airflow obstruction and airway plasma exudation in guinea-pig: role of thromboxane and its receptor. Br J Pharmacol 1993;110(1):127–132. doi: 10.1111/j.1476-5381.1993.tb13781.x.

Loïc Sentilhes, Hanane Bouchghoul, Aurélien Mattuizzi,
Alizée Froeliger, Hugo Madar

15 Obstetric Hemorrhage

15.1 Introduction

Postpartum hemorrhage (PPH) is the most common complication of childbirth and is responsible today for the deaths of 150,000 women a year, that is, 25% of the 600,000 annual maternal deaths worldwide [1]. PPH remains the leading cause of maternal mortality in developing countries and the second or third cause for direct maternal deaths, behind hypertensive and thromboembolic complications, in developed countries [1, 2]. In high-income countries, 80–90% of maternal deaths from PPH may be avoidable, for they appear to follow inadequate treatment or delays in diagnosis or management [2]. PPH is also the principal cause of acute severe maternal morbidity and resuscitation procedures of women during pregnancy or in the postpartum period in these countries, and exposes women to the complications of transfusion, resuscitation, infertility when treated by hysterectomy (1 case per 2,000–3,500 deliveries in developed countries), increased risks of thromboembolic complications, and greater psychological fragility [3, 4].

Numerous authorities have developed guidelines for the prevention and treatment of PPH to help professionals (obstetricians, anesthesiologists, hemostasis specialists, midwives, and nurses) care for the many women who bleed after giving birth and to try to reduce the maternal morbidity and the mortality associated with it [5–11]. The discrepancies among those sets of guidelines [12] underline our lack of knowledge. This review seeks to provide a global overview of PPH prevention, treatment, and key messages.

Main messages:

Postpartum hemorrhage is one of the leading causes of maternal death and severe maternal morbidity worldwide.

Because individual risk factors are poor predictors of postpartum hemorrhage, its prevention should be directed to all women giving birth.

Uterine atony is the main cause of postpartum hemorrhage.

Oxytocin, where available, is the first-line prophylactic drug that should be administered to all women after vaginal or cesarean delivery.

First-line measures to treat PPH should include calling in all relevant staff, noninvasive monitoring, estimating blood loss, securing venous access, taking initial blood samples, and performing plasma expansion by crystalloids, oxygen therapy, active skin warming, manual removal of the placenta, visual assessment of the genital tract, uterine massage, and uterotonic administration.

---

https://doi.org/10.1515/9783110615258-015

(continued)

If available, the first-line agent for treating PPH is oxytocin, for example, by a slow IV injection of 5–10 IU, followed by a maintenance infusion of 5–10 IU/h for 2 h.
If oxytocin fails to control bleeding, other uterotonics and tranexamic acids should be considered as well as transfusion of blood products, including the use of massive transfusion protocol.
If pharmacological treatment fails, balloon intrauterine tamponade, followed by vessel ligation or embolization, and peripartum hysterectomy – sooner rather than later – should be performed concomitantly with resuscitation.
The essential elements of a system that ensures the speed and effectiveness necessary to controlling PPH are a written up-to-date department protocol and trained staff who communicate correctly.
Critical retrospective study of the records of women with severe PPH should be encouraged.

15.2 Definitions and Thresholds for Intervention

Table 15.1 summarizes the various definitions of PPH, methods for assessing blood loss, and thresholds for intervention applied in the guidelines issued by the principal professional societies. PPH is generally defined as blood loss ≥500 mL from the genital tract after giving birth and severe PPH as ≥1,000 mL (see Table 15.1) [6–11]. Immediate or primary PPH, which occurs in the 24 h after delivery, is the most frequent form and the most likely to produce an acute, serious clinical state.

One of the pitfalls of the standard definition of PPH is that the method used to assess blood loss largely determines the result and, therefore, the reported incidence, and these methods vary [3, 11]. Several studies have shown that visual estimates of postpartum blood loss are not reliable; they lead to overestimation of low volumes and underestimation of high ones – an underestimation that increases with the quantity of bleeding, even for experienced clinicians [13, 14]. Objective methods to measure blood loss directly have been proposed, including a collection bag and the weighing of compresses (Table 15.1) [3, 5, 7, 10, 11]. Although these methods may enable better assessment of the blood volume actually lost, their practical implementation remains far from consistent. Moreover, their routine use for all deliveries is not associated with a diminution in the incidence of severe PPH [15]. As Table 15.1 shows, the United Kingdom [5], the WHO (World Health Organization) [9], and CNGOF (French college of obstetricians and gynecologists) [11] guidelines for PPH management do not apply different cutoff points for blood loss for vaginal and cesarean deliveries because no solid evidence justifies this difference. Nonetheless, the threshold for clinical intervention must take the blood flow rate and clinical context into account. Thus, it is reasonable to begin active management before the threshold of 500 mL is reached – when blood loss is rapid or clinical tolerance poor. Inversely, for cesarean deliveries, in view of the blood loss inherent in the surgical procedure, the threshold of action can be set at a level of blood loss higher than 500 mL, if clinical tolerance allows [3, 11] (Table 15.1).

Table 15.1: Different definitions of postpartum hemorrhage, methods for assessing blood loss, and thresholds of intervention recommended by the principal learned societies (modified from Sentilhes et al. [16]).

Variables	WHO (2012) [9]	FIGO (2012) [10]	RCOG (2016) [5]	ACOG (2017) [6]	SOGC (2009) [8]	RANZCOG (2016) [7]	CNGOF (2015) [11]
Definition							
Vaginal delivery	>500 mL Severe: >1,000 mL	>500 mL Any blood loss that has the potential to produce hemodynamic instability	Minor (500–1,000 mL). Major >1,000 mL	Despite this new characterization (see reVITALize program below), a blood loss greater than 500 mL in a vaginal delivery should be considered abnormal	>500 mL Any blood loss that has the potential to produce hemodynamic instability	>500 mL during puerperium Severe: >1,000 mL during puerperium	>500 mL Severe: >1,000 mL
Cesarean delivery	>500 mL Severe: >1,000 mL	>1,000 mL Any blood loss that has the potential to produce hemodynamic instability	Not specified	The American College of Obstetricians and Gynecologists' (ACOG) reVITALize program defines postpartum hemorrhage as cumulative blood loss greater than or equal to 1,000 mL or blood loss accompanied by signs or symptoms of hypovolemia within 24 h after the birth process (includes intrapartum loss) regardless of route of delivery	>1,000 mL Any blood loss that has the potential to produce hemodynamic instability	>500 mL during puerperium Severe: >1,000 mL during puerperium	>500 mL Severe: >1,000 mL

(continued)

Table 15.1 (continued)

Variables		WHO (2012) [9]	FIGO (2012) [10]	RCOG (2016) [5]	ACOG (2017) [6]	SOGC (2009) [8]	RANZCOG (2016) [7]	CNGOF (2015) [11]
Prevention								
Tools for assessment of blood loss		Not mentioned	Not mentioned	Clinicians should be aware that the visual estimation of peripartum blood loss is inaccurate and that clinical signs and symptoms should be included in the assessment of PPH.	Although visually estimated blood loss is considered inaccurate, use of an educational process, with limited instruction on estimating blood loss, has been shown to improve the accuracy of such estimates	Not mentioned	Not mentioned	Left to the clinician's discretion
Treatment								
Blood loss volume threshold to treat PPH	Vaginal delivery	Not specified	500 mL or 2 cups Any volume of blood loss for unstable woman	500–1,000 mL	Excessive blood loss	Not specified	500–1,000 mL	500 mL*
	Cesarean delivery		1,000 mL Any volume of blood loss for unstable woman	500–1,000 mL	Excessive blood loss	Not specified	500–1,000 mL	1,000 mL*

Tools for assessment of blood loss	Insufficient evidence to recommend the measurement of blood loss over clinical estimation of blood loss.	Sanitary napkin or other clean material put under the woman's buttocks. Collector bags are a promising tool for low-resource settings	Blood collection drapes for vaginal deliveries and weighing swabs	Not mentioned	Clinical markers rather than a visual estimation	Weighing drapes, pads, and swabs	Use of collector bag recommended

PPH, postpartum hemorrhage; WHO, World Health Organization; FIGO, International Federation of Gynaecology and Obstetrics; RCOG, Royal College of Obstetricians and Gynaecologists; ACOG, American College of Obstetricians and Gynecologists; SOGC, Society of Obstetricians and Gynaecologists of Canada; RANZOG, Royal Australian and New Zealand College of Obstetricians and Gynaecologists; CNGOF, French College of Gynecologists and Obstetricians

*Beginning active management before the threshold (of 500 mL for vaginal deliveries and 1,000 mL for cesarean deliveries) is reached is justified when the bleeding rate is high or clinical tolerance poor.

15.3 Incidence of Postpartum Hemorrhage (PPH)

PPH incidence is around 5% of deliveries when blood loss measurement is imprecise or when the data come from routine databases, and around 10% when blood loss is measured precisely and the data come from ad hoc or prospective studies [3, 11, 16]. The incidence of severe PPH (blood loss >1,000 mL) is around 2%, and that of PPH requiring transfusion is around 0.4% [3, 11, 16].

15.4 Causes of Postpartum Hemorrhage (PPH)

Uterine atony is the predominant cause of PPH, responsible for 50–80% of cases [11]. A defect in uterine contractility after delivery prevents the uterus from its normal postbirth contraction, which ensures mechanical hemostasis, by causing occlusion of the gaping arteries and drying up the bleeding. This mechanical hemostasis is flawed or does not occur at all in women with uterine atony, and abundant bleeding ensues, which secondarily can cause loss of coagulation factors, resulting in altered hemostasis, with hemodilution, if intravenous fluid resuscitation occurs concomitantly [3].

Placental retention is generally the second most common cause of PPH, involved in around 10–30% of cases, but its distinction from or coexistence with uterine atony is not always clear [3, 11, 16].

Lacerations and wounds are responsible for 15–20% of PPH; after vaginal delivery, these may be perineal, vaginal, or cervical tears or lacerations (including episiotomy) for PPH and, in cesareans, bleeding associated with the incision or the injury of a uterine pedicle [3, 11].

Other causes, each responsible for <1% of PPH cases, include constitutional or acquired coagulopathy (especially with an amniotic fluid embolism or HELLP syndrome), abruptio placentae, uterine rupture, and placental insertion abnormalities (placenta previa and accreta/percreta) [3, 11].

One PPH can be due to several causes, the distribution of which varies as a function of PPH severity [16]. The most frequent cause of PPH and severe PPH, regardless of mode of delivery, is uterine atony. But the proportion of PPH due to lacerations and wounds is higher among the severe PPH (29% after vaginal deliveries and 22% after cesareans) [16].

15.5 Risk Factors for PPH

Table 15.2 summarizes the principal risk factors of PPH, described consistently in recent observational studies, distinguishing those linked to mothers' prepregnancy characteristics from those related to the characteristics of pregnancy, labor, and delivery

[16–20]. On the whole, these factors and their various combinations do not predict PPH [3, 13].

Table 15.2: Principal risk factors for PPH in the most recent population-based studies [16–20] (modified from Sentilhes et al. [3]).

Mani risk factors for PPH	Range of reported OR for main risk factors
Mothers' characteristics before pregnancy	
Age ≥40 years*	Between 1 and 2
Primiparas	Between 1 and 2
Grand multiparas	Between 1 and 1.5
Previous cesarean	Between 1 and 2
Pregnancy characteristics	
Multiple pregnancy	Between 2 and 5
Pregnancy-related hypertensive disease	Between 1 and 2.5
Characteristics of labor and delivery	
Induction	Between 1 and 2
Prolonged labor	Between 1 and 2
Episiotomy	Between 1 and 2
Operative vaginal delivery**	Between 1 and 2.5
Cesarean before labor£	Between 1 and 2.5
Cesarean during labor£	Between 1 and 2.5
Macrosomia	Between 1 and 3.5

*Reference category (20–34 years).
**Reference category for mode of delivery: spontaneous vaginal delivery OR, odds ratio.

The risk factors for PPH most often reported are those for uterine atony, which is the dominant cause of PPH. They include grand multiparity, uterine overdistension in cases of multiple pregnancy, hydramnios and fetal macrosomia, labor induction with misoprostol, prolonged labor, and chorioamnionitis [11]. A history of PPH is one of the risk factors most closely associated with PPH, but its prevalence is low. Moreover, there is an association between the administration of oxytocin during labor and the onset of PPH. Effect of oxytocin appears to be independent of other risk factors, in particular, the mode of labor onset and its duration [21]. Finally, the risk of PPH does not increase at all for women receiving preventive anticoagulant treatment and only moderately for those receiving it as a curative dose [11]. The risk of recurrence triples in a subsequent pregnancy and increases even more with each PPH [3].

15.6 Prevention of Postpartum Hemorrhage

15.6.1 Active Management of the Third Stage of Labor

Because prediction models for PPH are not discriminatory, its prevention should be directed to all women giving birth [5–11].

Active management of the third stage of labor (AMTSL), first described in the United Kingdom and in Ireland, comprises a combination of three principal actions: prophylactic administration of an uterotonic immediately after delivery of the child, early cord clamping and cutting, and controlled cord traction (CCT). Some authors also include uterine massage [5–11]. According to the Cochrane review, active management for women at mixed levels of hemorrhage risk, compared to expectant management (i.e., signs of placental separation are awaited and the placenta is delivered spontaneously), reduces the rate of PPH > 500 mL and PPH > 1,000 mL, with similar findings for the subgroup of women at low risk of excessive bleeding [22].

A good level of evidence supports the specific and independent efficacy of preventive uterotonics, especially oxytocin [5–12, 23]. The meta-analysis of the trials testing the efficacy of prophylactic oxytocin administration concluded that it reduces the risk of blood loss >500 mL by 50% and the risk of blood loss >1,000 mL by 40% [24]. The situation is very different for CCT, even though it was inseparable from oxytocin administration in the initial concept of AMTSL. Two large randomized controlled trials (RCTs) recently showed that CCT for the management of placental expulsion has no significant effect on the incidence of PPH in either high- or low-resource settings [25, 26]. Moreover, early cord clamping is generally no longer included in AMTSL [8–11], as evidence now suggests that delayed clamping (performed approximately 1–3 min after birth) benefits the child [27]. Finally, blood loss does not differ in women with vaginal deliveries receiving oxytocin as well as transabdominal uterine massage, after placental delivery, compared with those receiving oxytocin alone [28]. In conclusion, among the four components of the AMTSL, only prophylactic uterotonic administration has been demonstrated to reduce blood loss and is, therefore, recommended by all authorities after all childbirths.

15.6.2 Uterotonics

The principal uterotonics evaluated in PPH prevention are oxytocin, ergot derivatives, misoprostol, and carbetocin [5–11].

Compared with placebo, oxytocin reduces the risk of PPH >500 mL (10% vs 23.9%, RR 0.53; 95% CI: 0.38–0.74), of severe PPH (>1,000 mL) (2.2% vs 10.9%, RR 0.62; 95% CI: 0.44–0.87), and of the need for supplementary uterotonics (5.1% vs 11.4%, RR 0.56; 95% CI: 0.36–0.87) [24]. The reduction of the risk of PPH > 500 mL was observed in all subgroups, whether administered intravenously (IV) or intramuscularly

(IM) and regardless of dose (which ranged from 3 to 10 IU) [24]. If oxytocin administration is not possible immediately after delivery of the child, in particular, after delivery of the anterior shoulder and before placental expulsion, it should nonetheless be administered afterwards [11]. Nevertheless, the principal disadvantage of oxytocin is that it requires cold storage (2–8 °C).

Administration of ergot derivatives reduces the incidence of PPH, compared with placebo for PPH > 500 mL (RR 0.49; 95% CI: 0.26–0.90) and for severe PPH (RR 0.32; 95% CI: 0.04–2.59) but at the cost of frequent adverse effects, most especially hypertension (RR 2.60; 95% CI: 1.03–6.57) [29]. In addition, reports of strokes, hypertensive encephalopathy, and myocardial infarction associated with methylergometrine call for extreme prudence in its use, especially among women with a predisposition for vascular disorders [30]. Finally, oxytocin is more effective than methylergometrine for reducing the risk of PPH > 500 mL (RR 0.76; 95% CI: 0.61–0.94) and better tolerated, inducing less nausea (RR 0.18; 95% CI: 0.06–0.53) and less vomiting (RR 0.07; 95% CI: 0.02–0.25) [31]. Syntometrine is a combination of ergometrine and oxytocin. It is not more effective than methylergometrine in preventing PPH > 500 mL or severe PPH [32]. Compared with oxytocin, syntometrine reduced the rate of PPH > 500 mL but had more frequent adverse effects, which raise serious questions about the routine use of syntometrine [33].

Oral or sublingual misoprostol, compared with other uterotonics (oxytocin IV or IM, methylergometrine, and syntometrine), is associated with an increased risk of severe PPH (RR 1.33; 95%CI: 1.16–1.52) [34], and more frequent side effects, including nausea, vomiting, and diarrhea [35]. There is some evidence that a lower dose of oral misoprostol (400 µg rather than 600 µg) may be as effective and associated with fewer side effects [34]. Besides, misoprostol, administered with prophylactic-routine oxytocin, did not reduce the rate of postpartum hemorrhage but increased the rate of adverse events [36].

Finally, carbetocin is a heat-stable synthetic analog of oxytocin, with a prolonged duration of action. The recommended dosage is 100 µg. Heat-stable carbetocin is noninferior to oxytocin for the prevention of blood loss of at least 500 ml, but not for the prevention of blood loss of at least 1,000 ml after vaginal delivery [37]. After cesarean delivery, carbetocin and oxytocin result in similar rates of PPH > 500 mL (RR 0.66; 95% CI: 0.42–1.06) and PPH > 1,000 mL (RR 0.91; 95% CI: 0.39–2.15), but complementary uterotonics and uterine massage were used less after carbetocin treatment (RR 0.64; 95% CI: 0.51–0.81 and RR 0.54; 95% CI: 0.31–0.96, respectively) [38].

Before the CHAMPION trial, there was a general consensus that oxytocin is the uterotonic of choice for all women after vaginal delivery, especially in light of the side effects associated with ergot alkaloids. Most authorities recommend 10 IU IM, because indirect comparisons suggest that 10 UI may be more effective than 5 IU, an IV line is not required, and oxytocin-related hemodynamic adverse are less frequent with IM than IV administration [24]. Oxytocin has a prominent vasodilation effect; IV oxytocin, like IV carbetocin [3], decreases systolic arterial pressure and systemic vascular resistance, and increases heart rate, stroke volume, and cardiac output. Nevertheless, no RCTs have compared the route and dosage of oxytocin for preventing PPH; indirect comparisons suggest that IV may be more effective than IM [24]. Consequently, the RCOG (UK Royal College of Obstetricians and Gynaecologists) and CNGOF suggest doses of either 5 or 10 IU (not only 10 IU), and CNGOF recommends slow IV rather than IM administration. If the IV route is chosen, however, providers must be aware that bolus administration is dangerous and that slow IV administration should be over about 1 min, and specifically in women with cardiac diseases to minimize the oxytocin-related hemodynamic adverse effects [5, 8, 11]. Evidence supporting the recommendation of oxytocin over ergot alkaloids or misoprostol in cesarean deliveries is mainly extrapolated from the literature on vaginal delivery [11].

15.6.3 Tranexamic Acid

Tranexamic acid, an antifibrinolytic agent, has failed to demonstrate in a large RCT (TRAAP trial) a reduction of blood loss ≥500 mL after vaginal delivery, in addition to prophylactic oxytocin administration (RR, 0.83; 95% CI, 0.68–1.01; $P = 0.07$) [39]. Even if the primary outcome was reduced among women at high risk of PPH (women who undergone operative vaginal delivery or episiotomy) and that relevant clinical secondary outcomes were reduced after the intravenous use of 1 g tranexamic acid (provider-assessed clinically significant postpartum hemorrhage, additional uterotonics, blood loss <500 mL) compared to placebo with no severe adverse events including thromboembolism events [39], no authority recommends today the systematic use of tranexamic acid for PPH prevention after vaginal deliveries [40]. Nevertheless, the results of the TRAAP trial do call into question whether, after a vaginal delivery, the benefit-harm ratio is in favor or against the routine use of tranexamic acid for all women worldwide, all women in low income countries with limited availability of resources and equipment such as blood transfusion and intensive resuscitation with inotrope drugs or surgery for PPH, or only in some women at higher risk of PPH such as those who will undergo an operative vaginal delivery and/or an episiotomy [40]. After cesarean deliveries, the large majority of the randomized controlled trials found tranexamic is associated with a reduction of blood loss [41]. But, as all published RCTs have major methodological deficiencies with no adequate assessment of adverse events and, in particular, thromboembolic events, there is today clearly no sufficient evidence to routinely use tranexamic acid for the prevention of postpartum hemorrhage after cesarean deliveries, even in women at "increased risk of PPH" [40, 41], contrary to the recommendation elaborated by the Royal College of Obstetricians and Gynecology [5], outside of the context of research.

15.6.4 Other Prevention Techniques

– **Management of retained placenta without bleeding:**

If bleeding occurs before placental delivery, immediate manual exploration and removal of the placenta is recommended (see below). A policy of CCT reduces the risk of manual removal of placenta (4.2% versus 6.1% (RR 0.69; 95% CI 0.53–0.90) [26]. When no bleeding occurs, there is no consensus about how long to await spontaneous detachment of placenta from the uterus before taking any action. Some authorities recommend action after 30 min [11], and others after 60 min [5, 10]. Injection of oxytocin solution into the umbilical vein did not reduce the need for manual removal, compared with expectant management [3].

– **Cord drainage**

Cord drainage, compared to no placental cord drainage, does not reduce the rate of PPH or of manual removal of the placenta [3].

– **Early suckling after birth**

Because no study has shown an association between early suckling (i.e., putting the baby's mouth to the mother's nipple) and reduction in PPH, its routine use for that purpose seems not relevant [11].

– **Methods of delivering the placenta after cesarean birth**

Manual removal of the placenta, compared with its spontaneous delivery, is associated with more blood loss, more severe blood loss (>1,000 mL), lower hematocrit after delivery, greater fall in hematocrit, more endometritis, and longer hospitalization [42]. Consequently, manual removal of the placenta during cesarean delivery should be avoided in the absence of hemorrhage [13].

– **Monitoring**

Early recognition of PPH is likely crucial for PPH management. All women should be ideally monitored every 15 min for two hours after childbirth, with abdominal palpation, to check uterine tonus for early identification of atony, estimated blood loss, vital signs such as blood pressure, heart rate, respiration (using an oximeter, electrocardiogram, and automated blood pressure recording), as well as general condition (i.e., color, level of consciousness, and anxiety) [5, 8, 10, 11].

15.7 Treatment of Postpartum Hemorrhage

Evidence to guide the management of PPH is sparse, but there is a global consensus among the various authorities about the major principles that should guide it [12].

To help caregivers in PPH management, authorities usually provide a PPH algorithm. For example, algorithm for PPH management after vaginal delivery, from the CNGOF is provided in Figure 15.1.

The RCOG has summarized the main measures that must be taken simultaneously: communication, resuscitation, monitoring, investigation, and treatment [5]. The steps for both management and monitoring must be recorded on a special monitoring form [11].

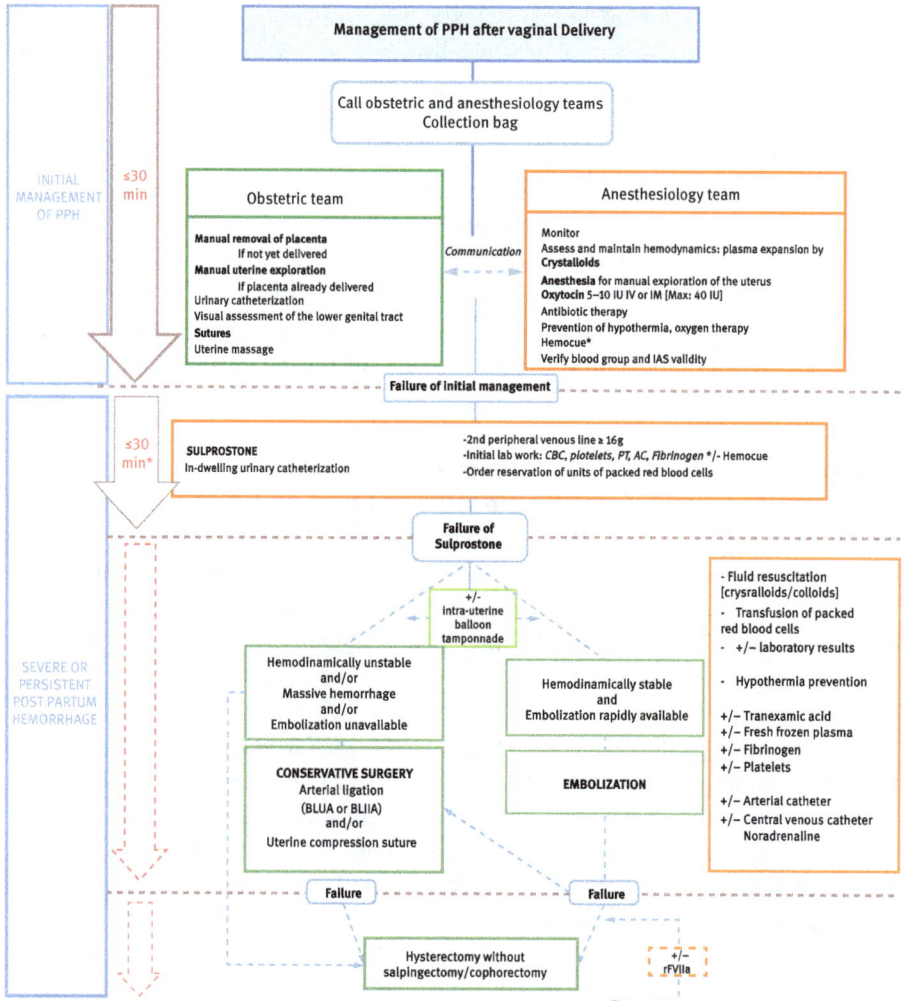

Figure 15.1: Algorithm for PPH management after vaginal delivery, from the French College of Gynecologists and Obstetricians (CNGOF). PPH, postpartum hemorrhage; Min, minute; slow IV, slow intravenous; IM, intramuscular; IU, international unit; IAS, irregular antibody screening; BLUA, bilateral ligation of the uterine arteries; BLIIA, bilateral ligation of the internal iliac arteries; CBC, complete blood count; PT, prothrombin time; ACT, activated clotting time; rFVIIa, recombinant activated factor VII.

15.7.1 First-Line Measures

All relevant staff (midwife, obstetrician, and anesthesiology/critical care team) must be called simultaneously. The medical team must immediately begin resuscitation, appropriate to the results of noninvasive monitoring (heart rate, blood pressure, and pulse oximetry) and estimated blood loss (CNGOF recommends the use of a collector bag [11], while RCOG recommends blood collection drapes and weighing swabs rather than clinical estimation [5]). Staff must then establish or secure venous access (two peripheral cannulae), take initial blood samples, if none are available (blood group and coagulation screen, both of which should normally be available before delivery, together with irregular antibody screening, complete blood count, platelets, and hemostasis including fibrinogen), initiate plasma expansion by crystalloids, oxygen therapy, and protection against hypothermia (active skin warming and, if needed, heating of infusion solutions and of blood products). Urinary output should also be assessed in all cases [12].

After adequate analgesia, the placenta/retained products of conception (retained placenta, cotyledon, or membranes) should rapidly be removed manually, and the genital tract should be assessed visually, as the perineum, vagina, and cervix are all potential sources of bleeding. Any areas of bleeding (i.e., episiotomy, vaginal, or cervical lacerations) must be repaired [12]. Some authorities recommend antibiotic prophylaxis after manual exploration of the uterus [11]. Uterine massage should also follow this exploration [12].

Uterotonic should be administered to strengthen uterine tone, constrict blood vessels, and decrease blood flow through the uterus. There is a wide consensus that oxytocin, if available, is the agent of choice for first-line PPH treatment, either IM or, preferably IV, by a short infusion, and then a continuing dose (Table 15.3). CNGOF, for example, suggests a slow IV injection of 5–10 IU oxytocin, followed by maintenance infusion of 5–10 IU/h for 2 h [11] (see Table 15.3). No evidence indicates that any given regimen is most effective or preferred.

15.7.2 Second-Line Measures for Persisting Hemorrhage

These second-line measures consist of intensifying resuscitation by using blood products mainly or uterotonic treatment, adding an additional or alternative uterotonic, and using tranexamic acid, a prohemostatic agent.

FIGO (the International Federation of Gynecology and Obstetrics), WHO, RCOG, and CNGOF have all chosen to recommend uterotonic administration in two steps: oxytocin first and then, only if oxytocin fails, other uterotonics (not in combination) (Table 15.3) [5, 9–11]. The aim of this two-step procedure is to help healthcare providers to prioritize or rank the uterotonic agents for bleeding women. Other authorities generally describe the drugs (ergot alkaloids, carboprost, sulprostone, misoprostol; all with

Table 15.3: Pharmacological measures for PPH treatment according to various international guidelines (modified from Sentilhes et al. [12]).

Pharmacologic PPH treatment	WHO (2012) [9]	FIGO (2012) [10]	RCOG (2016) [5]	ACOG (2017) [6]	SOGC (2009) [8]	RANZCOG (2016) [7]	CNGOF (2015) [11]
Temporal sequence of administration	Two-step administration of uterotonics, oxytocin first and, then, intravenous ergometrine, oxytocin-ergometrine fixed dose, or a prostaglandin drug (including sublingual misoprostol, 800 µg) if oxytocin fails.	Oxytocin should be preferred first. If oxytocin is not available, or if the bleeding does not respond to oxytocin or ergometrine, an oxytocin-ergometrine fixed dose combination, carbetocin, or misoprostol should be offered as second-line treatment; carboprost should be offered as the third-line treatment.	The following mechanical and pharmacological measures should be instituted, in turn, until the bleeding stops.	Not mentioned	Not mentioned	Uterotonics are commonly given in combination and, in the absence of individual contraindications, a patient may be given all four in the event of severe ongoing atonic bleeding.	Two-step administration of uterotonics, oxytocin first and then sulprostone if oxytocin fails.

Oxytocin	Intravenous oxytocin is the recommended uterotonic drug	Oxytocin 10 IU IM or 5 IU slow IV push, or 20–40 IU/L IV fluid infusion	Oxytocin 5 IU by slow intravenous injection (may have repeat dose) or oxytocin infusion (40 IU in 500 ml isotonic crystalloids at 125 mL/h) unless fluid restriction is necessary.	10–40 IU per 500–1,000 mL as continuous infusion (IV) or 10 IU IM	Oxytocin 10 IU IM or 5 IU IV or 20 to 40 IU at 500–1,000 mL/h	Oxytocin by slow IV or infusion, dose not specified	Slow IV or IM injection of 5–10 IU oxytocin followed by a maintenance infusion of 5–10 IU/h for 2 h. Cumulative dose must not exceed 40 IU.
Carbetocin	Not mentioned	100 µg IM or IV over 1 min	Not mentioned	Not mentioned	100 µg IM or IV over 1 min	Not mentioned	Not mentioned
Ergot alkaloids	See above	Ergometrine or methylergometrine 0.2 mg IM, every 2–4 h with a maximum of 5 doses (1 mg) per 24-h period or ergometrine 0.5 mg/oxytocin 5 IU IM (contraindicated in women with hypertension)	Ergometrine 0.5 mg by slow intravenous or intramuscular injection (contraindicated in women with hypertension)	Methylergonovine 0.2 mg IM every 2–4 h (contraindicated in women with hypertension; preeclampsia, cardiovascular disease, hypersensitivity to drug)	Ergonovine 0.25 mg IV or IM, can be repeated every 2 h (contraindicated in women with hypertension)	Ergometrine by slow IV, in the absence of a contraindication	Not recommended

(continued)

Table 15.3 (continued)

Pharmacologic PPH treatment	WHO (2012) [9]	FIGO (2012) [10]	RCOG (2016) [5]	ACOG (2017) [6]	SOGC (2009) [8]	RANZCOG (2016) [7]	CNGOF (2015) [11]
Injectable prostaglandins	See above	Carboprost 0.25 mg IM repeated at intervals of not less than 15 min to a maximum of 8 doses (contraindicated in women with asthma).	Carboprost 0.25 mg by intramuscular injection repeated at intervals of not less than 15 min to a maximum of eight doses (use with caution in women with asthma).	Carboprost 0.25 mg IM every 15–90 min with a maximum of 8 doses (contraindicated in women with asthma; relative contraindication for hypertension, active hepatic, headache, chills, pulmonary, or cardiac disease).	Carboprost 0.25 mg IM repeated at intervals of not less than 15 mins to a maximum of 8 doses (contraindicated in women with asthma).	Prostaglandin F2α (500 µg increments up to 3 mg) IM or intra-myometrially. The most potent uterotonic but also the most serious adverse effect profile (contraindicated in women with hypertension or asthma).	Sulprostone is recommended and must be administered within 30 min of the PPH diagnosis, should oxytocin be ineffective.
Misoprostol	See above	800 µg sublingually (4 × 200 µg tablets)	Misoprostol 800 µg sublingually	600–1,000 µg oral, sublingual, or rectal	400 to 800 µg sublingually or orally or 800–1,000 µg rectally	1,000 µg rectally	Not recommended if oxytocin available

| rFVIIa | Not recommended because although potentially life-saving, it is associated with life-threatening side effects. | Not mentioned | The routine use of rFVIIa is not recommended in the management of major PPH unless as part of a clinical trial. | Reserved for extenuating circumstances after multiple rounds of the standard massive transfusion agents and in consultation with a local or regional expert in massive hemorrhage. | Potential role. Not recommended as part of a routine practice. | For life-threatening hemorrhage. | For life-threatening hemorrhage. Fibrinogen should be above 1 g/L and platelets > 50,000/mm^3. |

PPH, postpartum hemorrhage; rFVIIa, recombinant activated factor VII; IM, intramuscular; IV, intravenous; IU, International Unit; WHO, World Health Organization; FIGO, International Federation of Gynaecology and Obstetrics; RCOG, Royal College of Obstetricians and Gynaecologists; ACOG, American College of Obstetricians and Gynecologists; SOGC, Society of Obstetricians and Gynaecologists of Canada; RANZOG, Royal Australian and New Zealand College of Obstetricians and Gynaecologists; CNGOF, French College of Gynecologists and Obstetricians.

similar dosages and route of administration in each set of guidelines) that may be used to treat PPH, alone or together, if appropriate; they do not, however, define a temporal sequence of administration [6–8] (Table 15.3). No evidence is available that this sequence is effective for the prompt management of early PPH. Moreover, there is no evidence for prioritizing one drug over the other if oxytocin fails [12]. Contrary to most other guidelines that recommend carboprost [11], CNGOF recommends only sulprostone as an injectable prostaglandin for PPH (Table 15.3). Moreover, only the French guidelines recommend against the use of both ergot alkaloids for treating PPH, because of the adverse effects associated with the ergot alkaloids (see above). Nevertheless, methylergonovine is the most commonly used second-line uterotonic in United States [43] and, reassuringly, Bateman et al. did not find a significant increase in the risk of methylergonovine acute coronary syndrome (ACS) and acute myocardial infarction (AMI) in women who received methylergonovine, compared with those who did not; estimates were increased only modestly or not at all [44]. Lastly, although no prospective study has compared ergot alkaloids with carboprost for the treatment of refractory uterine atony, Butwick et al. observed that the risk of hemorrhage-related morbidity was greater among those receiving carboprost than methergine [45].

Invasive monitoring of arterial blood pressure or central venous pressure may be necessary, depending upon the clinical situation. Urinary output should be monitored in all cases.

There is no data identifying optimal transfusion strategies for postpartum hemorrhage. Given these gaps in the evidence, obstetric societies, therefore, base their recommendations on expert opinion. They underline, however, that blood product use depends principally on clinical signs of PPH severity, without necessarily awaiting blood test results [5, 7, 11]. For example, the CNGOF guidelines state that the objective of RBC transfusion is to maintain a hemoglobin concentration (Hb) >8 g/dL. However, when severe PPH occurs, a massive transfusion protocol has attracted interest as a key therapeutic resource, by ensuring sustained availability of blood products to the labor and delivery units [46]. Guidelines also recommend maintaining a fibrinogen level >1–2 g/L [5, 7, 11], as fibrinogen <2 g/L is a strong marker of severe PPH (and even if a RCT found no evidence supporting the use fibrinogen concentrate as preemptive treatment for severe PPH in patients with normal fibrinogen levels [47]). Bedside hemoglobin monitoring may be useful for resuscitation, but there is currently not enough evidence to recommend routine thromboelastometry coagulation assessment for managing severe PPH [11], even if thromboelastometry can provide earlier data on the fibrinogen contribution to clot formation, compared to clauss-based fibrinogen tests [48], while it has never been demonstrated that its use was associated with an outcome improvement.

Finally, following the results of the WOMAN trial conducted mainly in middle and low income settings [49] (The generalizability of the WOMAN trial and the degree of effect in the high-income countries is uncertain, given the rate of maternal death due to bleeding is about 400 fold lower than the maternal death rate observed in the placebo group of the WOMAN trial [3, 6]), authorities recommend the administration of tranexamic acid (TXA) at a fixed dose of 1 g (100 mg/mL) intravenously (IV) at 1 mL per minute (i.e. administered over 10 min), with a second dose of 1 g IV, if bleeding continues after 30 min or if bleeding restarts within 24 h of completing the first dose [3]. Early use is likely to be superior to delayed treatment, as the benefit was primarily in women treated sooner than 3 h from the time of delivery [6]. Nevertheless, the impact of TXA on the renal function, in the context of maternal resuscitation with high resources (in particular massive fluid replacement and transfusion, inotrope drugs), even at low dose (<3 g), is likely null but not clearly demonstrated today [3].

15.7.3 Third-Line Measures for Refractory Hemorrhage

All guidelines propose the potentially life-saving procedures described below to stop bleeding. Their low level of evidence of efficacy results mainly from the lack of control groups.

Uterine balloon tamponade is the least invasive and the swiftest approach in the PPH life-saving therapeutic arsenal. The reported effectiveness of this method, defined by the absence of need for surgical management or interventional radiology, ranges from 60% to 100% [50]. Even when it is incomplete or not successful, intrauterine balloon tamponade can at least provide time for inter-hospital transfer to continue resuscitation at a more appropriate facility or for arterial embolization, when unavailable at the initial maternity ward [11].

Pelvic arterial embolization has become a reliable and safe alternative procedure for PPH. It is recommended especially in high-income countries, but only when the woman is hemodynamically stable and the embolization unit is located close to the delivery room. Its availability is limited by the specialized instrumentation and expertise required. Success rate is estimated to be about 90% and the serious complication rate, attributable to embolization, is approximately 5% [51]. Embolization for PPH, whether or not associated with a uterine-sparing surgical procedure, does not appear to compromise the woman's subsequent fertility and obstetric outcome [52].

Uterine-sparing surgical procedures are likely the ideal procedures for persistent, severe PPH during cesarean delivery. The first pelvic artery ligation reported, at the end of the nineteenth century, involved internal iliac arteries. However, many practitioners are only slightly familiar with this technique, which is associated with rare but severe complications, such as vascular or ureteral injury, transient buttock numbness, and ischemic nerve injury. Finally, the procedure has been found to be considerably less successful than previously thought (about 69%) [53]. Bilateral uterine ligation accomplishes the same goal and appears faster and easier to perform [54, 55], with a success rate >70% and a low risk of serious immediate complications

[56]. Uterine compression sutures, such as B-Lynch and Cho sutures, are another innovation developed in recent decades and promptly adopted throughout the world for PPH; their estimated success rate is 75% [57]. Pyometra and ischemic necrosis have been reported after uterine compression sutures [58]. Neither they nor uterine and/or iliac artery ligation seems to impair subsequent fertility and obstetric outcomes [11, 54, 55, 58]. No evidence suggests that any one of these methods is better than any other for the management of severe PPH and no technique for conservative surgery should be favored over any other [11].

In the case of massive PPH, very unstable hemodynamics, or failure of uterine-sparing procedures, peripartum hysterectomy should be promptly performed – sooner rather than later [5, 7]. Because total, compared with subtotal, hysterectomy is not associated with a significantly higher urinary tract injury rate, this choice is left to the operator's discretion [11].

Recombinant human activated factor VII (rFVIIa) activates coagulation to generate a thrombin burst and stabilize blood clots. It is considered a life-saving drug and is recommended by many authorities in cases of life-threatening hemorrhage [5–7, 11] (Table 15.3). It is also, however, associated with life-threatening side effects, which is why WHO was reluctant to recommend it [9]. The only open RCT in women with severe PPH refractory to uterotonics showed that rFVIIa reduces the need for specific second-line treatment (embolization, uterine-sparing procedures, or hysterectomy) in about one in three patients and that non-fatal venous thrombotic events occur in one in 20 patients [59]. These results confirm that rFVIIa should be limited to life-threatening hemorrhages. Before use, fibrinogen should ideally be >1 g/L and platelets >50,000/mm^3 [11].

In a UK population-based descriptive study, second-line treatment was used in about 2.2 cases per 10 000 women delivering, of whom 25% were managed with intrauterine tamponade to treat PPH, prior to the use of one of the specific second-line therapies. As the first second-line therapy, 73% had a uterine compression suture, 7% had a pelvic vessel ligation, 8% had an interventional radiological technique (embolization or intra-arterial balloon), and 11% received rFVIIa. Finally, 26% women had a hysterectomy [60]. In a French population-based observational study, second-line therapies were used in about 20 cases per 10,000 women delivering, that is, between six and eight times higher than in the UK. Among women who had a conservative procedure, 70% underwent arterial embolization and 30% had conservative surgery (about four arterial ligations for one uterine compression suture), and finally 14.5% had a hysterectomy [61]. These discrepancies between two countries in Europe regarding the use of second-line therapy indirectly reflect huge differences in management of PPH as well as in the content or organization of initial care.

15.8 After Postpartum Hemorrhage

Once the bleeding has been controlled and the initial resuscitation is completed, continuous close observation in either an intensive care or high-dependency unit on the labor ward is required. Staff should be aware that thromboembolic events may be considered PPH-related maternal morbidity, in cases of massive transfusion and/or surgery. There is a global consensus that thrombophylaxis should be recommended for blood loss >1,000 mL or after transfusion and surgery, once the acute situation is under control [5, 8, 11]. Finally, psychological assessment of the mother and her partner should be considered, after severe PPH, in either the immediate or late postpartum period [11], because of its potential long-term psychological impact [4].

The essential elements of a system ensuring the speed and effectiveness essential to controlling PPH are a department protocol that is regularly updated and trained staff members who communicate correctly. In particular, it has been demonstrated that instituting a comprehensive protocol for the treatment of maternal hemorrhage within a large health care system reduces the use of blood products and improves patient safety [62, 63]. Consequently, system-wide approaches are recommended to standardize care for improving outcomes in the form of bundles. For example, the National Partnership for Maternal Safety recommends the following for all US birthing facilities: a standard obstetric hemorrhage protocol and event checklist, a hemorrhage kit or cart with appropriate medication and equipment, partnership with the local blood bank for rapid and sustained availability of blood products, and universal use of AMTSL [64]. Each department is responsible for training all professionals likely to deal with patients with PPH, to manage this situation. Critical retrospective study of PPH files should be encouraged [11].

15.9 Conclusion

In conclusion, we have to underline that the level of evidence about preventing and managing PPH is globally low. Several key research questions about both prevention and treatment remain unanswered in low-, middle-, and high-income countries. Professionals should be aware that 80–90% of PPH-related maternal morbidity follows suboptimal care due to the late recognition of PPH or late or insufficiently aggressive management.

Financial disclosure: LS was a board member and carried out consultancy work and lecturer for Ferring. The other authors declare no relationships or activities that could appear to have influenced the submitted work.

References

[1] Khan KS, Wojdyla D, Say L et al. WHO analysis of causes of maternal death: a systematic review. Lancet 2006;367:1066–1074.

[2] Saucedo M, Deneux-Tharaux C, Bouvier-Colle MH. Ten years of confidential inquiries into maternal deaths in France, 1998–2007. Obstet Gynecol 2013;122:752–760.

[3] Sentilhes L, Merlot B, Madar H, Brun S, Sztark F, Deneux-Tharaux C. Postpartum haemorrhage: prevention and treatment. Expert Rev Hematol 2016;9:1043–1061.

[4] Sentilhes L, Gromez A, Clavier E et al. Long-term psychological impact of severe postpartum hemorrhage. Acta Obstet Gynecol Scand 2011;90:615–620.

[5] Mavrides E, Allard S, Chandraharan E et al. On behalf of the Royal College of Obstetricians and Gynaecologists. Prevention and management of postpartum haemorrhage. BJOG 2016;124:e106–e149.

[6] Committee on Practice Bulletins-Obstetrics. Practice Bulletin No. 183: postpartum hemorrhage. Obstet Gynecol 2017 Oct;130(4):e168–e186.

[7] Royal Australian and New Zealand College of Obstetricians and Gynaecologists. Management of postpartum hemorrhage. March 2011. Current: March 2014, amended in May 2015 & February 2016. Available at: http://www.ranzcog.edu.au/collegestatements-guidelines.html. Accessed May 1, 2019.

[8] Leduc D, Senikas V, Lalonde AB et al. Active management of the third stage of labour: prevention and treatment of postpartum hemorrhage. J Obstet Gynaecol Can 2009;31: 980–993. ** SOGC PPH guidelines.

[9] WHO recommendations for the prevention of postpartum haemorrhage. World Health Organisation, Geneva(Switzerland), 2012. http://apps.who.int/iris/bitstream/10665/75411/ 1/9789241548502_eng.pdf Accessed March 1, 2019

[10] FIGO safe motherhood and newborn health (SMNH) committee. Prevention and treatment of postpartum hemorrhage in low-resource settings. Int J Gynecol Obstet 2012;117: 108–118. ** FIGO PPH guidelines.

[11] Sentilhes L, Vayssière C, Deneux-Tharaux C et al. Postpartum Hemorrhage: guidelines for clinical practice from the French College of Gynaecologists and Obstetricians (CNGOF) in collaboration with the French Society of Anesthesiology and Intensive Care (SFAR). Eur J Obstet Gynecol Reprod Biol 2016;198:12–21.

[12] Sentilhes L, Goffinet F, Vayssière C et al. Comparison of postpartum haemorrhage guidelines: discrepancies underline our ignorance. BJOG 2017;124:718–72212.

[13] Legendre G, Richard M, Brun S et al. Evaluation by obstetric care providers of simulated postpartum blood loss using a collector bag: a French prospective study. J Matern Fetal Neonatal Med 2016;26:1–7.

[14] Brooks M, Legendre G, Brun S et al. Comparison between the use of a collector bag and the use of a visual aid in addition to a collector bag in the evaluation of postpartum blood loss by obstetrics providers: a French prospective simulation study. Sci Rep 2017;7:46333.

[15] Zhang WH, Deneux-Tharaux C, Brocklehurst P et al. Effect of a collector bag for measurement of postpartum blood loss after vaginal delivery: cluster randomised trial in 13 European countries. BMJ 2010;340:c293.

[16] Dupont C, Rudigoz RC, Cortet M et al. Frequency, causes and risk factors of postpartum haemorrhage: a population-based study in 106 French maternity units. J Gynecol Obstet Biol Reprod 2014;43:244–253.

[17] Al-Zirqi I, Vangen S, Forsen L et al. Prevalence and risk factors of severe obstetric haemorrhage. BJOG 2008;115:1265–1272.

[18] Sosa CG, Althabe F, Belizan JM et al. Risk factors for postpartum hemorrhage in vaginal deliveries in a Latin-American population. Obstet Gynecol 2009;113:1313–1319.

[19] Bateman BT, Berman MF, Riley LE et al. The epidemiology of postpartum hemorrhage in a large, nationwide sample of deliveries. Anesth Analg 2010;110:1368–1373.

[20] Kramer MS, Berg C, Abenhaim H et al. Incidence, risk factors, and temporal trends in severe postpartum hemorrhage. Am J Obstet Gynecol 2013;209:449 e441–447.

[21] Belghiti J, Kayem G, Dupont C et al. Oxytocin during labour and risk of severe postpartum haemorrhage: a population-based, cohort-nested case-control study. BMJ Open 2011;1:e000514.

[22] Begley CM, Gyte GM, Devane D et al. Active versus expectant management for women in the third stage of labour. Cochrane Database Syst Rev 2015;3:CD007412.

[23] Howard WF, McFadden PR, Keettel WC. Oxytocic drugs in fourth stage of labor. JAMA 1964;189:411–413.

[24] Westhoff G, Cotter AM, Tolosa JE. Prophylactic oxytocin for the third stage of labour to prevent postpartum haemorrhage. Cochrane Database Syst Rev 2013;10:CD001808.

[25] Gülmezoglu AM, Lumbiganon P, Landoulsi S et al. Active management of the third stage of labour with and without controlled cord traction: a randomised, controlled, non-inferiority trial. Lancet 2012;379:1721–1727.

[26] Deneux-Tharaux C, Sentilhes L, Maillard F et al. Effect of routine controlled cord traction as part of the active management of the third stage of labour on postpartum haemorrhage: multicentre randomised controlled trial (TRACOR). BMJ 2013;346:f1541.

[27] Hutton EK, Hassan ES. Late vs early clamping of the umbilical cord in full-term neonates: systematic review and meta-analysis of controlled trials. JAMA 2007;297:1241–1252.

[28] Hofmeyr GJ, Abdel-Aleem H, Abdel-Aleem MA. Uterine massage for preventing postpartum haemorrhage. Cochrane Database Syst Rev 2013;7:CD006431.

[29] Liabsuetrakul T, Choobun T, Peeyananjarassri K et al. Prophylactic use of ergot alkaloids in the third stage of labour. Cochrane Database Syst Rev 2007;CD005456. Qsd.

[30] Taylor GJ, Cohen B. Ergonovine-induced coronary artery spasm and myocardial infarction after normal delivery. Obstet Gynecol 1985;66:821–822.

[31] Poeschmann RP, Doesburg WH, Eskes TK. A randomized comparison of oxytocin, sulprostone and placebo in the management of the third stage of labour. Br J Obstet Gynaecol 1991;98: 528–530.

[32] Soltani H, Hutchon DR, Poulose TA. Timing of prophylactic uterotonics for the third stage of labour after vaginal birth. Cochrane Database Syst Rev 2010;8:CD006173.

[33] McDonald S, Abbott JM, Higgins SP. Prophylactic ergometrine-oxytocin versus oxytocin for the third stage of labour. Cochrane Database Syst Rev 2004;CD000201.

[34] Tuncalp O, Hofmeyr GJ, Gulmezoglu AM. Prostaglandins for preventing postpartum haemorrhage. Cochrane Database Syst Rev 2012;8:CD000494.

[35] Gulmezoglu AM, Villar J, Ngoc NT et al. WHO multicentre randomised trial of misoprostol in the management of the third stage of labour. Lancet 2001;358:689–695.

[36] Quibel GI, Goffinet F et al. Active management of the third stage of labor with a combination of oxytocin and misoprostol to prevent postpartum hemorrhage. Obstet Gynecol 2016;128: 805–811.

[37] Widmer M, Piaggio G, Nguyen TMH et al. Heat-stable carbetocin versus oxytocin to prevent hemorrhage after vaginal birth. NEJM 2018;379:743–752.

[38] Su LL, Chong YS, Samuel M. Carbetocin for preventing postpartum haemorrhage. Cochrane Database Syst Rev 2012;4:CD005457.

[39] Sentilhes L, Winer N, Azria E et al. for the Groupe de Recherche en Obstétrique et Gynécologie (GROG). Tranexamic acid for the prevention of blood loss after vaginal delivery. N Engl J Med 2018;379:731–742.

[40] Sentilhes L, Madar H, Mattuizzi A et al. Tranexamic acid for childbirth: why, when, and for who?. Expert Rev Hematol 2019;12:753–761.

[41] Sentilhes L, Lasocki S, Ducloy-Bouthors AS et al. Tranexamic acid for the prevention and treatment of post-partum hemorrhage. Brit J Anaesth 2015;114:576–587.

[42] Anorlu RI, Maholwana B, Hofmeyr GJ. Methods of delivering the placenta at caesarean section. Cochrane Database Syst Rev 2008;3:CD004737.

[43] Bateman BT, Tsen LC, Liu J et al. Patterns of second-line uterotonic use in a large sample of hospitalizations for childbirth in the United States: 2007–2011. Anesth Analg 2014;119: 1344–1349.

[44] Bateman BT, Huybrechts KF, Hernandez-Diaz S et al. Methylergonovine maleate and the risk of myocardial ischemia and infarction. Am J Obstet Gynecol 2013;209:459.e1–459.e13.

[45] Butwick AJ, Carvalho B, Blumenfeld YJ et al. Second-line uterotonics and the risk of hemorrhage-related morbidity. Am J Obstet Gynecol 2015;212:642 e1–7.

[46] Butwick AJ, Goodnough LT. Transfusion and coagulation management in major obstetric hemorrhage. Curr Opin Anaesthesiol 2015;28:275–284.

[47] Wikkelsø AJ, Edwards HM, Afshari A et al. Pre-emptive treatment with fibrinogen concentrate for postpartum haemorrhage: randomized controlled trial. Br J Anaesth 2015;114:623–633.

[48] Solomon C, Collis RE, Collins PW. Haemostatic monitoring during postpartum haemorrhage and implications for management.Br. J Anaesth 2012;109:851–863.

[49] WOMAN Trial Collaborators. Effect of early tranexamic acid administration on mortality, hysterectomy, and other morbidities in women with post-partum haemorrhage (WOMAN): an international, randomised, double-blind, placebo-controlled trial. Lancet 2017;389:2105–2116.

[50] Martin E, Legendre G, Bouet PE et al. Maternal outcomes after uterine balloon tamponade for postpartum hemorrhage. Acta Obstet Gynecol Scand 2015;94(4):399–404.

[51] Sentilhes L, Gromez A, Clavier E et al. Predictors of failed pelvic arterial embolization for severe postpartum hemorrhage. Obstet Gynecol 2009;113:992–999.

[52] Sentilhes L, Gromez A, Clavier E et al. Fertility and pregnancy following pelvic arterial embolisation for postpartum haemorrhage. BJOG 2010;117:84–93.

[53] Sentilhes L, Gromez A, Descamps P et al. Why stepwise uterine devascularization should be the first-line conservative surgical treatment to control severe postpartum hemorrhage?. Acta Obstet Gynecol Scand 2009;88:490–492.

[54] Bouet PE, Brun S, Madar H et al. Surgical management of postpartum haemorrhage: survey of French obstetricians. Sci Rep 2016;6:30342.

[55] Bouet PE, Madar H, Froeliger A et al. Surgical treatment of postpartum haemorrhage: national survey of French residents of Obstetrics and gynecology. BMC Pregnancy Childbirth 2019;19:91.

[56] Sentilhes L, Trichot C, Resch B et al. Fertility and pregnancy outcomes following uterine devascularization for postpartum hemorrhage. Hum Reprod 2008;23:1087–1092.

[57] Kayem G, Kurinczuk JJ, Alfirevic Z et al. Uterine compression sutures for the management of severe postpartum hemorrhage. Obstet Gynecol 2011;117:14–20.

[58] Sentilhes L, Gromez A, Razzouk K et al. B-Lynch suture for persistent massive postpartum hemorrhage following vessel ligation. Acta Obstet Gynecol Scand 2008;87:1020–1026.

[59] Lavigne-Lissalde G, Aya AG, Mercier FJ et al. Recombinant human FVIIa for reducing the need for invasive second-line therapies in severe refractory postpartum hemorrhage: a multicenter, randomized, open controlled trial. J Thromb Haemost 2015;13:520–529.

[60] Kayem G, Kurinczuk J, Alfirevic Z et al. Specific second-line therapies for postpartum haemorrhage: a national cohort study. BJOG 2011;118:856–864.

[61] Kayem G, Dupont C, Bouvier-Colle MH, Rudigoz RC, Deneux-Tharaux C. Invasive therapies for primary postpartum haemorrhage: a population-based study in France. BJOG 2016;123: 598–605.

[62] Shields LE, Wiesner S, Fulton J et al. Comprehensive maternal hemorrhage protocols reduce the use of blood products and improve patient safety. Am J Obstet Gynecol 2015;212:272–280.

[63] Shields LE, Smalarz K, Reffigee L et al. Comprehensive maternal hemorrhage protocols improve patient safety and reduce utilization of blood products. Am J Obstet Gynecol 2011;205:368 e1–8.

[64] D'Alton ME, Main EK, Menard MK et al. The national partnership for maternal safety. Obstet Gynecol 2014;123:973–977.

Dongmei Sun, Nadine Shehata
16 Anemia in Pregnancy

16.1 Introduction

Anemia in pregnant women is a global public health problem [1]. According to the World Health Organization (WHO), anemia affects 1.62 billion people. Forty-one percent of pregnant women, ranging from 6% in North America to 56% in Africa [2], are affected by anemia. The prevalence of anemia in women of childbearing age has been estimated to be 9.5% in Canada as of 2016, but can be as high as almost 80% of women at delivery in some regions of the world [3, 4]. Anemia has been associated with preterm delivery, low birth weight, and neurodevelopmental disorders in offspring [4–7]. The association of preterm delivery and neurodevelopmental disorders with anemia has been found to be of significance, with delivery at early gestational age (30 weeks or less) [7].

Accurate identification of the etiology of anemia and its management are integral to optimizing pregnancy and delivery.

16.2 Normal Hematological Physiological Changes

Hemodynamic changes in pregnancy occur as early as 8 weeks of gestational age. Hormonally induced reduction in peripheral vascular resistance leads to upregulation of the renin–angiotensin–aldosterone system, resulting in increased intravascular volume [8]. The increased intravascular volume has a physiological dilution effect, resulting in lower hemoglobin concentrations despite the increase of red cell mass that also ensues. Anemia is thus defined as a hemoglobin concentration less than 110 g/L in the first trimester, less than 105 g/L in the second and third trimesters, and less than 100 g/L in the postpartum period [9].

In addition to a lower hemoglobin criterion for the diagnosis of anemia in pregnancy, physiological macrocytosis may also occur due to increased reticulocytosis, making mean corpuscular volume less reliable to diagnose iron deficiency anemia [10, 11].

16.3 Iron Deficiency Anemia

The prevalence of iron deficiency anemia in North America is up to 20% in the pregnant population [2].

https://doi.org/10.1515/9783110615258-016

The total iron requirement during pregnancy is approximately 1.2 g, with the highest demand in the third trimester of up to 7.5 mg daily [12]. By diet alone, it is impossible to meet the daily requirement; thus, a prenatal vitamin and mineral supplement containing 27–35 mg of elemental iron is recommended for all pregnant women [13]. In the United States, iron deficiency anemia is the most common cause of anemia in pregnancy [14]. Iron deficiency occurs with increased frequency in the following groups: iron deficiency in a prior pregnancy, multiparity, low socioeconomic status, brief interval between pregnancies, poor nutritional status, or high blood loss at delivery [15].

16.3.1 Diagnosis

Diagnosis of iron deficiency anemia in pregnancy does not differ from the nonpregnant population. A ferritin value below 30 µg/L is highly suggestive of iron deficiency [16]. If the ferritin concentration is within a range not suggestive of iron deficiency, a transferrin saturation <15% suggests iron deficiency. However, as the calculation of transferrin saturation is affected by serum iron levels, a sample for transferrin saturation should be drawn in the morning after an overnight fast [15]. Serum hepcidin concentration and soluble transferrin receptor have been identified as useful diagnostic tests (serum hepcidin levels decrease and the soluble transferrin receptor level increases with iron deficiency); however, they are not readily available in some clinical settings [17, 18] and are not currently recommended to detect iron deficiency [19]. In the absence of an acute illness and with a normal ferritin and iron saturation levels, that is, over 50 µg/L and 15%, respectively, further investigation is needed for an anemic patient [15].

Screening with a complete blood count at 12 weeks and 28 weeks gestation to detect iron deficiency has been proposed [9]. Empirical treatment of anemia in pregnancies without a hemoglobin disorder, with oral iron with a resultant increase in hemoglobin concentration after 2 weeks, is suggestive of iron deficiency [9].

16.3.2 Management

The recommended daily allowance for iron intake in pregnancy is 27 mg per day, which is contained in most prenatal vitamin and mineral supplements [20]. However, the requirement is higher in patients who already have iron deficiency. Common oral iron formulations include iron salts, heme iron polypeptide, and polysaccharide-iron complex (Table 16.1) [21]. Iron absorption can be optimized when taken with vitamin C and reduced if taken with minerals like calcium or zinc, antacids, or beverages such as tea or coffee containing polyphenols [22]. In the absence of secondary causes of iron deficiency such as blood loss, an oral iron supplement containing elemental iron between 100 to 200 mg daily is recommended as the first-line therapy [9]. Oral iron supplement taken every other day may result in greater absorption and better tolerability than daily intake, and is an option for patients who are unable to tolerate daily iron supplements [9, 23]. The WHO recommends 120 mg of elemental iron (600 mg ferrous sulfate, 360 mg ferrous fumarate, or 1200 mg of ferrous gluconate) weekly for pregnant women unable to tolerate oral iron supplementation daily [24]. Intravenous iron has been shown to provide more substantial increase in hemoglobin levels in pregnancy [25, 26]. Beyond the second trimester, parenteral iron is recommended for women who do not respond to, or are intolerant of oral iron or are near delivery to reach the target hemoglobin of 110 g/L [9].

Table 16.1: Common iron preparations [21].

Preparation	Elemental iron (mg)	Dosage form
Polysaccharide-iron complex	150	Capsule/powder
Ferrous fumarate	100	Capsule/tablet
Ferrous sulfate	65	Tablet
Ferrous gluconate	35	Tablet
Prenatal vitamin (ferrous fumarate)	27–35 mg	Tablet
Heme-iron polypeptide	11 mg	Tablet

16.4 Hemoglobin Disorders in General

Adult hemoglobin predominantly consists of HbA, composed of α- and β-globins, regulated by four α-globin and two β-genes, respectively, a small proportion of HbA2 (α2δ2), and hemoglobin F (α2 γ2). Hemoglobin S stems from a single amino acid substitution (valine for glutamic acid) in position 6 of the β-globin protein and results in sickle cell trait, if inherited as a heterozygous mutation, and sickle cell disease (SCD), if homozygous. Thalassemia refers to the reduced production of α- and/or β-globin chains due to mutations in the α- and/or β-globin genes.

All women who are of ethnicities in which hemoglobin disorders (i.e., thalassemia and SCD) are prevalent (e.g., Mediterranean, African, Asian, and South American) should undergo screening for these conditions preconception or as early as possible in pregnancy [9]. Screening is to include a complete blood count, hemoglobin electrophoresis/hemoglobin genotyping, and ferritin to exclude concurrent iron deficiency.

16.5 Sickle Cell Disease

SCD is the most common hemoglobin disorder and includes the following geno-types – homozygous sickle cell disease (HbSS disease), HbSC disease, and sickle β-thalassemia (HbSβ° and HbSβ⁺). HbSS disease is the most common genotype in the United States [27]. Hemoglobin S polymerizes in relatively deoxygenated regions of the circulation, resulting in abnormal red cell morphology that leads to occlusion of the microvasculature, and acute and chronic organ dysfunction. Microvasculature occlusion occurs not only because of the rigidity of sickle cells but also because sickle cells adhere to other blood cells and the endothelium. Many women with sickle cell disease have recurrent vaso-occlusive events, functional asplenism, chronic anemia, and pulmonary hypertension [28].

Sickle cell trait is a carrier (heterozygote) state in which one β-globin gene is normal with one hemoglobin S allele (HbAS) [27]. Sickle cell trait is not associated with anemia.

16.5.1 Diagnosis

Women with SS disease predominantly have a normocytic anemia and those with SC and Sβ have a microcytic anemia. Sickle cells, target cells and Howell-Jolly bodies, if asplenic, are seen on a peripheral blood film. Diagnosis is confirmed by the presence of hemoglobin S using hemoglobin electrophoresis [27]. SCD is an autosomal recessive disease and genetic counseling is required, particularly if the partner has a hemoglobin disorder, to determine the risk of SCD in the fetus/neonate [9].

16.5.2 Fetal and Maternal Implications of Sickle Cell Disease

More women with SCD are entering pregnancy due to increased longevity and improved comprehensive and multidisciplinary care. Women with SCD can experience exacerbations of their underlying disease and pregnancy-related complications [29]. A recent systematic review and meta-analysis of 21 studies comparing pregnancies with and without SCD described a higher risk of maternal mortality with HbSS disease, relative risk (RR) 6.0, 95% confidence interval (CI) 1.9, 18.4. According to a population-based study on 8.8 million births, pregnant patients with SCD also have an increased risk of preeclampsia, thrombosis, and intrauterine fetal demise, compared to patients without SCD [29]. Mothers with SCD are more likely to be readmitted postpartum, compared to other pregnant patients [30]. Pregnancy-related complications also include increased stillbirth in women with HbSS disease RR 3.9, (95% CI 2.6, 6.0), and HbSC disease RR 1.8 (95% CI 1.0, 3.0), and preterm delivery with HbSS disease RR 2.2, (95% CI 1.5, 3.3) [31].

16.5.3 Management

Preconception counseling is imperative for women with SCD to reduce the risk of pregnancy complications. Considerations for prepregnancy management or the first visit during pregnancy are described in Table 16.2 [32]. The essential components are to optimize organ function (e.g., normal liver iron concentration) prior to pregnancy, discontinue potential therapy that can traverse the placenta, determine individual reference parameters (e.g., hemolytic indices), and reduce the risk of adverse events (e.g., vaccination to reduce the risk of infection, phenotyping red blood cells (RBCs) if transfusion is required to reduce the risk of alloimminization) (Table 16.2) [28, 32].

Acute vaso-occlusive pain is treated as in nonpregnant patients with hydration, oxygenation, and incentive spirometry, but with modification of analgesia such as limiting the use of nonsteroidal anti-inflammatory medication. The lowest effective narcotic dose is utilized to reduce the risk of neonatal abstinence syndrome [33]. RBC transfusion is restricted to patients who experience acute complications such as stroke or acute chest syndrome, previous intrauterine growth restriction (IUGR), or are on a regular transfusion regimen, and matched to recipient RBCs [34]. The use of prophylactic transfusion for all pregnancies with SCD to prevent maternal and pregnancy complications is debated. A recent meta-analysis concluded that prophylactic transfusion may improve maternal and fetal outcome; however, high-quality studies are lacking [35]. RBC transfusion also increases the risk of alloimmunization and its associated complications, including hemolytic transfusion reactions and iron overload [36].

Table 16.2: Management suggestions during pregnancy for sickle cell disease [32].

Preconception or first visit	
Assess baseline disease activities and control	Baseline hemoglobin, hemolytic indices and iron indices Frequency of vasooclusive pain and hospitalizations History of blood transfusion and red cell antibodies status
Genetic counseling	Clarify partner's status and obtain hemoglobin electrophoresis, if unknown. Discuss fetal implications, if any
Screening for chronic complications	Pulmonary hypertension Iron overload Red cell alloimmunization status Baseline proteinuria level Asplenia/Splenomegaly Sickle cell retinopathy
Assess drug therapy and safety	Discontinue hydroxyurea Begin folic acid supplementation at 5 mg/day Treat iron deficiency, if any Provide immunization due to functional asplenia Begin low dose aspirin to reduce risk of preeclampsia Consider calcium and vitamin D for osteopenia

Table 16.2 (continued)

In pregnancy: multidisciplinary approach	
	Fetal monitoring
	Formulate delivery plan
	Discuss blood transfusion strategy with red cell antigen matching (ABO, D, Cc, Ee, K at minimum)
	Optimize pain management
	Treatment of acute complications
Postpartum	VTE prophylaxis
	Resume disease-modifying medications, if indicated
	Discuss contraception

16.6 Thalassemia

Thalassemia is a hemoglobin disorder with reduced or absent synthesis of α- or β-globin chains as a result of gene deletions/mutations. Severe anemia, secondary to ineffective erythropoiesis and extramedullary hematopoiesis, characterizes individuals with β-thalassemia major who often begin a regular red blood cell (RBC) transfusion program in childhood. RBC transfusion is used to treat anemia and reduce the risk of morbidity from extramedullary hematopoiesis. RBCs are provided every 2–4 weeks to maintain a pretransfusion hemoglobin level of 9–10 g/dL [37, 38]. Because of the requirement for chronic transfusion, individuals are at risk of iron overload and resultant organ dysfunction, including liver cirrhosis and cardiomyopathy [39]. With iron chelation therapy, the survival rate has improved dramatically and many women enter reproductive age [40]. Individuals with thalassemia intermedia may also require chronic transfusion therapy and have similar organ dysfunction similar to β-thalassemia major. Environmental factors such as pregnancy may exacerbate the anemia associated with β-thalassemia intermedia, necessitating chronic transfusion therapy during pregnancy, if chronic transfusion therapy was not required previously.

16.6.1 Diagnosis

Many patients with β-thalassemia major and α-thalassemia are diagnosed in childhood by hemoglobin electrophoresis and hemoglobin gene sequencing for genes that control α-chain production respectively. Patients with β-thalassemia trait and alpha thalassemia minor (two α-genes deletion) have microcytosis and mild asymptomatic anemia [41], but in pregnancy, the anemia may become more severe [37]. Hemoglobin H disease, caused by three α-gene deletions, presents with more severe anemia, with hemolysis and hepatosplenomegaly [41]. Individuals with a single α-gene deletion usually do not have anemia or microcytosis.

16.6.2 Fetal and Maternal Implications of Thalassemia

Although fertility is reduced due to altered endocrine function from iron overload, successful pregnancies in patients with thalassemia major can be achieved [42]. In a small cohort of 32 women with 62 pregnancies in Iran, the majority with thalassemia intermedia and major, 45 pregnancies resulted in term delivery and 81% of total deliveries were vaginal [42]. There was one maternal death at the end of delivery and three women had evidence of cardiac failure [42]. Similarly, an Italian multicenter study of 46 women with thalassemia major and 11 women with thalassemia intermedia also showed favorable maternal and fetal outcomes [43]. The risk of intrauterine growth restriction in the latter study was not increased, compared to the general population [43]. However, because of iron deposition, maternal complications such as heart failure, liver disease, gestational diabetes, thyroid dysfunction, and osteopenia occur with increased frequency, and are screened during pregnancy.

16.6.3 Management

Preconception counseling is essential in women with thalassemia [44]. Partners are screened with a complete blood count, and hemoglobin electrophoresis and hemoglobin genotyping. Iron homeostasis and organ function (endocrine, hepatic, and cardiac) should be optimized preconception, particularly as cardiac iron deposition can lead to congestive heart failure during pregnancy. Iron chelation therapy is withheld because of the potential risk of teratogenicity in the first trimester, but may be resumed with deferoxamine in high-risk patients (e.g., those with cardiac iron deposition) in the later stages of gestation [45]. Anemia is exacerbated by pregnancy in patients with thalassemia major and thalassemia intermedia – RBC transfusion requirements routinely increase in frequency and/or volume during pregnancy. Providing phenotypically-matched RBCs reduces the risk of alloimmunization, similar to patients with SCD. Folic acid 5 mg is administered for chronic hemolysis [46]. Calcium and vitamin D are prescribed to reduce the risk of osteopenia, and gestational diabetes may be screened early in pregnancy and in the late second/third trimester. With careful management of thalassemia in a high-risk center with a multidisciplinary team, successful pregnancies are achieved.

16.7 Microangiopathic Hemolytic Anemia in General

The microangiopathic hemolytic anemia (MAHA) syndromes are characterized by endothelial dysfunction, leading to intravascular mechanical fragmentation of RBCs, with resultant hemolysis and schistocytes on the peripheral blood film: MAHA syndromes may be associated with organ dysfunction and thrombocytopenia, resulting from microvascular thrombosis [47]. The main disease entities that need to be considered in pregnancies with MAHA are listed in Table 16.3 [48]. Pregnancy is a known precipitant for MAHA syndromes associated with primary thrombotic microangiopathy (TMA); therefore, these syndromes are often difficult to differentiate from pregnancy-specific MAHA syndromes such as hemolysis, elevated liver enzymes, and low platelets (HELLP) [49].

Table 16.3: Disorders associated with microangiopathic hemolytic anemia in adults [48].

Pregnancy-unique disease entity	Thrombotic microangiopathy syndromes (TMA)	Other associated disorders
Severe preeclampsia, Eclampsia HELLP syndrome	Hereditary or acquired ADAMTS13 deficiency-mediated TMA (TTP) Complement-mediated TMA (atypical HUS) Metabolism-mediated TMA (e.g., B12 deficiency) Drug-induced TMA Shiga toxin–mediated HUS	Sepsis Malignancy Severe hypertension Systemic lupus erythematosus, Scleroderma Antiphospholipid syndrome Hematopoietic stem-cell or organ transplantation

ADAMTS13, a disintegrin and metalloproteinase with thrombospondin motifs 13; HELLP, hemolytic anemia, elevated liver enzymes, low platelets; HUS, hemolytic uremic syndrome; TTP, thrombotic thrombocytopenic purpura.

16.8 Pregnancy-Associated Microangiopathic Hemolytic Anemia Syndromes

16.8.1 HELLP Syndrome

Preeclampsia complicates 6% of pregnancies. HELLP syndrome occurs in 10–20% of patients with severe preeclampsia and 0.5–0.9% of all pregnancies [50]. HELLP syndrome is a variant of severe preeclampsia first described in 1982 by Weinstein [51]. In a prospective cohort of 442 pregnancies with HELLP syndrome, 70% of patients presented before delivery, with 11% before 27 weeks of gestational age [52]. Among the 30% of patients who developed HELLP syndrome postpartum, the majority developed symptoms within 48 h postpartum [52]. Common symptoms included abdominal pain, nausea, vomiting, and headaches [52]. Twenty percent of patients do not have any symptoms suggestive of preeclampsia [52].

HELLP syndrome is associated with increased maternal and perinatal morbidity and mortality. Approximately 8% of these patients develop acute kidney injury and 21% develop disseminated intravascular coagulopathy (DIC), which has a strong association with placenta abruption [52]. In addition to acute kidney injury and DIC, other serious maternal complications include hepatic rupture, pulmonary edema, and acute respiratory distress syndrome [52]. Maternal mortality is reported between 1% and 25% and perinatal mortality ranges from 8–34%, depending on the gestational age (50). Intrauterine growth restriction and intrauterine fetal death occur in 61% and 13.9% of pregnancies with HELLP [53].

Delivery is the only recommended intervention for HELLP syndrome if the gestational age is more than 34 weeks. High-dose dexamethasone has not been shown to be associated with a reduction in maternal complications or blood product use [54], and thus not recommended for treatment of HELLP syndrome [55].

Improvement of biochemical abnormalities should be seen within 24–36 h of delivery [47]. The average time for platelets to return to above $100 \times 10^9/\text{L}$ has been noted to be three days [56]. Blood pressure management is similar to preeclampsia. While optimal blood pressure for patients with HELLP syndrome or preeclampsia is unclear, treatment to avoid severe hypertension, defined as systolic blood pressure of 160 mmHg or more or diastolic blood pressure of 110 mmHg or more, is recommended [57]. For urgent blood pressure control, intravenous labetalol, hydralazine, and immediate-release tablet of nifedipine are the treatments of choice with close monitoring of maternal and fetal status [57]. Hepatic rupture, one of the rare complications of HELLP syndrome, requires prompt endovascular or surgical intervention [58].

16.8.2 Thrombotic Microangiopathies Associated with MAHA

Diagnosis of MAHA is established by the detection of new onset of anemia, elevated lactate dehydrogenase (LD), reduced haptoglobin concentration, and schistocytes on peripheral blood film. Thrombocytopenia is usually present in various degrees. Differentiating different disease entities that result in MAHA can be challenging in pregnancy. Other disorders such as sepsis or placental abruption that cause DIC will cause similar laboratory findings and need to be excluded before considering HELLP, TTP, or atypical HUS (Table 16.3) [48].

16.8.3 Thrombotic Thrombocytopenic Purpura

The thrombotic microangiopathies (TMAs) are a group of disorders characterized by MAHA, thrombocytopenia, and organ injury [49]. The TMAs are described in Table 16.3. Thrombotic thrombocytopenic purpura (TTP), due to a congenital or acquired deficiency in ADAMTS 13, a von Willebrand factor-cleaving protease that cleaves multimeric von Willebrand factor, results in ultra large von Willebrand factor multimers that lead to platelet thrombi in small vessels [49]. Hereditary or acquired TTP is infrequent, approximately 1 in 25,000 pregnancies [47, 59]. Hereditary TTP is predominantly diagnosed in childhood, but initial presentation can be during pregnancy [49]. Hereditary TTP during pregnancy generally occurs after 20 weeks gestation [60]. Acquired TTP, secondary to an autoantibody to ADAMTS 13, may also manifest in pregnancy [49].

16.8.4 Complement-Mediated Thrombotic Microangiopathy

Complement-associated TMA may also be triggered by pregnancy [61]. Complement activation may occur at uteroplacental interface, or triggered by postpartum bleeding, or infection in predisposed patients. The incidence of complement-mediated TMA, historically called atypical hemolytic uremic syndrome (HUS), is unknown in pregnancy but predominantly occurs postpartum. In a retrospective study of a European HUS registry of 87 women with complement-mediated TMA in pregnancy, 76% occurred postpartum [62]. Over 70% of patients required dialysis for acute kidney injury and more than 50% developed end-stage renal disease after seven years [62]. Fifty-six percent of patients had variants in complement genes in this study, which was associated with the risk of progression to end-stage renal disease [62]. While there were no maternal deaths in this cohort, the neonatal or fetal death rate was 14% [62]. Although the presence of complement gene variants is associated with poorer long-term outcomes, the lack of detectable complement gene-sequencing mutations does not exclude the diagnosis of atypical HUS [62].

During pregnancy, TTP may not necessarily manifest with the classic pentad, often described by hemolysis, thrombocytopenia, acute kidney injury, altered mental status, and fever as headaches, proteinuria, hypertension, and renal impairment can also herald TTP during pregnancy [60, 63]. Both TTP and HELLP tend to develop in the second to third trimester. In the first semester, TMA is highly likely to be TTP, as HELLP does not occur early in pregnancy. TTP and atypical HUS are much less common than HELLP syndrome. Hypertension and marked increased liver enzymes are more common with HELLP syndrome, with severe neurological symptoms including seizures or strokes more frequent with TTP. The platelet nadir with TTP tends to be lower than seen with the HELLP syndrome; platelet counts <20 × 10^9/L are suggestive of TTP [64]. An ADAMTS13 level below 10% supports a diagnosis of TTP; less severely reduced levels may occur with HELLP and atypical HUS [47]. The presence of an anti-body to ADAMTS 13 distinguishes acquired TTP. Progressive deterioration of renal function, following delivery, suggests atypical HUS. Renal failure is the most common organ dysfunction, although may not be severe in TTP as in HUS [65].

16.8.5 Management of TTP and HUS

Both TTP and atypical HUS are medical emergencies, as they carry a high risk of maternal mortality, if left untreated. Plasma infusion and plasma exchange, with selective immunosuppression, are the treatments of choice for hereditary and acquired TTP, respectively, and need to be initiated emergently, while an anti-complement therapy is needed for atypical HUS [47]. Eculizumab, a humanized monoclonal antibody to complement C5, is the treatment of choice for atypical HUS and can be used during pregnancy and with lactation [66, 67]. Seventy-five percent of women who received anti-complement therapy with eculizumab had complete renal recovery [62]. Plasma exchange is often used initially when TTP cannot be dif-ferentiated from atypical HUS. Plasma may be infused while waiting transport to centers with availability of exchange.

Without plasma exchange, the mortality in patients with acquired TTP is 90% [49]. Prompt treatment with plasma therapy for either early presentations (<20 weeks) or late presentations (>30 weeks) is associated with favorable outcomes [60]. There was no maternal mortality in a study of 47 women [60] who received plasma exchange or plasma infusion at the time of diagnosis, until remission [60]. For subsequent pregnancies in patients with congenital TTP, plasma infusion is pro-vided every 2 weeks in the first trimester and weekly in the second or early third trimester, or if the platelet count is less than 150×10^9/L, or if LD was increasing [60]. For women with acquired TTP, ADAMTS 13 levels are monitored regularly [60]. Normal ADAMTS 13 levels in successive pregnancies may indicate low risk of relapse [60]. Lev-els less than 10% are an absolute indication to initiate treatment [60]. Fetal survival is approximately 60% with the preponderance of fetal loss occurring when TTP occurs in the first or second trimester [60, 64, 68].

16.8.6 Conclusions

Anemia is highly prevalent in pregnancy and has been associated with increased maternal and fetal complications. While the most common etiology is iron defi-ciency anemia, the differential diagnoses can be broad. Management of pregnancies with underlying hemoglobin disorders requires a multidisciplinary approach. The MAHA-associated syndromes are associated with a substantial risk to mothers and fetuses. Preconception assessment and careful management of acute complications in pregnancy is imperative for all pregnancies.

References

[1]   Pasricha SR. Anemia: A comprehensive global estimate. Blood 2014;123(5):611–612.
[2]   B dB. Worldwide Prevalence of Anaemia 1993–2005. WHO Global Database on Anaemia Geneva. World Health Organization. 2008.
[3]   Prevalence of anemia among pregnant women (%) – North America. Available from: https://www.indexmundi.com/facts/indicators/SH.PRG.ANEM/map/north-america.
[4]   Kumari S, Garg N, Kumar A et al. Maternal and severe anaemia in delivering women is associated with risk of preterm and low birth weight: A cross sectional study from Jharkhand, India. One Health 2019;8:100098.
[5]   Adam I, Kheiri S, Sharif ME, Ahmed ABA, Rayis DA. Anaemia is associated with an increased risk for caesarean delivery. Int J Gynaecology Obstetrics the official organ of the International Federation of Gynaecology and Obstetrics 2019;147(2):202–205.
[6]   Rahmati S, Azami M, Badfar G, Parizad N, Sayehmiri K. The relationship between maternal anemia during pregnancy with preterm birth: A systematic review and meta-analysis. The journal of maternal-fetal & neonatal medicine: The official journal of the European association of perinatal medicine, the federation of Asia and Oceania Perinatal Societies. Int Soc Perinatal Obstet 2019;1–11.
[7]   Wiegersma AM, Dalman C, Lee BK, Karlsson H, Gardner RM. Association of prenatal maternal anemia with neurodevelopmental disorders. JAMA Psychiatry 2019;1–12.
[8]   Al-Sulttan S, Achary C, Odor PM, Bampoe S. Obstetric anaesthesia 1: Physiological changes in pregnancy. Br J Hosp Med (Lond) 2019;80(7):C107–C11.
[9]   Pavord S, Daru J, Prasannan N et al . UK guidelines on the management of iron deficiency in pregnancy. Br J Haematol 2019.
[10]   Chanarin I, McFadyen IR, Kyle R. The physiological macrocytosis of pregnancy. Br J Obstet Gynaecol 1977;84(7):504–508.
[11]   Milman N, Bergholt T, Byg KE, Eriksen L, Hvas AM. Reference intervals for haematological variables during normal pregnancy and postpartum in 434 healthy Danish women. Eur J Haematol 2007;79(1):39–46.
[12]   Milman N. Iron and pregnancy–a delicate balance. Ann Hematol 2006;85(9):559–565.
[13]   Canada H. Prenatal nutrition guidelines for health professionals – iron contributes to a healthy pregnancy 2009 [cited 2017 October 9th]. Available from: http://www.hc-sc.gc.ca/fn-an/pubs/nutrition/iron-fer-eng.php.
[14]   Mei Z, Cogswell ME, Looker AC et al. Assessment of iron status in US pregnant women from the national health and nutrition examination survey (NHANES), 1999–2006. Am J Clin Nutr 2011;93(6):1312–1320.
[15]   Breymann C, Auerbach M. Iron deficiency in gynecology and obstetrics: Clinical implications and management. Hematol Am Soc Hematol Educ Program 2017;2017(1):152–159.
[16]   Breymann C, Auerbach M. Iron deficiency in gynecology and obstetrics: Clinical implications and management. Hematology 2017;2017(1):152–159.
[17]   Bah A, Pasricha SR, Jallow MW et al. Serum hepcidin concentrations decline during pregnancy and may identify iron deficiency: Analysis of a longitudinal pregnancy cohort in the Gambia. J Nutr 2017;147(6):1131–1137.

[18] Zaman B, Rasool S, Jasim S, Abdulah D. Hepcidin as a diagnostic biomarker of iron deficiency anemia during pregnancy. The journal of maternal-fetal & neonatal medicine: The official journal of the European Association of Perinatal medicine, the federation of Asia and Oceania perinatal societies. Int Soc Perinatal Obstet 2019;1–9.

[19] Bah A, Muhammad AK, Wegmuller R et al. Hepcidin-guided screen-and-treat interventions against iron-deficiency anaemia in pregnancy: A randomised controlled trial in The Gambia. Lancet Global Health 2019;7(11):e1564–e74.

[20] Iron: Fact Sheet for Health Professionals National Institutes of Health. Available from: https://ods.od.nih.gov/factsheets/Iron-HealthProfessional/.

[21] Sun D, McLeod A, Gandhi S, Malinowski AK, Shehata N. Anemia in pregnancy: A pragmatic approach. Obstet Gynecol Surv 2017;72(12):730–737.

[22] Zeller MP, Verhovsek M. Treating iron deficiency. CMAJ: Can Med Assoc J = J De l'Assoc Med Can 2017;189(10):E409.

[23] Stoffel NU, Cercamondi CI, Brittenham G et al. Iron absorption from oral iron supplements given on consecutive versus alternate days and as single morning doses versus twice-daily split dosing in iron-depleted women: Two open-label, randomised controlled trials. Lancet Haematol 2017;4(11):e524–e33.

[24] WHO recommendations on antenatal care for a positive pregnancy experience. Geneva: World Health Organization; 2016(http://www.who.int/reproductivehealth/publications/maternal_perinatal_health/anc-positive-pregnancy-experience/en/

[25] Bhavi SB, Jaju PB. Intravenous iron sucrose v/s oral ferrous fumarate for treatment of anemia in pregnancy. A randomized controlled trial. BMC Pregnancy Childbirth 2017;17(1):137.

[26] Radhika AG, Sharma AK, Perumal V et al. Parenteral versus oral iron for treatment of iron deficiency anaemia during pregnancy and post-partum: A systematic review. J Obstet Gynaecol India 2019;69(1):13–24.

[27] Sickle Cell MAB. Disease. In: Adam MPAH, Pagon RA et al., editors. GenReviews®[Internet]. Seattle (WA): University of Washington; Seattle, 1993–2019; 2003 Sep 15 [Updated 2017 Aug 17].

[28] Jain D, Atmapoojya P, Colah R, Lodha P. Sickle cell disease and pregnancy. Mediterr J Hematol Infect Dis 2019;11(1):e2019040.

[29] Alayed N, Kezouh A, Oddy L, Abenhaim HA. Sickle cell disease and pregnancy outcomes: Population-based study on 8.8 million births. J Perinat Med 2014;42(4):487–492.

[30] Bae E, Tangel V, Liu N, Abramovitz SE, White RS. Inpatient mortality and postpartum readmission rates in sickle cell disease pregnancies: A multistate analysis, 2007–2014. The journal of maternal-fetal & neonatal medicine: The official journal of the European Association of Perinatal Medicine, the Federation of Asia and Oceania Perinatal Societies. Intl Soc Perinatal Obstet 2019;1–10.

[31] Oteng-Ntim E, Meeks D, Seed PT et al. Adverse maternal and perinatal outcomes in pregnant women with sickle cell disease: Systematic review and meta-analysis. Blood 2015;125(21):3316–3325.

[32] Smith-Whitley K. Complications in pregnant women with sickle cell disease. Hematol Am Soc Hematol Educ Program 2019;2019(1):359–366.

[33] Black E, Khor KE, Kennedy D et al. Medication use and pain management in pregnancy: A critical review. Pain Prac: Off J World Inst Pain 2019;19(8):875–899.

[34] Rees DC, Robinson S, Howard J. How I manage red cell transfusions in patients with sickle cell disease. Br J Haematol 2018;180(4):607–617.

[35] Malinowski AK, Shehata N, D'Souza R et al. Prophylactic transfusion for pregnant women with sickle cell disease: A systematic review and meta-analysis. Blood 2015;126(21). 2424–2435 quiz 37.

[36] Yazdanbakhsh K, Ware RE, Noizat-Pirenne F. Red blood cell alloimmunization in sickle cell disease: Pathophysiology, risk factors, and transfusion management. Blood 2012;120(3): 528–537.

[37] Rachmilewitz EA, Giardina PJ. How I treat thalassemia. Blood 2011;118(13):3479–3488.

[38] Goss C, Giardina P, Degtyaryova D, Kleinert D, Sheth S, Cushing M. Red blood cell transfusions for thalassemia: Results of a survey assessing current practice and proposal of evidence-based guidelines. Transfusion 2014;54(7):1773–1781.

[39] Cohen AR, Galanello R, Pennell DJ, Cunningham MJ, Vichinsky E. Thalassemia. In: Hematology American Society of Hematology Education Program. 2004, 14–34.

[40] Origa R, Comitini F. Pregnancy in Thalassemia. Mediterr J Hematol Infect Dis 2019;11(1): e2019019.

[41] Sayani FA, Kwiatkowski JL. Increasing prevalence of thalassemia in America: Implications for primary care. Ann Med 2015;47(7):592–604.

[42] Ansari S, Azarkeivan A, Tabaroki A. Pregnancy in patients treated for beta thalassemia major in two centers (Ali Asghar Children's Hospital and Thalassemia Clinic): Outcome for mothers and newborn infants. Pediatr Hematol Oncol 2006;23(1):33–37.

[43] Origa R, Piga A, Quarta G et al. Pregnancy and beta-thalassemia: An Italian multicenter experience. Haematologica 2010;95(3):376–381.

[44] Langlois S, Ford JC, Chitayat D et al. Carrier screening for thalassemia and hemoglobinopathies in Canada. J Obstet Gynaecol Can: JOGC = J D'Obstet Et Gynecol Du Can: JOGC 2008;30(10):950–971.

[45] Petrakos G, Andriopoulos P, Tsironi M Pregnancy in women with thalassemia: Challenges and solutions. Int J Women's Health 2016;8:441–451.

[46] Compernolle V, Chou ST, Tanael S et al. Red blood cell specifications for patients with hemoglobinopathies: A systematic review and guideline. Transfusion 2018;58(6):1555–1566.

[47] George JN, Nester CM, McIntosh JJ Syndromes of thrombotic microangiopathy associated with pregnancy. Hematology 2015;2015:644–648.

[48] Yan M, Malinowski AK, Shehata N. Thrombocytopenic syndromes in pregnancy. Obstet Med 2016;9(1):15–20.

[49] George JN, Nester CM. Syndromes of thrombotic microangiopathy. N Engl J Med 2014;371(19): 1847–1848.

[50] Haram K, Svendsen E, Abildgaard U The HELLP syndrome: Clinical issues and management. Rev BMC Pregnancy Childbirth 2009;9:8.

[51] Weinstein L. Syndrome of hemolysis, elevated liver enzymes, and low platelet count: A severe consequence of hypertension in pregnancy. Am J Obstet Gynecol 1982;142(2):159–167.

[52] Sibai BM. The HELLP syndrome (hemolysis, elevated liver enzymes, and low platelets): Much ado about nothing?. Am J Obstet Gynecol 1990;162(2):311–316.

[53] Aslan H, Gul A, Cebeci A. Neonatal outcome in pregnancies after preterm delivery for HELLP syndrome. Gynecol Obstet Invest 2004;58(2):96–99.

[54] Fonseca JE, Mendez F, Catano C, Arias F. Dexamethasone treatment does not improve the outcome of women with HELLP syndrome: A double-blind, placebo-controlled, randomized clinical trial. Am J Obstet Gynecol 2005;193(5):1591–1598.

[55] Magee LA, Pels A, Helewa M, Rey E, Von Dadelszen P, Committee SHG. Diagnosis, evaluation, and management of the hypertensive disorders of pregnancy: Executive summary. J Obstet Gynaecol Can: JOGC = J D'Obstet Et Gynecol Du Can: JOGC 2014;36(7):575–576.

[56] Chandran R, Serra-Serra V, Redman CW. Spontaneous resolution of pre-eclampsia-related thrombocytopenia. Br J Obstet Gynaecol 1992;99(11):887–890.

[57] ACOG. Practice Bulletin No. 202: gestational hypertension and preeclampsia. Obstet Gynecol 2019;133(1):e1–e25.

[58] Escobar Vidarte MF, Montes D, Perez A, Loaiza-Osorio S. Jose Nieto Calvache A. Hepatic rupture associated with preeclampsia, report of three cases and literature review. J Matern Fetal Neonatal Med 2019;32(16):2767–2773.

[59] Myers B. Diagnosis and management of maternal thrombocytopenia in pregnancy. Br J Haematol 2012;158(1):3–15.

[60] Scully M, Thomas M, Underwood M et al. Thrombotic thrombocytopenic purpura and pregnancy: presentation, management, and subsequent pregnancy outcomes. Blood 2014;124(2):211–219.

[61] George JN. The association of pregnancy with thrombotic thrombocytopenic purpura-hemolytic uremic syndrome. Curr Opin Hematol 2003;10(5):339–344.

[62] Bruel A, Kavanagh D, Noris M et al. Hemolytic uremic syndrome in pregnancy and postpartum. Clin J Am Soc Nephrol 2017;12(8):1237–1247.

[63] Gupta M, Felnberg BB, Burwick RM Thrombotic microangiopathies of pregnancy: differential diagnosis. Pregnancy Hypertens 2018;12:29–34.

[64] Scully M, Hunt BJ, Benjamin S et al. Guidelines on the diagnosis and management of thrombotic thrombocytopenic purpura and other thrombotic microangiopathies. Br J Haematol 2012;158(3):323–335.

[65] Brocklebank V, Wood KM, Thrombotic KD. Microangiopathy and the kidney. Clin J Am Soc Nephrol 2018;13(2):300–317.

[66] Kelly RJ, Hochsmann B, Szer J et al. Eculizumab in pregnant patients with paroxysmal nocturnal hemoglobinuria. N Engl J Med 2015;373(11):1032–1039.

[67] Sarno L, Tufano A, Maruotti GM, Martinelli P, Balletta MM, Russo D. Eculizumab in pregnancy: a narrative overview. J Nephrol 2019;32(1):17–25.

[68] Moatti-Cohen M, Garrec C, Wolf M et al. Unexpected frequency of Upshaw-Schulman syndrome in pregnancy-onset thrombotic thrombocytopenic purpura. Blood 2012;119(24):5888–5897.

Ann Kinga Malinowski, Emily Delpero

17 Sickle Cell Disease in Pregnancy

17.1 Introduction: Normal Hemoglobin

Hemoglobin (Hb), a protein found in red blood cells (RBCs) [1], is a tetramer composed of 4 polypeptide chains: 2 alpha (α)-like and 2 beta (β)-like globin subunits. Each chain is comprised of a heme group, containing iron molecules that reversibly bind to oxygen (O_2) for transport. Genes encoding the globin chains are found on two chromosomes: chromosome 16 for the α-like globin genes and chromosome 11 for the β-like globin genes (including β, epsilon (ϵ), gamma (γ), and delta (δ)) [2]. These globins are expressed in varying proportions throughout human development and distinguish embryonic, fetal and adult Hb:

1) Embryonic Hb (Hbϵ) – produced until 6–8 weeks' gestational age (GA) in the blood islands of the yolk sac [3, 4].
2) Fetal Hb (HbF – $\alpha2\gamma2$) [5] – synthesis from ~8 weeks' GA, with the bulk of erythropoiesis in the fetal liver and spleen. HbF's high O_2 affinity attracts O_2 from maternal blood and delivers it to the fetus. Its production wanes by ~32 weeks but continues to ~6 months after birth [6].
3) Adult Hb (HbA – $\alpha2\beta2$) – transition to HbA occurs with production of β-globins from ~32 weeks' GA and occurs in the bone marrow. At birth, Hb consists of ~75% HbF and 25% HbA. Eventually, adult Hb consists of ~97% HbA, 2.5% HbA$_2$ ($\alpha2\delta2$), and <1% HbF [5].

17.2 Sickle Hemoglobin

In sickle Hb, the two α chains are normal [7]. β-Chain variants occur due to a mutation in the sixth position on chromosome 11 [8], whereby valine or lysine is substituted for glutamic acid; the mutant β-chains are known as "S" chains or "C" chains, respectively [9]. While normal Hb molecules do not associate with one another allowing RBCs to maintain their shape and pliability regardless of circumstances, sickle Hb molecules interact with one another, and when de-oxygenated they polymerize, causing RBCs to lose their pliability and deformability, assuming a sickle shape [8].

https://doi.org/10.1515/9783110615258-017

17.3 Sickle Cell Trait Versus Sickle Cell Disease

The sickle cell gene is inherited in an autosomal recessive manner [10]. The sickle cell trait (HbAS) has evolved, as it confers resistance to falciparum malaria, and those who inherit it are less likely to contract the disease, express lower parasite counts, and incur less likelihood of death, should they become infected [11]. As such, high frequencies of HbAS are noted in areas where malaria is endemic.

Sickle cell disease (SCD), however, is the consequence of HbS inheritance in a homozygous (HbSS) fashion or in a compound heterozygote manner, alongside another Hb variant [11]. In addition to HbSS, common SCD genotypes include HbS/β^0-thalassemia (typically severe phenotype), HbS/β^+-thalassemia (wide clinical spectrum, depending on the molecular mutation of the β-globin gene and the amount of HbA produced, more prone to proliferative retinopathy), and HbSC (generally milder phenotype, more prone to proliferative retinopathy and splenic sequestration) [11]. Less common genotypes include HbS/HbD^{Punjab}, HbS/HbO^{Arab}, HbS/HbC^{Harlem}, and HbS/Hb^{Lepore} amongst others [10]. While each genotype is associated with a typical pattern of expression, significant variation in disease severity exists within each group, and the complications of SCD can occur in all. Phenotypic variability is also influenced by: co-inheritance of α^+-thalassemia, higher HbF levels, lower blood viscosity, and environmental factors (cold climate, nutrition, immunization status, etc.) [12, 13].

17.4 Pathophysiology of Sickle Cell Disease

Sickling of RBCs propagates hemolysis, vaso-occlusion, and hypercoagulability [11]. The complications of SCD are influenced by two distinct mechanisms: vaso-occlusion and hemolysis [8] (Figure 17.1), eventually resulting in diffuse end-organ damage. The subtype driven by hemolysis and low steady-state Hb is commonly characterized by pulmonary hypertension (PH), leg ulceration, sudden death, and stroke, likely as a consequence of endothelial dysfunction, influenced by a loss of nitric oxide, presence of free plasma Hb and reactive oxygen species, alongside arginine catabolism via plasma arginase [8]. Conversely, the subtype driven by vaso-occlusion and associated with high steady-state Hb and leukocyte counts, typically manifests in vaso-occlusive pain episodes (VOPE), acute chest syndrome (ACS), avascular necrosis, and retinopathy, likely secondary to microvasculature obstruction from sickled HbS cells and leukocytes (Figure 17.1) [8].

It is hypothesized that many of the complications of SCD can be divided into two overlapping subtypes, each driven by distinct mechanisms. ET-1 denotes endothelin 1, NOS nitric oxide synthase, O- superoxide, VCAM-1 vascular-cell adhesion molecule 1, and XO xanthine oxidase.

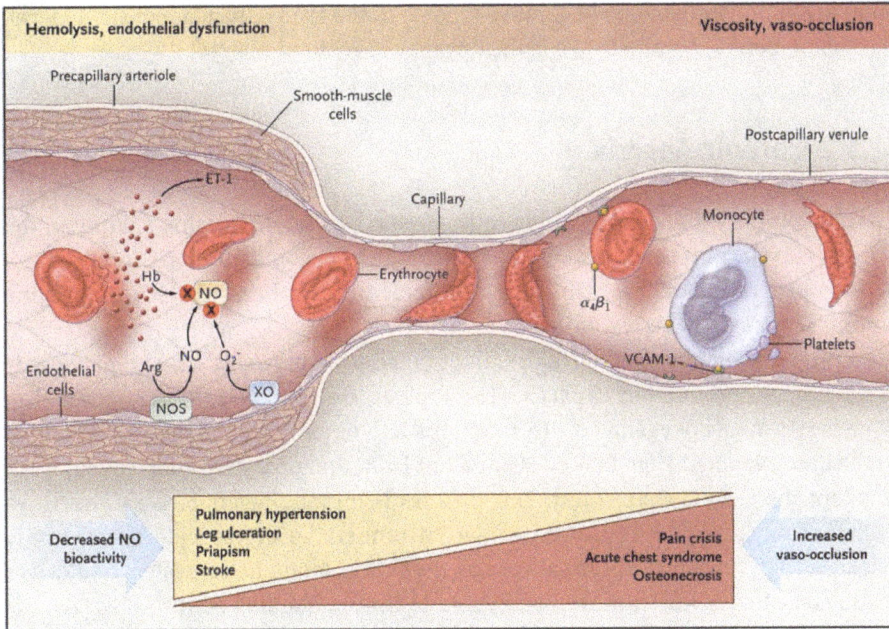

Figure 17.1: Hypothetical mechanisms of clinical subphenotypes of sickle cell disease [8].

17.5 Manifestations of Sickle Cell Disease and Influence of Pregnancy

17.5.1 SCD-Related Pain

Acute VOPEs are the most common manifestation of SCD and can be precipitated by infection, stress, dehydration, cold/damp environmental conditions, and pregnancy [11]. SCD-related pain often becomes chronic [14] and may be influenced by arthritis, avascular necrosis, leg ulcers, or vertebral body collapse [15]. Recurrent acute pain experiences may lead to development of neuropathic pain in the third or fourth life decade [15]. There are no studies on the optimal pain management in pregnant women with SCD, and guidelines typically follow recommendations for the nonpregnant population. Opiates remain the mainstay of treatment, with no teratogenicity concerns [16].

In a prospective cohort study, participants reported chronic SCD pain on over 50% of days surveyed [17]. Not surprisingly, SCD pain is frequently associated with mental health challenges including depression, anxiety, despair, insomnia, loneliness, and helplessness [14, 18]. Pain management in SCD thus requires a multipronged approach [14]. Consideration of curative therapy in the form of hematopoietic stem cell transplantation or, eventually, gene therapy may also play a role [14].

17.5.2 Chronic Anemia

Plasma volume expands, beginning in the first trimester, increasing sharply in the third trimester, ultimately peaking at 1 L [19]. The concomitant increase in red cell mass is proportionately less, resulting in hemodilutional anemia [20], amplifying chronic anemia in SCD.

Chronic anemia in SCD develops due to high erythrocyte turnover that exceeds bone marrow production capacity. The typical life span of RBC is shortened to 17 days [11]. While oxygenated HbS functions in a physiologic manner, its solubility in the deoxygenated state falls to 1/50 that of HbA, and polymerization causes RBCs to adopt the "sickle shape" [21]. This process is initially reversible, but repetitive cycles of oxygenation and de-oxygenation render the erythrocyte permanently "sickled." This prompts RBC clearance by the reticuloendothelial system and drives the higher rates of RBC turnover, compared to HbA-containing erythrocytes [22].

Systematic reviews of maternal anemia (Hb < 100–110 g/L) and birth outcomes have demonstrated inconsistent results regarding an association between anemia and preterm birth and growth restriction [23, 24]. A population-based cohort study of 515,270 pregnant women of whom 65,906 (12.8%) had an antenatal diagnosis of anemia reported an association between anemia and an array of adverse pregnancy outcomes, including potentially increased risk of preterm birth, small for gestational age (SGA) infants, and perinatal morbidity and mortality [25]. None of these studies, however, detail the etiology of anemia, (i.e., hemoglobinopathy vs. nutritional deficiency, etc.), which, in itself, can influence maternal and fetal/neonatal outcomes.

17.5.3 Cardiac Manifestations

Cardiac output (CO) increases 20% by 8 weeks' GA, primarily owing to peripheral vasodilatation [20], mediated by endothelium-dependent factors, including nitric oxide, up-regulated by estradiol and vasodilatory prostaglandins (PGI2), resulting in ~30% fall in systemic vascular resistance. To compensate, CO increases ~ 0–50% by the third trimester, predominantly via increased stroke volume, but also heart rate (10–20 bpm) [20].

Studies have demonstrated a wide range of structural and functional changes in cardiac function in patients with SCD [26, 27] with chronic anemia (and thus persistently increased CO) believed to be the primary driver [28]. Chamber dilatation and septal hypertrophy have been observed in stable SCD patients [26], as have diastolic dysfunction and restrictive cardiomyopathy [29]. Significant enlargement of the LV end-diastolic dimension, posterior wall, inter-ventricular septum, and ventricular mass (marked ventricular hypertrophy) have been observed in pregnant women with SCD, in comparison to healthy pregnant controls without SCD, without adverse effect on LV systolic function [30], However, diastolic function was lower, suggesting diminished ventricular compliance [30].

17.5.4 Pulmonary Manifestations

Lung volumes in patients with SCD tend to be reduced in comparison to controls, with total lung capacity (TLC) at $70.2 \pm 14.7\%$ predicted. The evolving view of lung function in SCD is that there is no predilection for a single pattern and while, among adults, the restrictive pattern tends to predominate, normal or obstructive patterns can also be seen [31]. Furthermore, a higher prevalence of airway hyperreactivity (31–83%) has been observed in SCD [31].

17.5.4.1 Acute Chest Syndrome (ACS)

ACS is the most common cause of maternal death in individuals with SCD [10]. It typically presents with cough, chest pain, dyspnea, fever, and hypoxia [32], often accompanied by worsening anemia, leukocytosis, and new infiltrates on chest x-ray (CXR) [13]. Imaging findings can lag 2–3 days behind clinical symptoms [33]. Three major triggers include: infection, bone marrow fat embolization, and intravascular RBC sequestration. Treatment consists of supplemental oxygen, intravenous (IV) hydration, and adequate analgesia. Incentive spirometry (IS) should be used at least every two hours for a minimum of 10 inspirations [33]. In a randomized trial, regular use of IS has been shown to reduce the rate of atelectasis and pulmonary infiltrates in comparison to nonusers (5.3% vs. 42.1%; $p = 0.019$) [34]. Given the challenges in identification of the precise etiology of ACS, presence of underlying infection must be presumed, and empiric antibiotic therapy for severe community acquired pneumonia is recommended, unless a specific microorganism has been isolated [33]. Ceftriaxone and azithromycin constitute a reasonable choice, with vancomycin for those with a significant penicillin allergy. Simple or exchange transfusion may also be indicated, particularly with signs of clinical deterioration, worsening CXR changes, or oxygen saturation below 90%, and always in consultation with hematology [33].

    ACS complicates 6–20% of pregnancies [35–37], most frequently in persons with HbSS (12.8/100 patient years), followed by HbS/β^0-thalassemia (9.4/100 patient years), HbSC (5.2/100 patient years), and HbS/β-plus-thalassemia (3.9/100 patient years) [37]. It is the most common reason for ICU admission, and of the most common reason for admission to the intensive care unit, and the most common cause of maternal death in this population [38]. The acute hemolytic anemia and hypoxia often seen with ACS have been noted in association with evidence of fetal stress, raising concern regarding the risk of intrauterine fetal demise [39].

17.5.4.2 Pulmonary Hypertension (PH)

PH has been identified in up to 11% of SCD-affected individuals and occurs at higher rates in those with severe hemolytic anemia [40, 41]. Its clinical presentation mirrors the underlying evolution of right heart failure: fatigue and dyspnea on exertion progressing to chest pain and syncope, with peripheral edema and RUQ pain secondary to hepatic congestion, in later stages [42]. Classically, pulmonary arterial hypertension (PAH) has been defined as pulmonary arterial pressure (PAP) of >25 mmHg on right heart catheterization; however, more recent WHO recommendations suggest a threshold of >20 mmHg [43]. Despite pressures much lower than those in idiopathic or hereditary forms of the condition, in SCD, borderline or mild PH is associated with up to a 50% 2-year mortality rate [44]. Right heart cardiac catheterization remains the gold standard for diagnosis; however, screening modalities are typically recommended initially, in view of its invasive nature [45]. Thus, regular echocardiography is advocated, with features like right atrial enlargement, right ventricle dilatation or hypertrophy, and tricuspid regurgitation suspicious for PH [40]. Furthermore, tricuspid regurgitant jet velocity (TRV) can be measured, elevation of which is suggestive of elevated RV systolic pressure [46]. A TRV threshold of >2.9 m/s has a specificity for PH of 81% [47]. Adding other parameters such as elevated serum N-terminal pro-B-type natriuretic peptide (NT-pro-BNP), indicative of ventricular strain, and abnormal 6 min walk test (6MWT) enhance TRV's predictive capacity [45].

Systematic reviews of pregnancy outcomes in the setting of pulmonary hypertension in non-SCD patients have reported maternal mortality rates as high as 25–50% [42]. In general, pregnancy in context of PH is strongly discouraged, and PH remains one of very few conditions where pregnancy termination is recommended [48]. While detailed discourse on PH management is beyond the scope of this chapter, for pregnancies that continue, supportive treatment includes consideration of anticoagulation, transfusion, supplemental oxygen, diuresis, and calcium channel blockade [42]. The aim of therapy is to promote vasodilation of the pulmonary vasculature to counteract the pathological effects of PH, and specific therapeutic agents include prostacyclin agonists (e.g., epoprostenol) and phosphodiesterase-5 inhibitors (e.g., sildenafil). There is no data on these agents in pregnant SCD patients. Endothelin receptor antagonists (e.g., bosentan) are contraindicated, owing to teratogenicity [49], while guidelines recommend against phosphodiesterase-5 inhibitor therapy in SCD patients [40], given early termination of a trial (Walk-PhaSST trial) of sildenafil vs. placebo for PH in SCD for higher adverse events in the sildenafil group, primarily hospitalization for VOE [50].

17.5.5 Splenic Manifestations

Autoinfarction is a common complication (particularly in HbSS and HbS/β⁰-thalassemia) and typically occurs by 5–6 years of age [11]. It confers a lifelong risk of infection, especially with encapsulated organisms including *Streptococcus pneumoniae, Haemophilus influenza*, and *Neisseria meningitidis*. Thus, maintenance of up-to-date immunization status is paramount [51].

Splenic sequestration is more commonly observed in childhood; however, it can also occur in individuals in whom splenic autoinfarction has not taken place (particularly in HbSC and HbS/β⁺-thalassemia) [52]. It is typically characterized by sudden severe anemia (Hb drop ≥ 20 g/L), reticulocytosis (indicative of active erythropoiesis), and rapid development of splenomegaly [53]. Thrombocytopenia is also often present. Treatment is supportive, aimed at restoring circulating blood volume, and may involve RBC transfusion [54].

17.5.6 Neurologic Manifestations

Stroke is a frequent SCD complication, with rates as high as 11% by age 20 and 24% by age 45, in the absence of screening and treatment [55]. While ischemic stroke is more frequently seen in children, hemorrhagic stroke is more common in adults [55]. Risk factors for the former include prior transient ischemic attacks, low steady-state Hb, recent ACS, and high systolic blood pressure, while for the latter they include low steady-state Hb and leukocytosis [10].

Moyamoya syndrome is another potential complication of SCD [56]. The characteristic angiographic appearance is akin to "a puff of smoke," which is moyamoya in Japanese. Abnormally dilated collateral vessels develop in response to progressive stenosis of the interior carotid arteries and diminished blood flow in the major vessels of the anterior circulation. Its progression is variable but inevitable, ultimately manifesting as: (a) brain ischemia, stroke, or seizures; or (b) a consequence of compensation to ischemia (including hemorrhage from fragile collaterals, or headache from dilated collaterals) [56].

17.5.7 Renal Manifestations

SCD nephropathy tends to develop insidiously and progress slowly [57]. Its pathogenesis is likely multifactorial [58]. The relative hypoxia of the inner medulla provides an environment conducive to sickling and recurrent cycles of sickling lead to ischemic injury and microinfarction, eventually resulting in diminished medullary blood flow [57]. Worsening hypoxia leads to local prostaglandin release and marked vasodilation, increasing renal blood flow and glomerular filtration rate. Over time, hyperfiltration contributes to microalbuminuria, proteinuria, glomerulosclerosis, and eventually chronic kidney disease [58]. Renal dysfunction is relatively more common and severe in patients with the HbSS or HbSβ^0 genotypes.

Renal papillary necrosis (RPN) is a condition characterized by microinfarcts in renal papillae, and can manifest with painless, gross hematuria [57]. Occasionally, patients present with painful "clot colic," stemming from larger areas of infarct and papillary necrosis. RPN is typically self-limiting and managed with hydration, analgesia, and Hb optimization, if needed. Rarely, hematuria may be the first sign of medullary cell carcinoma; thus, a thorough investigation to exclude this entity is warranted [57].

Management of renal complications entails monitoring the degree of proteinuria and, once pregnancy is completed, consideration of therapies, such as hydroxyurea or ACE inhibitors [59]. Effective management of hypertension is paramount, as is avoidance of NSAIDs, as they can decrease glomerular filtration rate and renal blood flow, potentially hastening progression to end-stage renal disease [58].

17.5.8 Hepatic Manifestations

Sickle hepatopathy encompasses a range of acute and chronic pathologies, including gallstones, hypoxic liver injury, hepatic sequestration, viral hepatitis, and sickle-cell intrahepatic cholestasis (SCIC) [60]. The prevalence of liver dysfunction in SCD is ~10% [61]. Assessment of liver damage can be challenging, as transaminitis may also be reflective of hemolysis. Nevertheless, elevated liver enzymes warrant a thorough evaluation for causes related and unrelated to SCD, including iron overload [60]. Clinical severity will dictate the extent of evaluation in the antenatal period. While deferral of full investigation of mild cases to the postpartum period could be reasonable, this would not be advised if the information gained by completing the full evaluation led to change of management or if deferral had the potential to result in a detrimental maternal outcome [62].

17.6 Pregnancy Outcomes

A systematic review of 21 studies (26,349 women with and 26,151,746 women without SCD), demonstrated that pregnancies in those with SCD carry a sixfold risk of maternal mortality, twofold risk of preeclampsia, fourfold risk of stillbirth, twofold risk of neonatal death, twofold risk of preterm delivery, and nearly a fourfold risk of SGA size [38]. Another systematic review of 16 studies, demonstrated nearly threefold risk of SGA and nearly fourfold risk of perinatal mortality in both high- and low-income countries [63].

Given such significant potential for adverse maternal and fetal outcomes, it is paramount that pregnant women with SCD are followed in centers with expertise in this area, which includes the multidisciplinary input of maternal–fetal medicine specialists, hematologists, obstetric medicine physicians, and neonatologists [64, 65].

17.7 Preconception Care

17.7.1 Fertility Preservation

Hematopoietic stem-cell transplantation (HSCT) and/or gene therapy are now a consideration for some individuals with SCD. Both require myeloablative conditioning regimens and radiation and, thus, have the potential to result in gonadal dysfunction and infertility. As such, fertility preservation should be offered to females with SCD prior to HSCT/gene therapy [66]. In postpubertal individuals, this would involve ovarian stimulation for oocyte preservation, while in prepubertal individuals, ovarian tissue cryopreservation may be considered, though is still somewhat experimental [67]. In women undergoing pelvic or abdominal radiation prior to HSCT, ovarian transposition may be an option, and preserving fertility in up to 50% of cases [66]. If a partner is available, ovarian stimulation, in vitro fertilization (IVF), and embryo cryopreservation may be attempted, as it is the most well-established method [68].

17.7.2 Determination of Fetal Risk

SCD is inherited in an autosomal recessive manner, with a single allele contributed by each parent [69]. Partner screening and genetic counselling of couples at risk is paramount [37]. If an SCD patient has a partner with SCD, every fetus they conceive will inherit SCD. If an SCD patient has a partner with sickle cell trait, 50% of their fetuses will inherit SCD, and 50% will inherit sickle cell trait. If both partners have sickle cell trait, 25% of their fetuses will inherit SCD, 50% will inherit sickle cell trait, while 25% will have a normal hemoglobin structure.

Consideration of risk prior to conception provides the opportunity for preimplantation genetic diagnosis (PGD) or prenatal diagnosis (discussed under antenatal care) following conception. PGD involves characterizing the genetic status of several cells biopsied from the trophectoderm of embryos created via IVF, prior to selection and transfer [70]. This preempts the need for termination of an affected pregnancy at the expense of the need for artificial reproductive technology even with intact fertility [70]. While a viable option for some, it is an invasive and expensive process likely not suitable for all.

17.7.3 Medical Optimization

Medical evaluation of SCD-related end-organ damage should include review of current medication, with attention to consideration of discontinuing potentially teratogenic agents, including hydroxyurea, angiotensin-converting enzyme inhibitors (ACE-I), angiotensin receptor blockers (ARB), and iron chelators [71]. Review of immunization status should be undertaken, especially vaccination against *H. influenzae* type B, meningococcus, pneumococcus (repeated every 5 years), hepatitis B, and influenza (yearly) [16, 51].

Laboratory investigations should include assessment of the degree of hemolysis (CBC, bilirubin, LDH, haptoglobin), hepatic (AST, ALT) and renal (creatinine, urine for protein to creatinine ratio) function, iron status (ferritin, iron studies), alloimmunization (group and screen), and RBC phenotype (to allow for extended cross-matching, in case transfusion is required) [16].

An echocardiogram to assess cardiac function and rule out pulmonary hypertension is recommended. Should the TRV exceed 2.5 m/s or should there be other echocardiographic findings suspicious for PH, further evaluation may be advised [42]. Ophthalmologic consultation may be considered, especially with HbSC and HbS/β-thalassemia, where particular risk of SCD-related proliferative retinopathy is noted [72]. Supplementation with folic acid 5 mg daily for prevention of ONTD and to support erythropoiesis with ongoing hemolysis is advised [73].

17.8 Antenatal Care

17.8.1 Prenatal Diagnosis

Once pregnancy is achieved, determination of fetal SCD risk can be secured through chorionic villus Sampling (CVS) or amniocentesis. CVS is a placental biopsy that allows evaluation of chorionic villi and is accomplished transvaginally or trans-abdominally with ultrasound guidance, from 10 to 13 weeks' GA. It carries a risk of pregnancy loss of ~1% [74]. Amniocentesis entails ultrasound-guided sampling of amniotic fluid, typically from 15–20 weeks' GA, with a risk of pregnancy loss of 1:400–1:900 [75]. A recent systematic review and meta-analysis quoted much lower procedure-related miscarriage risks of 0.2% for CVS and 0.3% for amniocentesis [76]. Noninvasive prenatal diagnosis, currently under evaluation, is an enticing option, as it would obviate the need for invasive testing. It utilizes fragmented DNA from apoptotic fetal cells (cell-free fetal DNA), obtained from a maternal blood sample as early as 9 weeks' GA [77]. At present, it is in the early stages of clinical application [78].

17.8.2 Fetal Surveillance

In addition to routine obstetric care, assessment of uterine artery blood flow and placental characteristics around 23 weeks' GA allows for stratification of the risk of placental insufficiency, which may manifest in the form of growth restriction or hypertensive disorders of pregnancy [79]. Subsequently, ultrasounds for fetal growth and well-being, including assessment of biophysical profile, amniotic fluid volume, umbilical and cerebral Doppler flow every 2–4 weeks from 28 weeks' GA, should be considered. Nonstress tests may be added, as needed. It should be noted that fetal assessment may be confounded by the effects of maternal opioid use. If regular opioids are required, an antenatal Pediatrics consultation is often useful to facilitate newborn assessment and monitoring for possible neonatal abstinence syndrome [19].

17.8.3 Maternal Management

17.8.3.1 General Approach

Prenatal care is preferably provided by a multidisciplinary team through a center with expertise in management of SCD in pregnancy [65]. Visits typically take place every 2–4 weeks in early pregnancy, every 2 weeks from 28 weeks' GA, and weekly from 36 weeks [16]. Folic acid supplementation (5 mg daily) is encouraged for the duration of pregnancy, initially to decrease the risk of myelomeningocele and, subsequently, to support erythropoiesis [73]. Education should be provided regarding avoidance of dehydration, vigorous physical activity, stress, and cold temperatures, which are common triggers for a vaso-occlusive event (VOE) [80]. Control of nausea is important in order to reduce the likelihood of dehydration precipitating a VOE. Additionally, monthly urine cultures should be considered to assess for bacteriuria, which should be treated promptly to avoid progression and potentially triggering a VOE [37, 81]. Assessment of iron status will allow determination of the utility of iron supplementation, whereby those replete with iron stores or evidence of iron overload should be advised to take prenatal vitamins without iron, and only those with iron deficiency should be prescribed iron supplementation [16]. Evaluation of end-organ damage should be arranged as discussed under Section 17.7.3, prior to conception.

17.8.3.2 Prevention of Preeclampsia

A multicenter, double-blind, placebo-controlled trial of 1,776 women with singleton pregnancies at high risk for preterm preeclampsia randomly assigned to receive aspirin 150 mg daily or placebo from 11 to 14 weeks' GA until 36 weeks' GA [82], noted a significant reduction of preterm preeclampsia in the aspirin group. Although there are no trials of low-dose aspirin in SCD, the favorable results of this RCT, alongside other data of the beneficial effects of low-dose aspirin in non-SCD women at risk [37], prompt the recommendation for its use in pregnant women with SCD. Given prior findings, commencement of therapy prior to 16 weeks' GA is needed, to observe benefit [83].

17.8.3.3 Acute Pain Crisis

It is the most common maternal SCD-associated complication, occurring in over 50% of pregnancies [83], encountered progressively more frequently with advancing gestation and postpartum. Despite its prevalence, there is a paucity of research addressing treatment approaches in pregnancy [84]. Maternal assessment should include evaluation of vital signs (including oxygen saturation) and urine output. Laboratory investigations should include CBC with reticulocyte count, LDH, haptoglobin, bilirubin, AST, ALT, creatinine, and consideration of an arterial blood gas, should hypoxia be present). If febrile, exclusion of infection is important and can be accomplished through urine, blood, and sputum (if appropriate) culture, as well as a chest x-ray [85]. Concurrent fetal assessment is likewise warranted, comprising Doptone fetal heart rate (FHR) check before 23 weeks' GA and nonstress tests (NST) thereafter, as well as obstetric ultrasound (including estimated fetal weight, amniotic fluid volume, biophysical profile, and umbilical/cerebral Doppler flow) [85]. Findings should be interpreted with caution in the context of opiate administration, which can transiently suppress fetal movements and heart rate variability [37]. Depending on maternal condition and GA, consideration may also be given to administration of steroids for fetal lung maturity [85]. Admission is typically warranted to accomplish the above assessment and institute treatment, which will often consist of: 1) hydration (oral if the VOE is mild and ability to drink is maintained, or intravenous, if this is not the case); 2) oxygenation (to maintain O_2 Sat above 95%) [37]; 3) incentive spirometry to decrease the likelihood of progression to ACS [34]; 4) analgesia (typically with opioids and acetaminophen); and 5) thromboprophylaxis with low molecular weight heparin to decrease VTE risk [37].

17.8.3.4 Analgesia during VOE

Input from the patient is paramount in terms of the degree of pain, current analgesics taken on a regular basis, previous effective pain control regimens, and past side effects [72]. Aggressive pain relief should be sought with opioid (morphine/hydromorphone) dosing every 2–3 h and orders for treating breakthrough pain. Acute Pain Service involvement may be considered for consideration of patient-controlled analgesia (PCA), if pain is not easily and quickly controlled. Once pain control is achieved, there should be no attempts at weaning until 24 h of adequate pain relief has passed. Thereafter, weaning by 10–20% daily, with frequent pain assessments has been advocated, with conversion to oral dosing once IV dosing has nearly reached typical home regimen [85]. A course of NSAIDs may be considered as an adjunct between 12 and 28 weeks' GA [72], owing to concerns regarding constriction and potential premature closure of the fetal ductus arteriosus after 28 weeks' GA, as well as fetal kidney injury and oligohydramnios with sustained use [86].

17.8.3.5 The Role of Transfusion

Given the transfusion burden potentially accrued over the lifetime by individuals with SCD, consideration of transfusion-related complications is paramount. These include viral infection, alloimmunization, hyperhemolysis, delayed hemolytic transfusion reactions, and iron overload [87]. Blood products given to patients with SCD should be cytomegalovirus-negative, leukocyte-depleted red cell units, phenotypically matched for at least the C, D, E, and Kell blood groups [88].

Simple transfusion is occasionally needed if acute anemia develops, though there is no evidence for a particular Hb level acting as a trigger. Some propose Hb <50–60 g/L or fall >20 g/L from baseline, especially if symptomatic [37, 89]. Exchange transfusion, on the other hand, allows HbS and irreversibly sickled cells to be removed from the circulation [90]. It may be completed via automated erythrocytapheresis or manually [85]. The automated process permits maintenance of isovolemia and monitoring of hematologic indices. Exchange/chronic transfusions are reserved for stroke [37], ACS [33], and, sometimes, for recurrent, nonresolving VOEs [90]. Transfusions can be on-demand (instituted to treat acute complications) or prophylactic. The approach to prophylactic transfusion remains uncertain [90]. In a systematic review of 12 studies involving 1,291 participants, prophylactic transfusions were associated with decreased maternal mortality, vaso-occlusive pain episodes, pulmonary complications, pulmonary embolism, perinatal mortality, and preterm birth [91]. However, the studies comprising the systematic review were at moderate to high risk of bias. Subsequently, a retrospective, cross-sectional study of 46 pregnancies in women with severe SCD phenotype investigated the role of early prophylactic erythrocytapheresis initiated at 5–6 weeks' GA and continued every 3–4 weeks, until delivery [92]. No hospitalizations for VOE and no hypertensive disorders were encountered in women who underwent the intervention. Fetal loss was experienced by three patients, all of whom were referred late and initiated the intervention after 20 weeks' GA. Both studies called for multicenter trials to conclusively address the impact of prophylactic exchange transfusion in pregnant women with SCD.

17.8.3.6 Intrapartum Care

Birth should occur in a hospital. There is no contraindication to labor or vaginal delivery solely based on SCD. To decrease the likelihood of peripartum VOE, assurance of: a) warm environment (blankets, warmed IV fluids); b) hydration (oral or IV); c) supplemental O_2 (if O_2 Sat < 95%); and d) adequate analgesia (e.g., early epidural) is particularly important [37, 71]. A retrospective review to determine the impact of anesthetic technique documented a postnatal sickling complication in 24% of patients [93]. General anesthesia and a leukocyte count at or above 15×10^9/L were identified as risk factors for postnatal complications, while neuraxial anesthesia and use of epinephrine were not shown to increase risk.

17.8.3.7 Postpartum Care

Routine postpartum care is appropriate, with particular attention to avoidance of VOE triggers. Supplementation with folic acid to support erythropoiesis should continue. Breastfeeding is encouraged, though the decision may be influenced by risks of delaying reintroduction of certain medication such as iron chelators [16]. Given the risk of VTE, prophylaxis with LMWH is recommended for 6 weeks postpartum [37]. Contraception should be discussed. Current guidelines suggest that progesterone-only contraceptive pills (POP) should be considered first [37, 72]. A Cochrane review identified one randomized trial, which demonstrated that women taking intramuscular depo-medroxyprogesterone acetate (DMPA) were less likely to experience painful episodes [94]. Although a systematic review recorded no increase in VOE with use of combined oral contraceptives (COC), the included studies did not specifically examine VTE risk [95]. An intrauterine contraceptive device (IUCD) is another safe and effective choice [96]. Given the theoretical nature of the increase in VTE risk for women with SCD on COC, and given the potential pregnancy-related morbidity of unintended pregnancies, the recommendations from the United States Medical Eligibility Criteria for Contraceptive Use suggest that long-acting and highly effective methods of contraception are indicated for women with SCD [97], with levonorgestrel-IUCD, DMPA, and POP as class 1 (no restriction for use), and copper-IUCD and COCs as class 2 (advantages of use generally outweigh theoretical or proven risks) [97].

17.9 Newborn Considerations

17.9.1 Genetic Testing

Genetic testing for SCD should be carried out if paternal hemoglobinopathy status was unknown, or if fetal risk has been identified antenatally, but there was no prenatal testing. In some jurisdictions (including Canada), SCD testing is part of the routine newborn screen performed at 24 h of life [72].

17.9.2 Neonatal Abstinence Syndrome (NAS)

NAS is a drug withdrawal syndrome that may result from chronic maternal opioid use during pregnancy – an expected and treatable condition seen in 30–80% of infants of women taking opioid agonists [98] – and may manifest as gastrointestinal, autonomic, and central nervous system disturbances, leading to a range of symptoms including irritability, high-pitched cry, or sleep and feeding disruptions [99]. Its onset may be noted anytime in the first 2 weeks of life, though typically it evolves within 72 h of birth and may last several days to weeks [99]. The American College of Obstetricians and Gynecologists underscores that pregnancy should not be the reason to withhold analgesia owing to concern for opioid misuse or NAS, and that concern for NAS alone should not result in nonprescription of opioids in pregnancy [19], as inadequate treatment of VOE may incite development of more significant maternal morbidity.

17.10 Conclusion

Sickle cell anemia is a hematological condition that can have multisystemic complications. Management in pregnancy requires close monitoring of both the mother and fetus by an experienced multidisciplinary team, in order to ensure optimal outcomes.

References

[1]   Hardison RC Evolution of hemoglobin and its genes. Cold Spring Harb Perspect Med. 2012;2(12):a011627.

[2]   Higgs D, Garrick D, Anguita E et al. Understanding α-globin gene regulation: aiming to improve the management of Thalassemia. Ann N Y Acad Sci. 2005;1054(1):92–102.

[3]   He Z, Russell JE Expression, purification, and characterization of human hemoglobins Gower-1 (zeta(2)epsilon(2)), Gower-2 (alpha(2)epsilon(2)), and Portland-2 (zeta(2)beta(2)) assembled in complex transgenic-knockout mice. Blood. 2001;97(4):1099–1105.

[4]   Al-mufti R, Hambley H, Farzaneh F, Nicolaides K Fetal and embryonic hemoglobins in erythroblasts of chromosomally normal and abnormal fetuses at 10–40 weeks of gestation. Haematologica. 2000;85:690–693.

[5]   Schechter AN Hemoglobin research and the origins of molecular medicine. Blood. 2008;112 (10):3927–3938.

[6]   Sankaran VG, Xu J, Orkin SH Advances in the understanding of haemoglobin switching. Br J Haematol. 2010;149(2):181–194.

[7]   Dean J, Schechter AN Sickle-cell anemia: molecular and cellular bases of therapeutic approaches. N Engl J Med. 1978;299(14):752–763.

[8]   Gladwin MT, Vichinsky E Pulmonary complications of sickle cell disease. N Engl J Med. 2008;359(21):2254–2265.

[9]   Hirsch RE, Raventos-Suarez C, Olson JA, Nagel RL Ligand state of intraerythrocytic circulating HbC crystals in homozygote CC patients. Blood. 1985;66(4):775–777.

[10] Serjeant GR The natural history of sickle cell disease. Cold Spring Harb Perspect Med. 2013;3(10):a011783.

[11] Oteng-Ntim E, Chase AR, Howard J, Khazaezadeh N, Anionwu EN Sickle cell disease in pregnancy. Obstet Gynaecol Reprod Med. 2008;18(10):272–278.

[12] Serjeant BE, Hambleton IR, Kerr S, Kilty CG, Serjeant GR Haematological response to parvovirus B19 infection in homozygous sickle-cell disease. Lancet. 2001;358(9295):17.

[13] Bonds DR Three decades of innovation in the management of sickle cell disease: the road to understanding the sickle cell disease clinical phenotype. Blood Rev. 2005;19(2):99–110.

[14] Ballas SK, Gupta K, Adams-Graves P Sickle cell pain: a critical reappraisal. Blood. 2012;120 (18):3647–3656.

[15] Uwaezuoke SN, Ayuk AC, Ndu IK, Eneh CI, Mbanefo NR, Ezenwosu OU Vaso-occlusive crisis in sickle cell disease: current paradigm on pain management. J Pain Res. 2018;11:3141–3150.

[16] Andemariam B, Browning SL. Current management of sickle cell disease in pregnancy. Clin Lab Med. 2013;33(2):293–310.

[17] Adam SS, Flahiff CM, Kamble S, Telen MJ, Reed SD, De Castro LM Depression, quality of life, and medical resource utilization in sickle cell disease. Blood Adv. 2017;1(23):1983.

[18] Smith WR, Penberthy LT, Bovbjerg VE, et al. Daily assessment of pain in adults with sickle cell disease. Ann Intern Med. 2008;148(2):94–101.

[19] De Haas S, Ghossein-Doha C, Van Kuijk SM, Van Drongelen J, Spaanderman ME Physiological adaptation of maternal plasma volume during pregnancy: a systematic review and meta-analysis. Ultrasound Obstet Gynecol. 2017;49(2):177–187.

[20] Soma-Pillay P, Nelson-Piercy C, Tolppanen H, Mebazaa A Physiological changes in pregnancy. Cardiovasc J Afr. 2016;27(2):89–94.

[21] White JG Ultrastructural features of erythrocyte and hemoglobin sickling. Arch Intern Med. 1974;133(4):545–562.

[22] Zipursky A, Chachula DM, Brown EJ The reversibly sickled cell. Am J Pediatr Hematol Oncol. 1993;15(2):219–225.

[23] Xiong X, Buekens P, Alexander S, Demianczuk N, Wollast E Anemia during pregnancy and birth outcome: a meta-analysis. Am J Perinatol. 2000;17(3):137–146.

[24] Badfar G, Shohani M, Soleymani A, Azami M Maternal anemia during pregnancy and small for gestational age: a systematic review and meta-analysis. J Matern Fetal Neonatal Med. 2019;32(10):1728–1734.

[25] Smith C, Teng F, Branch E, Chu S, Joseph KS Maternal and perinatal morbidity and mortality associated with anemia in pregnancy. Obstet Gynecol. 2019;134(6):1234–1244.

[26] Covitz W, Espeland M, Gallagher D, Hellenbrand W, Leff S, Talner N The heart in sickle cell anemia. The Cooperative Study of Sickle Cell Disease (CSSCD). Chest. 1995;108(5):1214–1219.

[27] Denenberg BS, Criner G, Jones R, Spann JF Cardiac function in sickle cell anemia. Am J Cardiol. 1983;51(10):1674–1678.

[28] Varat MA, Adolph RJ, Fowler NO Cardiovascular effects of anemia. Am Heart J. 1972;83(3): 415–426.

[29] Niss O, Quinn CT, Lane A, et al. Cardiomyopathy with restrictive physiology in sickle cell disease. JACC Cardiovasc Imaging. 2016;9(3):243–252.

[30] Veille JC, Hanson R Left ventricular systolic and diastolic function in pregnant patients with sickle cell disease. Am J Obstet Gynecol. 1994; 170 (1 Pt 1): 107–110.

[31] Koumbourlis AC Lung function in sickle cell disease. Paediatr Respir Rev. 2014;15(1):33.

[32] Vichinsky EP, Neumayr LD, Earles AN, et al. Causes and outcomes of the acute chest syndrome in sickle cell disease. National Acute Chest Syndrome Study Group. N Engl J Med. 2000;342(25):1855–1865.

[33] Howard J, Hart N, Roberts-Harewood M, Cummins M, Awogbade M, Davis B Guideline on the management of acute chest syndrome in sickle cell disease. Br J Haematol. 2015;169(4): 492–505.

[34] Bellet PS, Kalinyak KA, Shukla R, Gelfand MJ, Rucknagel DL Incentive spirometry to prevent acute pulmonary complications in sickle cell diseases. N Engl J Med. 1995;333(11):699–703.

[35] Smith JA, Espeland M, Bellevue R, Bonds D, Brown AK, Koshy M Pregnancy in sickle cell disease: experience of the cooperative study of sickle cell disease. Obstet Gynecol. 1996;87 (2):199–204.

[36] Serjeant GR, Loy LL, Crowther M, Hambleton IR, Thame M Outcome of pregnancy in homozygous sickle cell disease. Obstet Gynecol. 2004;103(6):1278–1285.

[37] Oteng-Ntim E, Howard J Royal College of Obstetricians & Gynaecologists Green-top Guideline No. 61: management of Sickle Cell Disease in Pregnancy. Available at: https://www.rcog.org. uk/globalassets/documents/guidelines/gtg_61.pdf Accessed on: 19 Dec 2019. London, UK.: Royal College of Obstetricians and Gynaecologists; 2011:1–20.

[38] Oteng-Ntim E, Meeks D, Seed PT, et al. Adverse maternal and perinatal outcomes in pregnant women with sickle cell disease: systematic review and meta-analysis. Blood. 2015;125(21): 3316–3325.

[39] Kavitha B, Hota BH Sickle cell disease complicating pregnancy: a retrospective study. J Dr NTR Univ Health Sci. 2017;6(4):242.

[40] Klings ES, Machado RF, Barst RJ, et al. An official American Thoracic Society clinical practice guideline: diagnosis, risk stratification, and management of pulmonary hypertension of sickle cell disease. Am J Respir Crit Care Med. 2014;189(6):727–740.

[41] Parent F, Bachir D, Inamo J, et al. A hemodynamic study of pulmonary hypertension in sickle cell disease. N Engl J Med. 2011;365(1):44–53.

[42] Martin SR, Edwards A. Pulmonary Hypertension and Pregnancy. Obstet Gynecol. 2019;134(5): 974–987.

[43] Simonneau G, Montani D, Celermajer DS, et al. Haemodynamic definitions and updated clinical classification of pulmonary hypertension. Eur Respir J. 2019;53(1).

[44] Gladwin MT, Sachdev V, Jison ML, et al. Pulmonary hypertension as a risk factor for death in patients with sickle cell disease. N Engl J Med. 2004;350(9):886–895.

[45] Mehari A, Klings ES Chronic Pulmonary Complications of Sickle Cell Disease. Chest. 2016;149 (5):1313–1324.

[46] Forfia PR, Vachiery JL Echocardiography in pulmonary arterial hypertension. Am J Cardiol. 2012;110(6 Suppl):16s–24s.

[47] Fitzgerald M, Fagan K, Herbert DE, Al-Ali M, Mugal M, Haynes J Jr. Misclassification of pulmonary hypertension in adults with sickle hemoglobinopathies using Doppler echocardiography. South Med J. 2012;105(6):300–305.

[48] Regitz-Zagrosek V, Blomstrom Lundqvist C, Borghi C, et al. ESC Guidelines on the management of cardiovascular diseases during pregnancy: the task force on the management of cardiovascular diseases during pregnancy of the European society of cardiology (ESC). Eur Heart J. 2011;32(24):3147–3197.

[49] Galie N, Channick RN, Frantz RP, et al. Risk stratification and medical therapy of pulmonary arterial hypertension. Eur Respir J. 2019;53(1).

[50] Machado RF, Barst RJ, Yovetich NA, et al. Hospitalization for pain in patients with sickle cell disease treated with sildenafil for elevated TRV and low exercise capacity. Blood. 2011;118(4): 855–864.

[51] Rubin LG, Levin MJ, Ljungman P, et al. 2013 IDSA clinical practice guideline for vaccination of the immunocompromised host. Clin Infect Dis. 2014;58(3):e44–100.

[52] Maia CB, Nomura RM, Igai AM, Fonseca GH, Gualandro SM, Zugaib M Acute splenic sequestration in a pregnant woman with homozygous sickle-cell anemia. Sao Paulo Med J. 2013;131(2):123–126.

[53] Solanki DL, Kletter GG, Castro O Acute splenic sequestration crises in adults with sickle cell disease. Am J Med. 1986;80(5):985–990.

[54] Naymagon L, Pendurti G, Billett HH Acute splenic sequestration crisis in adult sickle cell disease: a report of 16 cases. Hemoglobin. 2015;39(6):375–379.

[55] Stotesbury H, Kawadler JM, Hales PW, Saunders DE, Clark CA, Kirkham FJ Vascular instability and neurological morbidity in sickle cell disease: an integrative framework. Front Neurol. 2019;10:871.

[56] Scott RM, Smith ER Moyamoya disease and moyamoya syndrome. N Engl J Med. 2009;360 (12):1226–1237.

[57] Sharpe CC, Thein SL How I treat renal complications in sickle cell disease. Blood. 2014;123 (24):3720–3726.

[58] Ataga KI, Derebail VK, Archer DR The glomerulopathy of sickle cell disease. Am J Hematol. 2014;89(9):907–914.

[59] Roy NB, Fortin PM, Bull KR, et al. Interventions for chronic kidney disease in people with sickle cell disease. Cochrane Database Syst Rev. 2017;7:Cd012380.

[60] Gardner K, Suddle A, Kane P, et al. How we treat sickle hepatopathy and liver transplantation in adults. Blood. 2014;123(15):2302–2307.

[61] Schubert TT Hepatobiliary system in sickle cell disease. Gastroenterology. 1986;90(6): 2013–2021.

[62] American College of Obstetricians and Gynecologists Committee on Obstetric Practice. Committee Opinion No. 723: guidelines for diagnostic imaging during pregnancy and lactation. Obstet Gynecol. 2017;130(4):e210–e216.

[63] Boafor TK, Olayemi E, Galadanci N, et al. Pregnancy outcomes in women with sickle-cell disease in low and high income countries: a systematic review and meta-analysis. Bjog. 2016;123(5):691–698.

[64] Asare EV, Olayemi E, Boafor T, et al. Implementation of multidisciplinary care reduces maternal mortality in women with sickle cell disease living in low-resource setting. Am J Hematol. 2017;92(9):872–878.

[65] Elenga N, Adeline A, Balcaen J, et al. Pregnancy in sickle cell disease is a very high-risk situation: an observational study. Obstet Gynecol Int. 2016;2016.

[66] Ghafuri DL, Stimpson SJ, Day ME, James A, DeBaun MR, Sharma D Fertility challenges for women with sickle cell disease. Expert Rev Hematol. 2017;10(10):891–901.

[67] Oktay K, Bedoschi G Oocyte cryopreservation for fertility preservation in postpubertal female children at risk for premature ovarian failure due to accelerated follicle loss in Turner syndrome or cancer treatments. J Pediatr Adolesc Gynecol. 2014;27(6):342–346.

[68] Westphal LM, Massie JA Embryo and Oocyte Banking. 2012.

[69] Ashley-Koch A, Yang Q, Olney RS Sickle hemoglobin (Hb S) allele and sickle cell disease: a huge review. Am J Epidemiol. 2000;151(9):839–845.

[70] Vrettou C, Kakourou G, Mamas T, Traeger-Synodinos J Prenatal and preimplantation diagnosis of hemoglobinopathies. Int J Lab Hematol. 2018;40 Suppl 1:74–82.

[71] Jain D, Atmapoojya P, Colah R, Lodha P Sickle Cell Disease and Pregnancy. Mediterr J Hematol Infect Dis. 2019;11(1):e2019040.

[72] Canadian Haemoglobinopathy Association. Consensus statement on the care of patients with sickle cell disease in Canada. Ottawa, ON, Canada: The Canadian Haemoglobinopathy Association; 2015.

[73] American College of Obstetricians and Gynecologists (ACOG). ACOG Practice Bulletin No. 78: hemoglobinopathies in pregnancy. Obstet Gynecol. 2007;109(1):229–237.

[74] Bakker M, Birnie E, Robles De Medina P, Sollie KM, Pajkrt E, Bilardo CM. Total pregnancy loss after chorionic villus sampling and amniocentesis: a cohort study. Ultrasound Obstet Gynecol. 2017;49(5):599–606.

[75] Akolekar R, Beta J, Picciarelli G, Ogilvie C, D'Antonio F Procedure-related risk of miscarriage following amniocentesis and chorionic villus sampling: a systematic review and meta-analysis. Ultrasound Obstet Gynecol. 2015;45(1):16–26.

[76] Salomon LJ, Sotiriadis A, Wulff CB, Odibo A, Akolekar R Risk of miscarriage following amniocentesis or chorionic villus sampling: systematic review of literature and updated meta-analysis. Ultrasound Obstet Gynecol. 2019;54(4):442–451.

[77] Drury S, Hill M, Chitty LS Cell-Free Fetal DNA Testing for Prenatal Diagnosis. Adv Clin Chem. 2016;76:1–35.

[78] Lench N, Barrett A, Fielding S, et al. The clinical implementation of non-invasive prenatal diagnosis for single-gene disorders: challenges and progress made. Prenat Diagn. 2013;33 (6):555–562.

[79] Liston R, Sawchuck D, Young D. No. 197a-Fetal Health Surveillance: antepartum consensus guideline. J Obstet Gynaecol Can. 2018;40(4):e251–e271.

[80] McGann PT, Nero AC, Ware RE Current management of sickle cell anemia. Cold Spring Harb Perspect Med. 2013;3(8):a011817.

[81] Donkor ES, Osei JA, Anim-Baidoo I, Darkwah S Risk of asymptomatic bacteriuria among people with sickle cell disease in Accra, Ghana. Diseases. 2017;5(1):4.

[82] Rolnik DL, Wright D, Poon LC, et al. Aspirin versus Placebo in Pregnancies at High Risk for Preterm Preeclampsia. N Engl J Med. 2017;377(7):613–622.

[83] Roberge S, Nicolaides K, Demers S, Hyett J, Chaillet N, Bujold E The role of aspirin dose on the prevention of preeclampsia and fetal growth restriction: systematic review and meta-analysis. Am J Obstet Gynecol. 2017;216(2):110–120.e116.

[84] Marti-Carvajal AJ, Pena-Marti GE, Comunian-Carrasco G, Marti-Pena AJ Interventions for treating painful sickle cell crisis during pregnancy. Cochrane Database Syst Rev. 2009(1): Cd006786.

[85] Parrish MR, Morrison JC Sickle cell crisis & pregnancy. Semin Perinatol. 2013;37(4):274.

[86] Van Der Heijden BJ, Carlus C, Narcy F, Bavoux F, Delezoide AL, Gubler MC Persistent anuria, neonatal death, and renal microcystic lesions after prenatal exposure to indomethacin. Am J Obstet Gynecol. 1994;171(3):617–623.

[87] Chou ST Transfusion therapy for sickle cell disease: a balancing act. Hematology Am Soc Hematol Educ Program. 2013;2013:439–446.

[88] Josephson CD, Su LL, Hillyer KL, Hillyer CD Transfusion in the patient with sickle cell disease: a critical review of the literature and transfusion guidelines. Transfus Med Rev. 2007;21(2): 118–133.

[89] Society SC. Standards for the Clinical Care of Adults with Sickle Cell Disease in the UK. Sickle Cell Society; 2008.

[90] Howard J Sickle cell disease: when and how to transfuse. ASH Educ Prog Book. 2016;2016(1): 625–631.

[91] Malinowski AK, Shehata N, D'Souza R, et al. Prophylactic transfusion for pregnant women with sickle cell disease: a systematic review and meta-analysis. Blood. 2015;126(21): 2424–2435; quiz 2437.

[92] Vianello A, Vencato E, Cantini M, et al. Improvement of maternal and fetal outcomes in women with sickle cell disease treated with early prophylactic erythrocytapheresis. Transfusion. 2018;58(9):2192–2201.

[93] Camous J, N'da A, Etienne-Julan M, Stephan F Anesthetic management of pregnant women with sickle cell disease–effect on postnatal sickling complications. Can J Anaesth. 2008;55 (5):276–283.

[94] De Abood M, De Castillo Z, Guerrero F, Espino M, Austin KL Effect of Depo-Provera or Microgynon on the painful crises of sickle cell anemia patients. Contraception. 1997;56(5): 313–316.

[95] Haddad LB, Curtis KM, Legardy-Williams JK, Cwiak C, Jamieson DJ Contraception for individuals with sickle cell disease: a systematic review of the literature. Contraception. 2012;85(6):527–537.

[96] Legardy JK, Curtis KM Progestogen-only contraceptive use among women with sickle cell anemia: a systematic review. Contraception. 2006;73(2):195–204.

[97] Curtis KM, Tepper NK, Jatlaoui TC, et al. U.S. Medical eligibility criteria for contraceptive use, 2016. Available at: https://www.cdc.gov/mmwr/volumes/65/rr/pdfs/rr6503.pdf Accessed on: Dec. 19, 2019. MMWR Recomm Rep. 2016;65(3):1–103.

[98] McCarthy JJ, Leamon MH, Willits NH, Salo R The effect of methadone dose regimen on neonatal abstinence syndrome. J Addict Med. 2015;9(2):105–110.

[99] Nnoli A, Seligman NS, Dysart K, Baxter JK, Ballas SK Opioid utilization by pregnant women with sickle cell disease and the risk of neonatal abstinence syndrome. J Natl [Med] Assoc. 2018;110(2):163–168.

Kristin Harris, Mark Yudin

18 Human Immunodeficiency Virus and Pregnancy

18.1 Introduction

Acquired immunodeficiency syndrome (AIDS) was first described in 1981 and continues to be one of the worst global health pandemics in recorded history, with over 75 million people infected and 32 million deaths [1].

The human immunodeficiency viruses HIV-1 and HIV-2 are the causative agents of AIDS, with HIV-1 contributing to most cases worldwide. These RNA retroviruses primarily infect the T lymphocytes that express the CD4 antigen, resulting in impaired immunity. HIV is transmitted through direct contact with bodily fluids (i.e., sexual and perinatal transmission during pregnancy, delivery or breastfeeding, or from blood or blood-contaminated products). The Centers for Disease Control and Prevention (CDC) classifies HIV infection into five stages with increasing severity (0, 1, 2, 3, or unknown), according to both clinical and laboratory evaluations [2]. Stage 3 is characterized by the presence of an opportunistic infection and/or CD4 count <200/Ul [2].

The natural history of HIV infection and AIDS has changed dramatically, given advances in medical management, with particular credit to the introduction of combined antiretroviral therapy (cART). People living with HIV are now experiencing an improved quality of life, and in countries with financial and medical resources, life expectancy approaches that of the general population [3–5]. Advances in cART have also dramatically decreased perinatal transmission rates and the number of children worldwide who are living with HIV infection.

18.2 Epidemiology

In 2018, worldwide, there were 37.9 million people living with HIV, including 18.8 million women and 1.7 million children [1, 2]. Worldwide, women account for more than 52% of all adults living with HIV and 46% of new infections [1, 2]. In 2018, new infections among young women (aged 15–24 years) were 55% higher than men in the same age group, and in some regions, young women are twice as likely to be living with HIV compared to young men [2].

In 2018, 69,000 Canadians were living with HIV, with 2,561 new infections that year. Females account for approximately 29% of new cases, with the majority of exposures (64%) from heterosexual contact. One-third (33.7%) of these exposures are from sexual contact with a person originating from a HIV-endemic country [6]. Although great strides have been made in awareness and treatment programs,

https://doi.org/10.1515/9783110615258-018

some of the most troubling estimates continue to be that one in every seven Canadians living with HIV are undiagnosed and remain unaware of their infection and transmission risk [7].

Annually, there are 1.3 million pregnancies in women living with HIV, with the majority of childhood infections acquired through perinatal transmission [1]. Worldwide, in 2017, there were 180,000 new infections in children aged 0–14 years [1, 8]. However, advances in cART have dramatically decreased perinatal transmission rates and the number of children exposed to HIV who remain uninfected is on the rise, with 82% of pregnant women receiving antiretroviral therapy, globally [1]. In Canada, 259 infants were exposed to HIV in pregnancy in 2018, with 96.5% of mothers accepting perinatal antiretroviral therapy. Five infants contracted HIV, of which, two mothers were on antiretroviral therapy [6].

Although a majority of pregnant women are receiving antiretroviral therapy, there continues to be room for improvement. Further, shortfalls in coverage are evident in adolescents and children with low rates of follow-up testing and only 54% of those living with HIV receiving cART [1, 2].

18.3 Prenatal Testing

Most perinatal transmissions occur in women who are not screened [9]. Studies have revealed that targeted testing of women perceived to be at increased risk fails to identify a significant number of women living with HIV [9, 10]. Therefore, screening for HIV should be offered universally to pregnant women, early in pregnancy or at their first prenatal visit [11–13]. Although, screening is considered the standard of care, it is voluntary, and women must not be tested without their knowledge. Pretest counselling should be provided regarding the possible risks and benefits, unique to each individual situation, along with information regarding right of refusal. Women who test negative but continue to engage in high-risk behavior should be tested every trimester. Diagnosis is made with a combination immunoassay for HIV-1 and HIV-2 antibodies as well as HIV-1 p24 antigen [14]. Specimens that are reactive on antigen testing and nonreactive or indeterminate on antibody assay proceed to HIV-1 nucleic acid testing for conclusive results [14]. Women with no antenatal care and unknown HIV status should be offered rapid HIV testing, upon admission to labor and delivery, and consideration should be given regarding treatment and infant prophylaxis [15]. Testing should be offered in each pregnancy, regardless of previous negative serology [16].

High-risk behaviors:

Sharing needles or any other components during intravenous drug use
Condom-less intercourse with multiple partners
Condom-less intercourse with a partner known to be living with HIV
Condom-less intercourse with a partner who is from an HIV endemic area
Condom-less intercourse with a partner participating in known high-risk behaviors
Current or recent incarceration

18.4 Maternal and Perinatal Outcomes

18.4.1 Maternal Outcomes

Pregnancy has no significant effect on HIV progression. However, there are reports of increased risk of chorioamnionitis, postpartum endometritis, and wound infection, with maternal risk inversely proportional to CD4 count at the time of delivery [17]. Abnormal biochemical values have been reported with cART therapies (primarily, elevations in the alanine aminotransferase or creatinine level in 5% and 1% of women, respectively); however, there were no adverse outcomes associated with these values [18]. Concerns regarding decreased maternal bone mineral density in the postpartum period have been noted with the tenofovir protocol for mothers on cART, compared to mothers whose infants were on nevirapine alone ($p < 0.001$) [19].

18.4.2 Fetal Outcomes

The most important factor in preventing perinatal transmission in pregnancy is cART. The risk of perinatal transmission, without treatment, is 25%, which decreases to 1.8% with zidovudine alone and 0.5% with cART treatment regimens [18]. In Canada, perinatal transmission rates are reported at less than 0.4% with accessed care [20]. Factors that increase the risk of perinatal transmission include preterm birth, concurrent syphilis, chorioamnionitis, and maternal viral load >100,000 copies/mL [21]. Although prolonged ruptured membranes were felt to be in keeping with the elevated risk, a study by Mark et al. revealed that among women with undetectable viral loads, the length of time of rupture of membranes may not actually be associated with a higher risk of perinatal transmission [22]. Lastly, acquisition of HIV during pregnancy or lactation increases the risk of perinatal transmission by 15- and 4-fold, respectively, compared to women with chronic and well-managed HIV [23, 24].

A recent meta-analysis of prospective studies from 1980 to 2014 revealed that women living with HIV have a higher risk of preterm birth (RR 1.5, 95% CI 1.24–1.82), low birthweight (1.62, 1.41–1.86), small for gestational-age fetuses (1.31, 1.14–1.51), and stillbirth (1.67, 1.05–2.66) [25].

Regrettably, even with treatment, the incidence of perinatal complications is increased in women who are seropositive. A recent randomized control trial revealed increased rates of adverse pregnancy outcomes, low birthweight, and preterm delivery, in women on antiretroviral therapy, with higher rates in the cART regimens compared to zidovudine alone. There were no significant differences in stillbirth, spontaneous abortion, or congenital anomalies among the three groups [18].

Details regarding fetal outcomes with respect to the introduction of preconception cART are detailed in the following section.

18.5 Preconception Management

18.5.1 Counseling

Studies have consistently shown that the desire and intention of seropositive individuals to have children is high [26–28], and with continued positive strides in improving maternal health and decreasing perinatal transmission, many couples are seeking specialized counseling, services, and support regarding their unique fertility and pregnancy needs [29]. A referral to a health-care practitioner specializing in HIV care is important to ensure the appropriate steps are taken in pregnancy planning. Pre-pregnancy recommendations regarding healthy diet and lifestyle, abstinence of substances, and prenatal genetic screening are the same as for HIV-negative individuals. Recommendations for folic acid supplementation are consistent with low-risk couples (0.4–1 mg daily for 3 months prior to pregnancy and at least the first 3 months antenatally) [30]. However, there are a few considerations specific to seropositive individuals and serodifferent couples.

18.5.2 Medications

Prior to conception, a clinician should review all medications and complementary therapies taken by individuals living with HIV for safety in pregnancy. Treatment for hepatitis C is considered teratogenic and should be stopped by either partner at least six months prior to attempting to conceive. Global guidelines currently recommend cART for all individuals living with HIV, regardless of CD4 count [31]. Combined antiretroviral therapy with the greatest drug efficacy, tolerability, and least toxicity to the fetus/newborn should be selected and started in the preconception period or as early as possible in the first trimester [32]. Regardless of the method of conception, it is recommended that individuals living with HIV initiate cART and achieve viral suppression, prior to pregnancy. Full viral suppression for a minimum of three months preconception is advised, or, at minimum, two viral load measurements below the level of detection, at least 1 month apart [33].

Historically, cART was delayed until the second trimester for theoretical concerns regarding teratogenic effects; however, recent data reveals that early initiation is important for horizontal risk reduction [33–35] and decreasing perinatal transmission rates [36]. Current guidelines therefore recommend cART be started prior to pregnancy or as soon as possible, once pregnancy is confirmed [32].

Nevertheless, these benefits do not appear to be without consequence. A recent meta-analyses of 11 studies reported higher rates of preterm birth (<37 weeks) among women starting cART prior to conception [37]. A pooled analysis of three clinical trials (HPTN 052, ACTG A5208, and ACTG A5175) was also concerning for higher rates of preterm birth in women conceiving on ART (52% of all live births), with the median gestational age of live births being 35 weeks and 5 days (IQR: 35.1, 38.1) [38]. Further, the proportion of pregnancies ending in stillbirth (>20 weeks) was higher (4%) than previous studies in a similar population, with a higher median pre-pregnancy CD4 count significantly associated with live births (median 451 cell/mm^3) [38]. Lastly, a recent cohort study revealed nonsignificant trends with respect to preterm birth (OR 1.39, 0.94–1.92, $p = 0.06$); however, it did reveal a significant association of preconception cART with SGA (OR 1.35, 95% CI 1.03–1.77, $p = 0.03$) compared to women commencing cART after conception [39]. Given this emerging data, research is needed to understand the possible etiology and impact of these medications on maternal and infant outcomes, especially in early gestation. Adverse pregnancy outcomes, specifically increased risk of neural tube defects, have been associated with dolutegravir used at the time of conception, and regimens containing this drug should be discontinued prior to conception, if possible [40].

18.5.3 Conception and Fertility Treatment Considerations

Several large studies have shown that there is negligible risk of sexual HIV transmission if the plasma viral load is suppressed [33–35] and, therefore, condom-less timed intercourse or home insemination are now recommended options for conception in individuals with HIV [32]. The relative risk of transmission is dependent on the plasma viral load, length of time on cART, frequency of intercourse, and presence of sexually transmitted infections [41].

In serodifferent couples, pre-exposure prophylaxis (PrEP) is recommended for HIV-negative partners, when adherence to cART or viral suppression cannot be confirmed in the person living with HIV [42]. However, it does not appear to add significant advantage to cART in decreasing horizontal transmission when full viral suppression has already been achieved [31, 32, 43–45]. International guidelines differ in their recommendations for PrEP prior to conception and during pregnancy.

However, there is consensus that women should be informed of the availability of PrEP, as degree of risk is sometimes difficult to discern [46]. Pre-exposure prophylaxis is offered as tenofovir and emtricitabine in a single dailydose [46].

If conception is not achieved within 6–12 months, couples should be referred to a specialist for investigation. Infertility rates are higher in the seropositive population, with lower rates of implantation (10% vs 21%), pregnancy (12% vs 32%), and live-births (7% vs 19%), compared to uninfected controls [47]. Sperm washing followed by IUI, IVF, or ICSI is considered safe. A recent meta-analysis summarizing more than 40 trials in assisted reproductive cycles revealed no documented cases of HIV transmission [48]. Universal precautions should be applied to handling samples infected with HIV as well as processing in a separate laboratory or, at minimum, a designated area with designated equipment, to avoid cross-contamination [32]. Adoption, sperm or egg donation, and surrogacy should be explored as options, when applicable.

18.5.4 Immunizations/Infections

Lastly, individuals living with HIV are uniquely immunocompromised and, therefore, should be immunized and screened for infections as per their CD4 cell count. Universal recommendations for immunization in pregnancy, including diphtheria, tetanus toxoids, acellular pertussis (Tdap), and influenza should be respected [49]. Seropositive women with normal CD4 counts should also be offered immunizations for varicella, hepatitis, streptococcus pneumococcal, and human papillomavirus (HPV), prior to conception [50]. Women with CD4 cell counts <200 cells/mm^3 are at high risk of opportunistic infections, and treatment/prophylaxis should be given in addition to cART, with consideration of potential toxicities in pregnancy [50]. Detailed guidelines regarding immunizations as well as risks and treatment options for opportunistic infections are available elsewhere [49, 50].

18.6 Pregnancy Management: Antenatal Care

18.6.1 Schedule of Care

A multidisciplinary approach in obstetrical care is important for women living with HIV, given their unique and potentially complex medical, economic, social, and cultural needs. Care should be provided in a confidential and nonjudgmental fashion. Standard pregnancy investigations as well as HIV-specific history and examinations are detailed in Table 18.1.

Table 18.1: Proposed management algorithm for antepartum care for women living with HIV.

Antepartum management algorithm			
	TM1	**TM2**	**TM3**
History	– History of prior HIV-related illnesses – Past CD4 counts – Plasma HIV viral loads – Symptoms for opportunistic infections – Screening for sexually transmitted infections – Evaluation of immunization status	– Symptoms for opportunistic infections – Symptoms of preterm birth	– Symptoms for opportunistic infections – Symptoms of preterm birth – Plans for infant feeding
HIV-specific investigations	*At presentation and then q4–8 wks:* – CD4 count (absolute and fraction) – HIV viral load – HIV typing – CBC and differential – Liver functions tests – Renal function tests – Tuberculosis screen – HCV screen	*Every 4–8 weeks:* – CD4 cell count – HIV viral load – CBC – LFTs (AST, ALT, LDH, bilirubin) – Renal function (Cr, BUN)	*Every 4–8 weeks:* – CD4 cell count – HIV viral load – CBC – LFTs (AST, ALT, LDH, bilirubin) – Renal function (Cr, BUN) *Every 4 weeks:* – Well-being/growth US
Pregnancy-specific investigations	– Dating ultrasound – First-trimester screen – Urine culture – GC/CT screen – Serology testing – G&S ±PAP	– Anatomy US at 18–20 weeks – Glucose challenge ±Rhogam	– GBS

In the first trimester, a complete history and initial work-up in terms of HIV viral load, CD4 count, HIV genotyping, as well as liver and renal function is important for treatment and investigation planning through the remainder of pregnancy. Combined antiretroviral therapy should be initiated preconception or as early in pregnancy as possible. Nausea and vomiting should be treated aggressively, as this can interfere with initiation or continuation of antiviral medications. Alternative rare causes of vomiting (opportunistic infections, gastric lymphoma, pancreatitis, and elevated intracranial pressure) should be considered if nonresponsive to initial therapy [51].

Clinical, virologic, and immunologic status should be assessed regularly in the second trimester. A detailed anatomy scan is universally recommended at 18–20 weeks to assess fetal anatomy and growth. Invasive testing should be considered if aneuploidy is suspected on prenatal screening or, in some cases, with suspected fetal infection. In the pre-cART era, the risk of perinatal transmission with amniocentesis was twice as high as without (30% vs 16%, RR 1.85; 95% CI 0.69–4.98) [52]. However, there have been no documented transmissions when compliant with cART and a documented suppressed viral load [53–56]. Current recommendations are to begin cART at least 2 weeks prior to the procedure and delay the procedure until the viral load is undetectable [32]. Noninvasive prenatal testing should be considered in this population, when applicable, to avoid any theoretical risk of transmission with amniocentesis.

Even with good adherence to medications, the increased volume distribution of pregnancy can result in subtherapeutic levels of antiviral therapy and inadequate viral suppression. Nonadherence to therapy may also be a reason for inability to maintain viral suppression. In all cases, adherence, viral genotype history, drug levels, and viral load should be reassessed. Drug or dose adjustments may be required to achieve suppression. Serial growth ultrasound in the third trimester is recommended due to the risk of intrauterine growth restriction and oligohydramnios, associated with placental dysfunction and antiretroviral exposure. There is also a higher risk of preterm birth and, therefore, symptoms should be followed carefully with assessments mentioned earlier, if applicable (GBS testing and genital herpes prophylaxis). Delivery planning should be arranged and discussions regarding infant feeding should be discussed as below [32]. Figure 18.1 provides an approach to the evaluation and management of medications in pregnancy.

18.6.2 Antiretroviral Therapy

The selection of cART regimen in pregnancy requires careful consideration of a number of inter-related factors (outlined in Table 18.2) and should, therefore, be made in coordination with an infectious disease specialist. A cART regime should include a dual nonreverse transcriptase inhibitor (NRTI) backbone with an additional boosted protease inhibitor. The goal is a regimen with high transplacental passage, known safety and efficacy in pregnancy, and good maternal tolerability. In most cases, the preconception antiretroviral regimen can be continued. However, modifications should be considered in two populations. First, nevirapine initiation in pregnancy has been associated with life-threatening rash and hepatoxicity in 10% of patients. Patients tolerating this medication prior to pregnancy can be safely continued, but it should not be started in pregnancy, if an alternative is available [21]. Second, new antiretroviral regimes have little data regarding safety in pregnancy and, therefore, could be switched to a regimen with more evidence. Patients

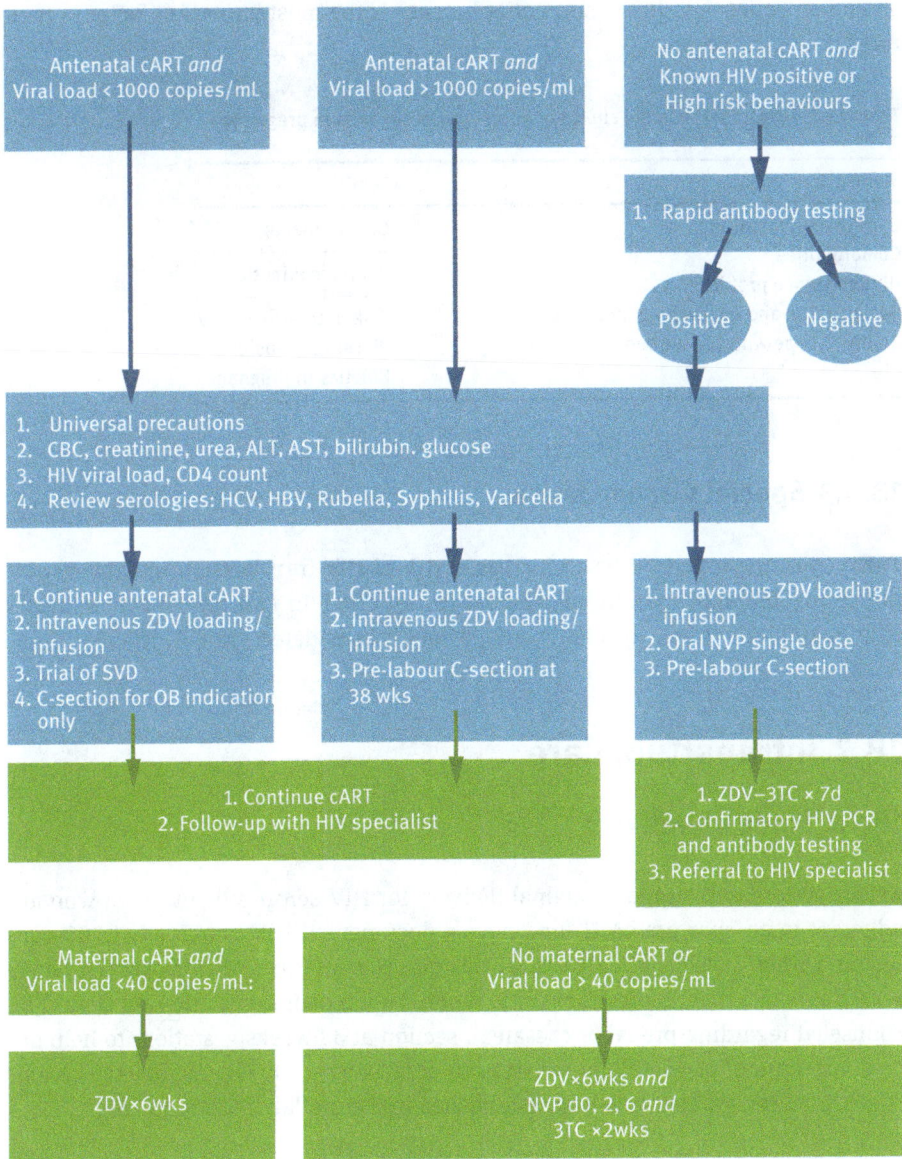

Antenatal cART *and* Viral load < 1000 copies/mL	Antenatal cART *and* Viral load > 1000 copies/ml	No antenatal cART *and* Known HIV positive or High risk behaviours

1. Rapid antibody testing

Positive   Negative

1. Universal precautions
2. CBC, creatinine, urea, ALT, AST, bilirubin. glucose
3. HIV viral load, CD4 count
4. Review serologies: HCV, HBV, Rubella, Syphillis, Varicella

1. Continue antenatal cART 2. Intravenous ZDV loading/ infusion 3. Trial of SVD 4. C-section for OB indication only	1. Continue antenatal cART 2. Intravenous ZDV loading/ infusion 3. Pre-labour C-section at 38 wks	1. Intravenous ZDV loading/ infusion 2. Oral NVP single dose 3. Pre-labour C-section

1. Continue cART 2. Follow-up with HIV specialist	1. ZDV–3TC × 7d 2. Confirmatory HIV PCR and antibody testing 3. Referral to HIV specialist

Maternal cART *and* Viral load <40 copies/mL:	No maternal cART *or* Viral load > 40 copies/mL

ZDV×6wks	ZDV×6wks *and* NVP d0, 2, 6 *and* 3TC ×2wks

Figure 18.1: Proposed management strategy for intrapartum and postpartum care for women living with HIV.

should be counseled that consistent adherence is the most important factor in perinatal transmission rates.

Table 18.2: Factors influencing choice of antiretroviral regimen in pregnancy.

Maternal	Fetal
Current health status	Gestational age
Comorbidities	
HIV resistance profile	**Pharmacokinetics**
Social status and intravenous drug use	Risk of teratogenicity
Ability to cope with pill burden	Placental transfer
	Kinetics in pregnancy

18.6.3 Special Circumstance

There does not appear to be an increased risk of HIV transmission in women with premature prelabor rupture of membranes on cART in two retrospective cohort studies and, therefore, expectant management is considered safe [57, 58].

18.7 Intrapartum Care

18.7.1 Mode of Delivery

Extensive research supports vaginal delivery for HIV seropositive women who are adherent to antepartum cART, and have a documented HIV viral load <1,000 copies/mL within 4 weeks of delivery. In this group, caesarean sections should be reserved for obstetrical indications only. Women not meeting this criterion should be counseled regarding pre-labor caesarean section at 38 weeks gestation, to help decrease the risk of perinatal transmission by at least 50% [51, 59]. Of note, the benefit of cesarean section has only been established in the pre-labor group [51, 59].

18.7.2 Antiretroviral Therapy

On admission to labor and delivery, bloodwork should be drawn for CBC, creatinine, urea, AST, ALT, bilirubin, glucose, HIV viral load, and CD4 count in women with seropositive status. Antepartum cART therapy should be continued in labor. The addition of intravenous zidovudine is recommended in labor for women with viral loads >400 copies/mL. However, there is discordance in guidelines regarding the benefit of zidovudine in women with <400 copies/mL. Canadian guidelines recommend zidovudine for all women, regardless of viral load, given the documented unpredictability of viral loads at time of delivery. A study by Money et al. revealed that 8.7% of women with previously undetectable viral loads had elevated viral loads at the time of delivery despite adequate adherence to therapy [60]. Intravenous zidovudine (2 mg/kg over 1 h, followed by 1 mg/kg/h) should be administered at time of active labor, rupture of membranes, or at least 2–3 h prior to caesarean section and continued until delivery [51].

Women with unknown HIV status or continued risk of HIV infection should be offered rapid HIV antibody testing, upon presentation to labor and delivery. If the test is positive, further serologies and standard HIV intrapartum bloodwork should be drawn. Women should be treated with intrapartum and postpartum prophylaxis to help decrease the risk of perinatal transmission from 25% to 10% [61–63]. Intrapartum therapy includes zidovudine as above, as well as a single-dose of nevirapine (200 mg) in labor and ideally 2–3 h prior to caesarean section [51]. Confirmatory HIV PCR and antibody testing should be organized.

18.7.3 Special Considerations

Invasive obstetrical procedures such as fetal electrodes, operative delivery, and episiotomy should be avoided, as they increase the risk of exposure of maternal blood to the fetus (see Table 18.3) [51]. Pre-antiretroviral data revealed increased rates of perinatal transmission with these procedures; however, further data is needed to understand whether this continues to be a risk with suppressed viral load on antepartum cART [64–67]. Prolonged rupture of membranes should be avoided, if possible, although recent data suggests this is not an independent predictor of transmission if viral load is undetectable [22]. General management strategies including epidurals, oxytocin augmentation, and Group B streptococcus prophylaxis should be offered as per standard guidelines. In the context of postpartum hemorrhage, ergonovine should be avoided, given the risk of exaggerating vasoconstriction in women receiving protease inhibitors.

Table 18.3: Obstetric management.

Safe	Avoid (if possible)
– Epidural	– Invasive procedures
– Oxytocin augmentation	– Prolonged rupture of membranes or artificial
– Group B streptococcus prophylaxis	rupture of membranes
– Preoperative antibiotic prophylaxis	– Ergonovine for management of postpartum
	hemorrhage

18.8 Postpartum Care

A number of complex issues should be addressed in the postpartum period, including contraception, antiretroviral therapy, infant feeding, pediatric care, mental health, and individual needs regarding social support services. Multidisciplinary care is important to ensure coordinated and comprehensive care for both mother and infant.

18.8.1 Antiretroviral Therapy

Women receiving antenatal cART should resume their regimen as soon as oral intake is tolerated, following delivery. If nevirapine is given in labor, women should receive zidovudine (300 mg) and lamivudine (150 mg) (Combivir) daily for 1 week to reduce the risk of developing resistance to nevirapine. Adherence in the postpartum period has proven to be challenging, which can contribute to virologic rebound [68, 69].

18.8.2 Infant Feeding

In low income settings, breastfeeding and cART is recommended as the morbidity and mortality from infection secondary to unclean water and lost protection from maternal antibodies in formula-fed infants have been considered to outweigh the risk of HIV transmission through breast milk. Historically, breastfeeding was contraindicated in developed countries, given the availability of clean water and a risk of up to 26% perinatal transmission, regardless of viral load, when not on cART [70]. Extended lactation accounted for up to one-third of all HIV transmission to infants in breastfeeding settings [70, 71]. However, recent data reveals no reported cases of mother-to-child transmission due to breastfeeding in women with an undetectable viral load and adherence to cART [72]. In the breastfeeding aspect of the IMPAACT PROMISE trial, mother-to-child transmission via breast milk at 6, 9, and 12 months were 0.3% (0.1–0.8), 0.6% (0.3–1.3), and 0.7% (0.3–1.4) in the maternal cART arms, respectively [73]. Interventional studies and systematic reviews have demonstrated that cART is efficacious in prevention of mother-to-child transmission of HIV through breast milk, with increased rates of infection when cART is stopped [74]. However, there are no formal studies of transmission rates on women fully suppressed on cART and given the potential lifelong consequences of transmission, the risks and benefits in each specific case should be reviewed. Modeling estimates place the postnatal transmission rate in women on cART as 0.2% per month of breastfeeding, which corresponds to 2.4% at 12 months, and greater if breastfeeding is extended [75].

Most recent guidelines suggest breastfeeding should not be actively recommended until more robust safety data is available; however, they no longer propose rigidly advising against breastfeeding in the optimal scenario of adherence to cART with a suppressed viral load in women who wish to breastfeed [72]. An open and unbiased discussion plans regarding infant feeding is important to help educate and empower women in their autonomous decisions, with a fulsome discussion of the risks, benefits, and current state of knowledge regarding this. It is important for providers and pregnant women to understand that blood viral load and breast milk viral load may not be perfectly correlated. There are no specific data to guide the frequency and source of virological monitoring, should a mother living with HIV choose to breastfeed. European and North American guidelines suggest monitoring of maternal viral load anywhere from twice monthly to every other month [76]. Infant cART prophylaxis is recommended in women who choose to breastfeed. The exact regimen may vary depending on the setting, and decision-making should involve a pediatrician specializing in infectious disease [77].

Data from the postpartum period in women living with HIV reveals that antiretroviral adherence frequently decreases after delivery due to the demands of caring for a newborn, and women benefit from additional support [78, 79]. Multidisciplinary care in the postpartum period, including family planning, women's health, and pediatric care should be integrated [78].

Should a woman choose to formula-feed, an early return to fertility can be expected and options surrounding contraception should be discussed. Condom use is recommended in serodifferent couples to reduce the risk of HIV transmission between partners. It is important to review potential interactions between individual antiretroviral medications and contraceptives as adverse events have been reported [80]. Further, classic therapies for lactation suppression were previously contraindicated with protease inhibitor use. A recent systematic review revealed that cabergoline, a dopamine receptor agonist, is a safe and well-tolerated medication for the indication of lactation inhibition or suppression [81]. More specifically, a review by Oladapo et al. described transient, mild-to-moderate adverse events with cabergoline in the HIV-positive population in clinical trials; however, there were no reported significant drug–drug interactions between cabergoline and any antiretroviral medications, including protease inhibitors [82]. However, prospective studies are needed regarding the safety, efficacy, and acceptability in women living with HIV, before it can be incorporated into perinatal guidelines and practice [83].

18.8.3 Infant Care

Infants with exposure to HIV infection should be offered prophylaxis according to their presumed level of risk, based on maternal viral load. Infants should be tested for HIV infection with HIV RNA PCR at birth, 4 weeks, and 3–4 months of age.

Negative testing includes two nonreactive tests, with one test at least 4 weeks after the end of prophylactic antiretroviral therapy. Confirmatory HIV EIA testing should be completed at 18 months. If reactive, a referral should be made to a pediatric HIV specialist as early initiation of cART has been shown to improve outcomes.

18.9 Conclusion

Concerted international efforts have helped to increase awareness of HIV status, improve access to treatment and continuation of therapy to achieve viral suppression with a goal of ending the AIDS epidemic by 2030. [1] HIV-related deaths fell by 45% between 2000 and 2018, which equivocates to 13.6 million lives saved due to cART [1]. The clinical outcomes for patients living with HIV on cART are considerably improved with prolonged life expectancy and superior quality of life. Further, perinatal transmission rates have dramatically decreased from one in three newborns infected to less than one in a hundred [21, 84], with elimination of mother-to-child transmission of HIV in a growing number of countries worldwide [85]. Gaps in knowledge and translation have been identified, and developments in these areas could further improve maternal and infant outcomes. The promise of a HIV-free generation is on the horizon and continued international efforts in preventing perinatal transmission are an important component of this achievement.

References

[1] World Health Organization. HIV/AIDS. https://www.who.int/news-room/factsheets/detail/hiv-aids. Accessed December 1, 2019.
[2] Centers for Disease Control and Prevention. Terms, Definitions and Calculations. https://www.cdc.gov/hiv/statistics/surveillance/terms.html. Accessed December 21, 2019.
[3] Palella FJ Jr, Baker RK, Moorman AC et al. HIV outpatient study investigators. Mortality in the highly active antiretroviral therapy era: Changing causes of death and disease in the HIV outpatient study. J Acquir Immune Defic Syndr 2006;43:27–34.
[4] Mocroft A, Ledergerber B, Katlama C et al. EuroSIDA study group. Decline in the AIDS and death rates in the EuroSIDA study: An observational study. Lancet 2003;362(9377):22–29.
[5] The Antiretroviral Therapy Cohort Collaboration. Life expectancy of individuals on combination antiretroviral therapy in high-income countries: a collaborative analysis of 14 cohort studies. Lancet 2008;372(9635):293–299.
[6] Public Health Agency of Canada. HIV in Canada: 2018 surveillance highlights. https://www.canada.ca/en/public-health/services/publications/diseases-conditions/hiv-2018-surveillance-highlights.html. Accessed December 19, 2019.
[7] Centers for Disease Control and Prevention. Terms, Definitions and Calculations. https://www.cdc.gov/hiv/statistics/surveillance/terms.html. Accessed December 21, 2019.

[8]   UNAIDS. UNAIDS calls on countries to accelerate efforts and close service gaps to end the
        AIDS epidemic among children and adolescents. https://www.unaids.org/en/keywords/
        pmtct. Accessed December 21, 2019.
[9]   Peckham CS, Newell M. Controversy in mandatory HIV screening of pregnant women. Curr
        Opin Infect Dis 1997;10:18e21.
[10]   Bitnum A, King SM, Arneson C et al. Failure to prevent perinatal HIV infection. CMAJ
        2002;166:904e5.
[11]   Canadian Paediatric Society. Testing for human immunodeficiency virus type I (HIV-1)
        infection in pregnancy. Paediatr Child Health 2001;6:685e9.
[12]   American Academy of Pediatrics and American College of Obstetricians and Gynecologists.
        Human immunodeficiency virus screening. Pediatrics 1999;104:128.
[13]   Institute of Medicine, National Research Council. Reducing the Odds: Preventing Perinatal
        Transmission of HIV in the United States. Washington, DC: National Academy Press; 1999.
[14]   Branson BM, Owen SM, Wesolowski LG et al. Centres for Disease Control and Prevention.
        Laboratory testing for the diagnosis of HIV infection: Updated recommendations. https://
        stacks.cdc.gov/view/cdc/23447 Accessed December 1, 2019.
[15]   Canada Communicable Disease Report. Point-of-Care HIV testing using rapid HIV test kits:
        Guidance for Health-care professionals. http://publications.gc.ca/collections/collection_
        2010/aspc-phac/H12-21-3-33-2-eng.pdf Accessed December 1, 2019.
[16]   Keenan-Lindsay L, Yudin MH. Society of obstetricians and gynaecologists of Canada. HIV
        screening in pregnancy, no 185. J Obstet Gynaecol Can 2017;39(7):e54ee58.
[17]   Calvert C, Ronsmans C. HIV and the risk of direct obstetric complications: A systematic review
        and meta-analysis. PLOS One 2013;8(10):e74848.
[18]   Fowler MG, Qin M, Fiscus SA et al. The IMPAACT 1077BF/1077FF PROMISE study team.
        Benefits and risks of antiretroviral therapy for perinatal HIV prevention. N Engl J Med
        2016;375:1726–1737.
[19]   Stranix-Chibanda L Impact of tenofovir-containing triple antiretroviral therapy (ART) on bone
        mineral density in HIV-infected breastfeeding women in sub-Saharan Africa. Oral
        presentation at the 8th International Workshop on HIV Pediatrics. Durban, South Africa.
        July 2016.
[20]   Forbes JC, Alimenti AM, Singer J et al. A national review of vertical HIV transmission. AIDS
        2012;26:757–763.
[21]   Cunningham FG, Leveno KJ, Bloom SL et al. Sexually Transmitted Infections, Williams
        Obstetrics 24th Edition. McGraw Hill Education, 2014; (65) 1279.
[22]   Mark S, Murphy KE, Read S et al. HIV mother-to-child transmission, mode of delivery, and
        duration of rupture of membranes: Experience in the current era. Infect Dis Obstet Gynecol
        2012;267969.
[23]   Birkhead GS, Pulver WP, Warren BL et al. Acquiring human Immunodeficiency virus during
        pregnancy and mother-to-child transmission in New York: 2002–2006. Obstet Gynecol
        2010;115:1247–1255.
[24]   Humphrey JH, Marinda E, Mutasa K et al. Mother to child transmission of HIV among
        Zimbabwean women who seroconverted postnatally: Prospective cohort study. BMJ 2010;341:
        c6580.
[25]   Wedi CO, Kirtley S, Hopewell S et al. Perinatal outcomes associated with maternal HIV
        infection: A systematic review and meta-analysis. Lancet HIV 2016;3:e33–48.
[26]   Loutfy MR, Hart TA, Mohammed SS et al. Ontario HIV fertility research team. Fertility desires
        and intentions of HIV-positive women of reproductive age in Ontario, Canada: a
        crosssectional study. PLoS ONE 2009;4(12):e7925.

[27]   Ogilvie GS, Palepu A, Remple VP et al. Fertility intentions of women of reproductive age living with HIV in British Columbia, Canada. AIDS 2007;21(Suppl 1):583–588.

[28]   Oladapo OT, Daniel OJ, Odusoga OL, Ayoola-Sotubo O. Fertility desires and intentions of HIV-positive patients at a suburban specialist center. J Natl Med Assoc 2005;97:1672–1681.

[29]   Tharao W, Logie C, James L, Loutfy M. "These are some of the things we need": women living with HIV discuss issues in their daily lives as research priorities. Oral abstract presented at Canadian Association for AIDS Researchers Conference Toronto 2011.

[30]   Moore A, Mundle W, O'Connor et al. Pre-conception folic acid and multivitamin supplementation for the primary and secondary prevention of neural tube defects and other folic acid-sensitive congenital anomalies, no 324. J Obstet Gynaecol Can 2015;37(6):534–549.

[31]   World Health Organization. Consolidated guidelines on the use of antiretroviral drugs for treating and preventing HIV infection. Recommendations for a public health approach. 2nd ed. http://apps.who.int/iris/bitstream/10665/208825/1/9789241549684_eng.pdf Accessed December 1, 2019.

[32]   Loutfy M, Kennedy VL, Poliquin V et al. Society of obstetricians and gynaecologists of Canada. Canadian HIV pregnancy planning guidelines, no 354. J Obstet Gynaecol Can Jan 2018;40(1):94–114.

[33]   Cohen MS, Chen YQ, McCauley M et al. Antiretroviral therapy for the prevention of HIV-1 transmission. N Engl J Med 2016;375:830–839.

[34]   Loutfy MR, Wu W, Letchumanan M et al. Systematic review of HIV transmission between heterosexual serodiscordant couples where the HIV-positive partner is fully suppressed on antiretroviral therapy. PLoS ONE 2013;8:e55747.

[35]   Rodger AJ, Cambiano V, Bruun T et al. Sexual activity without condoms and risk of HIV transmission in serodifferent couples when the HIV-positive partner is using suppressive antiretroviral therapy. JAMA 2016;316:171–181.

[36]   Mandelbrot L, Tubiana R, Le Chenadec J et al. No perinatal HIV-1 transmission from women with effective antiretroviral therapy starting before conception. Clin Infect Dis 2015;61: 1715–1725.

[37]   Uthman OA, Nachega JB, Anderson J et al. Timing of initiation of antiretroviral therapy and adverse pregnancy outcomes: A systematic review and meta-analysis. Lancet HIV 2017;4(1): e21–e30.

[38]   Stringer EM, Kendall MA, Lockman S et al. Pregnancy outcomes among HIV-infected women who conceived on antiretroviral therapy. PLoS One 2018;13(7):e0199555.

[39]   Snijdewind IJM, Smit C, Godfried MH et al. Preconception use of cART by HIV-positive pregnant women increases the risk of infant being born small for gestational age. PLoS ONE 2018;13(1):e0191389.

[40]   Zash R, Holmes L, Diseko M et al. Neural-tube defects and antiretroviral treatment regimens in Botswana. NEJM 2019;381(9):827–840.

[41]   Barreiro P, Castilla JA, Labarga P et al. Is natural conception a valid option for HIV-serodiscordant couples?. Hum Reprod 2007;22:2353–2358.

[42]   Fonner VA, Dalglish SL, Kennedy CE et al. Effectiveness and safety of oral HIV pre-exposure prophylaxis (PrEP) for all populations: A systematic review and meta-analysis. AIDS 2016;30 (12):1973–1983.

[43]   Van Damme L, Corneli A, Ahmed K et al. FEM-PrEP study group. pre-exposure prophylaxis for HIV infection among African women. N Engl J Med 2012;367:411–422.

[44]   Marrazzo JM, Ramjee G, Richardson BA et al. VOICE study team. tenofovir-based preexposure prophylaxis for HIV infection among African women. N Engl J Med 2015;372:509–518.

[45] Centers for Disease Control and Prevention. Provider information sheet – PrEP during conception, pregnancy, and breastfeeding. https://www.cdc.gov/hiv/pdf/prep_gl_clinician_factsheet_pregnancy_english.pdf. Accessed on December 1, 2019.

[46] Seidman DL, Weber S, Timoney MT et al. Use of HIV pre-exposure prophylaxis during the preconception, antepartum and postpartum periods at two United States medical centers. Am J Obstet Gynecol 2016;215:632e1–7.

[47] Stora C, Epelboin S, Devouche E et al. Women infected with human immunodeficiency virus type 1 have poorer assisted reproduction outcomes: A case-control study. Fertil Steril 2016;105(5):1193–1201.

[48] Zafer M, Horvath H, Mmeje O et al. Effectiveness of semen washing to prevent human immunodeficiency virus (HIV) transmission and assist pregnancy in HIV-discordant couples: A systematic review and meta-analysis. Fertil Steril 2016;105(3):645–655.

[49] Gruslin A, Steben M, Halperin et al. Immunization in pregnancy, no 236. J Obstet Gynaecol Can 2009;31(11):1085–1092.

[50] Panel on Opportunistic Infections in HIV-Infected Adults and Adolescents. Guidelines for the prevention and treatment of opportunistic infections in HIV-infected adults and adolescents: recommendations from the Centers for Disease Control and Prevention, the National Institutes of Health, and the HIV Medicine Association of the Infectious Diseases Society of America. http://aidsinfo.nih.gov/contentfiles/lvguidelines/adult_oi.pdf Accessed December 1, 2019.

[51] Money D, Tulloch K, Boucoiran I et al. Guidelines for the care of pregnant women living with HIV and interventions to reduce perinatal transmission, no 310. J Obstet Gynaecol Can 2014;36(8eSuppl A):S1–S46.

[52] Maiques V, Garcia-Tejedor A, Perales A et al. HIV detection in amniotic fluid samples. amniocentesis can be performed in HIV pregnant women?. Eur J Obstet Gynecol Reprod Biol 2003;108:137–141.

[53] Somigliana E, Bucceri AM, Tibaldi C et al. Italian collaborative study on HIV infection in pregnancy. early invasive diagnostic techniques in pregnant women who are infected with the HIV: A multicenter case series. Am J Obstet Gynecol 2005;193:437–442.

[54] Coll O, Suy A, Hernandez S et al. Prenatal diagnosis in human immunodeficiency virus-infected women: A new screening program for chromosomal anomalies. Am J Obstet Gynecol 2006;194:192–198.

[55] Ekoukou D, Khuong-Josses MA, Ghibaudo N et al. Amniocentesis in pregnant HIV-infected patients. absence of mother-to-child viral transmission in a series of selected patients. Eur J Obstet Gynecol Reprod Biol 2008;140:212–217.

[56] Mandelbrot L, Jasseron C, Ekoukou D et al. Amniocentesis and mother-to-child human immunodeficiency virus transmission in the agence Nationale de Recherches sur le SIDA et les hepatites virales French Perinatal Cohort. Am J Obstet Gynecol 2009;200(2):160e1–9.

[57] Aagaard-Tillery KM, Lin MG, Lupo V et al. Preterm premature rupture of membranes in human immunodeficiency virus-infected women: a novel case series. Infect Dis Obstet Gynecol 2006;2006:53234.

[58] Alvarez JR, Bardeguez A, Iffy L et al. Preterm premature rupture of membranes in pregnancies complicated by human immunodeficiency virus infection: A single centre's five-year experience. J Matern Fetal Neonatal Med 2007;20(12):853–857.

[59] The international perinatal HIV group. The mode of delivery and the risk of vertical transmission of human immunodeficiency virus type 1. NEJM 1999;340(13):977–987.

[60] Money D, Van Schalkwyk J, Alimenti A et al. HIV viral rebound near delivery in previously suppressed, combination antiretroviral therapy (cART) treated pregnant women. paper presented at: 20th conference on retroviruses and opportunistic infections; March 2013;

Atlanta and at the 22nd Annual Canadian Conference on HIV/AIDS Research; April 2013. Vancouver Can J Infect Dis Med Microbio 2013;24(Suppl A):20.

[61] Wiktor SZ, Ekpini E, Karon JM et al. Short-course oral zidovuidine for prevention of mother-to-child transmission of HIV-1 in Abidjan, Cote d'Ivoire: A randomized trial. Lancet 1999;353:781e5.

[62] Shaffer N, Chuachoowong R, Mock PA et al. Short-course zidovudine for perinatal HIV-1 transmission in Bangkok, Thailand: A randomized controlled trial. Lancet 1999;353:773e80.

[63] Guay LA, Musoke P, Fleming T et al. Intrapartum and neonatal single-dose nevirapine compared with zidovudine for prevention of mother-to-child transmission of HIV-1 in Kampala, Uganda: HIVNET 012 randomised trial. Lancet 1999;354:795e802.

[64] Boyer PJ, Dillon M, Navaie M et al. Factors predictive of maternal-fetal transmission of HIV-1. Preliminary analysis of zidovudine given during pregnancy and/or delivery. JAMA 1994;271: 1925–1930.

[65] Mandelbrot L, Mayaux MJ, Bongain A et al. Obstetric factors and mother-to-child transmission of human immunodeficiency virus type 1: The French perinatal cohorts. SEROGEST French pediatric HIV infection study group. Am J Obstet Gynecol 1996;175:661–667.

[66] Mofenson LM, Lambert JS, Stiehm ER et al. Risk factors for perinatal transmission of human immunodeficiency virus type 1 in women treated with zidovudine. pediatric AIDS clinical trials group study 185 team. N Engl J Med 1999;341:385–393.

[67] Shapiro DE, Sperling RS, Mandelbrot L et al. Risk factors for perinatal human immunodeficiency virus transmission in patients receiving zidovudine prophylaxis. pediatric AIDS clinical trials group protocol 076 study group. Obstet Gynecol 1999;94:897–908.

[68] Nachega JB, Uthman OA, Anderson J et al. Adherence to antiretroviral therapy during and after pregnancy in low-income, middle-income, and high-income countries: a systematic review and meta-analysis. AIDS 2012;26:2039–2052.

[69] Kaida A, Forrest J, Money D et al. Antiretroviral adherence during pregnancy and postpartum among HIV-positive women enrolled in the drug treatment program in British Columbia, Canada. Paper presented at: 18th Annual Canadian Conference on HIV/AIDS Research; April 23–26, 2009. Vancouver Can J Infect Dis Med Microbiol 2009;20(B):25B.

[70] Decock KM, Fowler MG, Mercier E et al. Prevention of mother-to-child transmission in resource poor countries: Translating research into policy and practice. JAMA 2000;283: 1175–1182.

[71] Coutsoudis A, Dabis F, Fawzi W et al. Breastfeeding and HIV international transmission study group. late postnatal transmission of HIV-1 in breast-fed children: An individual patient data meta-analysis. J Infect Dis 2004;189(12):2154.

[72] Kahlert C, Aebi-Popp K, Bernasconi E et al. Is breastfeeding an equipoise option in effectively treated HIV-infected mothers in a high-income setting?. Swiss Med Weekly 2018;148:w14648.

[73] Flynn PM, Taha TE, Cababasay M et al. The PROMISE study team. prevention of HIV-1 transmission through breastfeeding: efficacy and safety of maternal antiretroviral therapy versus infant nevirapine prophylaxis for duration of breastfeeding in HIV-1-infected women with high CD4 cell count (IMPAACT PROMISE): a randomized, open label, clinical trial. J Acquired Immune Defic Syndrome 2018;77(4):383–39.

[74] Bispo S, Chikhungu L, Rollins N et al. Postnatal HIV transmission in breastfed infants of HIV-infected women on ART: A systematic review and meta-analysis. J Int AIDS Soc 2017;20 (1):21251.

[75] Rollins N, Mahy M, Becquet R, Kuhn L, Creek T, Mofenson L. Estimates of peripartum and postnatal mother-to-child transmission probabilities of HIV for use in spectrum and other population-based models. Sex Transm Infect 2012;356(Suppl 2):i44–51. doi: 10.1136/sextrans-2012-050709. pmid: 23172345.

[76] Waitt C, Low N, Van De Perre P et al. Does U=U for breastfeeding mothers and infants? breastfeeding by mothers on effective treatment for HIV infection in high-income settings. Lancet HIV 2018;5(9):e531–e536.

[77] Van De Perre P, Kankasa C, Nagot N et al. Pre-exposure prophylaxis for infants exposed to HIV through breastfeeding. BMJ 2017;356:j1053.

[78] Nachega JB, Uthman OA, Anderson J et al. Adherence to antiretroviral therapy during and after pregnancy in low-income, middle-income, and high-income countries: A systematic review and meta-analysis. AIDS 2012;26:2039–2052.

[79] Kaida A, Forrest J, Money D et al. Antiretroviral adherence during pregnancy and postpartum among HIV-positive women enrolled in the drug treatment program in British Columbia, Canada. Paper presented at: 18th Annual Canadian Conference on HIV/AIDS research; April 23–26, 2009. Vancouver Can J Infect Dis Med Microbiol 2009;20(B):25B.

[80] Panel on Treatment of HIV-Infected Pregnant Women and Prevention of Perinatal Transmission. Recommendations for use of antiretroviral drugs in pregnant HIV-1-infected women for maternal health and interventions to reduce perinatal HIV transmission in the United States. https://aidsinfo.nih.gov/guidelines/html/3/perinatal/224/whats-new-in-the-guidelines. Accessed December 25, 2019.

[81] Harris K, Murphy KE, Horn D et al. Safety of cabergoline for postpartum lactation inhibition or suppression: A systematic review. J Obstet Gynaecol Can 2019. epud ahead of print.

[82] Oladapo OT, Fawole B. Treatments for suppression of lactation. Cochrane Database Syst Rev 2012(9):CD005937.

[83] Tulloch KJ, Dodin P, Tremblay-Racine FM et al. Cabergoline: A review of its use in the inhibition of lactation for women living with HIV. J Int AIDS Soc 2019;22(6):e25322.

[84] Fowler MG, Flynn P, Aizire J. Current opinion: what's new in perinatal HIV prevention?. Curr Opin Pediatric 2018;30(1):144–151.

[85] World Health Organization. Global guidance on criteria and processes for validation: Elimination of Mother-to-Child Transmission of HIV and Syphilis (2nd edition). https://apps.who.int/iris/bitstream/handle/10665/259517/9789241513272-eng.pdf?sequence=1. Accessed December 1, 2019.

Moran Shapira, Yoav Yinon

19 Congenital Cytomegalovirus Infection

19.1 Introduction

Human cytomegalovirus (CMV) is a large enveloped virus that belongs to the herpesvirus family. CMV infects most of the human population at some stage in their lives, with seroprevalence ranging between 40% and 100% in different populations [1, 2]. Seroprevalence tends to be higher in lower socioeconomic groups, racial/ethnic minorities, women of higher parity and advanced maternal age, and women with close contact with young children [2–7].

Being a member of the herpesvirus family, CMV has biologic properties of latency and reactivation; after primary infection, defined as CMV infection in a previously seronegative person, the virus is not cleared from the host, but rather persists throughout life in a latent state, from which it can be reactivated. Reactivation of the virus results in secondary infection and may occur after various stimuli such as inflammation or immune impairment due to pregnancy, various diseases and requires medical treatment with immunomodulating agents [8]. In addition, due to extensive viral strain diversity [9], secondary infection may also occur following infection of a seropositive person with another strain of CMV. In healthy immunocompetent adults, CMV infection is usually asymptomatic, but may occasionally result in mononucleosis syndrome characterized by prolonged fever, flu-like symptoms, lymphadenopathy, hepatosplenomegaly, and arthralgia.

19.2 Congenital CMV Infection

Congenital CMV infection is the most common intrauterine infection and the leading infectious cause of sensorineural hearing loss and mental retardation [10]. As expected, the prevalence of congenital CMV varies according to geography, ethnicity, and socioeconomic status, with a prevalence of 0.6–0.7% in developed countries [11, 12], as opposed to 0.6–6% in developing countries [13].

Intrauterine infection with CMV results from transplacental transmission of the virus, either during primary or non-primary infection. Due to the absence of preconceptional immunity, transmission rate is much higher following primary infection (30–40%), as compared to secondary infection (1%) [14]. However, secondary infections are the main source of congenital CMV cases, owing to the high prevalence of seropositivity around the world [15] and a relatively low seroconversion rate among pregnant women (0.7–4.1%) [16]. When primary infection is considered, the risk of in utero transmission increases with gestational age – from 30% in the first trimester,

https://doi.org/10.1515/9783110615258-019

40% in the second trimester, up to 60% in the third trimester [17–21]. Preconception infection (up to 8 weeks before conception) carries no risk for transmission whereas periconceptional infection (defined as maternal infection between 8 weeks before and 6 weeks after conception) is associated with a smaller, yet non-negligible risk for transmission of 5% [21]. While the risk for transmission increases with gestational age, the likelihood of severe sequelae appears to be lower; it is estimated at 15–20% following first-trimester infection, decreasing to 2–5% after second-trimester infection. Following third-trimester infection, chances of sequelae are especially slim [22, 23].

Indeed, congenital infection with CMV infection may result in a wide array of obstetric, fetal, neonatal, and long-term consequences ranging over a wide spectrum of severity. Possible obstetric complications include intrauterine fetal growth restriction [24, 25], preterm delivery [24], preeclampsia [26], and intrauterine fetal death, with the latter estimated to occur in 0.5% of cases [27, 28]. At birth, 5–15% of first-trimester infected newborns are symptomatic and may suffer unilateral/bilateral sensorineural hearing loss, microcephaly, seizures, chorioretinitis, optic atrophy, vision loss, hepatosplenomegaly, petechiae, jaundice, thrombocytopenia, and anemia [8]. Up to 30% of these affected newborns will ultimately die due to disseminated intravascular coagulation, hepatic dysfunction, or bacterial superinfection [29]. In addition, of those who are initially asymptomatic at birth, approximately 10% develop long-term neurological sequelae such as hearing loss and more rarely, visual impairment and delayed psychomotor development [30, 31].

19.3 Prenatal Diagnosis of Maternal CMV Infection

Maternal infection cannot be established on clinical grounds, as over 95% of pregnant women infected with CMV are asymptomatic [32]. Therefore, serology testing provides the primary tool for diagnosis of primary infection, which can be established when seroconversion occurs, or when a positive CMV-IgM emerges along with a low-avidity CMV-IgG result, indicating recent infection. Seroconversion relates to the detection of CMV-IgG in a previously seronegative woman. However, this approach is mostly irrelevant in the absence of pregestational screening programs allowing the identification of seronegative women [33]. When a baseline serologic testing in unavailable, detection of CMV-IgM may point to a recent maternal infection.

Typically, CMV infection results in an IgM response, followed by an IgG production shortly after. Therefore, serology of isolated CMV-IgM is not often encountered. Rather, a combination of CMV-IgM and CMV-IgG more frequently raises the suspicion for an acute infection. However, only about 50% of CMV-IgM-positive individuals have primary infection [34]; CMV-IgM can persist over a year after infection [35, 36] and may also occur during recurrent infection [37]. Moreover, false-positive results may occur due to cross-reactivity with other viral strains. Therefore, in the presence of positive CMV-IgM, CMV-IgG avidity assay should be used to date the timing of the infection. Antibody avidity indicates the strength with which an antibody binds to an antigen and can be used to distinguish recent primary infection from remote or secondary infection. An avidity index <30% indicates a primary infection of less than 3 months, with sensitivity and specificity of more than 90% [38], while an avidity index> 60% suggests a past or secondary infection. The latter is commonly diagnosed when a significant rise in IgG levels occurs in an already seropositive patient [39].

19.4 Prenatal Diagnosis of Fetal CMV Infection

Once maternal infection has been serologically proven, it is important to determine whether fetal infection occurred in order to provide further surveillance and counseling, accordingly. At present, both invasive and noninvasive modalities can be offered to pregnant women who are at risk for fetal CMV Infection. Ultrasound represents the primary noninvasive tool, enabling the detection of fetal morphologic abnormalities compatible with CMV infection. Practically, since maternal infection is commonly asymptomatic and routine screening is not customary, the first sign leading to the diagnosis of fetal infection could be abnormalities detected during routine ultrasound examination. These include numerous intracranial findings such as ventriculomegaly, microcephaly, increased periventricular echogenicity, calcifications, periventricular pseudocysts, intraventricular synechiae, lenticulostriate vasculopathy (LSV), and cortical migration abnormalities [40] (Figures 19.1 and 19.2). Extracranial sonographic features may also appear, including bowel hyperechogenicity, ascites, oligohydramnios/polyhydramnios, hydrops fetalis, pleural effusion, hepatosplenomegaly, liver calcifications, and fetal growth restriction [41]. Nonetheless, sonographic signs for CMV can be detected in up to 14–38% of infected fetuses [42–45], depending on timing of maternal infection, and can initially appear at the late stages of pregnancy [46]. Moreover, many of the sonographic features associated with fetal CMV infection are not specific and may arise in the context of other intrauterine infections or chromosomal disorders [40]. In view of these limitations, ultrasound should be regarded as an adjunctive rather than the primary tool for the diagnosis of fetal CMV infection.

Compared to ultrasound, isolation of CMV from amniotic fluid requires much higher sensitivity and specificity. Amniocentesis is indicated following detection of primary maternal CMV infection during pregnancy, or when fetal abnormalities suggestive of infection are present [47]. When secondary infection is considered, the risk for fetal transmission is much lower, and consensus regarding the optimal management in absent [29]. Amniotic fluid can be tested either by viral culture or PCR, with the latter being preferred due to a higher sensitivity of 90–100%, depending upon the PCR method used [48]. To minimize false negative results, amniocentesis should be performed after 21 weeks of gestation and at least 7 weeks following maternal infection

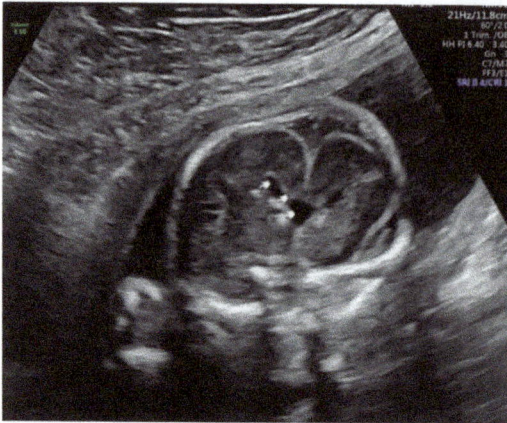

Figure 19.1: Periventricular calcifications at 23 weeks of gestation in a CMV-infected fetus following first-trimester infection.

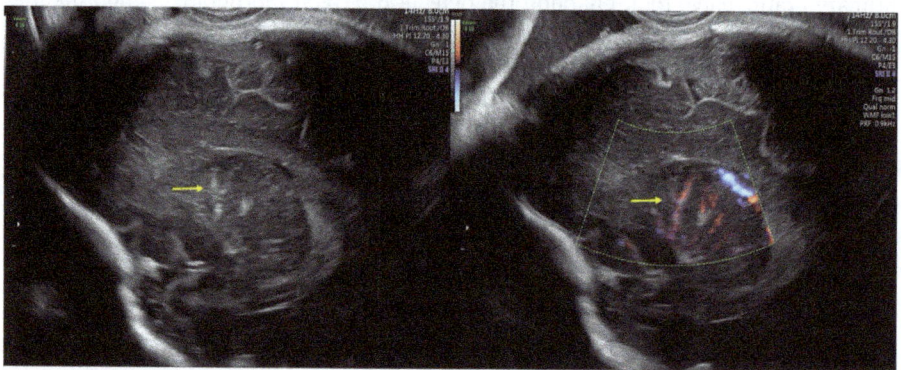

Figure 19.2: Lenticulostriate vasculopathy (LSV) at 37 weeks of gestation in a CMV-infected fetus following first-trimester infection.

[22, 49]. At this time point, fetal urination is well established, and a sufficient amount of the virus is secreted to the amniotic fluid [50, 51]. False-positive results are rare and are mostly explained by contamination of amniotic fluid with maternal blood. Cordocentesis can also provide evidence for fetal infection. However, fetal blood test for both CMV DNA and serology has reduced sensitivities compared to amniotic fluid analysis [52]. Thus, and especially because cordocentesis carries a higher risk compared to amniocentesis, this procedure is not recommended for prenatal diagnosis of fetal infection.

19.5 Prognostic Markers of CMV Disease

Since fetal infection does not necessarily result in clinical sequelae for the infant, identification of prognostic markers could significantly assist in patients' management and counseling. Fetal imaging, DNA counts in amniotic fluid, and fetal blood parameters have all been suggested to have a role in predicting neonatal and long-term outcome. However, limitations of each of these modalities should be acknowledged.

19.5.1 Fetal Imaging

Once fetal infection is diagnosed, serial ultrasound examinations should be done every 3–4 weeks to look for signs that may assist in evaluating the severity of fetal disease. It is generally agreed that demonstration of intracranial anomalies carry an ominous neurodevelopmental prognosis [53]. Specifically, microcephaly at birth was found to predict mental retardation and major motor disability with a specificity of 100% and 92%, respectively [54]. Extracranial sonographic manifestations carry a lower risk for clinical sequela, estimated at a range of 20–60% [20, 44]. It is important to note that symptomatic disease at birth has been described in spite of normal sonographic assessment during pregnancy. Thus, the absence of sonographic anomalies cannot guarantee the absence of symptomatic infection. According to current studies, normal serial targeted US scan performed from the second trimester onward can rule out a clinical sequela with a negative predictive value (NPV) of 72–93% [43, 55, 56]. Fetal MRI can be incorporated into the imaging evaluation. However, when combined with serial sonographic assessment, its added value remains questionable. According to some studies, the contribution of MRI is limited, resulting in a negligible increase in NPV [43, 55], while increasing the chance of detection of findings with no clinical significance [55]. In contrast, other studies found fetal MRI to provide additional valuable information to sonographic evaluation, especially with regard to the presence of intracranial anomalies [57–59]. The role of fetal MRI in evaluation of CMV-infected fetuses still needs to be determined, but should be encouraged to be part of the routine evaluation of pregnancies complicated by fetal CMV infection. Meanwhile, MRI should most definitely be considered when ultrasound is technically limited or to provide equivocal results [43, 55].

19.5.2 DNA Counts in Amniotic Fluid

High CMV viral loads have been associated with a higher risk for symptomatic infection in several studies [60, 61], but not in others [56, 62, 63]. Moreover, much overlapping existed between values of symptomatic and asymptomatic fetuses. This may be attributed to differences in gestational age and time interval between maternal infection and amniocentesis.

19.5.3 Fetal Blood Parameters

Low fetal platelet counts, high CMV-IgM levels, and DNA loads have all been associated with increased risk for adverse fetal outcome [64–67]. In a recent study [56], both platelet counts and viral DNA load in fetal blood have been found to be superior to amniotic fluid DNA load in predicting symptomatic infection at birth. When fetal blood parameters were added to sonographic assessment, the negative predictive value for symptomatic infection improved from 93% to 100%. Whether this data justifies cordocentesis remains to be determined.

19.6 Prevention and Treatment of Intrauterine CMV Infection

During the last 15 years, studies have focused on interventions aiming to prevent transmission of CMV from mother to fetus or to treat fetal infection in case it has already occurred, in order to decrease the risk of long-term sequelae.

19.6.1 Prevention of Transmission

In their prospective non-randomized observational study, Nigro et al. were the first to evaluate CMV hyperimmune globulin (CMV HG) for prevention of mother-to-fetus transmission [68]. Monthly 100 U/Kg CMV HG was found to reduce viral transmission to 16%, compared to 40% in women who did not receive CMV HG. Subsequent retrospective studies reported mixed results; however, these studies lacked comparison groups and relied on transmission rates obtained from previous publications [69, 70]. In a phase II randomized controlled double-blind trial enrolling patients with first/second-trimester maternal infection, participants received either 100 U/kg CMV HG or a placebo, every 4 weeks, until 36 weeks gestation [71]. The rates of fetal infection were 30% (18/61) and 44% (27/62), respectively, a difference which was not statistically significant. The authors noticed six preterm deliveries and two growth-restricted uninfected newborns in the treatment group, versus none in the placebo group, but this observation was not substantiated by further studies [72]. Interestingly, in a recent prospective study, women with first-trimester CMV infection, who were given 200 U/kg CMV HG every 2 weeks, had a transmission rate of 7.5%, which was significantly lower than a rate of 35%, observed in a historic cohort [73]. The authors attributed the lower transmission rate to a shorter time interval between diagnosis of primary infection and first HG administration, increased frequency of HG administration, and doubling of the dose to 200 U/kg. Currently, results of a large phase III randomized placebo-controlled double-blinded trial (NCT01376778) are awaited. Also of interest, is a recent double-blind placebo-controlled study of 90 patients with evidence of primary CMV infection during the periconceptional period and the first trimester, who were randomly assigned to treatment with 8 g/day of valacyclovir or a placebo. Treatment was initiated at the time of serologic detection and continued until amniocentesis. Among the valacyclovir group, 5 (11.1%) had evidence of fetal infection in amniocentesis compared to 14 (29.8%) in the placebo group (p = 0.03), corresponding with an odds ratio of 0.29 (95% CI: 0.09–0.90) for vertical CMV transmission [74]. For now, considering the current lack of demonstrated definitive efficacy, neither CMV HG nor Valacyclovir should be routinely administered with the aim of preventing congenital CMV.

19.6.2 Treatment of Intrauterine Infection

CMV HG was first introduced as a therapeutic agent for fetal infection back in 1999 [75]. Since then, few studies have been performed to evaluate the role of intravenous CMV HG in treating infected fetuses, occasionally with the aid of intra-amniotic, intraperitoneal or intra-umbilical fetal HG administration (Table 19.1). Most of these small, non-randomized studies suggest beneficial effect for HG treatment during pregnancy of CMV-infected fetuses, as demonstrated by lower rates of symptomatic disease as well as higher rates of resolution of CMV-related sonographic findings. However, these studies suffer from methodological concerns and are limited by the small number of CMV HG-treated women. Furthermore, the studies vary considerably from one another with regard to HG dosing, route of administration, treatment duration, and time interval between maternal infection and HG treatment. Thus, antenatal CMV HG treatment for fetal infection cannot be recommended at this stage.

19.6.3 Antiviral Drugs

Antiviral drugs are natural candidates for the treatment of CMV infection. However, their use, especially during pregnancy, is hindered by questionable safety and efficacy. Among the antiviral drugs available, acyclovir and its oral prodrug valacyclovir have the best safety profile [78]. However, data to support the efficacy of these drugs in treating fetal infection are very limited. An observational small study found that 8 g/day valacyclovir reached therapeutic concentration in fetal compartments and reduced viral load in fetal blood [79]. No maternal or fetal adverse effects were reported. In a more recent, open-label, phase II study, 8 g/day valacolvir

Table 19.1: Studies evaluating the role of CMV HG in treating infected fetuses.

Author	N	Design	Primary/secondary infection	Gestational age at maternal infection	Treatment	Outcome measure	Newborn follow-up	Result
Nigro 2005 [68]	45	Prospective	Primary	Median 12; IQR 8–15	200 u/kg every 2–6 weeks, 1–3 doses + 400 u/fkg IU/IA in 9 pts	Resolution of sonographic findings; CMV disease at birth	2 year	14/15 (93%) vs 0/7 (0%); 1/31 (3%) vs 7/14 50% (p < 0.001)
Visentin 2012 [76]	68	Prospective	Primary	<17 weeks	200 u/kg, 1 dose	Resolution of sonographic findings; poor outcome at 1 year	1 year	0/4 vs 0/5; 4/31 (13%) vs 16/37 (41%) (p < 0.01)
Nigro 2012 [77]	16	Prospective	13 primary, 3 secondary infection	12 patients – first trimester	200 u/kg, monthly, 1–3 doses	Resolution of hyperechogenic bowel; infant with sequela	2–8 years	7/9 (78%) vs 3/8 (38%), p = 0.15; 1/9 (11%) vs 8/8 (100%), p < 0.01
Blanquez-gamero 2019 [69]	16	Retrospective, uncontrolled	Primary	≤30 weeks	200 u/kg 1–2 doses	CMV disease at birth; CMV disease at 1 year	1 year	8/16 (50%) 4/15 (26.7%)

was given to 43 pregnant women carrying a moderately symptomatic infected fetus (extracerebral or mild cerebral ultrasound findings). Valacyclovir was well tolerated and increased the proportion of asymptomatic neonates (82%) compared to a historical cohort (43%) [80]. Further studies should be conducted to validate the encouraging results of this preliminary study.

19.7 Prevention of Maternal CMV Infection

In the absence of definite therapeutic interventions, prevention of CMV infection during pregnancy is an important goal. The ultimate prevention strategy would be vaccination of seronegative women of childbearing age, and the development of such a vaccine has already been recognized as a priority public healthcare goal, about 20 years ago [81]. Although there is currently no licensed CMV vaccine, a significant progress toward this goal has been made in clinical trials. Multiple vaccine candidates have been developed during the past decades [82], but their review is beyond the scope of this chapter.

At this time, the only mean available to prevent maternal CMV infection is limiting exposure to the virus. CMV infection occurs through direct contact with infectious biological fluids. Simple hygiene measures such as handwashing and avoidance of intimate contact with urine and salivary secretions of young children, may assist in preventing maternal infection. Such behavioral interventions that are devoid of any risks or costs have been evaluated in several studies, showing effectiveness of up to 85% in preventing primary CMV infection in pregnant patients [10, 83–86].

19.8 Screening for CMV

Routine serologic screening for CMV is very controversial and has not been implemented worldwide. A major argument against screening is that an effective, safe CMV vaccine is not available and cannot be provided for seronegative women who contemplate pregnancy. Moreover, no effective treatment to prevent fetal transmission following maternal infection or to decrease the rate of neurological impairment has been established, to date. In addition, screening programs aim at identifying seronegative patients or seroconversion, but maternal and, consequently, fetal infection can occur in seropositive patients as well. Arguments to support screening include the opportunity to educate seronegative women about behavioral precautions that can prevent infection. Additionally, screening may assist in differentiating between primary and secondary infection, especially if performed before pregnancy.

From an economic standpoint, the cost-effectiveness of a universal CMV screening program depends on the incidence of primary CMV infection during pregnancy and on the effectiveness and cost of preventive and therapeutic measures. In a recent study, universal screening was found cost effective only at a primary CMV incidence higher than 0.89% and behavioral intervention effectiveness higher than 75% [87]. At this moment, routine CMV screening of all pregnant women is not recommended. Serological testing for CMV should be used only in women who develop influenza-like symptoms or in case CMV-related sonographic findings are detected during pregnancy.

19.9 Conclusion

Being the most frequent nongenetic cause of severe malformations in newborns and the leading cause of childhood hearing loss, congenital CMV infection remains a significant concern in pregnant women. Diagnosis of primary maternal infection can be made by serology testing, and if confirmed, should be followed by amniocentesis to evaluate for fetal infection. Fetal imaging, DNA counts in amniotic fluid, and fetal blood parameters may assist in predicting the outcome of the infected fetuses, all to a limited extent. To date, no pharmacological intervention has been proven to prevent or treat congenital infection, although recent data suggest that valacyclovir may decrease the rate of vertical transmission of the virus. Whil these results are awaited, efforts should be taken to educate women of childbearing age about basic hygiene measures for prevention of congenital infection.

References

[1] Bate SL, Dollard SC, Cannon MJ. Cytomegalovirus seroprevalence in the United States: the national health and nutrition examination surveys, 1988–2004. Clin Infect Dis 2010;50(11): 1439–1447.

[2] Cannon MJ, Schmid DS, Hyde TB. Review of cytomegalovirus seroprevalence and demographic characteristics associated with infection. Rev Med Virol 2010;20(4):202–213.

[3] Basha J, Iwasenko JM, Robertson P, Craig ME, Rawlinson WD. Congenital cytomegalovirus infection is associated with high maternal socio-economic status and corresponding low maternal cytomegalovirus seropositivity. J Paediatr Child Health 2014;50(5):368–372.

[4] Mustakangas P, Sarna S, Ammala P, Muttilainen M, Koskela P, Koskiniemi M. Human cytomegalovirus seroprevalence in three socioeconomically different urban areas during the first trimester: a population-based cohort study. Int J Epidemiol 2000;29(3):587–591.

[5] Staras S, Dollard SC, Radford KW, Flanders WD, Pass RF, Cannon MJ. Seroprevalence of cytomegalovirus infection in the United States, 1988–1994. Clin Infect Dis 2006;43(9): 1143–1151.

[6] Pass RF, Hutto C, Lyon MD, Cloud G. Increased rate of cytomegalovirus infection among day care center workers. Pediatr Infect Dis J 1990;9(7):465–470.

[7]   Adler SP. Cytomegalovirus and child day care. Evidence for an increased infection rate among day-care workers. N Engl J Med 1989;321(19):1290–1296.

[8]   Van Zuylen WJ, Hamilton ST, Naing Z, Hall B, Shand A, Rawlinson WD. Congenital cytomegalovirus infection: clinical presentation, epidemiology, diagnosis and prevention. Obstet Med 2014;7(4):140–146.

[9]   Pignatelli S, Dal Monte P, Rossini G, Landini MP. Genetic polymorphisms among human cytomegalovirus (HCMV) wild-type strains. Rev Med Virol 2004;14(6):383–410.

[10] Revello MG, Tibaldi C, Masuelli G et al. Prevention of primary cytomegalovirus infection in pregnancy. EBioMedicine 2015;2(9):1205–1210.

[11] Goderis J, De Leenheer E, Koenraad S, Van Hoecke H, Keymeulen A, Dhooge I. Hearing loss and congenital CMV infection: a systematic review. Pediatrics 2014;134(5):972–982.

[12] Kenneson A, Cannon MJ. Review and meta-analysis of the epidemiology of congenital cytomegalovirus (CMV) infection. Rev Med Virol 2007;17(4):253 276.

[13] Lanzieri TM, Dollard SC, Bialek SR, Grosse SD. Systematic review of the birth prevalence of congenital cytomegalovirus infection in developing countries. Int J Infect Dis 2014;22:44–48.

[14] Stagno S, Pass RF, Cloud GC et al. Primary cytomegalovirus infection in pregnancy. Incidence, transmission to fetus, and clinical outcome. JAMA 1986;256(14):1904–1908.

[15] Wang C, Zhang X, Bialek S, Cannon MJ. Attribution of congenital cytomegalovirus infection to primary versus non-primary maternal infection. Clin Infect Dis 2011;52(2):e11–3.

[16] Nigro G. Maternal-fetal cytomegalovirus infection: from diagnosis to therapy. J Matern Fetal Neonatal Med 2009;22(2):169–174.

[17] Revello MG, Fabbri E, Furione M et al. Role of prenatal diagnosis and counseling in the management of 735 pregnancies complicated by primary human cytomegalovirus infection: a 20-year experience. J Clin Virol 2011;50(4):303–307.

[18] Bodeus M, Kabamba-Mukadi B, Zech F, Hubinot C, Bernard P, Goubau P. Human cytomegalovirus in utero transmission: follow-up of 524 maternal seroconversions. J Clin Virol 2010;47(2):201–202.

[19] Pass RF, Fowler KB, Boppana SB, Britt WJ, Stagno S. Congenital cytomegalovirus infection following first trimester maternal infection: symptoms at birth and outcome. J Clin Virol 2006;35(2):216–220.

[20] Picone O, Vauloup-Fellous C, Cordier AG et al. A series of 238 cytomegalovirus primary infections during pregnancy: description and outcome. Prenat Diagn 2013;33(8):751–758.

[21] Feldman B, Yinon Y, Tepperberg Oikawa M, Yoeli R, Schiff E, Lipitz S. Pregestational, periconceptional, and gestational primary maternal cytomegalovirus infection: prenatal diagnosis in 508 pregnancies. Am J Obstet Gynecol 2011;205(4):342 e1–6.

[22] Liesnard C, Donner C, Brancart F, Gosselin F, Delforge ML, Rodesch F. Prenatal diagnosis of congenital cytomegalovirus infection: prospective study of 237 pregnancies at risk. Obstet Gynecol 2000;95(6 Pt 1):881–888.

[23] Gindes L, Teperberg-Oikawa M, Sherman D, Pardo J, Rahav G. Congenital cytomegalovirus infection following primary maternal infection in the third trimester. BJOG 2008;115(7): 830–835.

[24] Lorenzoni F, Lunardi S, Liumbruno GF et al. Neonatal screening for congenital cytomegalovirus infection in preterm and small for gestational age infants. J Matern Fetal Neonatal Med 2014;27(15):1589–1593.

[25] Pereira L, Petitt M, Fong A et al. Intrauterine growth restriction caused by underlying congenital cytomegalovirus infection. J Infect Dis 2014;209(10):1573–1584.

[26] Xie F, Hu Y, Magee LA et al. An association between cytomegalovirus infection and pre-eclampsia: a case-control study and data synthesis. Acta Obstet Gynecol Scand 2010;89(9): 1162–1167.

[27] Iwasenko JM, Howard J, Arbuckle S et al. Human cytomegalovirus infection is detected frequently in stillbirths and is associated with fetal thrombotic vasculopathy. J Infect Dis 2011;203(11):1526–1533.

[28] McMullan BJ, Palasanthiran P, Jones CA et al. Congenital cytomegalovirus–time to diagnosis, management and clinical sequelae in Australia: opportunities for earlier identification. Med J Aust 2011;194(12):625–629.

[29] Yinon Y, Farine D, Yudin MH. No. 240-Cytomegalovirus Infection in Pregnancy. J Obstet Gynaecol Can 2018;40(2):e134–e141.

[30] Boppana SB, Pass RF, Britt WJ, Stagno S, Alford CA. Symptomatic congenital cytomegalovirus infection: neonatal morbidity and mortality. Pediatr Infect Dis J 1992;11(2):93–99.

[31] Dollard SC, Grosse SD, Ross DS. New estimates of the prevalence of neurological and sensory sequelae and mortality associated with congenital cytomegalovirus infection. Rev Med Virol 2007;17(5):355–363.

[32] Lazzarotto T, Guerra B, Lanari M, Gabriella L, Landini MP. New advances in the diagnosis of congenital cytomegalovirus infection. J Clin Virol 2008;41(3):192–197.

[33] Revello MG, Gerna G. Diagnosis and management of human cytomegalovirus infection in the mother, fetus, and newborn infant. Clin Microbiol Rev 2002;15(4):680–715.

[34] Prince HE, Lape-Nixon M. Role of cytomegalovirus (CMV) IgG avidity testing in diagnosing primary CMV infection during pregnancy. Clin Vaccine Immunol 2014;21(10):1377–1384.

[35] Grazia Revello M, Percivalle E, Zannino M, Rossi V, Gerna G. Development and evaluation of a capture ELISA for IgM antibody to the human cytomegalovirus major DNA binding protein. J Virol Methods 1991;35(3):315–329.

[36] Stagno S, Tinker MK, Elrod C, Fucillo DA, Cloud G, O'Beirne AJ. Immunoglobulin M antibodies detected by enzyme-linked immunosorbent assay and radioimmunoassay in the diagnosis of cytomegalovirus infections in pregnant women and newborn infants. J Clin Microbiol 1985;21 (6):930–935.

[37] Griffiths PD, Stagno S, Pass RF, Smith RJ, Alford CA. Infection with cytomegalovirus during pregnancy: specific IgM antibodies as a marker of recent primary infection. J Infect Dis 1982;145(5):647–653.

[38] Kilby MD, Ville Y, Acharya G. Screening for cytomegalovirus infection in pregnancy. BMJ 2019;367:l6507.

[39] Yinon Y, Yagel S, Tepperberg-Oikawa M, Feldman B, Schiff E, Lipitz S. Prenatal diagnosis and outcome of congenital cytomegalovirus infection in twin pregnancies. BJOG 2006;113(3): 295–300.

[40] Malinger G, Lev D, Lerman-Sagie T. Imaging of fetal cytomegalovirus infection. Fetal Diagn Ther 2011;29(2):117–126.

[41] Masini G, Maggio L, Marchi L et al. Isolated fetal echogenic bowel in a retrospective cohort: the role of infection screening. Eur J Obstet Gynecol Reprod Biol 2018;231:136–141.

[42] Lipitz S, Achiron R, Zalel Y, Mendelson E, Tepperberg M, Gamzu R. Outcome of pregnancies with vertical transmission of primary cytomegalovirus infection. Obstet Gynecol 2002;100(3): 428–433.

[43] Lipitz S, Yinon Y, Malinger G et al. Risk of cytomegalovirus-associated sequelae in relation to time of infection and findings on prenatal imaging. Ultrasound Obstet Gynecol 2013;41(5): 508–514.

[44] Guerra B, Simonazzi G, Puccetti C et al. Ultrasound prediction of symptomatic congenital cytomegalovirus infection. Am J Obstet Gynecol 2008;198(4):380 e1–7.

[45] Leyder M, Vorsselmans A, Done E et al. Primary maternal cytomegalovirus infections: accuracy of fetal ultrasound for predicting sequelae in offspring. Am J Obstet Gynecol 2016;215(5):638 e1–638 e8.

[46] Malinger G, Lev D, Zahalka N et al. Fetal cytomegalovirus infection of the brain: the spectrum of sonographic findings. AJNR Am J Neuroradiol 2003;24(1):28–32.

[47] Society For Maternal-fetal M, Hughes BL, Gyamfi-Bannerman C. Diagnosis and antenatal management of congenital cytomegalovirus infection. Am J Obstet Gynecol 2016;214(6): B5–B11.

[48] Saldan A, Forner G, Mengoli C, Gussetti N, Palu G, Abate D. Testing for cytomegalovirus in pregnancy. J Clin Microbiol 2017;55(3):693–702.

[49] Lipitz S, Yagel S, Shalev E, Achiron R, Mashiach S, Schiff E. Prenatal diagnosis of fetal primary cytomegalovirus infection. Obstet Gynecol 1997;89(5 Pt 1):763–767.

[50] Revello MG, Gerna G. Pathogenesis and prenatal diagnosis of human cytomegalovirus infection. J Clin Virol 2004;29(2):71–83.

[51] Nigro G, Mazzacco M, Anceschi MM, La Torre R, Antonelli G, Cosmi EV. Prenatal diagnosis of fetal cytomegalovirus infection after primary or recurrent maternal infection. Obstet Gynecol 1999;94(6):909–914.

[52] Lazzarotto T, Guerra B, Gabrielli L, Lanari M, Landini MP. Update on the prevention, diagnosis and management of cytomegalovirus infection during pregnancy. Clin Microbiol Infect 2011;17(9):1285–1293.

[53] Ancora G, Lanari M, Lazzarotto T et al. Cranial ultrasound scanning and prediction of outcome in newborns with congenital cytomegalovirus infection. J Pediatr 2007;150(2):157–161.

[54] Noyola DE, Demmler GJ, Nelson CT et al. Early predictors of neurodevelopmental outcome in symptomatic congenital cytomegalovirus infection. J Pediatr 2001;138(3):325–331.

[55] Birnbaum R, Ben-Sira L, Lerman-Sagie T, Malinger G. The use of fetal neurosonography and brain MRI in cases of cytomegalovirus infection during pregnancy: a retrospective analysis with outcome correlation. Prenat Diagn 2017;37(13):1335–1342.

[56] Leruez-Ville M, Stirnemann J, Sellier Y et al. Feasibility of predicting the outcome of fetal infection with cytomegalovirus at the time of prenatal diagnosis. Am J Obstet Gynecol 2016;215(3):342 e1–9.

[57] Averill LW, Kandula V, Akyol Y, Epelman M. Fetal brain magnetic resonance imaging findings in congenital cytomegalovirus infection with postnatal imaging correlation. Semin Ultrasound CT MR 2015;36(6):476–486.

[58] Doneda C, Parazzini C, Righini A et al. Early cerebral lesions in cytomegalovirus infection: prenatal MR imaging. Radiology 2010;255(2):613–621.

[59] Picone O, Simon I, Benachi A, Brunelle F, Sonigo P. Comparison between ultrasound and magnetic resonance imaging in assessment of fetal cytomegalovirus infection. Prenat Diagn 2008;28(8):753–758.

[60] Lazzarotto T, Varani S, Guerra B, Nicolosi A, Lanari M, L. Prenatal indicators of congenital cytomegalovirus infection. J Pediatr 2000;137(1):90–95.

[61] Guerra B, Lazzarotto T, Quarta S et al. Prenatal diagnosis of symptomatic congenital cytomegalovirus infection. Am J Obstet Gynecol 2000;183(2):476–482.

[62] Goegebuer T, Van Meensel B, Beuselinck K et al. Clinical predictive value of real-time PCR quantification of human cytomegalovirus DNA in amniotic fluid samples. J Clin Microbiol 2009;47(3):660–665.

[63] Picone O, Costa JM, Leruez-Ville M, Ernault P, Olivi M, Ville Y. Cytomegalovirus (CMV) glycoprotein B genotype and CMV DNA load in the amniotic fluid of infected fetuses. Prenat Diagn 2004;24(12):1001–1006.

[64] Fabbri E, Revello MG, Furione M et al. Prognostic markers of symptomatic congenital human cytomegalovirus infection in fetal blood. BJOG 2011;118(4):448–456.

[65] Benoist G, Salomon LJ, Jacquemard F, Daffos F, Ville Y. The prognostic value of ultrasound abnormalities and biological parameters in blood of fetuses infected with cytomegalovirus. BJOG 2008;115(7):823–829.

[66] Enders G, Bader U, Lindemann L, Schalasta G, Daiminger A. Prenatal diagnosis of congenital cytomegalovirus infection in 189 pregnancies with known outcome. Prenat Diagn 2001;21(5): 362–377.

[67] Revello MG, Zavattoni M, Baldanti F, Sarrasini A, Paolucci S, Gerna G. Diagnostic and prognostic value of human cytomegalovirus load and IgM antibody in blood of congenitally infected newborns. J Clin Virol 1999;14(1):57–66.

[68] Nigro G, Adler SP, La Torre R, Best AM et al. Passive immunization during pregnancy for congenital cytomegalovirus infection. N Engl J Med 2005;353(13):1350–1362.

[69] Blazquez-Gamero D, Izquierdo AG, Del Rosal T et al. Prevention and treatment of fetal cytomegalovirus infection with cytomegalovirus hyperimmune globulin: a multicenter study in Madrid. J Matern Fetal Neonatal Med 2019;32(4):617–625.

[70] Buxmann H, Stackelberg OM, Schlober RL et al. Use of cytomegalovirus hyperimmunoglobulin for prevention of congenital cytomegalovirus disease: a retrospective analysis. J Perinat Med 2012;40(4):439–446.

[71] Revello MG, Lazzarotto T, Guerra B et al. A randomized trial of hyperimmune globulin to prevent congenital cytomegalovirus. N Engl J Med 2014;370(14):1316–1326.

[72] Nigro G, Capretti I, Manganello AM, Best AM, Adler SP. Primary maternal cytomegalovirus infections during pregnancy: association of CMV hyperimmune globulin with gestational age at birth and birth weight. J Matern Fetal Neonatal Med 2015,28(2):168–171.

[73] Kagan KO, Enders M, Schampera MS et al. Prevention of maternal-fetal transmission of cytomegalovirus after primary maternal infection in the first trimester by biweekly hyperimmunoglobulin administration. Ultrasound Obstet Gynecol 2019;53(3):383–389.

[74] Shahar-Nissan K et al. Valacyclovir to prevent vertical transmission of cytomegalovirus after maternal primary infection during pregnancy: a randomised, double-blind, placebo-controlled trial. Lancet 2020;396(10253):779–785.

[75] Nigro G, La Torre R, Anceschi MM, Mazzocco M, Cosmi E. Hyperimmunoglobulin therapy for a twin fetus with cytomegalovirus infection and growth restriction. Am J Obstet Gynecol 1999;180(5):1222–1226.

[76] Visentin S, Manara R, Milanese L et al. Early primary cytomegalovirus infection in pregnancy: maternal hyperimmunoglobulin therapy improves outcomes among infants at 1 year of age. Clin Infect Dis 2012;55(4):497–503.

[77] Nigro G, Adler SP, Gatta E, Mascaretti G et al. Fetal hyperechogenic bowel may indicate congenital cytomegalovirus disease responsive to immunoglobulin therapy. J Matern Fetal Neonatal Med 2012;25(11):2202–2205.

[78] Leruez-Ville M, Ville Y. Fetal cytomegalovirus infection. Best Pract Res Clin Obstet Gynaecol 2017;38:97–107.

[79] Jacquemard F, Yamamoto M, Costa JM et al. Maternal administration of valacyclovir in symptomatic intrauterine cytomegalovirus infection. BJOG 2007;114(9):1113–1121.

[80] Leruez-Ville M, Ghout I, Bussieres L et al. In utero treatment of congenital cytomegalovirus infection with valacyclovir in a multicenter, open-label, phase II study. Am J Obstet Gynecol 2016;215(4):462 e1–462 e10.

[81] Anderholm KM, Bierle CJ, Schleiss MR. Cytomegalovirus vaccines: current status and future prospects. Drugs 2016;76(17):1625–1645.

[82] Xia L, Su R, An Z, Fu TM, Luo W. Human cytomegalovirus vaccine development: immune responses to look into vaccine strategy. Hum Vaccin Immunother 2018;14(2):292–303.

[83] Reichman O, Miskin I, Sharoni L et al. Preconception screening for cytomegalovirus: an effective preventive approach. Biomed Res Int 2014;2014:135416.

[84] Vauloup-Fellous C, Picone O, Cordier AG et al. Does hygiene counseling have an impact on the rate of CMV primary infection during pregnancy? Results of a 3-year prospective study in a French hospital. J Clin Virol 2009;46(Suppl 4):S49–53.

[85] Picone O, Vauloup-Fellous C, Cordier AG et al. A 2-year study on cytomegalovirus infection during pregnancy in a French hospital. BJOG 2009;116(6):818–823.

[86] Adler SP, Finney JW, Manganello AM, Best AM. Prevention of child-to-mother transmission of cytomegalovirus among pregnant women. J Pediatr 2004;145(4):485–491.

[87] Albright CM, Werner EF, Hughes BL. Cytomegalovirus screening in pregnancy: a cost-effectiveness and threshold analysis. Am J Perinatol 2019;36(7):678–687.

Valentine Faure Bardon, Yves Ville
20 Fetal Toxoplasmosis

20.1 Introduction

Congenital toxoplasmosis (CT) results from fetal infection with the protozoa *Toxoplasma gondii*. There are several strains of this parasite, with different geographic predispositions, and there seems to be a good correlation between the type of strain and the severity of CT, explaining the differences in outcomes of infected children between countries [1, 2]. The WHO has reported a global annual incidence of CT of 190,100 cases and has highlighted that CT poses a substantial burden of poor health, globally [3].

20.2 Maternal Infection

Maternal infection is acquired by ingestion of viable tissue cysts in meat or oocysts excreted by cats that contaminate the environment [4].

In recent decades, there has been a drop in seroprevalence in many countries. In the population of French pregnant women, it decreased from 54% in 1995 to 37% in 2010 [5]. The same decrease was observed among women of childbearing age in the United States, where the last estimate of seroprevalence was 9.1% [6]. Almost all fetal infections are related to primary maternal infection with *Toxoplasma gondii*, but it should be kept in mind that in pregnant women with immunosuppression caused by AIDS or immunosuppressive therapies, a reactivation of a preexisting latent toxoplasma infection could occur and lead to CT [7, 8]. In France, the rate of seroconversion during pregnancy was between 0.2% and 0.25%, in 2015 [9]. Toxoplasmosis infection in immunocompetent pregnant women is generally subclinical (lymphadenopathy, fever, fatigue, malaise) or unapparent [10].

Maternal risk factors for acute toxoplasmosis in pregnancy have been identified, and they are divided into three areas: cat hygiene, food hygiene, and personal hygiene. In the European Research Network on CT, consumption of inadequately cooked or raw meat was the main risk factor for infection with toxoplasma [4].

Centers for Disease Control and Prevention have published eight specific recommendations for prevention where pregnant women, health-care providers, and governments all have a role to play in reducing the risk of primary maternal infection [10]. To go further in primary prevention, the Society of Obstetricians and Gynecologists of Canada (SOGC) has recommended advising a nonpregnant woman, who has been diagnosed with an acute Toxoplasma gondii infection, to wait at least 6 months before attempting to become pregnant [11]. However, surprisingly, when looking at

https://doi.org/10.1515/9783110615258-020

the only two randomized trials that specifically studied the impact of health education approaches, no significant difference in seroconversion rates and no change in food hygiene and personal hygiene behavior were found [12, 13].

Only a few countries around the world have decided to offer routine screening for toxoplasmosis during pregnancy. The two countries most involved are France and Austria, which have been providing serological screening to pregnant women since the 1970s [14, 15]. However, some differences remain in the sequential serological follow-up which is, respectively, in these countries monthly and 3-monthly. In both, these screening programs have been associated with a decline in the incidence of congenital infection, as well as a decline in fetal and child injuries [16, 17]. In countries where routine universal screening during pregnancy is not recommended, such as Canada [11], the arguments put forward are the low incidence of the disease, the price of such screening, and the lack of evidence regarding the effectiveness of antenatal treatment. In both France and Austria, recent publications have suggested that prenatal screening for prevention was cost-saving and led to maintain their current policies [15, 16].

Maternal primary infection is detected by the appearance of specific G immunoglobulins (IgG) in a previously seronegative patient or by marked elevation of specific IgG in the presence of specific immunoglobulin M (IgM). The difficulty rests in the interpretation of positive IgM. Indeed, IgM may persist for years following acute infection and so, when isolated, positive IgM should not be considered as an absolute evidence of recent toxoplasmosis [18]. Algorithms of interpretation, using different assays to measure immunoglobulin titers, IgG avidity, and sequential serological testing should be used to date maternal infection within expert laboratories [15].

20.3 Fetal Infection

The fetus is infected with *Toxoplasma gondii* by vertical transmission via its mother.

Transmission from mother to child is by transplacental passage of the parasite, and the rate increases significantly with gestational age at seroconversion (odds ratio [OR], 1.17 for each additional week higher; 95% CI, 1.08–1.27) [19]. In one meta-analysis, the rate of mother-to-child transmission by gestational age at seroconversion was 15%, 44%, and 71% at 13, 26, and 36 weeks, respectively [20]. In case of maternal seroconversion in the first weeks of pregnancy, the rate appears to be <5% [21, 22].

The diagnosis of CT can be suspected either in the presence of a biologically identified maternal seroconversion or in the presence of ultrasound features suggestive of CT visualized during screening ultrasounds. The diagnosis is confirmed by amniocentesis, performed at least 4 weeks after maternal seroconversion for better sensitivity, and not before 18 weeks with detection of *Toxoplasma gondii* by positive PCR on amniotic fluid [9, 11].

Several PCR kits exist depending on the laboratory, and the interpretation of the results must be done in the light of their performance and limitations. Most published data were obtained in conventional PCR assays, frequently based on targeting the B1 gene, and this routine PCR analysis showed a sensitivity and specificity of 87.2% and 99.7%, respectively [23]. More recently, new techniques have been developed to increase the performances of PCR tests through real-time amplification method [24]. Indeed, using the 529 base-pairs (bp), PCR assay improved the sensitivity up to 100.0% [25]. Whichever PCR technique is used, a negative PCR cannot completely exclude a congenital infection, particularly because transmission can be delayed [19, 26].

The antenatal clinical manifestations are variable. The infected fetus can be asymptomatic, suffers multi-system damage including damage to the brain, and can sometimes be so severely affected that in utero fetal death occurs [27]. Most often, the fetus is asymptomatic at birth, but a risk of long-term sequelae persists, particularly, neurodevelopmental impairment and visual disorder (chorioretinitis).

In France, since 2007, between 200 and 300 cases of CT have been notified each year to the National Reference Center, that is, an overall prevalence estimated at around 3 to 4 cases per 10,000 live births (prevalence of severe forms: 0, 1 in 10,000), causing symptomatic forms at birth in 10% of the cases (including a quarter of severe forms) and more than 10% leading to medical terminations of pregnancy [9].

20.4 Prognostic Markers of Fetal Infection

20.4.1 Timing of Maternal Primary Infection (MPI)

Gestational age at maternal seroconversion is the major prognostic factor in cases of CT concerning the risk of morphological abnormalities visible on ultrasound and concerning the overall risk of sequelae.

First, the number of fetuses showing morphological abnormalities on ultrasound scans is higher in cases of early fetal infection during pregnancy with a rate as high as 78% in case of maternal infection in the first trimester [28].

Second, the risk of developing clinical signs before the age of 3 years falls from an estimated 61% risk when MPI occurred at 13 weeks to 25% and 9% when seroconversion occurred at 26 and 36 weeks, respectively [29]. However, the Systematic Review on Congenital Toxoplasmosis (SYROCOT) group reported that gestational age at seroconversion was indeed strongly associated with a decreased risk of intracranial lesions, but not with eye lesions [20]. Moreover, early maternal toxoplasmosis may cause severe fetoplacental infections that generally lead to a spontaneous abortion.

20.4.2 Findings on Imaging

As previously stated, CT is most often asymptomatic during antenatal period but, in some cases, this multisystemic disease may lead to fetal symptoms resulting in brain and noncerebral lesions. The ultrasound images of fetal brain damage most commonly found are ventriculomegaly, echogenic nodular foci in multiple brain areas, diffuse periventricular echogenicity, and abnormal echogenicity and thickening of the germinal matrix below the frontal horns. Ventricular dilatation is the most common sign and is classically bilateral, symmetrical with a rapid evolution over a period of few days. It has been reported that cerebral anomalies were usually detected after a long period of time between the onset of fetal infection and the appearance of the first brain anomalies [26, 30].

Extracerebral ultrasound abnormalities which can be detected are: hepatosplenomegaly, liver echogenicities, ascites (generally moderate), hydrops, and an increased thickness of the placenta. Intrauterine growth restriction (IUGR) is rarely reported.

20.5 Prognostic Value of Imaging Findings

20.5.1 Neurodevelopmental

In a recent French cohort, 1.5% of women (10/676), decided to terminate the pregnancy because of severe fetal hydrocephaly suspected of initiating neurological prognosis. Otherwise, in this cohort, prospective ultrasound screening showed only minor abnormalities in 5% (6/112) of the fetuses. Those six children had long-term follow-up (23–238 months), and all of them had normal psychomotor development, except for 2:1 had a slight language delay and the other had a second developed epilepsy [22].

When looking at prenatal cohorts, ventriculomegaly associated with multiple echo-dense nodules seems to be characteristic of severe fetal toxoplasmosis and carries a poor prognosis with a high risk of developmental delay, seizures, and blindness [31]. Histological analyses show that this hydrocephaly seen on ultrasound was the result of necrotizing lesions of the Sylvius duct [28].

In case of strictly isolated prenatal echogenic nodular foci of the brain, neurodevelopmental prognosis is debated. For some authors, it was favorable in the living population of children [30], but in studies looking at postmortem examinations of terminated cases, these lesions corresponded to limited areas of cerebral necrosis [28].

The major limitations of those prenatal studies were the small sample size and short follow-up.

In case of normal antenatal ultrasound follow-up, the risk of neurological disorder is almost nil, even in the high-risk population of fetuses infected in the first trimester [22, 32].

20.5.2 Chorioretinitis

In case of CT, an overall 26% (28/107) risk of chorioretinitis was reported in a population of infected children who were treated prenatally. In those infected children, 10% (3/28) had prenatal ultrasound features described as mild (ventricular dilatation <12 mm, mild ascites, IUGR). Visual impairment was infrequently severe, as chorioretinitis was peripheral with normal visual acuity in 82% [22]. For congenitally infected children, a long-term follow-up is recommended to monitor ocular prognosis, since only 39% of cases of chorioretinitis are diagnosed at birth; 85% and 96% are diagnosed before 5 and 10 years, respectively [22].

Prenatally, the risk of ocular damage is difficult to assess. Ocular damages were found in living children who had presented strictly isolated echoic parenchymal cerebral nodules on prenatal ultrasound follow-up [30]. Normal ultrasound monitoring throughout pregnancy also does not protect against the risk of chorioretinitis [32].

20.5.3 Contribution of Fetal Head MRI

Very few studies have evaluated the contribution of fetal brain MRI in case of CT, and they all concluded that MRI did not contribute any additional information, compared to ultrasound exams [28, 29].

20.6 Prenatal Treatment

The interest of setting up an antenatal treatment in congenital toxoplasma infection is still very controversial. In the teams that favor setting up antenatal treatment, two indications were retained. On the one hand, it can be established with the aim of reducing the risk of mother-to-child transmission in the event of biologically proven maternal primary infection. On the other hand, it can be established in order to reduce the risk of complications, especially once the diagnosis of fetal infection is made (positive PCR in amniotic fluid). Even within these same teams, there are different treatment protocols. In France, spiramycin is introduced from the diagnosis of maternal primary infection and is either changed to pyrimethamine-sulfadiazine in case of positive amniocentesis or left in case of negativity; in both cases, the treatments are continued throughout the pregnancy until term. In Austria, women are initially treated with pyrimethamine-sulfamide (PS) that is changed to spiramycin, in case of negative amniocentesis.

20.6.1 Drugs

For the use of PS, two different regimens are being used: the molecules are given separately or as a combination therapy [15]. In both cases, supplementation with folinic acid is required, as pyrimethamine is a dihydrofolate reductase inhibitor. The combination of PS seems to be well tolerated in neonates and fetuses, if used after 14 weeks of gestation, with a few exceptions [19, 33–35]. In women, good tolerance has also been reported, in general, but checking blood cell counts is still mandatory during pregnancy because of the risk of bone marrow toxicity [15, 19, 36].

Spiramycin is given as 3 million units (1 g), 3× per day. The drug accumulates in the placenta but does not cross it, that is, spiramycin is not effective on established CT. Maternal tolerance is good. Some minor maternal gastrointestinal intolerance may occur, but taking the medication during meal reduces this adverse effect.

The role of other anti-Toxoplasma therapies (atovaquone, pyrimethamine-clindamycin, pyrimethamine-azithromycin, etc.) in pregnancy is not established, and these should not be used [37].

20.6.2 Prevention of Mother-to-Fetus Transmission

In a large prospective cohort of European centers offering prenatal screening for toxoplasmosis, the authors were unable to demonstrate a beneficial effect of the timing or type of prenatal treatment on the risk of vertical transmission. In this cohort, of 1,208 women analyzed, 72% were first given spiramycin, 19% PS, and 9% (mostly infected during the last trimester) were untreated [38]. More recently, the SYROCOT study group, in a review of 26 cohorts with 1,438 treated women identified by prenatal screening, found weak evidence that treatment started within 3 weeks of seroconversion reduced mother-to-child transmission, compared with treatment started after 8 or more weeks ($p = 0.05$). The group also noticed that the type of prenatal treatment did not seem to have a significant effect, but drug regimens differed according to gestational age [20].

When taking into account gestational age, a recent German study reported that the rate of vertical transmission was lower than expected (4.8%) when using Spiramycin from the time of diagnosis of acute acquisition of infection by the pregnant woman until week 16, followed by PS and folinic acid for at least 4 weeks. However, there was no control group [36].

Only one randomized study has been conducted to date to compare the efficacy and tolerance of PS vs. Spiramycin in reducing placental transmission. The transmission rate was twofold lower when using PS vs. Spiramycin, but the difference did not reach statistical significance, probably for lack of statistical power [19].

To conclude, none of these studies reported a significant effect of treatment on mother-to-child transmission, but none could exclude clinically significant effects.

20.6.3 Antiparasitic Therapy to Reduce Fetal Complications

In the SYROCOT study group review, in 550 infected live-born infants identified by prenatal or neonatal screening, they found no evidence that prenatal treatment significantly reduced the risk of clinical manifestations [20]. However, severe cases and fetal demises were excluded from analysis.

In contrast, and more recently, the European Multicenter Study on Congenital Toxoplasmosis (EMSCOT) found that prenatal treatment reduced the risk of serious neurological sequelae (SNSD) by three-quarters in infected fetuses (OR: 0.24). The limitations of the study were the small number of SNSD cases and uncertainty about the timing of maternal seroconversion. In a retrospective French study conducted on 300 infants with congenital toxoplasmosis, a delay of > 8 weeks between maternal infection and treatment initiation increased the risk for retinochoroiditis in congenitally infected children during the first two years of life [39]. With the German treatment scheme, the rate of clinical manifestations in newborns (1.6%) was also lower than expected in natural history [36].

In the only randomized, controlled trial, the incidence of prenatal cerebral signs of toxoplasmosis following prophylactic therapy was significantly lower in the PS than in the spiramycin group. Indeed, all of the cerebral signs appeared in the spiramycin group, suggesting that starting PS very early may be beneficial for fetuses with congenital toxoplasmosis. Since then, a French multidisciplinary working group has published guidelines on the prenatal management of CT [15] in 2019.

20.7 Neonates Born to women with Toxoplasmosis Infection

In the event of proven maternal seroconversion, the newborn should undergo a standardized evaluation including a complete clinical examination, a fundoscopic eye examination, and a cranial ultrasound cerebral imaging (evaluation of cerebral ventricles and search for intracranial calcifications).

In case of negative amniocentesis or when prenatal diagnosis was not performed, a test for specific IgM and IgA in neonates and a comparative mother–infant Western blot should be done. PCR for parasite detection can also be performed on the placenta, cord blood, or in amniotic fluid on delivery. Serological follow-up should be performed at 1 month and every 2 months thereafter, showing a decreasing antibody titer, until complete disappearance of anti-toxoplasma IgG (of maternal origin), confirming the absence of CT. If the diagnosis of CT is proven by serological evolution (synthesis of IgG, IgM and/or IgA), a treatment and surveillance should be initiated [15].

In case of positive antenatal and/or neonatal testing, treatment for 12 months should be started, as soon as possible [15].

These infected neonates/children must then benefit from close clinical and ophthalmic monitoring. The duration of this follow-up remains debated [22].

20.8 Comparison of Various Approaches

Figures 20.1–20.3 depict various approaches to the evaluation and management of congenital toxoplasmosis.

*Prenatal treatment given is as follows:
- Spiramycin = 1 g 3×/day
- PS combinations:

1) Pyrimethamine: 50 mg/day + sulfadiazine 2× 1,500/day + folinic acid 2× 25 mg/week
2) Or fansidar® (sulfadoxine 500 mg/pyrimethamine 25 mg) 2×/week + folinic acid 2× 25 mg/week
** Amniocentesis: performed before 18 weeks of gestation not less than 4 weeks after the estimated date of maternal infection.
*** The indication and duration of therapy may be discussed in case of asymptomatic toxoplasmosis, but the treatment is imperative in the presence of neurological and ophthalmological signs.
**** The duration of the follow-up is subject to discussion.

ASAP, as soon as possible; PS, pyrimethamine–sulfamide; BCC, blood cell count; US, ultrasound examination; PCR, polymerase chain reaction; Ig, immunoglobulin; CT, congenital toxoplasmosis; kg, kilogram; mg, milligram; D, day.

*Prenatal treatment is given as follows:
- Spiramycin = 1 g 3×/day
- PS combination: combination of pyrimethamine (day 1: 50 mg; thereafter: 25 mg/day) + sulfadiazine (<80 kg body weight: 3 g/day; ≥80 kg body weight: 4 g/day) + folinic acid (10–15 mg/week)

ASAP, as soon as possible; PS, pyrimethamine–sulfamide; PCR, polymerase chain reaction; Ig, immunoglobulin; CT, congenital toxoplasmosis; kg, kilogram; mg, milligram; D, day.

*Prenatal treatment is given as follows:
- Spiramycin = 2.3 g per day in 3 dosages
- PS combination: pyrimethamine (50 mg first dose, then 25 mg daily) in combination with sulfadiazine (1.5 g first dose, then 0.75 g daily) and folinic acid (15 mg 3× a week)

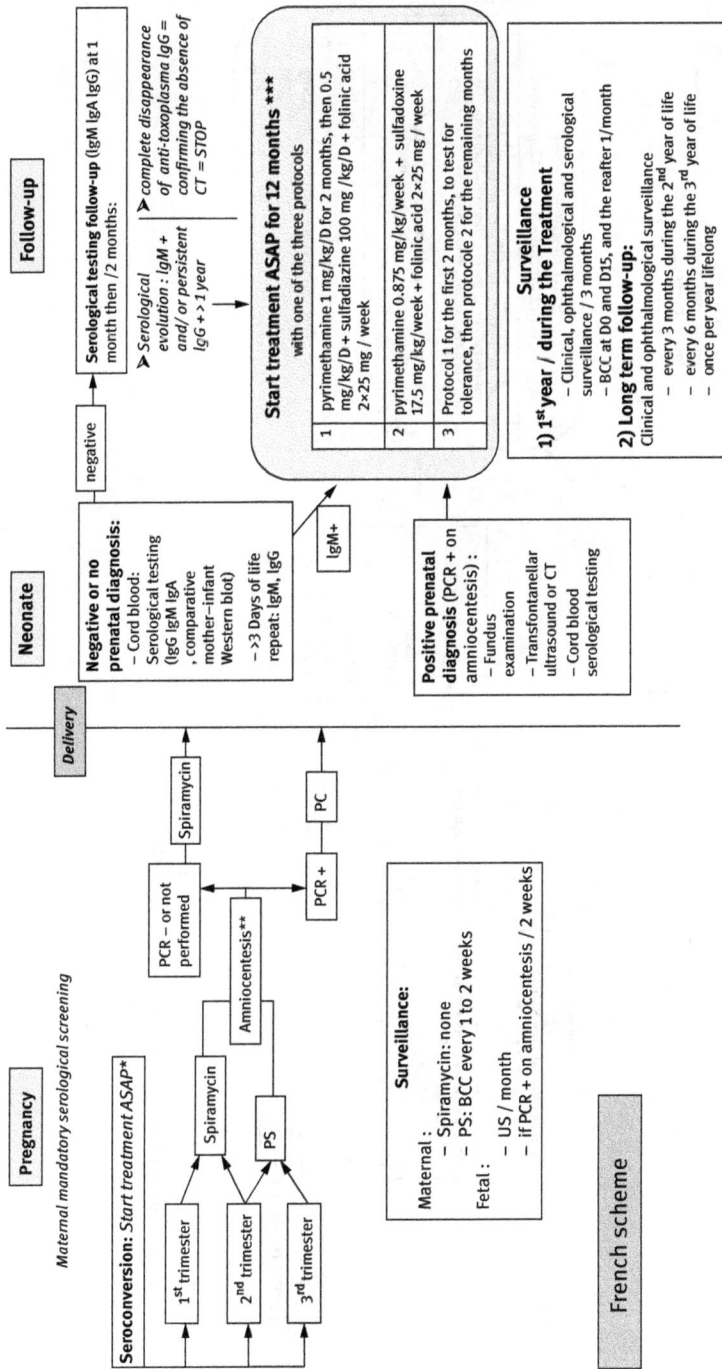

Figure 20.1: French scheme: prenatal and postnatal treatment[15]. ASAP, as soon as possible; PS, pyrimethamine–sulfamide; BCC, blood cell count; US, ultrasound examination; PCR, polymerase chain reaction; Ig, immunoglobulin; CT, congenital toxoplasmosis; kg, kilogram; mg, milligram; D, day.

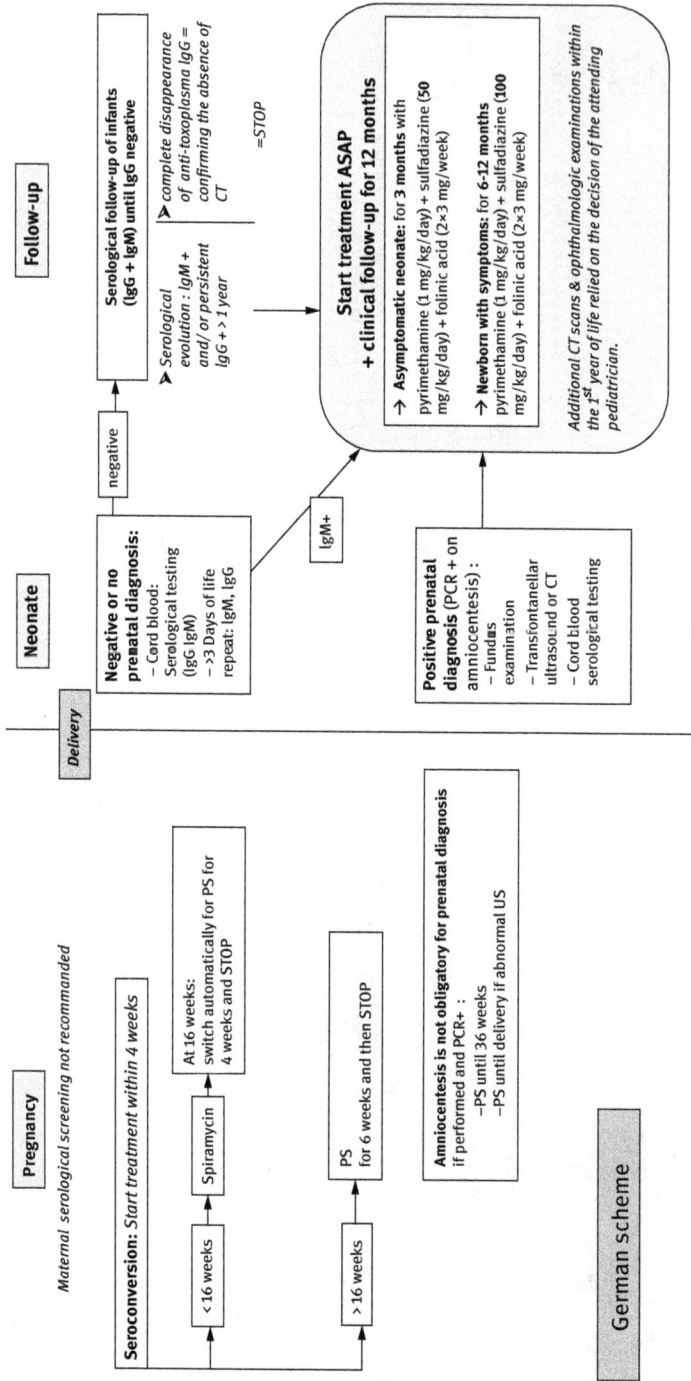

Figure 20.2: German scheme: prenatal and postnatal treatment [36].

Pregnancy

Maternal mandatory serological screening

Seroconversion: *Start treatment ASAP**

< 16 weeks → Spiramycin

At 16 weeks: switch automatically for PS

PS for 4 weeks

< 16 weeks → PS for 4 weeks

Amniocentesis

PCR − → Spiramycin

PCR + or Not performed → PS 4 weeks ⇄ Spiramycin 4 weeks

Austrian scheme

Delivery

Neonate

Negatie or no prenatal dianosis:
– Cord blood: Serological testing (IgG IgM)
– >3 Days of life repeat: IgM, IgG

negative → (Follow-up)

IgM+ →

Positive prenatal diagnosis (PCR + on amniocentesis)
– Fundus examination
– transfontanellar ultrasound or CT
– Cord blood serological testing

Follow-up

Serological follow-up of infants (IgG + IgM 3 months) until IgG negative

➤ *Serological evolution : IgM+ and/ or persistent IgG + 1 year*

➤ *complete disappearance of anti-toxoplasma IgG = confirming the absence of CT*

= STOP

Start treatment ASAP + clinical follow-up for 12 months

→ **Asymptomatic neonate:**
Combination for 6 weeks, followed by the alternating treatment: 6 weeks spiramycin and 4 weeks combination

→ **Newborn with symptoms :**
– For 6 months : combination
– For additional 6 months : alternating treatment scheme: 6 weeks and 4 weeks combination

– *Combination = pyrimethamine (1 mg/kg/D) + sulfadiazine (85 mg/kg/D) + folinic acid (2×5 mg/week)*
– *Spiramycin = 100 mg/kg/D*

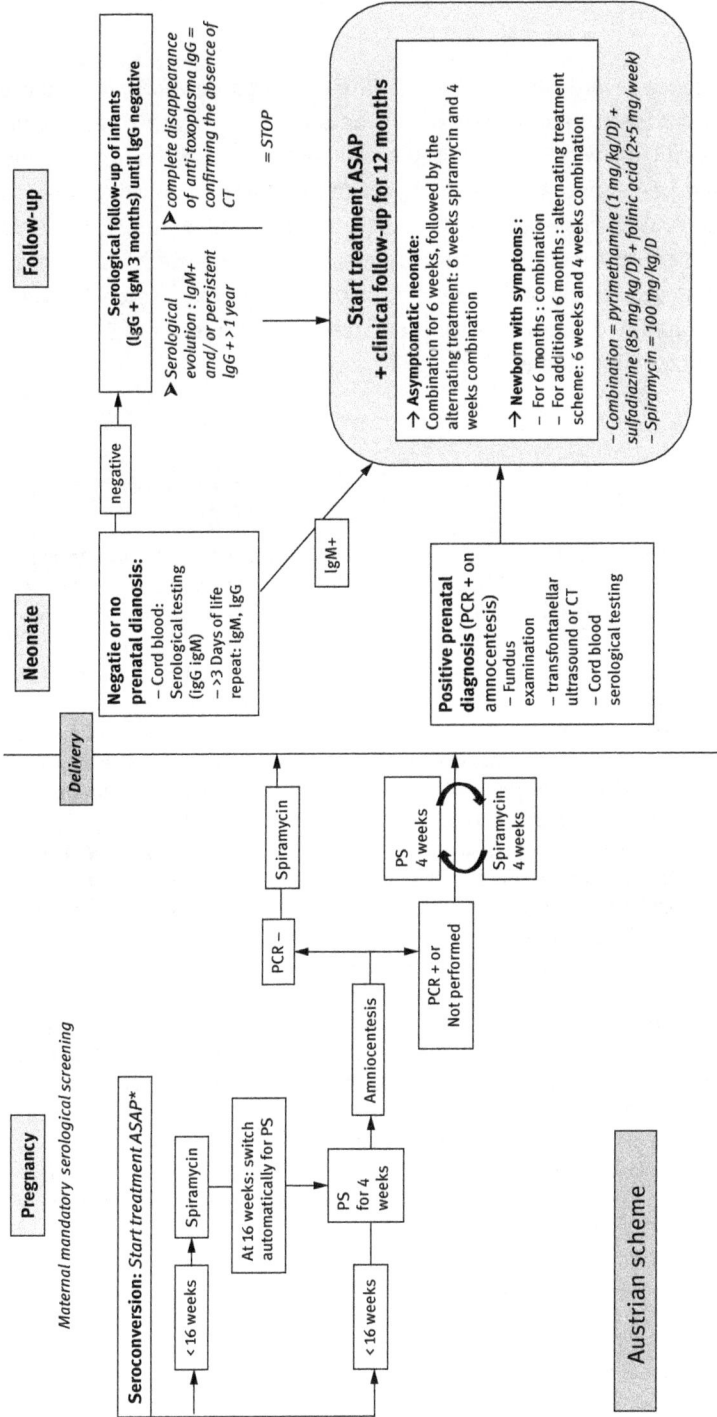

Figure 20.3: Austrian scheme: prenatal and postnatal treatment [14].

20.9 Conclusion

Although CT can cause severe complications in the fetus and newborn, its decline in prevalence and incidence and controversial data on the efficacy of antenatal therapy mean that only a few countries in the world continue to screen for it during pregnancy. Primary prevention and screening for toxoplasmosis, however, remain simple to implement, with cost–benefit studies going in this direction. The caring antenatal management of a maternal seroconversion must especially pass by an identification and precise dating of the infection, a multidisciplinary care within expert centers, and a mature discussion with the patient on the interest of an antenatal treatment, despite its limitations.

References

[1]   McLeod R, Boyer KM, Lee D et al. Prematurity and severity are associated with Toxoplasma gondii Alleles (NCCCTS, 1981–2009). Clin Infect Dis [Internet] 1juin 2012cité 23 févr 2020;54 (11):1595-605. Disponible sur:https://academic-oup-com.sirius.parisdescartes.fr/cid/article/ 54/11/1595/323276.

[2]   Gilbert RE, Freeman K, Lago EG et al. Ocular Sequelae of Congenital Toxoplasmosis in Brazil Compared with Europe. PLoS Negl Trop Dis 13août 2008cité 23 févr 2020;2(8):e277. Disponible sur:https://journals.plos.org/plosntds/article?id=10.1371/journal.pntd.0000277.

[3]   Torgerson PR, Mastroiacovo P. The global burden of congenital toxoplasmosis: A systematic review. Bull World Health Organ 1juill 2013cité 24 févr 2020;91(7):501Disponible sur:https:// www-ncbi-nlm-nih-gov.sirius.parisdescartes.fr/pmc/articles/PMC3699792/.

[4]   Cook AJC, Holliman R, Gilbert RE et al. Sources of toxoplasma infection in pregnant women: European multicenter case-control study Commentary: Congenital toxoplasmosis – further thought for food. BMJ [Internet] 15juill 2000cité 24 févr 2020;321(7254):142–7. Disponible sur:https://www-bmj-com.sirius.parisdescartes.fr/content/321/7254/142.

[5]   Article – Bulletin épidémiologique hebdomadaire . cité 26 févr 2020Disponible sur:http:// beh.santepubliquefrance.fr/beh/2015/15-16/2015_15-16_5.html.

[6]   Price C, Wilkins PP, Kruszon-Moran D, Jones JL, Rivera HN. Toxoplasma gondii Seroprevalence in the United States 2009–2010 and Comparison with the Past Two Decades. Am J Trop Med Hyg [Internet] 4juin 2014cité 26 févr 2020;90(6):1135–9Disponible sur:http://www.ajtmh. org/content/journals/10.4269/ajtmh.14-0013.

[7]   De Azevedo KML, Setúbal S, Lopes VGS, Camacho LAB, De Oliveira SA. Congenital toxoplasmosis transmitted by human immunodeficiency-virus infected women. Braz J Infect Dis 1mars 2010cité 24 févr 2020;14(2):186-9Disponible sur:http://www.sciencedirect.com/sci ence/article/pii/S1413867010700362.

[8]   D'Ercole C, Boubli L, Franck J et al. Recurrent congenital toxoplasmosis in a woman with lupus erythematosus. Prenat Diagn 1 déc 1995cité 24 févr 2020;15(12):1171–5. Disponible sur: https://obgyn-onlinelibrary-wiley-com.sirius.parisdescartes.fr/doi/abs/10.1002/pd. 1970151216.

[9]   Diagnostic biologique de la toxoplasmose acquise du sujet immunocompétent (dont la femme enceinte), la toxoplasmose congénitale (diagnostic pré- et postnatal) et la toxoplasmose oculaire . Haute Autorité De Santé cité 24 févr 2020Disponible sur:https://

www.has-sante.fr/jcms/c_2653655/fr/diagnostic-biologique-de-la-toxoplasmose-acquise-du-sujet-immunocompetent-dont-la-femme-enceinte-la-toxoplasmose-congenitale-diagnostic-pre-et-postnatal-et-la-toxoplasmose-oculaire.

[10] Preventing Congenital Toxoplasmosis [Internet]. cité 22 févr 2020Disponible sur:https:// www.cdc.gov/mmwr/preview/mmwrhtml/rr4902a5.htm.

[11] Paquet C, Yudin MH, Allen VM et al. Toxoplasmosis in Pregnancy: Prevention, Screening, and Treatment. J Obstet Gynaecol Can 1janv 2013cité 22 févr 2020;35(1):78–9. Disponible sur: http://www.sciencedirect.com/science/article/pii/S1701216315310537.

[12] Gollub EL, Leroy V, Gilbert R, Chêne G, Wallon M. Effectiveness of health education on Toxoplasma-related knowledge, behavior, and risk of seroconversion in pregnancy. Eur J Obstet Gynecol Reprod Biol 1févr 2008cité 22 févr 2020;136(2):137–45Disponible sur:http:// www.sciencedirect.com/science/article/pii/S0301211507004307.

[13] The effectiveness of a prenatal education programme for the prevention of congenital toxoplasmosis. – PubMed – NCBI [Internet]. cité 22 févr 2020Disponible sur:https://www-ncbi-nlm-nih-gov.sirius.parisdescartes.fr/pubmed/2606162.

[14] Prusa A-R, Kasper DC, Pollak A, Gleiss A, Waldhoer T, Hayde M. The Austrian Toxoplasmosis Register, 1992–2008. Clin Infect Dis 15janv 2015cité 24 févr 2020;60(2):e4–10Disponible sur: https://academic-oup-com.sirius.parisdescartes.fr/cid/article/60/2/e4/2895402.

[15] Peyron F, L'ollivier C, Mandelbrot L et al. Maternal and Congenital Toxoplasmosis: Diagnosis and Treatment Recommendations of a French Multidisciplinary Working Group. Pathogens mars 2019cité 24 févr 2020;8(1):24. Disponible sur:https://www.mdpi.com/2076-0817/8/1/24.

[16] Congenital toxoplasmosis in Austria: Prenatal screening for prevention is cost-saving [Internet]. cité 19 févr 2020Disponible sur:https://journals.plos.org/plosntds/article?id=10. 1371/journal.pntd.0005648.

[17] Wallon M, Peyron F, Cornu C et al. Congenital toxoplasma infection: monthly prenatal screening decreases transmission rate and improves clinical outcome at age 3 years. Clin Infect Dis 1mai 2013cité 24 févr 2020;56(9):1223–31. Disponible sur:https://academic-oup-com.sirius.parisdescartes.fr/cid/article/56/9/1223/293975.

[18] Goldstein EJC, Montoya JG, Remington JS. Management of Toxoplasma gondii Infection during Pregnancy. Clin Infect Dis [Internet] 15août 2008cité 24 févr 2020;47(4):554–66Disponible sur:https://academic-oup-com.sirius.parisdescartes.fr/cid/article/47/4/554/304753.

[19] Mandelbrot L, Kieffer F, Sitta R et al. Prenatal therapy with pyrimethamine + sulfadiazine vs spiramycin to reduce placental transmission of toxoplasmosis: A multicenter, randomized trial. Am J Obstet Gynecol 1oct 2018cité 22 févr 2020;219(4):386.e1–386.e9Disponible sur: http://www.sciencedirect.com/science/article/pii/S0002937818304411.

[20] Effectiveness of prenatal treatment for congenital toxoplasmosis: A meta-analysis of individual patients' data. The Lancet . 13janv 2007cité 19 févr 2020;369(9556): 115–22Disponible sur:http://www.sciencedirect.com/science/article/pii/ S0140673607600725.

[21] Rabilloud M, Wallon M, Peyron F. In Utero and at Birth Diagnosis of Congenital Toxoplasmosis: Use of Likelihood Ratios for Clinical Management. Pediatr Infect Dis J mai 2010cité 24 févr 2020;29(5):421–425Disponible sur:http://journals.lww.com/pidj/Abstract/ 2010/05000/In_Utero_and_at_Birth_Diagnosis_of_Congenital.9.aspx.

[22] Berrébi A, Assouline C, Bessières M-H et al. Long-term outcome of children with congenital toxoplasmosis. Am J Obstet Gynecol 1déc 2010cité 22 févr 2020;203(6):552. e1–552.e6Disponible sur:http://www.sciencedirect.com/science/article/pii/ S0002937810007027.

[23] Prusa A-R, Kasper DC, Pollak A, Olischar M, Gleiss A, Hayde M. Amniocentesis for the detection of congenital toxoplasmosis: Results from the nationwide Austrian prenatal

screening program. Clin Microbiol Infect 1fév 2015cité 24 févr 2020;21(2):191.
e1–191.e8Disponible sur:http://www.sciencedirect.com/science/article/pii/
S1198743X14000548.

[24] Wallon M, Franck J, Thulliez P et al. Accuracy of real-time polymerase chain reaction for
Toxoplasma gondii in amniotic fluid. Obstet Gynecol 2010cité 22 févr 2020;115(4):727–33.
Disponible sur:insights.ovid.com.

[25] Kasper DC, Sadeghi K, Prusa A-R et al. Quantitative real-time polymerase chain reaction for
the accurate detection of Toxoplasma gondii in amniotic fluid. Diagn Microbiol Infect Dis
1janv 2009cité 24 févr 2020;63(1):10–5. Disponible sur:http://www.sciencedirect.com/sci
ence/article/pii/S0732889308004094.

[26] Gay-Andrieu F, Marty P, Pialat J, Sournies G, De Laforte TD, Peyron F. Fetal toxoplasmosis and
negative amniocentesis: Necessity of an ultrasound follow-up. Prenat Diagn 1juill 2003cité 22
févr 2020;23(7):558–60Disponible sur:https://obgyn-onlinelibrary-wiley-com.sirius.parisdes
cartes.fr/doi/abs/10.1002/pd.632.

[27] Desmonts G, Couvreur J. Congenital toxoplasmosis. N Engl J Med 16mai 1974cité 24 févr
2020;290(20):1110–6Disponible sur: https://doi.org/10.1056/NEJM197405162902003.

[28] Hohlfeld P, MacAleese J, Capella-Pavlovski M et al. Fetal toxoplasmosis: Ultrasonographic
signs. Ultrasound Obstet Gynecol 1juill 1991cité 22 févr 2020;1(4):241–4. Disponible sur:
https://obgyn-onlinelibrary-wiley-com.sirius.parisdescartes.fr/doi/abs/10.1046/j.1469-
0705.1991.01040241.x.

[29] Dunn D, Wallon M, Peyron F, Petersen E, Peckham C, Gilbert R. Mother-to-child transmission
of toxoplasmosis: Risk estimates for clinical counselling. THE LANCET 1999;353:5.

[30] Dhombres F, Friszer S, Maurice P et al. Prognosis of fetal parenchymal cerebral lesions
without ventriculomegaly in congenital toxoplasmosis infection. Fetal Diagn Ther 2017cité 22
févr 2020;41(1):8–14. Disponible sur:https://www-karger-com.sirius.parisdescartes.fr/Arti
cle/FullText/445113.

[31] Malinger G, Werner H, Rodriguez Leonel JC et al. Prenatal brain imaging in congenital
toxoplasmosis. Prenat Diagn 1sept 2011cité 22 févr 2020;31(9):881–6. Disponible sur:
https://obgyn-onlinelibrary-wiley-com.sirius.parisdescartes.fr/doi/full/10.1002/pd.2795.

[32] Berrebi A, Bardou M, Bessieres M-H et al. Outcome for children infected with congenital
toxoplasmosis in the first trimester and with normal ultrasound findings: A study of 36 cases.
Eur J Obstet Gynecol Reprod Biol 1nov 2007cité 22 févr 2020;135(1):53–7. Disponible sur:
http://www.sciencedirect.com/science/article/pii/S0301211506006336.

[33] McLeod R, Boyer K, Karrison T et al. Outcome of treatment for congenital toxoplasmosis,
1981–2004: the national collaborative Chicago-based, congenital toxoplasmosis study. Clin
Infect Dis 15mai 2006cité 26 févr 2020;42(10):1383-94. Disponible sur:https://academic-oup-
com.sirius.parisdescartes.fr/cid/article/42/10/1383/277874.

[34] DRESS compliqué d'un syndrome d'activation macrophagique chez un nourrisson traité pour
une toxoplasmose congénitale – ScienceDirect [Internet]. cité 26 févr 2020Disponible sur:
https://www-sciencedirect-com.sirius.parisdescartes.fr/science/article/pii/
S0151963817302430?via%3Dihub.

[35] Teil J, Dupont D, Charpiat B et al. Treatment of congenital toxoplasmosis: safety of the
sulfadoxine–pyrimethamine combination in children based on a method of causality
assessment. Pediatr Infect Dis J [Internet] juin 2016cité 26 févr 2020;35(6):634–638.
Disponible sur:http://journals.lww.com/pidj/Abstract/2016/06000/Treatment_of_Congeni
tal_Toxoplasmosis__Safety_of.8.aspx.

[36] Hotop A, Hlobil H, Groß U. Efficacy of rapid treatment initiation following primary Toxoplasma
gondii infection during pregnancy. Clin Infect Dis 1juin 2012cité 26 févr 2020;54

(11):1545-52Disponible sur:https://academic-oup-com.sirius.parisdescartes.fr/cid/article/54/11/1545/321395.

[37] Dunay IR, Gajurel K, Dhakal R, Liesenfeld O, Montoya JG. Treatment of toxoplasmosis: historical perspective, animal models, and current clinical practice. Clin Microbiol Rev 1oct 2018cité 26 févr 2020;31(4):Disponible sur:https://cmr-asm-org.sirius.parisdescartes.fr/content/31/4/e00057-17.

[38] European Multicenter Study on Congenital Toxoplasmosis, Participants are listed on page 119. Effect of timing and type of treatment on the risk of mother to child transmission of Toxoplasma gondii. BJOG Int J Obstet Gynaecol 1févr 2003cité 26 févr 2020;110(2):112-20. Disponible sur:https://obgyn-onlinelibrary-wiley-com.sirius.parisdescartes.fr/doi/full/10.1046/j.1471-0528.2003.02325.x.

[39] Kieffer F, Wallon M, Garcia P, Thulliez P, Peyron F, Franck J. Risk factors for retinochoroiditis during the first 2 years of life in infants with treated congenital toxoplasmosis. Pediatr Infect Dis J janv 2008cité 26 févr 2020;27(1):27–32Disponible sur:http://journals.lww.com/pidj/Fulltext/2008/01000/Risk_Factors_for_Retinochoroiditis_During_the.6.aspx.

Daniela N. Vasquez, Maria-Teresa Pérez

21 Sepsis in Pregnancy

21.1 Introduction

Sepsis represents approximately 11% of maternal deaths and is the third most common cause of deaths directly attributable to pregnancy worldwide. Almost all of these deaths occur in low-income countries [1]. However, in the recent past, an upsurge in maternal deaths due to sepsis has been observed in high-income countries as well [2–4]. In England, from 2006 to 2008, genital tract sepsis was the most common cause of direct maternal death, especially due to group A *Streptococcus* (GAS) [4]. In the national inpatient sample (NIS) of approximately 45,000 pregnant patients in the USA, the probability of acquiring severe sepsis and sepsis-related mortality increased 10% per year over a 10-year period (1998–2008) [3]. Furthermore, sepsis is also associated with severe maternal morbidity, which can also lead to fetal morbidity and mortality [5]. Improvement in patient care could lead to a reduction in maternal mortality associated with sepsis up to 50% [3, 6]. Thus, continuing medical education and training are key factors to improve outcomes.

21.2 Risk Factors

Pregnant women are at increased risk of acquiring certain infections, such as listeriosis or malaria, and suffer more severe complications due to a few viruses, such as influenza, hepatitis E, or herpes simplex. The 2009 H_1N_1 influenza pandemic is a perfect example of this situation, as many pregnant women suffered severe complications, some ending in death [7]. Cell-mediated immunity seems to be especially compromised during pregnancy [7].

Other factors associated with higher incidence of sepsis in pregnancy or with progression from less severe to more severe forms are: demographics (age >35, ethnic minority status, type of health insurance, etc.), preexisting medical conditions (cardiovascular disease, diabetes, chronic liver or renal disease, systemic lupus erythematosus (SLE), HIV, etc.), obstetric history (preterm premature rupture of membranes (PPROM), retained products of conception, primiparity, multiple pregnancy, etc.), or management (cesarean section, history of transfusion, etc.) [2, 3, 8–10]. Noticeably, the risk associated with a priori factors is significantly cumulative [8]. The obstetric and comorbidity factors with the highest population-attributable fractions were: congestive heart failure (5.9%), PPROM (2.6%), retained products of conception (1.5%), and SLE (1.4%) [3].

https://doi.org/10.1515/9783110615258-021

Any patient with the aforementioned risk factors has an increased risk of developing infection. Therefore, the physician not only needs to be aware of these factors but also understand that, when present, patients are more likely to develop sepsis. A high level of suspicion will allow medical personnel to detect and treat sepsis promptly. However, population-attributable fractions for factors independently associated with severe sepsis were low [3], which means that most diseases cannot be attributed to these exposures and thus cannot be prevented, even if the risk factors are eliminated. This context highlights the importance of early recognition, close monitoring, and urgent treatment of sepsis in the entire pregnant/postpartum population, as most patients will not have risk factors to alert medical staff of the possibility of sepsis.

21.3 Diagnosis

Recognition of sepsis during pregnancy or in early puerperium may be challenging. Physiological changes of pregnancy can prompt either overestimation or underestimation of sepsis. In the former, pregnant patients normally have higher heart rates (HR) (up to 107 bpm), respiratory rate (RR) (up to 25), and white blood cells (WBC) (up to $17,500/mm^3$) as well as lower levels of mean arterial pressure (MAP) during the first and especially the second trimesters, leading to an overestimation of sepsis [11]. In the latter, creatinine values are usually lower in pregnant patients compared to nonpregnant patients (<0.9 vs 1.2 mg/dL) [12], often resulting in overlooking renal dysfunction and, consequently, underdiagnosing sepsis.

The previous definition of sepsis included the presence of infection in addition to systemic inflammatory response syndrome (SIRS), which, in turn, was considered when any two of the four SIRS criteria were present: HR > 90 bpm, RR > 20 pm or pCO_2 < 32 mmHg, WBC <4,000 or >12,000/mm^3, or temperature > 38 °C or < 36 °C [13]. However, this definition was proven to be inaccurate due to its high sensitivity and low specificity, especially in pregnant patients, as mentioned above [11].

In 2016, the Critical Care Medical Society and the European Society of Critical Care Medicine launched a new definition of sepsis and septic shock. Sepsis is now considered a life-threatening organ dysfunction due to dysregulated host response to infection. Organ dysfunction was defined according to a Sequential Organ Failure Assessment score (SOFA) ≥2 (Table 21.1). On the other hand, septic shock was defined according to the presence of sepsis, hypotension requiring vasopressors to maintain an MAP ≥ 65 mmHg and lactate level >2 mmol/L or 18 mg/dL [14]. However, the SOFA score was not calibrated for pregnant patients. For example, the normal cutoff for creatinine was set at 1.2 mg/dL and MAP at 70 mmHg, which are high values for pregnant patients [15].

Table 21.1: Sequential Organ Failure Assessment (SOFA) score.

System	Score				
	0	1	2	3	4
Respiration: PaO_2/FiO_2	>400	≤400	≤300	≤200 (with respiratory support)	≤100 (with respiratory support)
Coagulation: Platelets $(x10^3/mm^3)$	>150	≤150	≤100	≤50	≤20
Liver: Bilirubin (mg/dL) (μmol/L)	<1.2 <20	1.2–1.9 20–32	2–5.9 33–101	6–11.9 102–204	>12 >204
Cardiovascular: Hypotension	No hypotension	MAP <70 mmHg	Dopamine ≤5 or dobutamine (any dose)*	Dopamine >5 or epinephrine ≤0.1 or norepinephrine ≤0.1*	Dopamine > 15 or epinephrine > 0.1 or norepinephrine >0.1 *
Central nervous system: Glasgow Coma Scale	15	13–14	10–12	6–9	<6
Renal: Creatinine (mg/dL) (μmol/L) Or urine output (mL/day)	<1.2 <110	1.2–1.9 110–170	2–3.4 171–299	3.5–4.9 300–440 or <500	>5 > 440 or <200

*Adrenergic agents administered for at least 1 h (doses given in μg/kg/min) [15].

Similarly, the same task force developed the quickSOFA (qSOFA) for use outside the ICU, in order to recognize patients with suspected infection as well as those that may develop poor outcomes, thereafter [14]. Recognizing sepsis outside the ICU is not a simple task, as fewer tests are run on a daily basis. The qSOFA is a simple tool that does not require laboratory analysis and has predictive validity outside the ICU that is statistically greater than the SOFA score. The qSOFA components are: systolic blood pressure (SBP) ≤ 100 mmHg, RR > 22 bpm, and altered mentation. The presence of any two of these three variables in non-ICU settings was associated with increased in-hospital mortality. However, like SOFA, the qSOFA was not calibrated for pregnant patients, either. And in these patients, as mentioned earlier, blood pressure can be lower and RR can be higher than in nonpregnant patients.

Although not specific to sepsis, the maternal early warning (MEW) score is a tool explicitly designed for obstetric patients to identify higher risk of morbidity and mortality. In this chart, a complete set of physiological parameters are adjusted for pregnancy, and abnormalities are identified by a number and color score combination. Continued monitoring of changes in *all* parameters and totaling them into a score allows for early detection of deterioration; and this, along with standardizing procedures, helps eliminate errors related to staff management [16]. The performance of MEW in identifying cases of impending sepsis was evaluated in a case–control multicenter study comprised of pregnant or recently postpartum women hospitalized for delivery [17]. The presence of SBP < 90 mmHg, HR > 120 bpm, RR > 30 pm, or neurological changes indicated a sensitivity of 82% and a specificity of 87% for identifying sepsis. While the accuracy of MEW was superior, on average, to SIRS and qSOFA, it still missed 18% of patients with sepsis [17]. Similar drawbacks were reported by Lappen et al., whose study of an obstetric population also indicated poor accuracy for SIRS and a MEW of ≥5 for predicting ICU transfer, sepsis, or death [18].

Another tool designed to evaluate sepsis-associated morbidity in obstetric patients in the ER is the Sepsis in Obstetric Score (S.O.S.). S.O.S. criteria are adjusted for the natural changes occurring during pregnancy. S.O.S. ≥6 was independently associated with ICU admission and positive blood cultures [19]. In the same group of patients, increasing levels of lactic acid were also associated with transfer to the ICU or telemetry unit [20].

In view of the abovementioned limitations for defining sepsis and evaluating its associated morbidity in obstetric patients, the Society of Obstetric Medicine of Australia and New Zealand (SOMANZ) guidelines have proposed a modified qSOFA and SOFA, specifically for obstetrics. The modification involves adjusting cutoff points for pregnancy (e.g., qSOFA-SBP < 90 mmHg, RR > 25 bpm, and SOFA-creatinine = 1); however, these modified scores have not been validated, yet [21].

The World Health Organization (WHO) has proposed a new maternal sepsis definition as: a life-threatening condition defined as organ dysfunction resulting from infection during pregnancy, childbirth, post abortion, or postpartum period. The parameters adjusted for pregnancy are currently being addressed in the Global Maternal Sepsis Study (GLOSS) [22].

21.4 Sources of Sepsis in Pregnant and Postpartum Patients

Causes of sepsis in pregnant and postpartum patients can be classified into obstetric – those occurring *during* pregnancy or in the postpartum period, and nonobstetric – those that can also occur in nonpregnant patients. The most common causes of obstetric sepsis are puerperal sepsis, chorioamnionitis, and septic abortion, while the most common nonobstetric causes are urinary tract infection and pneumonia [3, 9, 10, 17, 23–25].

Puerperal sepsis is defined by WHO as an infection of the genital tract occurring at any time between the onset of membrane rupture or labor and the 42nd day postpartum; it is characterized by fever and at least one of the following: pelvic pain, abnormal vaginal discharge, and/or delay in the rate of reduction of uterine size [26]. Chorioamnionitis is usually suspected when fever cannot be attributed to any identifiable cause of sepsis. It usually presents with maternal and fetal tachycardia, uterine tenderness, foul-smelling amniotic fluid, and maternal leukocytosis [27]. In countries with restrictive abortion laws, septic abortion should be suspected in any woman of reproductive age complaining of lower abdominal pain, fever, and vaginal bleeding or abnormal vaginal discharge [28].

A particular clinical presentation of puerperal sepsis is toxic shock syndrome (TSS) due to GAS, which is potentially fatal. It is characterized by fever, abdominal pain, hypotension, and rapid progression to organ dysfunction [29]. It mostly presents in the postpartum period (85%), where maternal mortality rates can be as high as 25% for cases developing within the first 2 days postpartum. Although presentation during the last trimester is less frequent (15%), it is associated with the highest maternal and fetal mortality rates (56% and 71%, respectively) [30]. Early detection, prompt treatment, and advanced clinical support are key in improving related outcomes.

Urinary tract infections are common during pregnancy due to increased bladder volume, decreased bladder and ureteral tone with ureteral dilation, and urinary stasis causing vesicoureteral reflux. Bacterial growth is also facilitated by the presence of glycosuria. Decreased peristalsis and ureteral dilation are due to the effects of both progesterone and compression by the enlarged uterus [31]. Pyelonephritis mainly occurs during the second and third trimester [31–33] and is associated with significant morbidity, such as increased risk of: sepsis (OR 108), pneumonia (OR 18.5), ARDS (OR 11.6), acute renal failure (OR 15), pulmonary edema (OR 11.3), mechanical ventilation (OR 10.9), preterm labor, and chorioamnionitis (OR 1.7 each) [34].

Community-acquired pneumonia (CAP) also commonly presents during the second and third trimester [35–40]. The most common microorganism isolated was *S. pneumoniae* [35, 36]. CAP incidence in pregnant patients is not higher than in nonpregnant patients [36]; however, it is associated with bad maternal and fetal outcomes and needs to be recognized early to avoid delays in treatment [9]. Pandemic 2009 influenza A (H_1N_1) virus infection was associated with a disproportionately high mortality rate in this group of patients [37, 38]. Pregnant patients have reduced oxygen reserve (due to reduced functional residual capacity) and increased oxygen consumption (due to increased maternal and fetal metabolic demands), placing them at a respiratory disadvantage [39].

21.5 Microorganisms Responsible for Maternal Sepsis

In a 10-year study with approximately 45 million patients hospitalized for delivery taken from NIS, 4,158 patients developed severe sepsis. Of these, 40% presented bacteremia due to the following microorganisms: *E. coli* 26.7%, *Staphylococcus* 22.2%, *Streptococcus* 20.1%, other gram-negatives 19.3%, and others [3].

The most common origins of *E. coli* bacteremia during pregnancy or postpartum are the urinary and genital tracts (55.2% and 44.8%, respectively). In general, bacteremia during pregnancy can be associated with fetal mortality up to 27%; and in 83% of these fetal deaths, the origin of bacteremia was the genital tract [40].

E. coli is an incredibly common microorganism in the general population, classified into different phylogenetic groups. However, in pregnant patients, certain strains of *E. coli* appear more frequently than in the nonpregnant population, such as B2 (72%) and D phylogroups (17%) [40, 41]. The B2 phylogroup was shown to possess high intrinsic extraintestinal virulence in a mouse model [40]. Still, the impact of virulence scores on outcomes in human studies continues to be controversial. For example, one study of reproductive age women showed more virulent strains in samples taken from pregnant versus nonpregnant patients, but did not measure the virulence impact on clinical outcomes [41]. Another study found lower virulence scores in the group of obstetric patients with fetal deaths compared to those with surviving fetuses [40]. In addition, variations in bactericidal activity of the genital tract secretions in pregnant versus nonpregnant patients and among pregnant women, in general, could explain the disparity in colonization rates associated with preterm birth and neonatal sepsis [42].

GAS is another pathogen that deserves special attention for postpartum patients, because it has marked predisposition to cause severe infections – in fact, it is associated with twice the risk of mortality compared to other causes of obstetric sepsis [10]. The risk of acquiring GAS infection among postpartum patients is 20 times higher than in nonpregnant patients. Emm 28 is the most frequent GAS subtype identified among pregnant and postpartum patients compared to nonpregnant patients [43]. TSS due to GAS is related to the presence of bacterial superantigens that, through a series of interactions, cause a massive cytokine release provoking severe illness [29].

21.6 Management

Effective sepsis management for obstetric patients will follow the same protocols as for critically ill patients; however, some adjustments and/or special considerations need to be taken into account for this population. Recognition is the key component in sepsis management, especially in obstetric patients where the progression of symptoms is accelerated [10]; however, this cannot occur without first contemplating the *possibility* of sepsis. Early recognition will result in prompt treatment and hopefully reduced maternal mortality due to sepsis.

Approximately 20 years ago, the early goal-directed therapy for sepsis was developed [44]. This approach was implemented globally and was proven to reduce sepsis-related mortality up to 25%, even in nonresearch settings [45, 46]. The original surviving sepsis bundle (2004) targeted the first 6 h after diagnosing sepsis as the *golden period* for treatment in order to improve survival [47]. However, the current recommendation (2018) reduced the following set of actions to be completed within a 1-h period [48]:

- Lactate should be measured immediately and then remeasured, if the initial value is >2 mmol/L.
- Broad-spectrum antibiotics should be administered.
- Blood cultures should be taken before antibiotics are started; but if this is impossible, antibiotics must still be administered within the hour, and blood cultures should be done as soon as possible.
- Fluid resuscitation should be started *immediately* and 30 ml/kg of crystalloids (Ringer's lactate or normal saline) should be administered, if hypotension or lactate ≥4 mmol/L is present.
- Vasopressors should be applied to maintain a MAP ≥ 65 mmHg, if the patient is hypotensive during, or after fluid resuscitation.

Lactate should be measured as it is an early indicator of tissue hypoperfusion; it is part of the definition of septic shock, and it is a marker of prognosis [14, 48]. Lactate-guided resuscitation has been associated with lower mortality in patients with elevated lactate [48].

Antibiotics should be administered within 1 hour of diagnosing sepsis. This is imperative because each hour's delay in administering appropriate antibiotics is associated with a measurable increase in mortality [49]. Given the wide range of potential sources of sepsis and possible organisms in pregnant/postpartum patients, broad spectrum antibiotics should be indicated. Notwithstanding, studies worldwide frequently describe delays in administering antibiotics [50] or inappropriate coverage, indicating that these goals are rarely achieved [40, 51]. Empirical antibiotic choices should be guided by suspected source and local antibiotic resistance patterns; however, in most studies, *E. coli* resistance to amoxicillin/ampicillin and cephalotin was high enough to recommend avoiding them as a single first-line empirical treatment (50–60% and 35%, respectively) [32, 33, 40]. *E. coli* presented high resistance to amoxicillin-clavulanate in only one study from France [40], whereas its resistance was between 1.5% and 14% in studies elsewhere [32, 33, 52]. Clindamycin should be indicated in puerperal sepsis, because it has been shown to inhibit the production of some exotoxins associated with GAS infections [53]. Various antibiotic regimens are presented in Table 21.2 [27, 30, 54–57]. Once pathogens are isolated, antibiotics should be narrowed to avoid bacterial resistance, minimize adverse effects, decrease costs, etc.

Table 21.2: Frequent microorganisms and antibiotic regimens for obstetric and nonobstetric sepsis [27, 30, 57–59, 78].

Type of sepsis	Microorganisms	Antibiotics
Obstetric sepsis		
Puerperal sepsis	Gram-negative (*E. coli*, Enterobacteriaceae, etc.) gram-positive (beta-hemolytic streptococcus group A, B and D, *Staphylococcus*, etc.), and anaerobes (*Peptococcus*, bacteroides, etc.) [3, 42, 58]	Clindamycin 900 mg IV every 8 h + gentamicin 5 mg/kg IV once daily [58, 59] Ampicillin-sulbactam[a] 3 g IV every 6 h Piperacillin/tazobactam 4.5 g IV every 6 h
	Group A *Streptococcus* (GAS) confirmed	Clindamycin [a] 600–900 mg IV every 8 h + penicillin [a] 2–4 million units IV every 4–6 h Penicillin allergy: clindamycin [a] 600–900 mg IV every 8 h + vancomycin 1 g IV every 12 h [a] or daptomycin [a]
Chorioamnionitis	Gram-negative (*E. coli*, Enterobacteriaceae, etc.) gram-positive (beta-hemolytic *Streptococcus*- group A, B, and D, *Staphylococcus*, etc.) and anaerobes[27]	Ampicillin[a] 2 g IV every 6 h + gentamicin [b] 5 mg/kg IV once daily Cefazolin [a] 1 g IV every 8 h + gentamicin[b] 5 mg/kg IV once daily Ampicillin-sulbactam[a] 3 g IV every 6 h Piperacillin/tazobactam [a] 4.5 g IV every 6 h Penicillin allergy: clindamycin[a] 600–900 mg IV every 8 h + vancomycin 1 g every 12 h [a]
Nonobstetric sepsis		
Urinary tract infection	Gram-negative (*E. coli. Klebsiella, Proteus*, etc.), gram-positive (*Enterococcus faecalis*) [31–33, 54]	Ampicillin-sulbactam[a] 3 g IV every 6 h Piperacillin/tazobactam[a] 4.5 g IV every 6 h Ceftriaxone [a] 1–2 g IV once daily Ampicillin[a] 2 g IV every 6 h + gentamicin[b] 5 mg/kg IV once daily

| Community acquired pneumonia | Streptococcus pneumoniae, H. influenzae, Mycoplasma, etc. [35, 37], respiratory viruses (influenza, etc.) | If **no** comorbidities, use single agent:
Amoxicillin[a] 1 g IV every 8 h OR ampicillin[a] 2 g IV every 6 h
Azithromycin[a] 500 mg IV day 1, 250 mg IV days 2–5
Clarithromycin[c] 500 mg IV every 12 h
If **comorbidities** (diabetes, chronic heart disease, etc.), use combination therapy:
B-lactams (ampicillin-sulbactam[a] 3 g IV every 6 h OR cefuroxime 500 mg IV every 12 h OR cefatoxime[a], etc.) **+** macrolide (azithromycin[a] 500 mg IV day 1, 250 mg IV days 2–5 OR clarithromycin[c] 500 mg IV every 12 h):
During influenza season: add oseltamivir[c] 75 mg PO every 12 h[79] OR oseltamivir 150 mg PO every 12 h[40] |

[a] The following antibiotics are considered FDA Pregnancy Category B: penicillins (including beta-lactam/beta-lactamase inhibitor combinations), vancomycin, daptomycin, clindamycin, azithromycin, and cephalosporins (caution in the use of ceftriaxone at term due to risk of kernicterus) [57] – the ORACLE I study described a higher incidence of necrotizing enterocolitis with the use of co-amoxiclavulanate; however, other studies have not corroborated this data [80, 81].

[b] aminoglycosides, as a class, are considered FDA Pregnancy Category D, because streptomycin use was associated with hearing loss in newborns and should be avoided; but short-term use of other amynoglycosides is acceptable with monitoring, according to risk–benefit ratio [57].

[c] Clarithromycin and oseltamivir are considered FDA Pregnancy Category C; this means choose azithromycin over clarithromycin when available; however, oseltamivir is still recommended for influenza as the risk is so great. Fluoroquinolones should be avoided during pregnancy (FDA Pregnancy Category C), because they were associated with fetal harm (renal, cardiac, CNS, and bone) in animal studies, especially considering that other options are available [57]. Tetracyclines are considered FDA Pregnancy Category D, because they are proven to be toxic in humans [57].

Fluid resuscitation should be started immediately to avoid or correct tissue hypoperfusion. Crystalloids are preferred over colloids as they are widely available and less expensive; furthermore, the hemodynamic profile advantage of colloids is not as beneficial, as originally proposed. Moreover, in some studies, the colloid hydroxyethyl starch was associated with increased risk of mortality and renal replacement therapy in septic patients [58, 59]. Noradrenaline is the vasopressor of choice, if blood pressure is not restored after fluid resuscitation. An important consideration for resuscitating pregnant patients is correct positioning. After mid-pregnancy, compression of the inferior vena cava (IVC) by the gravid uterus impairs venous return and consequently reduces cardiac output. Elevation of the right hip by at least 10 cm off the bed will displace the uterus to the left and relieve IVC compression, thereby improving cardiac output. Resuscitation goals are: MAP $\geq$ 65 mmHg, urinary output $\geq$ 0.5 mL/kg/h, and normalizing lactate [60].

As noted above, sepsis bundles were created for the general population. Depending on the trimester – if the patient is pregnant – or during the postpartum period, conditions for sepsis can vary. For example, blood cultures would still be drawn during the first hour, but if pharyngitis is suspected, throat swabs should also be taken, given that GAS infections can be fatal for obstetric patients. The same is true for H_1N_1 influenza, wherein, when suspected, it should be promptly treated ($\leq$2 days from symptom onset), without waiting for confirmation, in order to reduce ICU admission and mortality rates [38, 61]. For this reason, the pregnant population is considered a target population to receive the influenza vaccination [37, 38].

Fetal monitoring is another aspect of maternal sepsis management. Fetal tachycardia may be the first indicator of chorioamnionitis, before any other maternal sign of sepsis develops. Furthermore, fetal monitoring may help detect fetal compromise and the ability to respond to treatment [62]. Nonstress testing or a biophysical profile may assist in the evaluation of fetal hypoxia or acidosis in viable fetuses; however, the performance and indications of each test may vary or be deemed inadequate, depending on gestational age [62]. Antenatal corticosteroids should be indicated for women at risk of preterm delivery (<37 weeks) to decrease neonatal respiratory complications [63]. For fetal neuroprotection, antenatal magnesium sulphate should be considered for women with imminent preterm birth (from viability to $\leq$33 + 6 weeks) [64].

A particular aspect that must be considered in pregnant patients is fever management. Hyperthermia $\geq$38.8 °C for more than 24 h, especially during the first 4 weeks gestation but also after, was associated with fetal malformations [65]. Therefore, it is important to treat the source of sepsis as well as to reduce maternal temperature promptly.

In terms of vasopressors, norepinephrine is the drug of choice for treating hypotension in critically ill patients in the general population as compared to dopamine, based on documented outcomes [66]. As norepinephrine increases systemic vascular resistance and also cardiac output, it would also be a good option for pregnant patients with sepsis. Similarly, in pregnant patients under spinal anesthesia, norepinephrine has shown good maternal and fetal performance, although its effect on umbilical artery pH is still controversial [67, 68]. The takeaway is that there is evidence on vasopressor use inpregnancy, while limited; therefore, if hypotension does not improve after fluids, norepinephrine should be started, without hesitation, to increase MAP, assure appropriate uterine flow, and increase oxygen delivery to fetal and maternal tissues. It should be noted that phenylephrine is commonly used for treating or preventing hypotension during scheduled C-sections, but it would not be suitable for managing blood pressure in patients with septic shock, because it is associated with decreased cardiac output.

Source control is a key aspect of obstetric sepsis. Chorioamnionitis indicates prompt delivery. Postpartum endomyometritis requires assessment for retained products of conception and may necessitate uterine evacuation. Septic abortion requires urgent removal of infected products of conception, which can be safely performed through either sharp or suction curettage [69, 70]. In most patients, source control via uterine curettage will be enough [28]. However, some cases will still require laparotomy: clostridial myometritis, uterine perforation with suspected bowel injury, pelvic abscess needing open surgical drainage, and lack of response to curettage and antibiotics [70]. Hysterectomy is reserved for uterine gas gangrene (crepitation of pelvic tissue or abdominal CT scan showing air within the uterine wall) and a discolored, woody appearance of the uterus [70].

21.7 Delivery Considerations

Delivery should be indicated without hesitation if the source of sepsis is obstetric, such as chorioamnionitis [27]. In nonobstetric sepsis, for example pneumonia or urinary tract infection, evidence is scarce. In a case series study including 30 patients with severe sepsis and septic shock, most patients with severe sepsis did not require immediate delivery – 70% delivered at term; whereas almost all patients with septic shock delivered immediately [71]. Delivery decisions must take into consideration gestational age and maternal and fetal status. The objective should be to stabilize the mother — fetal improvement will follow. As delivery does not appear to improve maternal outcomes, the objective should be to continue the pregnancy for as long as possible and base delivery decisions on obstetric indications [72].

21.8 Outcomes: Maternal Morbidity and Mortality due to Sepsis

Mortality associated with septic shock during pregnancy or postpartum is lower than in the general population (7.7–14% vs. 46.5%, respectively), even after adjusting for age and chronic comorbidities [8, 10, 73, 74]. This could be related to myriad factors, such as physiological advantages related to pregnancy (increased oxygen delivery to tissue, increased glomerular filtration rate, etc.), more diligent clinical care for obstetric patients, easy access to source control, and the lower mortality associated with genitourinary tract infections, which are the most frequent causes of sepsis in obstetric patients [73, 75].

In a national cohort study from the UK, factors found to be associated with maternal mortality due to sepsis were maternal deprivation, body mass index ≥25, and ≥3 organ system dysfunctions, especially respiratory, renal, and hematological [9]. Sepsis is also associated with increased morbidity in these patients; for example, in a case–control study, the presence of infection on admission was associated with stroke during hospitalization, even after adjusting for hypertensive disease of pregnancy, race, or insurance [76].

21.9 Conclusion

Women in pregnancy and postpartum are still susceptible to infections and subsequent sepsis. The most important challenge remains early recognition, and more work is required to develop an ideal scoring and detection tool. Prompt initiation of therapy and IV fluids remain the cornerstone of management.

References

[1]   Say L, Chou D, Gemmill A et al. Global causes of maternal death: A WHO systematic analysis. Lancet Glob Health 2014;2(6):e323–333.
[2]   Al-Ostad GKA, Spence AR, Abenhaim HA Incidence and risk factors of sepsis mortality in labor, delivery, and after birth: Population-based study in the USA. J Obstet Gynaecol Res 2015;41:1201–1206.
[3]   Bauer MEBB, Bauer ST, Shanks AM, Mhyre JM Maternal sepsis mortality and morbidity during hospitalization for delivery: Temporal trends and independent associations for severe sepsis. Anesth Analg 2013;117:944–950.
[4]   Cantwell R, Clutton-Brock T, Cooper G et al. Saving mothers' lives: reviewing maternal deaths to make motherhood safer: 2006-2008. the eighth report of the confidential enquiries into maternal deaths in the united kingdom. BJOG 2011;118(Suppl 1):1–203.

[5]   Knowles SJ, O'Sullivan NP, Meenan AM et al. Maternal sepsis incidence, aetiology and outcome for mother and fetus: A prospective study. BJOG 2015;122(5):663–671.

[6]   Kinght M, Tuffnell D, J K, et al. Message from the prevention and treatment of sepsis. Saving Lives, Improving Mothers Care Lessons learned to inform maternity care from the UK and Ireland Confidential Enquiries into Maternal Deaths and Morbidity 2013-2015. *University of Oxford* 2017.

[7]   Kourtis AP, Read JS, Jamieson DJ. Pregnancy and infection. N Engl J Med 2014;370(23): 2211–2218.

[8]   Acosta CDKM, Lee HC, Kurinczuk JJ, Gould JB, Lyndon A. The continuum of maternal sepsis severity: Incidence and risk factors in a population-based cohort study. PLoS One 2013;8(7).

[9]   Acosta CD, Harrison DA, Rowan K et al. Maternal morbidity and mortality from severe sepsis: A national cohort study. BMJ Open 2016;6(8):e012323.

[10] Kramer HMC SJ, Zwart JJ, Shuitemaker NEW, Steegers EAP, Van Roosmalen J Maternal mortality and severe morbidity from sepsis in the Netherlands. Acta Obstet Gynecol Scand 2009;88:647–653.

[11] Bauer MEBS, Rajala B, MacEachern MP et al. Maternal physiologic parameters in relationship to systemic inflammatory response syndrome criteria: A systematic review and meta-analysis. Obstet Gynecol 2014;124:535–541.

[12] Larsson A, Palm M, Hansson LO et al. Reference values for clinical chemistry tests during normal pregnancy. BJOG 2008;115(7):874–881.

[13] Bone RCBR, Cerra FB, Dellinger RP et al. Members of the American College of Chest Physicians/Society of Critical Care Medicine Consensus Conference Committee. American College of Chest Physicians/Society of Critical Care Medicine Consensus Conference: Definitions for sepsis and organ failure and guidelines for the use of innovative therapies in sepsis. Crit Care Med 1992;20:864–874.

[14] Singer MDC, Seymour CW, Shankar-Hari M et al. For the sepsis definitions task force. The third international consensus definitions for sepsis and septic shock (sepsis-3). JAMA 2016;315(8):801–810.

[15] Vincent JL, De Mendonca A, Cantraine F et al. Use of the SOFA score to assess the incidence of organ dysfunction/failure in intensive care units: Results of a multicenter, prospective study. Working group on "sepsis-related problems" of the European Society of Intensive Care Medicine. Crit Care Med 1998;26(11):1793–1800.

[16] Carle C, Alexander P, Columb M et al. Design and internal validation of an obstetric early warning score: Secondary analysis of the Intensive Care National Audit and Research Centre Case Mix Programme database. Anaesthesia 2013;68(4):354–367.

[17] Bauer ME, Housey M, Bauer ST et al. Risk factors, etiologies, and screening tools for sepsis in pregnant women: a multicenter case-control study. Anesth Analg 2018.

[18] Lappen JR, Keene M, Lore M et al. Existing models fail to predict sepsis in an obstetric population with intrauterine infection. Am J Obstet Gynecol 2010;203(6):573 e571–575.

[19] Albright CM, Ali TN, Lopes V et al. The sepsis in obstetrics score: a model to identify risk of morbidity from sepsis in pregnancy. Am J Obstet Gynecol 2014;211(1):39 e31–38.

[20] Albright CM, Ali TN, Lopes V et al. Lactic acid measurement to identify risk of morbidity from sepsis in pregnancy. Am J Perinatol 2015;32(5):481–486.

[21] Bowyer L, Robinson HL, Barrett H et al. SOMANZ guidelines for the investigation and management sepsis in pregnancy. Aust N Z J Obstet Gynaecol 2017;57(5):540–551.

[22] Bonet M, Souza JP, Abalos E et al. The global maternal sepsis study and awareness campaign (GLOSS): Study protocol. Reprod Health 2018;15(1):16.

[23] Aarvold AB, Ryan HM, Magee LA et al. Multiple organ dysfunction score is superior to the obstetric-specific sepsis in obstetrics score in predicting mortality in septic obstetric patients. Crit Care Med 2017;45(1):e49–e57.

[24] Timezguid N, Das V, Hamdi A et al. Maternal sepsis during pregnancy or the postpartum period requiring intensive care admission. Int J Obstet Anesth 2012;21(1):51–55.

[25] Vasquez DN, Das Neves AV, Vidal L et al. Characteristics, outcomes, and predictability of critically ill obstetric patients: a multicenter prospective cohort study. Crit Care Med 2015;43 (9):1887–1897.

[26] Maharaj D. Puerperal pyrexia: A review. Part I. Obstet Gynecol Surv 2007;62(6):393–399.

[27] Fahey JO. Clinical management of intra-amniotic infection and chorioamnionitis: A review of the literature. J Midwifery Womens Health 2008;53(3):227–235.

[28] Vasquez DN, Das Neves AV. Unsafe abortion: The silent endemic; an avoidable cause of maternal mortality. A review. Curr Women's Health Rev 2011;7(2):151163.

[29] McCormick JK, Yarwood JM, Schlievert PM Toxic shock syndrome and bacterial superantigens: An update. Annu Rev Microbiol 2001;55:77–104.

[30] Hamilton SM, Stevens DL, Bryant AE. Pregnancy-related group a streptococcal infections: Temporal relationships between bacterial acquisition, infection onset, clinical findings, and outcome. Clin Infect Dis 2013;57(6):870–876.

[31] Sharma P, Thapa L. Acute pyelonephritis in pregnancy: A retrospective study. Aust N Z J Obstet Gynaecol 2007;47(4):313–315.

[32] Artero A, Alberola J, Eiros JM et al. Pyelonephritis in pregnancy. How Adequate Is Empirical Treatment? Rev Esp Quimioter 2013;26(1):30–33.

[33] Zanatta DAL, Rossini MM, Trapani Junior A. Pyelonephritis in pregnancy: clinical and laboratorial aspects and perinatal results. Rev Bras Ginecol Obstet 2017;39(12):653–658.

[34] Dotters-Katz SK, Heine RP, Grotegut CA Medical and infectious complications associated with pyelonephritis among pregnant women at delivery. Infect Dis Obstet Gynecol 2013;2013:124102.

[35] Benedetti TJ, Valle R, Ledger WJ. Antepartum pneumonia in pregnancy. Am J Obstet Gynecol 1982;144(4):413–417.

[36] Shariatzadeh MR, Marrie TJ. Pneumonia during pregnancy. Am J Med 2006;119(10):872–876.

[37] Estenssoro E, Rios FG, Apezteguia C et al. Pandemic 2009 influenza A in Argentina: A study of 337 patients on mechanical ventilation. Am J Respir Crit Care Med 2010;182(1):41–48.

[38] Siston AM, Rasmussen SA, Honein MA et al. Pandemic 2009 influenza A(H1N1) virus illness among pregnant women in the United States. JAMA 2010;303(15):1517–1525.

[39] Hegewald MJ, Crapo RO. Respiratory physiology in pregnancy. Clin Chest Med 2011;32(1): 1–13.

[40] Surgers L, Bleibtreu A, Burdet C et al. Escherichia coli bacteraemia in pregnant women is life-threatening for fetuses. Clin Microbiol Infect 2014;20(12):O1035–1041.

[41] Guiral E, Bosch J, Vila J et al. Prevalence of Escherichia coli among samples collected from the genital tract in pregnant and nonpregnant women: Relationship with virulence. FEMS Microbiol Lett 2011;314(2):170–173.

[42] Ghartey JP, Carpenter C, Gialanella P et al. Association of bactericidal activity of genital tract secretions with Escherichia coli colonization in pregnancy. Am J Obstet Gynecol 2012;207 (4):297 e291–298.

[43] Deutscher M, Lewis M, Zell ER et al. Incidence and severity of invasive Streptococcus pneumoniae, group A Streptococcus, and group B Streptococcus infections among pregnant and postpartum women. Clin Infect Dis 2011;53(2):114–123.

[44] Rivers E, Nguyen B, Havstad S et al. Early goal-directed therapy in the treatment of severe sepsis and septic shock. N Engl J Med 2001;345(19):1368–1377.

[45] Levy MM, Rhodes A, Phillips GS et al. Surviving sepsis campaign: association between performance metrics and outcomes in a 7.5-year study. Crit Care Med 2015;43(1):3–12.

[46] Rhodes A, Phillips G, Beale R et al. The surviving sepsis campaign bundles and outcome: results from the international multicenter prevalence study on sepsis (the IMPreSS study). Intensive Care Med 2015;41(9):1620–1628.

[47] Dellinger RP, Carlet JM, Masur H et al. Surviving Sepsis Campaign guidelines for management of severe sepsis and septic shock. Intensive Care Med 2004;30(4):536–555.

[48] Levy MM, Evans LE, Rhodes A. The surviving sepsis campaign bundle: 2018 update. Crit Care Med 2018;46(6):997–1000.

[49] Kumar A, Roberts D, Wood KE et al. Duration of hypotension before initiation of effective antimicrobial therapy is the critical determinant of survival in human septic shock. Crit Care Med 2006;34(6):1589–1596.

[50] Albright CM, Has P, Rouse DJ et al. Internal validation of the sepsis in obstetrics score to identify risk of morbidity from sepsis in pregnancy. Obstet Gynecol 2017;130(4):747–755.

[51] Bauer ME, Lorenz RP, Bauer ST et al. Maternal deaths due to sepsis in the state of Michigan, 1999–2006. Obstet Gynecol 2015;126(4):747–752.

[52] Taye S, Getachew M, Desalegn Z et al. Bacterial profile, antibiotic susceptibility pattern and associated factors among pregnant women with Urinary Tract Infection in Goba and Sinana Woredas, Bale Zone, Southeast Ethiopia. BMC Res Notes 2018;11(1):799.

[53] Tanaka M, Hasegawa T, Okamoto A et al. Effect of antibiotics on group A Streptococcus exoprotein production analyzed by two-dimensional gel electrophoresis. Antimicrob Agents Chemother 2005;49(1):88–96.

[54] Leiner S, Mays M. Pharmacologic management of common lower respiratory tract disorders in women. J Midwifery Womens Health 2002;47(3):167–181.

[55] Bookstaver PB, Bland CM, Griffin B et al. A review of antibiotic use in pregnancy. Pharmacotherapy 2015;35(11):1052–1062.

[56] Mackeen AD, Packard RE, Ota E et al. Antibiotic regimens for postpartum endometritis. Cochrane Database Syst Rev 2015;(2):CD001067.

[57] Rac H, Gould A, Eiland LS et al. Common bacterial and viral infections: Review of management in the pregnant patient. Annals of Pharmacotherapy 2018;1–13.

[58] Myburgh JA, Mythen MG. Resuscitation fluids. N Engl J Med 2013;369(13):1243–1251.

[59] Perel P, Roberts I, Ker K. Colloids versus crystalloids for fluid resuscitation in critically ill patients. Cochrane Database Syst Rev 2013;(2):CD000567.

[60] Rhodes A, Evans LE, Alhazzani W et al. Surviving sepsis campaign: international guidelines for management of sepsis and septic shock: 2016. Crit Care Med 2017;45(3):486–552.

[61] Louie JK, Acosta M, Jamieson DJ et al. Severe 2009 H1N1 influenza in pregnant and postpartum women in California. N Engl J Med 2010;362(1):27–35.

[62] Chau A, Tsen LC. Fetal optimization during maternal sepsis: Relevance and response of the obstetric anesthesiologist. Curr Opin Anaesthesiol 2014;27(3):259–266.

[63] Gyamfi-Bannerman C, Thom EA. Antenatal betamethasone for women at risk for late preterm delivery. N Engl J Med 2016;375(5):486–487.

[64] Magee LA, De Silva DA, Sawchuck D et al. No. 376-Magnesium Sulphate for Fetal Neuroprotection. J Obstet Gynaecol Can 2019;41(4):505–522.

[65] Graham JM Jr., Edwards MJ, Edwards MJ. Teratogen update: Gestational effects of maternal hyperthermia due to febrile illnesses and resultant patterns of defects in humans. Teratology 1998;58(5):209–221.

[66] Gamper G, Havel C, Arrich J et al. Vasopressors for hypotensive shock. Cochrane Database Syst Rev 2016;2:CD003709.

[67] Mohta M, Garg A, Chilkoti GT et al. A randomized controlled trial of phenylephrine and noradrenaline boluses for treatment of postspinal hypotension during elective caesarean section. Anaesthesia 2019;74(7):850–855.

[68] Ngan Kee WD, Lee SW, Ng FF et al. Randomized double-blinded comparison of norepinephrine and phenylephrine for maintenance of blood pressure during spinal anesthesia for cesarean delivery. Anesthesiology 2015;122(4):736–745.

[69] Eschenbach DA. Treating spontaneous and induced septic abortions. Obstet Gynecol 2015;125(5):1042–1048.

[70] Stubblefield PG, Grimes DA. Septic abortion. N Engl J Med 1994;331(5):310–314.

[71] Snyder CC, Barton JR, Habli M et al. Severe sepsis and septic shock in pregnancy: Indications for delivery and maternal and perinatal outcomes. J Matern Fetal Neonatal Med 2013;26(5): 503–506.

[72] Society for Maternal-Fetal Medicine. Electronic address pso Plante LA, Pacheco LD et al. SMFM Consult Series #47: Sepsis during pregnancy and the puerperium. Am J Obstet Gynecol 2019;220(4):B2–B10.

[73] Kidson KM, Henderson WR, Hutcheon JA. Case Fatality and Adverse Outcomes Are Reduced in Pregnant Women With Severe Sepsis or Septic Shock Compared With Age-Matched Comorbid-Matched Nonpregnant Women. Crit Care Med 2018;46(11):1775–1782.

[74] Shankar-Hari MPG, Levey MM, Seymour CW et al. for the Sepsis Definitions Task Force. Developing a new definition and assessing new clinical criteria for septic shock. For the Third International Consensus Definitions for Sepsis and Septic Shock (Sepsis-3). JAMA 2016;318(8):775–787.

[75] Knaus WA, Sun X, Nystrom O et al. Evaluation of definitions for sepsis. Chest 1992;101(6): 1656–1662.

[76] Miller EC, Gallo M, Kulick ER et al. Infections and risk of peripartum stroke during delivery admissions. Stroke 2018;49(5):1129–1134.

[77] Metlay JP, Waterer GW, Long AC et al. Diagnosis and treatment of adults with community-acquired pneumonia. an official clinical practice guideline of the American thoracic society and infectious diseases society of America. Am J Respir Crit Care Med 2019;200(7):e45–e67.

[78] Ehsanipoor RM, Chung JH, Clock CA et al. A retrospective review of ampicillin-sulbactam and amoxicillin + clavulanate vs cefazolin/cephalexin and erythromycin in the setting of preterm premature rupture of membranes: Maternal and neonatal outcomes. Am J Obstet Gynecol 2008;198(5):e54–56.

[79] ACOG Committee Opinion. No. 753: Assessment and treatment of pregnant women with suspected or confirmed influenza. Obstet Gynecol 2018;132(4):e169–e173.

[80] Reed BD, Schibler KR, Deshmukh H et al. The impact of maternal antibiotics on neonatal disease. J Pediatr 2018;197(97–103):e103.

[81] Tang P, Wang J, Song Y. Characteristics and pregnancy outcomes of patients with severe pneumonia complicating pregnancy: A retrospective study of 12 cases and a literature review. BMC Pregnancy Childbirth 2018;18(1):434.

Mónica Centeno, Diogo Ayres-de-Campos

22 Thyroid Disease in Pregnancy

22.1 Introduction

Thyroid disease is the second most common endocrine disorder of pregnancy, after gestational diabetes. Pregnancy-induced hormonal changes have a marked impact on thyroid gland function. Even more importantly, thyroid dysfunction is associated with an increased risk of adverse obstetrical and perinatal outcomes [1–3].

Universal screening of thyroid gland dysfunction during pregnancy is a controversial subject [4, 5], but there is reasonable body of evidence on which to support the recommendation of early serum TSH testing in high-risk cases, such as when any of the following are present [6]:

1. Previous history of hypothyroidism/hyperthyroidism or current symptoms/ signs of thyroid dysfunction
2. Known thyroid antibody positivity or presence of a goiter
3. History of head and neck radiation or prior thyroid surgery
4. Type 1 diabetes or other autoimmune disorders
5. History of pregnancy loss, preterm delivery or infertility
6. Family history of autoimmune thyroid disease or thyroid dysfunction
7. Body mass index $\geq$ 40 Kg/m2
8. Current treatment with amiodarone or lithium, or recent administration of iodinated radiologic contrast
9. Residing in an area of known moderate to severe iodine insufficiency

22.2 Thyroid Physiology During Pregnancy

22.2.1 Maternal Thyroid Gland

Pregnant women have increased metabolic requirements, and thyroid hormones are heavily involved in the physiologic changes necessary for these needs to be met. The size of the thyroid gland increases between 10 and 40% during pregnancy, depending on previous iodine status of the population [6]. Similarly, thyroid hormone production increases by around 50%. Serum thyroxine-binding globulin (TBG) concentration roughly doubles during pregnancy, and there is a *circa* 50% increase in total triiodothyronine (T3) and tetraiodothyronine (T4) concentrations. Levels of the latter two hormones peak at approximately 16 to 20 weeks [7]. These modifications naturally require increased total daily iodine requirements.

https://doi.org/10.1515/9783110615258-022

Due to the structural similarity between human chorionic gonadotropin (hCG) and thyroid stimulating hormone (TSH), the rising level of hCG during the first trimester leads to a stimulation of TSH receptors, an increase in thyroid hormone production, and a subsequent suppression of TSH levels [8–12]. Increases in renal clearance of iodine, secondary to pregnancy-induced increased glomerular filtration rate, causes a reduction in circulating iodine, which constitutes an additional challenge for thyroid gland hormone production [11, 12].

During the first trimester, total T4 and T3 level are high, free T4 (fT4) and free T3 (fT3) levels are usually within the normal range or slightly increased, and TSH levels are low. Around 15% of healthy women during the first trimester of pregnancy have TSH levels below 0.4 mU/L [13]. This transient subclinical hyperthyroidism should be considered a normal physiological finding. Conditions associated with very high levels of HCG (i.e. multiple pregnancy, gestational trophoblastic disease) are likely to cause an even higher thyroid hormone production and suppression of TSH [14].

Because T4 measurements are conditioned by changing levels of thyroxin binding globulin and albumin, serum TSH is considered the most reliable measure of thyroid function in early pregnancy [15]. Total T4 (tT4) is a reliable marker for thyroid function only in late pregnancy [6]. According to the American Thyroid Association (ATA), normal serum TSH levels during pregnancy should be defined using population and trimester-specific based reference ranges. When these are not available, ATA guidelines recommend using general population values, reducing the lower limit of TSH by 0.4 mU/L and the upper limit by 0.5 mU/L. This corresponds to a normality range of around 0.1 to 4.0 mU/L during the first trimester, with a gradual return to non-pregnant ranges during the second and third trimesters [6, 16].

Accuracy of fT4 measurements during pregnancy varies significantly with the laboratory method used. Method-specific and trimester-specific reference ranges should also be used to measure fT4 levels. When these are unavailable, ATA suggests calculating the normality range by increasing non-pregnant limits by 50%, after 16 weeks of pregnancy. Before the 16th week of pregnancy, the upper reference range can be calculated by increasing the nonpregnant limit by 5% per week, beginning at week 7.

22.2.2 Fetal Thyroid Gland

The fetus starts to produce thyroid hormones from approximately the 12th week of gestation, but synthesis only becomes relevant after the 18–20th week and increases gradually until term [17]. Therefore, the fetus depends totally on maternal thyroid hormones during the first half of pregnancy. Fetal nervous system development is strongly mediated by thyroid hormones, and these hormones are involved in key processes such as neuronal migration, neuronal proliferation, axonal growth, dendritic branching and myelination [18]. For these reasons, thyroid function in early pregnancy can strongly affect future neurodevelopment.

22.3 Hypothyroidism

22.3.1 Definition

Hypothyroidism is a condition characterized by insufficient thyroid hormone production. It can be subclassified into primary hypothyroidism if the thyroid gland itself is the cause, or central hypothyroidism (secondary when there is decreased pituitary stimulus, tertiary if the etiology is hypothalamic) [19].

In pregnancy, maternal hypothyroidism is defined as the detection of an elevated TSH level, above the upper limit of a pregnancy-specific reference range. As referred to above, when these reference values are unavailable an upper limit of 4.0 mU/L can be used [6]. Depending on the severity of thyroid function abnormalities it can be classified as:

1. Overt primary hypothyroidism: Elevated TSH and decreased fT4 values
2. Subclinical hypothyroidism: Elevated TSH and normal fT4 values
3. Isolated hypothyroxinemia: Normal TSH and decreased fT4 values

22.3.2 Incidence

The incidence of overt hypothyroidism in pregnancy ranges between 0.3 and 0.5% of all pregnancies [20, 21]. Subclinical hypothyroidism is more frequent, affecting between 0.25 and 2.5% of pregnancies [21, 22]. The incidence of all types of hypothyroidism in patients with type 1 diabetes is much higher, affecting between 5 and 8% of all pregnant women [23].

22.3.3 Etiology

The most common cause of hypothyroidism worldwide is iodine deficiency. In iodine-rich countries the most common cause is autoimmune thyroiditis [24]. Other causes include previous thyroid surgery and treatment with radioactive iodine.

22.3.4 Clinical Manifestations

Although many patients are asymptomatic, manifestations are similar to those occurring in nonpregnant adults and include dry skin, generalized weakness, weight gain, cold intolerance, constipation, hair loss, intellectual slowness, edema, and voice changes [25]. As many of these symptoms are relatively common in normal pregnant women, clinical diagnosis can be more difficult.

22.3.5 Diagnosis

Because universal screening is not recommended by most scientific organizations, and because clinical manifestations are difficult to distinguish from those referred by normal pregnant women, the diagnosis of hypothyroidism in pregnancy relies heavily on early serum TSH screening in high risk women.

When serum TSH levels are above the upper limit of the reference range (or above 4.0 mU/L), serum fT4 levels should be measured. For TSH values above 2.5 mU/L it is also recommended to measure anti-thyroid peroxidase (anti-TPO) antibodies, as these have a closer association with adverse obstetric and perinatal outcome (see below).

Primary overt hypothyroidism is diagnosed when TSH levels are above the upper limit of the reference range (or above 4.0 mU/L) and fT4 are lower than the reference range, or when TSH levels are above 10 mU/L independently of fT4 levels.

Subclinical hypothyroidism is assumed when TSH levels are between 4 and 10 mU/L and fT4 levels are in the normal range [6]. With central hypothyroidism (secondary and tertiary), serum THS levels are low and fT4 levels are also decreased.

22.3.5.1 Hypothyroidism Diagnosed in Pregnancy

The ATA guidelines (B) recommend the following approach for management of thyroid dysfunction diagnosed in pregnancy (Figure 22.1): start levothyroxine treatment if TSH values > 10.0 mU/L, or if TSH values 4.0–10.0 mU/L and anti-TPO antibodies are positive. Consider levothyroxine treatment if TSH values between 2.5–4.0 mU/L and anti-TPO antibodies are positive or if TSH values between 4.0–10.0 mU/L, even if anti-TPO antibodies are negative. After delivery, levothyroxine can be discontinued if therapy was initiated during pregnancy and the dose is ≤50 mcg/day. Thyroid function should be evaluated 6 weeks post-partum [26].

22.3.6 Complications

Overt hypothyroidism in pregnancy is associated with increased risks of miscarriage (30%), hypertensive diseases of pregnancy (22%), placental abruption (3%), preterm delivery (20%), and perinatal mortality (12%) [27–30]. Children born of mothers with overt hypothyroidism have higher risks of neuropsychological and cognitive impairment [31], and have an 8 to 10 point decrease in intelligence scores, when compared to the general population [31].

The association between subclinical hypothyroidism and adverse pregnancy outcomes is much more subtle, and the risk magnitudes are lower than that of overt

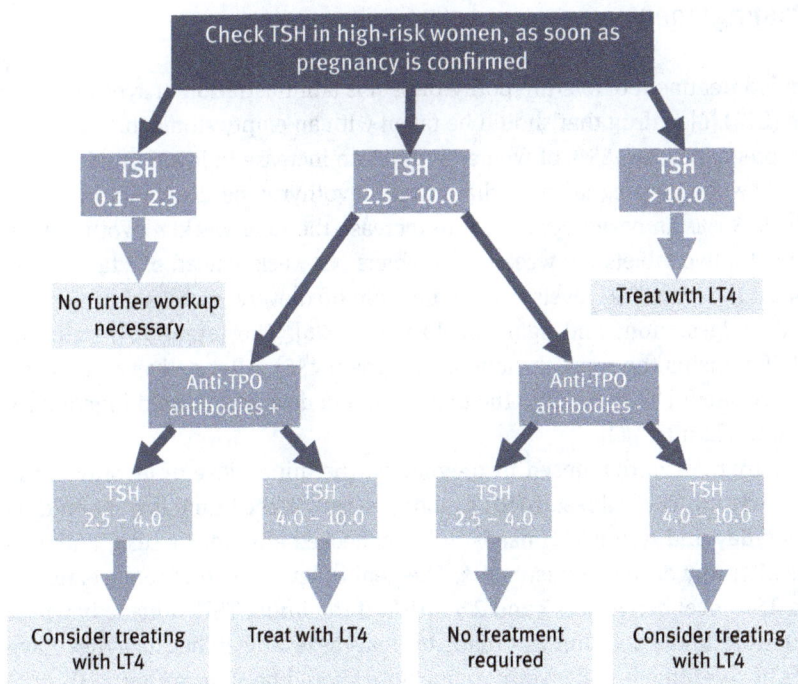

Figure 22.1: Management of thyroid dysfunction in pregnancy. Adapted from [6].

hypothyroidism. A recent systematic review and meta-analysis of observational studies shows that women with subclinical hypothyroidism have higher risks of pregnancy loss (RR = 2.01, 95% CI 1.66–2.44), placental abruption (RR = 2.14, 95% CI 1.23–3.7) and neonatal death (RR = 2.58, 95% CI 1.41–4.7), when compared with euthyroid women. The risks of preterm delivery and preeclampsia do not seem to be statistically different between the two populations [32]. Some studies suggest an association between subclinical hypothyroidism and impaired cognitive development in children [3, 31, 33, 34], but this association has not always been found. Interpretation of results is frequently limited by differences in TSH cut-off values and cognitive tests that were selected.

Measurement of anti-thyroid peroxidase (anti-TPO) antibodies appears to be useful in women with TSH values in the high normal range (i.e. 2.5–4.0 mU/L) and in those with subclinical hypothyroidism, as positive anti-TPO antibodies doubles the risk of early pregnancy loss [6, 35, 36]. The relation between these antibodies and increased risks of preterm delivery, placental abruption and perinatal death is still unclear [37–40].

22.3.7 Management

Recommended treatment of overt hypothyroidism is administration of synthetic levothyroxine (LT4) [6], a drug that should be taken with an empty stomach.

During pregnancy, 50–85% of women require an increase in levothyroxine dose [6, 30, 41]. As soon as pregnancy is diagnosed, levothyroxine dose should be increased by 25–30%. An easy approach is to increase the total weekly levothyroxine dose by an extra two tablets per week (i.e. 9 tablets per week instead of 7 tablets per week) [6, 42, 43]. Serum TSH levels need to be monitored every 4 weeks during pregnancy until midgestation, and again at 30 weeks [26]. The target TSH value of 0.5–2.5 mU/L remains the same throughout pregnancy [8]. After delivery, the levothyroxine dose should be reduced to the preconception dose and thyroid function rechecked 4–6 weeks after [43].

For hypothyroidism diagnosed in pregnancy, the initial dose of levothyroxine depends on existing TSH values: if TSH is above 4.0 mU/L the initial dose should be 100–150 mcg/day and serum TSH needs to be rechecked after four weeks, and also four weeks after any dosage adjustments. The goal of levothyroxine replacement is to obtain a TSH level between 0.5 and 2.5 mU/L. If the initial TSH value is between 2.6 and 4.0 mU/L and a decision was made to treat these women because they have anti-TPO antibodies, the initial levothyroxine dose should be 50 mcg/day.

22.4 Iodine Deficiency

Women have increased iodine requirements during pregnancy and lactation, due to the previously described increase in thyroid hormone production, renal iodine excretion, and fetal iodine requirements [8]. The World Health Organization (WHO) estimates that around 2 billion people are iodine deficient worldwide, and more than 20 million have adverse neurological sequelae secondary to *in utero* iodine deprivation. The resulting neurological handicap, also known as cretinism, affects 2–10% of the population in iodine deficient areas and causes mild mental handicap in a further 10–50% [44, 45].

Both WHO and ATA recommend that women during pregnancy and lactation should have a daily iodine intake of 250 mcg. There are also recommendations that it should not exceed 500 mcg [46]. Iodine is present in high concentrations in most fish, vegetables and dairy products. Some countries have implemented national strategies to iodinate flour, salt or water. Unfortunately, these strategies are difficult to implement in other parts of the world [44]. The benefits of generalized supplementation with potassium iodine during pregnancy have yet to be conclusive, but a recent meta-analysis showed that it improves some maternal thyroid indices and may benefit cognitive function in school-age children [47]. Iodine supplementation is strongly recommended in iodine-deficient areas, in women who do not include iodine-rich foods in their diet, and in those who do not have regular access to iodinated flour, salt or water.

22.5 Hyperthyroidism

22.5.1 Definition and Incidence

Hyperthyroidism is a thyroid dysfunction consequent to excessive production of thyroid hormones. The term thyrotoxicosis refers to increased amounts of thyroid hormones in circulation. Overt hyperthyroidism is defined by suppressed TSH levels and elevated fT4 levels. In pregnancy it has a prevalence of 0.1–0.4% [1, 48].

22.5.2 Etiology

Graves' disease, an autoimmune condition caused by antibodies that bind to TSH receptors, is the most common cause of clinical hyperthyroidism in pregnancy (85%) [1, 49]. An additional etiology is transient hCG-mediated hyperthyroidism (also known as gestational transient thyrotoxicosis). As described before, this is caused by circulating hCG activating TSH receptors, due to the structural similarity between the two, and it affects 1–5% of all pregnancies [9]. Other less common causes of hyperthyroidism include toxic multinodular goiter, toxic adenoma and thyroiditis.

22.5.3 Clinical Manifestations

Symptoms of hyperthyroidism mimic those of the hypermetabolic state of pregnancy, and include palpitations, excessive sweating, heat intolerance, anxiety, insomnia, weight loss and tremors. Physical examination may show tachycardia, diaphoresis, hyperreflexia, exophthalmos, diffuse goiter or pretibial myxedema.

22.5.4 Diagnosis

Women with symptoms or signs of hyperthyroidism should be evaluated with serum TSH and fT4 levels [9, 17]. Overt hyperthyroidism is diagnosed when TSH levels are < 0.1 mU/L and fT4 levels are above the upper limit of pregnancy reference values (see above). Subclinical hyperthyroidism is diagnosed when TSH levels are

< 0.1 mU/L and serum fT4 are in the normal range. The diagnosis of Graves' disease is based on the clinical history of goiter or hyperthyroidism symptoms occurring before pregnancy, and on the presence of TSH receptor antibodies (TRAbs), characteristic of this disease.

22.5.5 Complications

Uncontrolled hyperthyroidism in pregnancy is associated with increased risks of abortion, pregnancy-induced hypertension, prematurity, fetal grow restriction, stillbirth, and serious maternal complications such as thyroid storm and congestive heart failure [50–52].

Circulating TRAbs cross the placenta and can lead to fetal hyperthyroidism [53]. Persistent maternal TRAb levels > 5 IU/L (approximately three times the upper limit of normality) in the latter half of pregnancy can predict neonatal hyperthyroidism with a 100% sensitivity and 43% specificity [50, 53].

22.5.6 Management

Pregnant women with hyperthyroidism require management by a multidisciplinary team, including endocrinologists, obstetricians and neonatologists. TSH, fT4 and tT4 levels need to be monitored every 4 weeks in pregnancy [26], and TRAb levels should be checked when pregnancy is confirmed, at 18–22 weeks, and again at 30–34 weeks, to evaluate the need for postnatal monitoring [8]. The goal of treatment is to maintain mild maternal hyperthyroidism levels, while avoiding fetal hypothyroidism [54].

Medical treatment is recommended in women with overt hyperthyroidism due to Graves' disease, toxic adenoma, and toxic multinodular goiter [42]. The aim is to use the lowest possible dose of antithyroid drugs, so that maternal and fetal adverse effects can be minimised. This dose should be adjusted to maintain maternal serum fT4 in the upper limit of the normality range [55].

Methimazole and propylthiouracil are the two most commonly used antithyroid drugs in pregnancy. Both drugs cross the placenta and can have potential implications in fetal development. Risks include fetal malformations, fetal goiter and transient hypothyroidism [2]. Propylthiouracil is the preferred drug before 16 weeks, as methimazole is associated with an increased risk of congenital anomalies [8, 26]. After 16 weeks of pregnancy both drugs can be used. Antithyroid drugs cause maternal adverse effects in 3 to 5% of women, with allergic reactions being the most common. More severe side effects are rare agranulocytosis (0.15%), and liver failure (<1%) [56, 57]. Short-term treatment with beta-blockers (propranolol or metoprolol) can be used to control troublesome symptoms such as palpitations, heat intolerance, anxiety, insomnia, and tremors.

Thyroidectomy is rarely needed to treat hyperthyroidism in pregnancy, and should be reserved for patients who do not respond to large doses of antithyroid drugs or cannot tolerate them, because of side effects. If necessary, it should preferably be performed during the second trimester [58]. Radioactive iodine ablation is contraindicated during pregnancy.

Subclinical hyperthyroidism and gestational thyrotoxicosis do not require treatment during pregnancy, however, monitoring of thyroid function every 4 to 6 weeks should be considered, to confirm the diagnosis and evolution of the disease.

22.5.7 Management of Fetal and Neonatal Effects

Offspring of mothers with Graves' disease have a 1–5% risk of fetal and neonatal hyperthyroidism due to transplacental transfer of TRAbs. The risk may be even higher when mothers have high TRAb levels. When pregnant women are taking antithyroid drugs, neonates can also be born with hypothyroidism. Some of the potential effects of fetal hyperthyroidism can be detected on ultrasound: tachycardia, fetal growth restriction, fetal goiter, congestive heart failure and hydrops [26]. Neonatologists need to be informed of antithyroid drugs taken by the mother and of existing TRAb levels, as the neonate is likely to require thyroid function monitoring [55].

22.6 Thyroid Nodules

In countries with mild to moderate iodine deficiency, the prevalence of thyroid nodules during pregnancy varies between 3 and 21% [59–61]. Personal and family history of benign or malignant thyroid disease caries an important weight in risk assessment of these cases. Physical examination should include inspection and palpation of the thyroid gland and neck [62]. Additional workup usually involves thyroid ultrasound and TSH measurement. Fine-needle aspiration has the same clinical indications as in non-pregnant patients, and surgery may be indicated when there is rapid growth of the nodule, compression of adjacent organs or suspicious cytologic findings. As occurs with all surgical interventions in pregnancy, it should preferably be performed in the second trimester [63].

22.7 Thyroid Cancer

Thyroid cancer occurs in 1/1000 pregnant women with a palpable thyroid nodule, and 5–10% of all thyroid tumors are malignant. Management of this situation requires a multidisciplinary team, involving thyroid surgeons, endocrinologists and obstetricians. Most cases of thyroid cancer are well differentiated and have an indolent course [64], so surgical treatment can usually be delayed until after delivery. In rare circumstances, when rapid growth occurs or when metastases are detected, surgery is indicated during pregnancy, and again the second trimester is the safest period. The prognosis of thyroid cancer does not seem to be greatly influenced by the advent of pregnancy [65].

References

[1]   Lazarus JH. Thyroid function in pregnancy. Br Med Bull 2011;137–148.
[2]   Abalovich M, Amino N, Barbour LA et al. Management of thyroid dysfunction during pregnancy and postpartum: an endocrine society clinical practice guideline. J Clin Endocrinol Metab 2007;92(Suppl):s1–47.
[3]   Fan X, Wu L. the impact of thyroid abnormalities during pregnancy on subsequent neuropsychological development of the offspring: a meta-analiysis. J Matern Fetal Neonatal Med 2016;29:3971–3976.
[4]   Lazarus JH, Bestwick JP, Shannon S et al. Antenatal thyroid screening and childhood cognitive function. N Engl J Med 2012;366:493.
[5]   Negro R, Schwartz A, Gismondi R et al. Universal screening versus case finding for detection and treatment of thyroid hormonal dysfunction during pregnancy. J Clin Endocrinol Metal 2010;95:1699.
[6]   Alexander EK, Pearce EN, Brent GA, Brown RS, Chen H, Dousiou C et al. Guidelines of the American thyroid association for the diagnosis and management of thyroid disease during pregnancy and postpartum. Thyroid 2017;27:315–389.
[7]   Weeke J, Dybkjaer L, Granline K et al. A longitudinal study of serum TSH, and total and free iodothyronines during normal pregnancy. Acta Endocrinol (Copenh) 1982;101(4):531–537.
[8]   Smith A, Eccles-Smith J, Lust K. Thyroid disorders in pregnancy and postpartum. Aust Prescr 2017;41:214–219.
[9]   Glinoer D. The regulation of thyroid function in pregnancy: pathways of endocrine adaptation from physiology to pathology. Endocr Rev 1997;18(3):404–433.
[10]   Teng W, Shan Z, Patil-Sisoda K, Cooper DS. Hypothyroidism in pregnancy. Lancet Diabetes Endocrinol 2013;1:228–237.
[11]   Yazbeck CF, Sullivan SD. Thyroid disorders during pregnancy. Med Clin N Am 2012;96: 235–256.
[12]   Fantz CR, Daggo-Jack S, Ladenson JH, Gronowski AM. Thyroid function during pregnancy. Clin Chem 1999;45:2250–2258.
[13]   Soldin OP, Tractenberg RE, Hollowell JG, Jonklaas J, Janicic N, Soldin SJ. Trimester-specific changes in maternal thyroid hormone, thyrotropin, and thyroglobulin concentrations during gestation: trends and associations across trimesters in iodine sufficiency. Thyroid 2004;14 (12):1084–1090.
[14]   Sapin R, D'Herbomez M, Schilienger JL. Free thyroxine measured with equilibrium dialysis and nine immunoassays decreases in late pregnancy. Clin Lab 2004;50:581–584.
[15]   Glinoer D, Spencer CA. Serum TSH determinations in pregnancy: how, when nd why?. Nat Rev Endocrinol 2010;6:526–529.
[16]   Lambert-Messerlian G, McClain M, Haddow JE et al. First and second-trimester thyroid hormone reference data in pregnant woman: a FASTER (First and Second- Trimester

Evaluation of Risk for aneuploidy). Research consortium study. Am J Obstet Gynecol 2008;199:62 e1.

[17] Burrow GN, Fisher DA, Larsen PR. Maternal and fetal thyroid function. N Engl J Med 1994;331: 1072–1078.

[18] Williams GR. Neurodevelopmental and neurophysiological actions of thyroid hormone. J Neuroendocrinol 2008;20:784–794.

[19] Brenta G, Vaisman M, Sgarbi JA et al. Clinical practice guidelines for the management of hypothyroidism. Arq Bras Endocrinol Metabol 2013;57:265–291.

[20] Montoro MN. Management of hypothyroidism during pregnancy. Clin Obstet Gynecol 1997;40:65–80.

[21] Klein RZ, Haddow JE, Faix JD et al. Prevalence of thyroid deficiency in pregnant women. Clin Endocrinol 1991;35:41–46.

[22] Allan WC, Haddow JE, Palomaki GE et al. Maternal thyroid deficiency and pregnancy complications; implications for population screening. J Med Screen 2000;7:127.

[23] Alvarez-Marfany M, Roman SH, Drexler AJ, Robertson C, Stagnaro-Green A. Long-term prospective study of postpartum thyroid dysfunction in women with insulin dependent diabetes mellitus. J Clin Endocrinol Metab 1994;79:10–16.

[24] Ban Y, Greenberg DA, Davies TF, Jacobson E, Conception E, Tomer Y. Linkage analysis of thyroid antibody production: evidence for shared susceptibility to clinical autoimmune thyroid disease. J Clin Endocrinol Metabol 2008;93:3589–3596.

[25] Rakel RE. Textbook of Family Practice. 6th ed. Philadelphia: WB Saunders;2002.

[26] Kalra B, Sawhney K, Kalra S. Management of thyroid disorders in pregnancy: recommendations made simple. J Pak Med 2017;67(9):1452–1455.

[27] Reid SM, Middleton P, Cossich MC, Crowther CA. Interventions for clinical and subclinical hypothyroidism in pregnancy. Cochrane Database Syst Rev 2010;CD007752.

[28] Leung AS, Millar LK, Koonings PP, Montoro M, Mestman JH. Perinatal outcome in hypothyroid pregnancies. Obstet Gynecol 1993;81:349–353.

[29] Davis LE, Leveno KJ, Cunningham FG. Hypothyroidism complicating pregnancy. Obstet Gynecol 1988;72:108–112.

[30] Abalovich M, Gutierrez S, Alcaraz G, Maccallini G, Garcia A, Levalle O. Overt and subclinical hypothyroidism complicating pregnancy. Thyroid 2002 Jan;12(1):63–68.

[31] Haddow JE, Palomaki GE, Allan WC et al. Maternal thyroid deficiency during pregnancy and subsequent neuropsychological development of the child. N Engl J Med 1999;341:549.

[32] Maraka S, Ospina NM, O'Keeffe D et al. Subclinical hypothyroidism in pregnancy: a systematic review and meta-analysis. Thyroid 2016;26:580.

[33] Li Y, Shan Z, Teng W et al. Neurologic development affect neuropsychological development of their children at 25–30 months. Clin Endocrinol (Oxf) 2010;72:825.

[34] Smit BJ, Kok JH, Vulsma T et al. Neurologic development of thew newborn and young child in relation to maternal thyroid function. Acta Paediatr 2000;89:291.

[35] Liu H, Shan Z, Li C et al. Maternal subclinicv hypothyroidism, thyroid autoimmunity, and the risk of miscarriage: a prospective cohort study. Thyroid 2014;24:1642.

[36] Chen L, Hu R. Thyroid autoimmunity and miscarriage: a meta-analysis. Clin Endocrinol 2011;74:513–519.

[37] Abbassi-Ghanavati M, Casey BM, Spong CY, McIntire DD, Halvorson LM, Cunningam FG. Pregnancy outcomes in women with thyroid peroxidase antibodies. Obstet Gynecol 2010;116: 381–386.

[38] Wasserman EE, Nelson K, Rose NR, Eaton H, Pillion JP et al. Maternal thyroid autoantibodies during the third trimester and hearing deficits in children: an epidemiologic assessment. Am J Epidemiol 2008;167:701–710.

[39] Haddow JE, Cleary-Goldman J, Mc Clain MR et al. First and second trimester risk of aneuploidy (FaSTER) research consortium. Thyroperoxidase and thyroglobulin antibodies in early pregnancy and preterm delivery. Obstet Gynecol 2010;116:58–62.

[40] Negro R, Schwartz A, Gismondi R, Tinelli A, Mangieri T, Stagnaro-Green A. Thyroid antibody positivity in first trimester of pregnancy is associated with negative pregnancy outcomes. J Clin Endocrinol Metab 2011;96:E920–24.

[41] Mandel SJ, Larsen PR, Seely EW, Brent GA. Increased need for thyroxine during pregnancy in women with primary hypothyroidism. N Eng J Med 1990;323:91–96.

[42] Alexander EK, Marqusse E, Lawrence J, Jarolim P, Fischer GA, Larsen PR. Timing and magnitude of increases in levothyroxine requirements during pregnancy in women with hypothyroidism. N Engl J Med 2004;351:241–249.

[43] Yassa L, Narqusse E, Fawcett R, Alexander EK. Thyroid hormone early adjustment in pregnancy (the THERAPY) trial. J Clini Endocrinol Metab 2010;95:3234–3241.

[44] Girling J. Review Thyroid disease in pregnancy. RCOG 2008;10:237–243.

[45] World Health Organization. WHO Global Database on iodine deficiency www.who.int/vmnis/iodine/data/en/

[46] Shi X, Han C, Li C et al. Optimal and safe upper limits of iodine intake for early pregnancy in iodine-sufficient regions: a cross-sectional study of 7190 pregnant woman in Chin. J Clin Endocrinol Metab 2015Apr;10084:1630–1638.

[47] Taylor PN, Okosieme OE, Dayan CM, Lazarus JH. Therapy of endocrine disease: impact of iodine supplementation in mild-to-moderate iodine deficiency: systematic review and meta-analysis. Eur J Endocrinol 2013;170:R1–15.

[48] Krassas GE, Poppe K, Glinoer D. Thyroid function and human reproductive health. Endocr Rev 2010;31:702.

[49] Coopee DS, Laurberg P. Hyperthyroidism in pregnancy. Lancet Diabetes Endocrinol 2013 Nov;1(3):238–249.

[50] Davis LE, Lucas MJ, Hankins GD, Roark ML, Cunniningham FG. Thyrotoxicosis complicating pregnancy. Am J Obstet Gynecol 1989;160:63–70.

[51] Laurberg P, Bournaud C, Karmisholt J, Orgiazzi J. Management of Graves' hyperthyroidism in pregnancy: focus on both maternal and foetal thyroid function, and caution against surgical thyroidectomy in pregnancy. Eur J Endocrinol 2009;160:1–8.

[52] Abeillon-du Payrat J, Chikh K, Bossard N et al. Predictive value of maternal second-generation thyroids-binding inhibitory immunoglobulin assay for neonatal autoimmune hyperthyroidism. Eur J Endocrinol 2014;171:451–460.

[53] Nguyen C, Sasso E, Barton L, Mestman J. Graves' hyperthyroidism in pregnancy: a clinical review. Clin Diab and Endocrinol 2018;4:4.

[54] Momotani N, Noh J, Oyanagi H, Ishikawa N, Ito K. Antithyroid drug therapy for Graves' disease during pregnancy. Optimal regimen for fetal thyroid status. N Eng J Med 1986;315(1):24–28.

[55] Earl R, Crowther CA, Middleton P. Interventions for hyperthyroidism pre-pregnancy and during pregnancy. Cochrane Database Syst Rev 2013;CD008633.

[56] Nakamura H, Miyauchi A, Miyawaki N, Imagawa J. Analysis of 754 cases of antithyroid drug-induced agranulocytosis over 30 years in Japan. J Clin Endocrinol Metab 2013;98–4776–83.

[57] Watanabe N, Narimatsu H, Noh JY et al. Antithyroid drug-induced hematopoietic damage: a retroapective cohort study of agranulocytosis and pancytopenia involving 50,385 patients with Graves' disease. J Clin Endocrinol Metab 2013;98–4776–53.

[58] Patil-ssisodia K, Mestman JH. Graves hyperthyroidism and pregnancy: a clinical update. Endocr Pract 2010;16:118–129.

[59] Glinoer D, Soto MF, Bourbdoux P et al. Pregnancy in patients with mild thyroid abnormalities: maternal and neonatal repercussions. J Clin Endocrinol Metab 1991;73:421–427.

[60] Struve CW, Haupt S, Ohlen S. Influence of frequency of previous pregnancies on the prevalence of thyroid nodules in women without clinical evidence of thyroid disease. Thyroid 1993;3:7–9.

[61] Kung AW, Chau MT, Lao TT, Tam SC, Low LC. The effect of pregnancy on the prevalence of thyroid nodule formation. J Clin Endocrinol Metab 2002;87:1010–1014.

[62] Tan GH, Gharib H, Reading CC. Solitary thyroid nodule. Comparison between palpation and ultrasonography. Arch Intern Med 1995;155:2418–2423.

[63] Tan GH, Gharib H, Goellner JR, Van Heerden JA, Bahn RS. Management of thyroid nodules in pregnancy. Arch Intern Med 1996;156:2317–2320.

[64] ACOG practice bulletin 148. Thyroid disease in pregnancy. 2015.

[65] Moosa M, Mazzaferri EL. Outcome of differentiated thyroid cancer diagnosed in pregnant women. J Clin Endocrinol Metab 1997 Sep;82(9):2862–2866.

Sawyer Huget-Penner, Denice S. Feig

23 Preexisting Diabetes in Pregnancy

23.1 Introduction

The prevalence of preexisting diabetes (type 1 and type 2 diabetes diagnosed prior to pregnancy) is increasing as more women of reproductive age are being diagnosed with diabetes [1]. In Ontario, Canada, the age-adjusted rate of preexisting diabetes in pregnancy doubled from 1996 to 2010 [1]. This is primarily due to the younger age of onset of type 2 diabetes and the rise in maternal age and obesity [1, 2]. Women with preexisting diabetes in pregnancy have increased pregnancy complications, including preeclampsia, congenital malformations, large-for-gestational age neonates, perinatal mortality, preterm birth and C-section deliveries, as well as maternal complications such as worsening retinopathy and nephropathy [1, 3–7]. Given the increasing frequency of preexisting diabetes in pregnancy and the associated risks, it is important to understand the effect of preexisting diabetes on pregnancy outcomes and interventions that have been shown to improve outcomes.

23.2 Maternal Risks of Preexisting Diabetes in Pregnancy

Preexisting diabetes in pregnancy increases the risk of developing hypertension in pregnancy, preeclampsia and worsening of diabetic microvascular complications [3]. Hypertension may already be present prior to pregnancy or may develop during pregnancy [8, 9]. Chronic hypertension is diagnosed prepregnancy or prior to 20 weeks of gestation [10]. Gestational hypertension is elevated blood pressure first diagnosed after 20 weeks of gestation [10]. Please refer to Chapter 4 on chronic hypertension for more details.

One study looking at 100 pregnancies in women with type 2 diabetes and 100 pregnancies in women with type 1 diabetes showed that the incidence of hypertension in pregnancy was similar in the two groups, with 41% of those with type 2 diabetes and 45% of those with type 1 diabetes having hypertension in pregnancy [8]. However, it was more likely to be chronic hypertension in the type 2 diabetes patients, compared to gestational hypertension (i.e., induced by pregnancy) in type 1 diabetes patients [8]. In comparison, the baseline risk of gestational hypertension is about 17% of healthy nulliparous women [11]. The major maternal risk of hypertension in pregnancy is the increased risk of preeclampsia [9]; in addition, severe hypertension puts women at risk of hemorrhagic stroke in pregnancy [12].

https://doi.org/10.1515/9783110615258-023

Women with preexisting diabetes have an increased risk of developing pre-eclampsia. Preeclampsia is diagnosed when there is new-onset hypertension with proteinuria or end-organ dysfunction [10]. It can also be superimposed on chronic hypertension [10]. One meta-analysis showed that women with preexisting diabetes have a 3.7 times higher risk of developing preeclampsia compared to nondiabetic women [13]. While both women with types 1 and 2 diabetes have an increased risk of preeclampsia, women with type 1 diabetes have a higher risk [8]. In one study, 19% of those with type 1 diabetes compared to 7% of those with type 2 diabetes developed preeclampsia [8]. It has also been shown that the risk in type 1 diabetes is similar in nulliparous and multiparous women which is unlike the general population where the risk of preeclampsia is higher in nulliparous women [14]. Women with type 1 diabetes who have preeclampsia or gestational hypertension also have an increased risk of severe diabetic retinopathy later in life [15].

Patients with preexisting diabetes are also at risk of microvascular complications including retinopathy, neuropathy, and nephropathy and these can worsen in pregnancy [16]. An analysis of the DCCT trial, which looked at patients with type 1 diabetes and intensive (average HbA1c 7.2%) versus conventional therapy (average HbA1c 9.1%), all of whom had intensive therapy once pregnant, showed that pregnant women with type 1 diabetes had a 1.63-fold greater risk of worsening retinopathy in the intensive group compared to nonpregnant women, but a 2.48-fold greater risk in the conventional group during pregnancy compared to nonpregnant women [16, 17]. This increased risk persisted for as long as 12 months post-partum [16]. Despite this transient worsening of retinopathy in pregnancy, at the end of the DCCT trial the mean levels of retinopathy were the same in those who had become pregnant compared to those who had not [16].

A prospective cohort study of 155 women with preexisting diabetes showed an increased risk of retinopathy with worsening progression if they had a higher HbA1c at baseline as well as a larger magnitude of improvement of glucose control in the first trimester [18]. It was hypothesized that the increased risk was either due to the hyperglycemia itself or the rapid improvement in glycemic control in pregnancy [18]. Progression of retinopathy was seen in 10.3% of the patients with no baseline retinopathy, 21.1% of those with microaneurysms only, 18.8% of those with mild nonproliferative retinopathy, and 54.8% of those with moderate-to-severe nonproliferative retinopathy [18]. Proliferative retinopathy occurred in 6.3% of those with mild baseline retinopathy and 29% with moderate-to-severe retinopathy [18]. Having had diabetes for over 15 years, having poor glycemic control and having hypertension are all risk factors for progression of retinopathy in pregnancy [19, 20].

Retinopathy is typically treated with laser photocoagulation and with anti-vascular endothelial growth factor (anti-VEGF); however, anti-VEGF therapy may not be safe in pregnancy as it is not known if it crosses the placenta [3]. Treatment of severe nonproliferative retinopathy or early proliferative retinopathy is possible during pregnancy; however, photocoagulation done prior to pregnancy may better protect against progression during pregnancy [19]. Visual impairment in pregnancy can be prevented with aggressive photocoagulation treatment [19, 20]. There does not seem to be a risk of worsening retinopathy or vision loss in type 1 diabetes patients with the Valsalva that occurs during vaginal delivery and an active second stage of labor [21].

Women with preexisting diabetes and albuminuria may have a transient increase in albuminuria in pregnancy [22, 23]. If their kidney function is normal prepregnancy, pregnancy does not appear to have any long-term impact on kidney function or survival in those with microalbuminuria, especially if they have good glucose and blood pressure control in pregnancy [22–24]. There is however an increased risk of preeclampsia in women with albuminuria and/or decreased renal function [25]. As well, those with a marked decrease in renal function prepregnancy can have progression of nephropathy through pregnancy [26, 27]. One study of 67 women and 82 pregnancies in which the women had a baseline Cr >124 µmol/L showed that 43% had further loss of renal function and 10% progressed to end-stage renal disease [26]. Another study in which there were 11 patients with diabetic nephropathy of moderate to severe renal dysfunction (Cr >124 µmol/L at baseline) showed that 27% had stable renal function, 27% had transient worsening and 45% had a permanent decline [27]. Overall, long-term data is limited in this high-risk group.

23.3 Neonatal Risks of Preexisting Diabetes in Pregnancy

Pre-existing diabetes in pregnancy increases the risk of congenital malformations, preterm delivery, large for gestational age infants, neonatal hypoglycemia, cesarean section (C-section) delivery, and perinatal mortality.

Preexisting diabetes increases the risk of both major and minor congenital malformations. The most common major malformations in women with diabetes are cardiac but can also include anencephaly, urogenital anomalies, and neural tube defects [28]. Minor malformations reported in patients with type 1 diabetes include hypospadias, vertebral anomalies, and club foot [28]. Major malformations have been shown to have a 2- to 3-fold increased incidence in patients with type 1 diabetes compared to the general population and have been reported at 13% of type 1 diabetes pregnancies [28–30]. Hyperglycemia is teratogenic; the higher the HbA1c is in the first trimester, the higher the incidence of congenital malformations [28–30]. One study showed congenital malformations in 6.3% of those with HbA1c 4.0–6.0%, 6.4% in those with HbA1c 6.1–7% and 12.9% in those with HbA1c >7% [28]. Major malformations were the leading cause of neonatal death in one study, being responsible for 10 out of 36 neonatal deaths in 5,089 type 1 diabetes pregnancies [29]. Type 2 diabetes also has an increased risk of congenital anomalies [31]. Again, the higher the initial glucose and HbA1c, the more likely the chance of both major and minor anomalies [31]. There is also a higher likelihood of a baby having multiple organ systems involved the higher the initial glucose levels are [31]. For every 1% decrease in HbA1c there is a decrease in the risk of congenital malformations [32].

The risk of preterm delivery is increased in diabetic pregnancies. Preterm deliveries occur before 37 weeks of gestation and very preterm delivery occurs before 32 weeks of gestation [29]. One population-based study noted that 21% of those born to type 1 diabetes patients were born at <37 weeks and 2.3% were born <32 weeks compared to 5.1% and 0.7% of controls respectively [29]. In another prospective cohort study of pregnant patients with type 1 diabetes, 32.3% had a spontaneous preterm delivery and 20.4% had an induced delivery before 37 weeks [28]. The main reasons for early induction were preeclampsia, fetal distress, and macrosomia [28]. The increased risk of very preterm deliveries also increases morbidity in offspring, such as respiratory distress syndrome, hyperbilirubinemia, and asphyxia [28, 29].

Neonatal hypoglycemia is not uncommon in newborns of mothers with diabetes. This is thought to be from maternal hyperglycemia during pregnancy and at the time of labor and delivery crossing the placenta and resulting in increased fetal insulin secretion [33, 34]. A retrospective study of postpartum women with type 1 and type 2 diabetes reported a neonatal hypoglycemia rate (neonatal glucose <2.2 mmol/L) in 69% of newborns [34]. There was a correlation with maternal glucose >6.5 mmol/L at time of delivery [34]. In the Continuous Glucose Monitoring in Type 1 Diabetes Pregnancy Trial (CONCEPTt), neonatal hypoglycemia was reported in 25.3% of newborns and was higher in those whose mothers had higher second (6.6% vs 6.2%) and third trimester (6.7% vs 6.3%) HbA1cs and lower continuous glucose monitor time-in-range (46% vs 53%) [33].

There is an 8-fold increased risk of fetal macrosomia in type 1 diabetes patients [29]. One population-based study noted a 31% risk of large for gestational age infants compared to 3.6% of controls [29]. Another prospective cohort study showed that 52.5% of infants born to type 1 diabetes patients had macrosomia, with 28.4% being severely macrosomic [28]. Those with a mean HbA1c of 6.4% in pregnancy had a significantly higher likelihood of macrosomia compared to those with an average HbA1c of 6% [28]. In women with type 2 diabetes, studies have reported the rate of large for gestational age infants (birth weight >90th percentile) to be between 17% and 56% and the rate of infants with a birth weight >4,500 g to be 8% [35, 36].

C-section rates are increased in those with preexisting diabetes and have been shown to have an increased odds ratio of 5.31 compared to the general population [29]. One population study showed a C-section rate of 46% in patients with type 1 diabetes compared to 12% in controls [29]. Fetal distress was 3 times more common in this population and often the indication for C-section [29]. Another cohort study reported a 44.3% rate of C-section deliveries which was close to a 4-fold increase risk compared to controls [28]. The main indications were fetal distress, preeclampsia, macrosomia, and breech presentation [28].

There is an increase in perinatal mortality in people with preexisting diabetes with perinatal mortality including stillbirth and mortality within the first 28 days of life [28, 29]. It has been reported at a 2–2.8% rate in those with type 1 diabetes, which is about a 4-time higher risk than controls [28, 29, 37]. The incidence has not been shown to be different between those with type 1 diabetes and those with type 2 diabetes [37]. Stillbirth alone has been reported at 1.4% in those with preexisting diabetes, and this is significantly higher at all gestations >32 weeks compared to controls [38]. Increased HbA1c preconception >6.6% and third trimester HbA1c >6.1% have been shown to be independently associated with an increased risk of fetal and newborn death [32, 37].

23.4 Management of Preexisting Diabetes in Pregnancy

23.4.1 Preconception Management

Excellent glycemic control preconception and during pregnancy improves both maternal and fetal outcomes and decreases the risks noted above. It is important to discuss with women the importance of optimal control before proceeding with pregnancy planning. One meta-analysis showed that preconception care for those with preexisting diabetes resulted in a relative risk reduction of congenital malformations of 25% with a NNT of 17 [39]. The American Diabetes Association recommends aiming for an HbA1c of <6.5% preconception and the Canadian Diabetes Association recommends aiming for a HbA1c ≤7.0% or ≤6.5% if it can be safely achieved [3, 40]. It is also recommended that women take a multivitamin with 1 mg of folic acid starting at least 3 months prior to conception to decrease the risk of congenital anomalies, and stop any medications that may be teratogenic, including ACE inhibitors, ARBs, and statins, and certain diabetes agents such as SGLT2 inhibitors, GLP-1 agonists, and DPP-IV inhibitors [3]. Women should also have an ophthalmologic assessment prior to conception [3]. A multidisciplinary approach and specific pre-pregnancy care programs have been shown to improve outcomes, decrease congenital anomalies, and improve preconception HbA1c levels [41, 42]. Once pregnant, a focused diabetes in pregnancy clinic, in which a multidisciplinary approach is used (diabetes educators, dieticians, endocrinologists, and obstetricians), is also recommended to improve outcomes [3].

23.4.2 Pregnancy Management

In pregnancy it is important for women to have tight glycemic control to improve outcomes and decrease the risks of malformations, perinatal death, macrosomia, neonatal hypoglycemia, preeclampsia, and C-section. It is recommended that women maintain an HbA1c <6.5% throughout pregnancy [3]. If possible, an HbA1c of ≤6.1% should be targeted by the third trimester as an HbA1c >6.1% has been shown to increase the risk of stillbirth [37]. The optimal preprandial and postprandial blood glucose levels for women with preexisting diabetes are not known as there have not been any randomized controlled studies. Therefore, the mean blood glucose in those without diabetes plus 2 standard deviations is what is currently recommended [3, 43]. Both the Canadian Diabetes Association and the American Diabetes Association recommend fasting and preprandial glucose levels of ≤ 5.3 mmol/L, 1 h postprandial glucose levels of ≤7.8 mmol/L and 2 h postprandial glucose levels of ≤6.7 mmol/L [3, 40]. However, for those women with preexisting diabetes using continuous glucose monitoring, an international panel of experts have recommended that women aim for a target range of 3.5–7.8 mmol/L for >70% of the time, with <25% of the time spent above this target, and <4% spent below this target [44].

Glucose in pregnancy is monitored by SMBG (self-monitoring of blood glucose). This can be done using a glucometer. There is also the option to use continuous glucose monitors (CGMs) or flash glucose monitors. The flash glucose monitors are approved for use in pregnancy in Europe but have not been approved for use in Canada or the USA. One study looked at the accuracy of the FreeStyle Libre flash glucometer system in pregnancy in which 74 women with type 1 diabetes ($n = 24$), type 2 diabetes ($N = 11$), or gestational diabetes ($N = 39$) were given masked sensors to wear for 14 days and the results were compared to SMBG values done at least 4 times per day [45]. There was good agreement in the results of the flash glucometer and the SMBG results with clinical accuracy of 88.1%–99.8% with a mean absolute difference (MARD) of 11.8% [45]. The use of CGMs in women with type 1 diabetes has been shown to improve maternal and neonatal outcomes [46, 47]. The Continuous Glucose Monitoring in Women with Type 1 Diabetes in Pregnancy (CONCEPTT trial) randomized 325 women to a CGM or SMBG testing [46]. Those who used CGM in pregnancy had more glucose readings in target, less hyperglycemia, lower large for gestational age (LGA) infants, less NICU admissions >24 h, and less neonatal hypoglycemia [46].

Treatment for preexisting diabetes in pregnancy is typically done with insulin therapy. This can be done with basal-bolus multiple daily injections (MDI) or with continuous subcutaneous insulin infusion (CSII) with an insulin pump. CSII therapy has not been shown to be superior to MDI therapy in pregnancy [48]. The CONCEPTT trial noted that those on MDI actually had better outcomes with lower HbA1c levels, rates of gestational hypertension, neonatal hypoglycemia, and NICU admissions and therefore it is possible that MDI may be the preferred management in pregnancy [46, 49]. This study randomized participants to CGM, but the participants chose the mode of insulin delivery and therefore there may be cofounders to explain the difference in outcome between MDI and CSII in the CONCEPTT trial.

Overall, regular short-acting insulin as well as rapid insulins (lispro and aspart) are felt to be safe in pregnancy [3]. One study of 635 pregnant women with type 1, type 2, or gestational diabetes assessed both lispro and regular insulin with no difference in maternal or fetal outcomes, although those using lispro had a lower predelivery HbA1c and had improved patient satisfaction [50]. Lispro has been shown to have less severe hypoglycemia than regular insulin during pregnancy [51, 52]. Another meta-analysis of 24 studies concluded that aspart and lispro were safe in pregnancy but lispro was shown to possibly result in a higher birth weight and increased rates of LGA [52]. Lispro has not been shown to cross the placenta except at doses above 50 units, and aspart has not been looked at for placental transfer [53]. For basal insulin, NPH, glargine, and detemir can all be used with no increase in poor outcomes [3, 52, 54]. In one randomized controlled trial, there was less maternal hypoglycemia with detemir compared to NPH with otherwise similar outcomes in pregnancy [55]. There is no data on ultra-rapid insulin analogues, glargine U-300, lispro U-200, or degludec in pregnancy [3].

Insulin is the preferred treatment for women with preexisting diabetes in pregnancy. However, metformin and glyburide are felt to be safe in pregnancy for those with type 2 diabetes or gestational diabetes as they have not been shown to result in congenital malformations [56–58]. One small randomized study looked at 28 women with either type 2 diabetes or gestational diabetes starting treatment before 20 weeks of gestation [59]. Women were randomized to metformin or insulin and both groups had similar glycemic control; however, 43% of those randomized to metformin required supplemental insulin to achieve glucose targets [59]. In another study of 206 women with type 2 diabetes randomized in an open-label trial to receive metformin or insulin, those receiving metformin (plus insulin if needed) had improved maternal and neonatal outcomes; however, several methodological flaws and the fact that women already on insulin were excluded make this study less generalizable [60]. A large randomized placebo-controlled trial (Metformin in Women with Type 2 Diabetes in Pregnancy (MiTy)) is currently underway to see if the addition of metformin to insulin will be beneficial in women with type 2 diabetes [61].

In addition to excellent glycemic control, appropriate weight gain is also recommended [3]. Excess weight gain in pregnancy increases the risk for LGA infants independent of glycemic control [62, 63]. The Institute of Medicine (IOM) guidelines are usually recommended in pregnancy and are based on prepregnancy BMI [64]. Some small studies have looked at targeting lower than the IOM guidelines in those with type 2 diabetes and obesity. These have shown conflicting results from no harm, to benefit of improved perinatal morbidity with less LGA and also an increased risk of small for gestational age (SGA) [64–66].

It is also recommended that aspirin (ASA) be given to all women with preexisting diabetes starting at 12–16 weeks of gestation, as it has been shown to decrease the incidence of preeclampsia in those at high risk [67]. This study did not look at patients specifically with preexisting diabetes, although a subset did have type 1 and type 2 diabetes. We know this population is at high risk for preeclampsia, and therefore, this recommendation has been extrapolated to this population [3, 67].

It is recommended that those with preexisting diabetes have an eye exam in the first trimester of pregnancy for assessment of retinopathy and then further visits determined by their retinal specialist [3]. Those with albuminuria or CKD should be followed closely for hypertension and preeclampsia [3]. Creatinine should be used for monitoring and not eGFR, given renal hyperfiltration in pregnancy [68].

23.4.3 Antepartum and Intrapartum Monitoring and Management

While monitoring a patient with preexisting diabetes in pregnancy it is important to watch for changes in insulin requirements. Given the increasing insulin resistance during pregnancy, it is normal to have increasing requirements. One study of women with type 1 diabetes using pumps in pregnancy showed a 50% increase in basal insulin, and a 400% increase in the bolus insulin doses [69]. Near the end of pregnancy, there is some evidence that decreasing insulin requirements may be a sign of placental insufficiency and a cause for concern [70]. One study showed an increased risk of stillbirth, SGA, increased preeclampsia, preterm delivery, and NICU admissions with decreasing insulin requirements over 15% [70]. However, this was a small retrospective study and other studies have not shown an association with decreased insulin requirements and poor outcomes [71]. Therefore, it is not clear if dropping insulin requirements are actually clinically significant and at what level one should be concerned.

Given the increased perinatal morbidity and mortality with preexisting diabetes in pregnancy it is recommended to have fetal surveillance starting at 34–36 weeks of gestation [3]. This may include nonstress tests, amniotic fluid index, or biophysical profile [3]. Induction of labor at 38–39 weeks of gestation in patients with diabetes has been shown to improve outcomes with decreased macrosomia and may decrease C-section rates [72, 73]. However, if induction is done at 38 weeks and not 39 weeks, there is a higher rate of NICU admissions [72, 73].

There are no large RCTs to determine optimal labor management for those with preexisting diabetes. Intravenous insulin or subcutaneous insulin can be used, and the labor plan should be individualized to the specific care center as well as the patient [3]. The American College of Obstetricians and Gynecologists recommends using IV insulin infusion for management in labor [74]. Continuing CSII therapy in labor is also safe and may actually be beneficial in comparison to switching to IV insulin [75]. Management in labor of glucose is important to avoid maternal hypoglycemia, maternal hyperglycemia, and neonatal hypoglycemia [76]. It is recommended to maintain maternal glucose between 4.0 and 7.0 mmol/L in labor [3, 76].

After delivery a woman's insulin sensitivity increases, and it is recommended to decrease IV insulin and CSII insulin dosing by at least 50% with the first few days after delivery having a decreased requirement of about 30–50% compared to the prepregnancy insulin requirements [3, 77].

Breastfeeding has been shown to be more difficult in those with preexisting diabetes [78, 79]. Good glycemic control improves milk production in type 1 diabetes [78]. It is recommended to encourage breastfeeding in this population. In addition, breastfeeding is beneficial for the newborn in decreasing the risk of neonatal hypoglycemia and the risk of diabetes and obesity development in the future if done for at least four months [80–82].

23.5 Conclusion

Preexisting diabetes in pregnancy can result in increased complications in pregnancy for both the pregnant individual and baby, including preeclampsia, worsening retinopathy and nephropathy, congenital malformations, large-for-gestational-age neonates, perinatal mortality, preterm birth, neonatal hypoglycemia, and C-section deliveries. Given this, it is important to closely monitor and manage these patients to achieve the best pregnancy outcomes possible.

References

[1]   Feig DS, Hwee J, Shah BR et al. Trends in incidence of diabetes in pregnancy and serious perinatal outcomes: a large; population-based study in Ontario, Canada, 1996–2010. Diabetes Care 2014;37:1590–1596.

[2]   Lascar N, Brown J, Pattison H, Barnett AH, Bailey CJ, Bellary S. Type 2 diabetes in adolescents and young adults. Lancet Diabetes Endocrinol 2018;6:69–80.

[3]   Feig DS, Berger H, Donovan L et al. Diabetes Canada 2018 clinical practice guidelines for prevention and management of diabetes in Canada: diabetes and pregnancy. Can J Diabetes 2018;42(Suppl 1):S255–S282.

[4]   CEMACH. Pregnancy in Women with Type 1 and Type 2 Diabetes in 2002–03, England, Wales and Northern Ireland. London, UK: Confidential Enquiry into Maternal and Child Health (CEMACH); 2005 http://www.bathdiabetes.org/resources/254.pdf.

[5]   Feig DS, Razzaq A, Sykora K et al. Trends in deliveries, prenatal care, and obstetrical complications in women with pregestational diabetes: a population-based study in Ontario, Canada, 1996–2001. Diabetes Care 2006;29:232–235.

[6]   Macintosh MC, Fleming KM, Bailey JA et al. Perinatal mortality and congenital anomalies in babies of women with type 1 or type 2 diabetes in England, Wales, and Northern Ireland: population based study. BMJ 2006;333:177.

[7]   Cundy T, Gamble G, Neale L et al. Differing causes of pregnancy loss in type 1 and type 2 diabetes. Diabetes Care 2007;30(10):2604–2607.

[8]   Cundy T, Slee F, Gamble G and Neale L. Hypertensive disorders of pregnancy in women with type 1 and type 2 diabetes. Diabetic Med 2002;19(6):482–489.

[9]   American College of Obstetricians and Gynecologists, Task Force on Hypertension in Pregnancy. Hypertension in pregnancy. Report of the American college of obstetricians and gynecologists' task force on hypertension in pregnancy. Obstet Gynecol 2013;122:1122–1131.

[10] Brown MA, Lindheimer MD, De Swiet M et al. The classification and diagnosis of the hypertensive disorders of pregnancy: statement from the international society for the study of hypertension in pregnancy. Hypertension in Pregnancy 2001;20(1):9–14.

[11] Hauth JC, Ewell MG, Levine RJ et al. Pregnancy outcomes in healthy nulliparas who developed hypertension. Calcium for preeclampsia prevention study group. Obstet Gynecol 2000;95: 24–28.

[12] Clark SL, Christmas JT, Frye DR et al. Maternal mortality in the United States: predictability and the impact of protocols on fatal postcesarean pulmonary embolism and hypertension-related intracranial hemorrhage. Am J Obstet Gynecol 2014;211(32):1–9.

[13] Bartsch E, Medcalf KE, Park AL et al. Clinical risk factors for pre-eclampsia determined in early pregnancy: systematic review and meta-analysis of large cohort studies. BMJ 2016;353.

[14] Castiglioni MT, Valsecchi L, Cavoretto P et al. The risk of preeclampsia beyond the first pregnancy among women with type 1 diabetes parity and preeclampsia in type 1 diabetes. Pregnancy Hypertens 2014;4:34–40.

[15] Gordin D, Kaaja R, Forsblom C et al. Pre-eclampsia and pregnancy-induced hypertension are associated with severe diabetic retinopathy in type 1 diabetes later in life. Acta Diabetol 2013;50:781–787.

[16] Diabetes Control and Complications Trial Research Group, The Diabetes Control and Complications Trial Research Group. Effect of pregnancy on microvascular complications in the diabetes control and complications trial. Diabetes Care 2000;23:1084–1091.

[17] The Diabetes Control and Complications Trial Research Group. The effect of intensive treatment of diabetes on the development and progression of long-term complications in insulin-dependent diabetes mellitus. N Engl J Med 1993;329:977–986.

[18] Chew EY, Mills JL, Metzger BE et al. Metabolic control and progression of retinopathy. The diabetes in early pregnancy study. National institute of child health and human development diabetes in early pregnancy study. Diabetes Care 1995;18:631–637.

[19] Rahman W, Rahman FZ, Yassin S et al. Progression of retinopathy during pregnancy in type 1 diabetes mellitus. Clin Exp Ophthalmol 2007;35:231–236.

[20] Ramussen KL, Laugesen CS, Ringholm L et al. Progression of diabetic retinopathy during pregnancy in women with type 2 diabetes. Diabetologia 2010;53(6):1076–1083.

[21] Feghali M, Khoury JC, Shveiky D et al. Association of vaginal delivery efforts with retinal disease in women with type I diabetes. J Matern Fetal Neonatal Med 2012;25:27–31.

[22] Rossing K, Jacobsen P, Hommel E et al. Pregnancy and progression of diabetic nephropathy. Diabetologia 2002;45:36–41.

[23] Leguizamon G, Reece EA. Effect of medical therapy on progressive nephropathy: influence of pregnancy, diabetes and hypertension. J Matern Fetal Med 2000;9:70–78.

[24] Nielsen LR, Damm P, Mathiesen ER. Improved pregnancy outcome in type 1 diabeticwomen with microalbuminuria or diabetic nephropathy: effect of intensified antihypertensive therapy?. Diabetes Care 2009;32:38–44.

[25] Ekbom P, Damm P, Feldt-Rasmussen B et al. Pregnancy outcome in type 1 diabetic women with microalbuminuria. Diabetes Care 2001;24:1739–44.

[26] Jones DC, Hayslett JP. Outcome of pregnancy in women with moderate or severe renal insufficiency. N Engl J Med 1996;335(4):226.

[27] Purdy LP, Hantsch CE, Molitch ME et al. Effect of pregnancy on renal function in patients with moderate-to-severe diabetic renal insufficiency. Diabetes Care 1996;19:1067–1074.

[28] Evers IM, De Valk HW, Visser GH. Risk of complications of pregnancy in women with type 1 diabetes: nationwide prospective study in the Netherlands. BMJ 2004;328:915.

[29] Persson M, Norman M, Hanson U. Obstetric and perinatal outcomes in type 1 diabetic pregnancies: a large, population-based study. Diabetes Care 2009;32:2005–2009.

[30] Miller E, Hare JW, Cloherty JP et al. Elevated maternal hemoglobin A1c in early pregnancy and major congenital anomalies in infants of diabetic mothers. N Engl J Med 1981;304(22):1331.

[31] Schaefer-Graf U, Buchanan TA, Xiang A et al. Patters of congenital anomalies and relationships to initial maternal fasting glucose levels in pregnancies complicated by type 2 and gestational diabetes. AJOG 2000;182(2):313–320.

[32] Inkster ME, Fahey TP, Donnan PT et al. Poor glycated haemoglobin control and adverse pregnancy outcomes in type 1 and type 2 diabetes mellitus: systematic review of observational studies. BMC Pregnancy Childbirth 2006;6:30.

[33] Yamamoto JM, Corcoy R, Donovan LE et al. Maternal glycaemic control and risk of neonatal hypoglycaemia in type 1 diabetes pregnancy: a secondary analysis of the conceptt trial. Diabet Med 2019;36:1046–1053.

[34] Kline GA, Edwards A. Antepartum and intra-partum insulin management of type 1 and type 2 diabetic women: impact on clinically significant neonatal hypoglycemia. Diabetes Res Clin Pract 2007;77(2):223–230.

[35] Alexander LD, Tomlinson G, Feig DS. Predictors of large-for-gestational-age birthweight among pregnant women with type 1 and type 2 diabetes: a retrospecitve cohort study. Canadian J Diabetes 2019;43(8):560–566.

[36] Clausen TD, Mathiesen E, Ekbom P et al. Poor pregnancy outcome in women with type 2 diabetes. Diabetes Care 2005;28(2):323–328.

[37] Tennant PW, Glinianaia SV, Bilous RW et al. Pre-existing diabetes, maternal glycated haemoglobin, and the risks of fetal and infant death: a populationbased study. Diabetologia 2014;57:285–294.

[38] Holman N, Bell R, Murphy H et al. Women with pre-gestational diabetes have a higher risk of stillbirth at all gestations after 32 weeks. Diabet Med 2014;31:1129–1132.

[39] Wahabi HA, Alzeidan RA, Bawazeer GA et al. Preconception care for diabetic women for improving maternal and fetal outcomes: a systematic review and meta-analysis. BMC Pregnancy Childbirth 2010;10:63.

[40] Management of diabetes in pregnancy: standards of medical care in diabetes-2019. American diabetes association. Diabetes Care 2019;42(Suppl1):S165.

[41] Owens LA, Egan AM, Carmody L et al. Ten years of optimizing outcomes for women with type 1 and type 2 diabetes in pregnancy-The Atlantic dip experience. J Clin Endocrinol Metab 2016;101:1598–605.

[42] Murphy HR, Roland JM, Skinner TC et al. Effectiveness of a regional prepregnancy care program in women with type 1 and type 2 diabetes: benefits beyond glycemic control. Diabetes Care 2010 Dec;33(12):2514–2520.

[43] Hernandez TL, Friedman JE, Van Pelt RE et al. Patterns of glycemia in normal pregnancy: should the current therapeutic targets be challenged? Diabetes Care 2011;34:1660–1668.

[44] Danne T, Nimri R, Battelino T et al. International consensus on use of continuous glucose monitoring. Diabetes Care 2017;40:1631–1640.

[45] Scott E, Bilous RW and Kaurzky-Willer A. Accuracy, User Acceptability. Safety evaluation for the freestyle libre flash glucose monitoring system when used by pregnant women with diabetes. Diabetes Technol Ther 2018;20(3):180–188.

[46] Feig DS, Donovan LE, Corcoy R et al. Continuous glucose monitoring in pregnant women with type 1 diabetes (CONCEPTT): a multicentre international randomised controlled trial. The Lancet 2017;390:2347–2359.

[47] Murphy HR, Rayman G, Lewis K et al. Effectiveness of continuous glucose monitoring in pregnant women with diabetes: randomised clinical trial. BMJ 2008;337:a1680.

[48] Ranasinghe PD, Maruthur NM, Nicholson WK et al. Comparative effectiveness of continuous subcutaneous insulin infusion using insulin analogs and multiple daily injections in pregnant women with diabetes mellitus: a systematic review and meta-analysis. J Womens Health 2015;24:237–249.

[49] Feig DS, Corcoy R, Donovan LE et al. Pumps or multiple daily injections in pregnancy involving type 1 diabetes: a prespecified analysis of the CONCEPTt randomized trial. Diabetes Care 2018;41(12):2471–2479.

[50] Bhattacharyya A, Brown S, Hughes S, Vice PA. Insulin lispro and regular insulin in pregnancy. QJM: An Int J Med 2001;94:255–260.

[51] Brunelle RL, Llewelyn J, Anderson JH Jr, Gale EAM, Koivisto VA. Meta-analysis of the effect of insulin lispro on severe hypoglycemia in patients with type 1 diabetes. Diabetes Care 1998;21:1726–1731.

[52] Lv S, Wang J, Xu Y. Safety of insulin analogs during pregnancy: a metaanalysis. Arch Gynecol Obstet 2015;292:749–756.

[53] Boskovic R, Feig DS, Derewlany L et al. Transfer of insulin lispro across the human placenta: in vitro perfusion studies. Diabetes Care 2003;26:1390–4.

[54] Pollex E, Moretti ME, Koren G et al. Safety of insulin glargine use in pregnancy: a systematic review and meta-analysis. Ann Pharmacother 2011;45:9–16.

[55] Herrera KM, Rosenn BM, Foroutan J et al. Randomized controlled trial of insulin detemir versus NPH for the treatment of pregnant women with diabetes. Am J Obstet Gynecol 2015;213(426):e1–7.

[56] Gutzin SJ, Kozer E, Magee LA et al. The safety of oral hypoglycemic agents in the first trimester of pregnancy: a meta-analysis. Can J Clin Pharmacol 2003;10:179–183.

[57] Cassina M, Dona M, Di Gianantonio E et al. First-trimester exposure to metformin and risk of birth defects: a systematic review and meta-analysis. Hum Reprod Update 2014;20:656–669.

[58] Glueck CJ, Bornovali S, Pranikoff J et al. Metformin, pre-eclampsia and pregnancy outcomes in women with polycystic ovary syndrome. Diabet Med 2004;21(8):829–836.

[59] Hickman MA, McBride R, Boggess KA et al. Metformin compared with insulin in the treatment of pregnant women with overt diabetes: a randomized controlled trial. Am J Perinatol 2013;30:483–490.

[60] Ainuddin JA, Karim N, Zaheer S, Ali SS, Hasan AA. Metformin treatment in type 2 diabetes in pregnancy: an active controlled, parallel-group, randomized, open label study in patients with type 2 diabetes in pregnancy. J Diabetes Res 2015;2015:325851.

[61] Feig DS, Murphy K, Asztalos E et al. Metformin in women with type 2 diabetes in pregnancy (MiTy): a multi-center randomized, controlled trial. BMC Pregnancy and Childbirth (Study Protocol) 2016;16:173.

[62] Secher AL, Parellada CB, Ringholm L et al. Higher gestational weight gain is associated with increasing offspring birth weight independent of maternal glycemic control in women with type 1 diabetes. Diabetes Care 2014;37:2677–2684.

[63] Parellada CB, Asbjornsdottir B, Ringholm L et al. Fetal growth in relation to gestational weight gain in women with type 2 diabetes: an observational study. Diabet Med 2014;31:1681–1689.

[64] Yee LM, Cheng YW, Inturrisi M et al. Effect of gestational weight gain on perinatal outcomes in women with type 2 diabetes mellitus using the 2009 institute of medicine guidelines. Am J Obstet Gynecol 2011;205(257):e1–6.

[65] Harper LM, Shanks AL, Odibo AO et al. Gestational weight gain in insulin resistant pregnancies. J Perinatol 2013;33:929–933.

[66] Asbjörnsdóttir B, Rasmussen SS, Kelstrup L et al. Impact of restricted maternal weight gain on fetal growth and perinatal morbidity in obese women with type 2 diabetes. Diabetes Care 2013;36:1102–1106.

[67] Rolnik DL, Wright D, Poot LC et al. Aspirin versus placebo in pregnancies at high risk for preterm preeclamsia. NEJM 2017;377(7):613–623.

[68] Koetje PM, Spaan JJ, Kooman JP et al. Pregnancy reduces the accuracy of the estimated glomerular filtration rate based on cockroft-gault and MDRD formulas. Reprod Sci 2011;18: 456–462.

[69] Mathiesen JM, Secher AL, Ringholm L et al. Changes in basal rates and bolus calculator settings in insulin pumps during pregnancy in women with type 1 diabetes. Fetal Neonatal Med 2014;27(7):724–728.

[70] Padmanabhan S, McLean M, Cheung NW. Falling insulin requirements are associated with adverse obstetric outcomes in women with preexisting diabetes. Diabetes Care 2014;37: 2685–2692.

[71] Achong N, Callaway L, d'Emden M et al. Insulin requirements in late pregnancy in women with type 1 diabetes mellitus: a retrospective review. Diabetes Res Clin Pract 2012;98: 414–421.

[72] Kjos SL, Henry OA, Montoro M et al. Insulin-requiring diabetes in pregnancy: a randomized trial of active induction of labor and expectant management. Am J Obstet Gynecol 1993;169: 611–615.

[73] Melamed N, Ray JG, Geary M et al. Induction of labor before 40 weeks is associated with lower rate of cesarean delivery in women with gestational diabetes mellitus. Am J Obstet Gynecol 2016;214(364):e1–8.

[74] ACOG Practice bulletin no. 201: pregestational diabetes mellitus. Obstet Gynecol 2018;132 (6):e228.

[75] Drever E, Tomlinson G, Bai AD et al. Insulin pump use compared with intravenous insulin during labour and delivery: the inspired observational cohort study. Diabet Med 2016;33(9): 1253–1259.

[76] Ryan EA, Al-Agha R. Glucose control during labor and delivery. Curr Diab Rep 2014;14:450.

[77] Ringholm L, Mathiesen ER, Kelstrup L et al. Managing type 1 diabetes mellitus in pregnancy–from planning to breastfeeding. Nat Rev Endocrinol 2012;8:659–667.

[78] Neubauer SH, Ferris AM, Chase CG et al. Delayed lactogenesis in women with insulin-dependent diabetes mellitus. Am J Clin Nutr 1993;58:54–60.

[79] Riddle SW, Nommsen-Rivers LA. A case control study of diabetes during pregnancy and low milk supply. Breastfeed Med 2016;11:80–85.

[80] Yan J, Liu L, Zhu Y et al. The association between breastfeeding and childhood obesity: a meta-analysis. BMC Public Health 2014;14:1267.

[81] Cordero L, Ramesh S, Hillier K et al. Early feeding and neonatal hypoglycemia in infants of diabetic mothers. Sage Open Med 2013;1:2050312113516613.

[82] Al Mamun A, O'Callaghan MJ, Williams GM et al. Breastfeeding is protective to diabetes risk in young adults: a longitudinal study. Acta Diabetol 2015;52:837–844.

Maya Ram, Yariv Yogev

24 Gestational Diabetes Mellitus

24.1 Introduction

Gestational diabetes mellitus (GDM) is one of the most common pregnancy complications. It is a state of carbohydrate intolerance which is defined as any degree of
hyperglycemia that is recognized for the first time during pregnancy [1, 2]. However,
the definition of the degree of hyperglycemia has varied between experts and associations, and the diagnosis of GDM still lacks uniformity. In the past, GDM has been
regarded as benign [3] and was even questioned if a disease at all. Nowadays, irrespective of diagnostic criteria, it is well established that GDM increases the risk of
adverse pregnancy outcome for both the mother and fetus and that effective treatment can improve outcome [4–6]. Moreover, GDM diagnosis identifies a group of
women and their offspring which are at higher risk for long-term future type 2 diabetes (T2D), obesity, and future cardiovascular disease [7–9].

The prevalence of GDM has been increasing over time, possibly due to the increasing rates of obesity in the general population and the trend toward advanced
maternal age in pregnancy [10–12]. The prevalence is now estimated to affect from
3% to more than 30% of pregnancies worldwide [12, 13]. Differences in the geographic
location, ethnic groups, characteristics of the population screened, and the diagnostic criteria that are applied are responsible for the wide reported range [12–14]. Attention has been drawn to the increasing prevalence of GDM and has stimulated many
debates in the last decades regarding its etiology, pathophysiology, diagnosis, treatment, and long-term consequences to the mother and fetus. Unfortunately, consider-
able controversies and many gaps in knowledge still exist.

24.2 Risk Factors for GDM

Epidemiological studies of risk factors for GDM are limited and typically afflicted by
confounding factors. Non-modifiable risk factors include advanced maternal age [15],
ethnicity, and being overweight or obese prior to pregnancy [13]. The latter was
reported as the most significant modifiable risk factor for the development of GDM
[16, 17]. The observed association between obesity and GDM is biologically plausible.
Normal pregnancy is associated with metabolic changes, including increased insulin
resistance, which is further enhanced by the chronic insulin resistance in obese
women. Therefore, obesity plays a central role in the development of GDM [18–20].

Other reported risk factors include, excessive gestational weight gain [21], western-
ized diet [21], ethnicity [22], genetic mutation and polymorphisms [23, 24], family and

https://doi.org/10.1515/9783110615258-024

personal history of GDM [25], previous macrosomia in the newborn [24], and other diseases of insulin resistance, such as polycystic ovarian syndrome (PCOS) [26].

24.3 Pathophysiology of GDM

Pregnancy by itself is a state of increased metabolic activity, in which maintaining glucose homeostasis is of upmost importance. Many factors play a role in controlling euglycemia state, and it is likely that a combination of genetic, epigenetic, and environmental factors all contribute to the development of GDM [27].

In normal pregnancy, several changes in glucose regulation occur to facilitate nutrient supply to the developing fetus. The placenta releases a variety of molecules with physiological effects on the metabolism of both mother and fetus [28, 29], thereby controlling insulin sensitivity [28]. In the first trimester, maternal insulin sensitivity is frequently increased, subsequently with lipogenesis and lipid storage at the adipose tissue [30], leading to fasting and postprandial glucose that are lower than in nonpregnant women [31, 32]. However, by the second half of pregnancy, along with the fast growth of the fetus, a decrease in insulin sensitivity, increased hepatic glucose production, and an induction of lipolysis are observed [30]. The pancreatic β-cells adapt to the physiologic changes by expanding their mass, thereby producing increased amounts of insulin to maintain an euglycemic state [33, 34]. Inability of pancreatic β-cells to respond adequately to the increased insulin requirements results in varying degrees of hyperglycemia in the pregnant mother [35]. In populations with preexisting hyper-insulinemic conditions such as obesity, PCOS, or metabolic syndrome, the defect in β-cell function most likely existed before conception [36, 37]. Pregnancy appears to unmask the asymptomatic β-cell dysfunction [36] due to both widespread testing of glucose levels [13] and the metabolic adaptations that increase the stress on β-cells, thus exacerbating preexisting insulin resistance [35]. The resulting hyperglycemia directly contributes to β-cells failure in a process described as glucotoxicity [38]. Thus, once β-cell dysfunction begins, a vicious cycle of hyperglycemia, insulin resistance, and further β-cell dysfunction is set in motion (see Figure 24.1)

In addition to β-cell dysfunction and chronic insulin resistance, tissue inflammation and neurohormonal dysfunction play an important role in failure of adaptive mechanisms maintaining glucose homeostasis [27]. Not less important is the genetic role which links T2D susceptibility genes to GDM development including variants in GCK, CDKAL1, KCNQ1, etc. [39].

All play a role in the maternal adverse outcomes, including development of T2D as for the pathogenesis described above and hypertensive-related disorders both during and following pregnancy.

Maternal hyperglycemia starts a cascade that can lead to maternal b-cell failure and metabolic syndrome later in life. From the fetus point of view, maternal

Table 24.1: Summary of major societies' guidelines on controversial aspects of GDM diagnosis and management.

	ACOG [1]	ADA [32, 101]	IADPSG [98]	FIGO [37][1]	WHO [31]	CDA [102]
Early screening[2]	Risk factor based	Risk factor based	Risk factor based or universal	Universal	Risk factor based or universal	Risk factor based
Early pregestational diabetes diagnosis	Standard WHO criteria[3]	Standard WHO criteria[3] or A1C ≥6.5%	A1C ≥6.5% or FPG ≥126 or RPG ≥200[5]	Standard WHO criteria[3]	Standard WHO criteria[3]	A1C ≥6.5% or FPG ≥126
Early GDM diagnosis	NA	NA	FPG >92mg/dL	FPG or 2-h glucose load[4]	FPG or 2-h glucose load[4]	NA
GDM diagnostic criteria						
Universal/selective screening/testing	Universal screening	Universal screening or testing	Universal testing	Universal testing	Universal testing	Universal screening
When	24–28 weeks	24–28 weeks	Any time	Any time	Any time	24–28 weeks
Approach	2 steps	2 steps/1 step	1 step	1 step	1 step	2 steps
Screening	GCT[6]	GCT[6]	–	–	–	GCT[6]
Screening thresholds(mg/dL)	130, 135, 140[7]	130, 135, 140[7]	–	–	–	140[8]

(continued)

Table 24.1 (continued)

	ACOG [1]		ADA [32, 101]		IADPSG [98]	FIGO [37][1]	WHO [31]	CDA [102]
Test: OGTT[9]	3 h, 100 g: C&C/NDDG		3 h, 100 g/ 2 h, 75 g		2 h, 75 g	2 h, 75 g	2 h, 75 g	2 h, 75 g[10]
	C&C	NDDG	3 h, 100 g	2 h, 75 g				
Number of abnormal values	2	2	2	1	1	1	1	1
Fasting glucose (mg/dL)	≥95	≥105	≥95	≥92	≥92	≥92	≥92	≥95
1 h glucose (md/dL)	≥180	≥190	≥180	≥180	≥180	≥180	≥180	≥190
2 h glucose (md/dL)	≥155	≥165	≥155	≥153	≥153	≥153	≥153	≥162
3 h glucose (md/dL)	≥140	≥145	≥140	–	–	–	–	–
Glucose targets (mg/dL):	Fasting <95 1 h post meal <140 2 h post meal <120				NA	Same as for ACOG and ADA	NA	Same as for ACOG and ADA

When to initiate pharmacological treatment?	Failing to achieve glycemic control with lifestyle intervention	Failing to achieve glycemic control with lifestyle intervention	NA	Failing to achieve glycemic control with lifestyle intervention	NA	Glycemic targets are not achieved within 2 weeks of lifestyle intervention
First line pharmacologic treatment	**Insulin**	**Insulin**	NA	**Insulin, metformin, glyburide[11]**	NA	**Insulin or metformin**
Alternative treatment	**Metformin**	**Metformin or Glyburide**	NA	**Insulin[12]**	NA	**Glyburide only as third option**
When to deliver well-controlled GDM?	**GDMA1: 41 weeks** **GDMA2: 39–39 + 6 weeks**	NA	NA	GDMA1/2 ± EFW ≤ 3,800 g: **40–41 weeks** GDMA1/2 ± EFW ≥ 3,800 g: **38–39 weeks**	GDMA1/2: **41 weeks**	GDMA1/2: **38–40 weeks**

GDM= Gestational Diabetes Mellitus; ACOG= American College of Obstetricians and Gynecologists; ADA= American Diabetes Association; IADPSG= International Association of Diabetes and Pregnancy Study Groups; FIGO= Federation of International of Gynecologists and Obstetricians; WHO= World Health Organization; CDA= Canadian Diabetes Association; FPG= Fasting Plasma Glucose; RPG= Random Plasma Glucose; A1C= Glycated hemoglobin; C&C= Carpenter and Coustan; NDDG= National Diabetes Data Group; GCT= Glucose challenge test; OGTT= Oral glucose tolerance test; GDMA1= GDM controlled with diet; GDMA2= GDM controlled with pharmacologic treatment

1. FIGO recommends various diagnostic strategies based on available resources at country level and local practice. The recommendations in this table are for fully resourced settings only.
2. At first prenatal visit
3. WHO 2006 criteria [31] for diagnosis of overt diabetes include any of the following:
   1. Fasting plasma glucose≥ 126 mg/dl (7.0 mmol/L). Fasting is defined as no caloric intake for at least 8 h. or
   2. 2-hour plasma glucose≥ 200 mg/dl (11.1 mmol/L) during an OGTT.
   3. Random plasma glucose≥ 200 mg/dl (11.1 mmol/L) in a patient with diabetic symptoms

4. WHO 2006 criteria [31] for diagnosis of gestational diabetes mellitus should include any of the following:
   1. Fasting plasma glucose: 92–125 mg/dL (5.1–6.9 mmol/l)
   2. 1-h-post 75 gram glucose >180 mg/dL (<10 mmol/l)
   3. 2-h-post 75 gram glucose: 153–199 mg/dL (8.5–11.0 mmol/l)
5. If RPG is the initial measure, the tentative diagnosis of overt diabetes in pregnancy should be confirmed by FPG or A1C
6. GCT Screening test is based on oral intake of 50 g glucose solution, given to the non-fasting women followed by venous glucose examination 1 h later.
7. Any of the following thresholds are accepted as positive screening ≥130 mg/dL, ≥135 mg/dL, or ≥140 mg/dL (7.2 mmol/L, 7.5 mmol/L, or 7.8 mmol/L)
8. GDM is diagnosed if the glucose level 1 h after the 50 g GCT is ≥ 200 mg/dL (11.1 mmol/L) without the need to perform the full 2-h-OGTT
9. OGTT is the diagnostic approach for GDM which is performed following fasting of 8–12 h, oral glucose solution of either 75 g or 100 g glucose and 2 or 3 blood samples every hour respectively. For diagnosis 2 values need to meet or exceed thresholds in the 100 g or 1 value in the 75 g load.
10. The "preferred" approach for sequential screening consists of a 50 g GCT followed by a 75 g OGTT using the glucose thresholds that result in an OR of 2.0 for the increased risk of LGA and cord C-peptide. A diagnostic strategy consistent with the IADPSG approach of a 1-step 75 g OGTT using the glucose thresholds that result in an OR of 1.75 for the risk of LGA and cord C-peptide was added as an "alternative" method
11. In the second or third trimester each is approved and effective for GDM. FIGO suggest that Metformin might be better choice than Glyburide.
12. Insulin should be considered as the first-line treatment in women with GDM who are at high risk of failing on OAD therapy such as: GDM diagnosis < 20 weeks, need for pharmacologic treatment >30 weeks, FPG >110 mg/dL, pregnancy weight gain >12 kg, 1 h post-prandial glucose >140 mg/dL

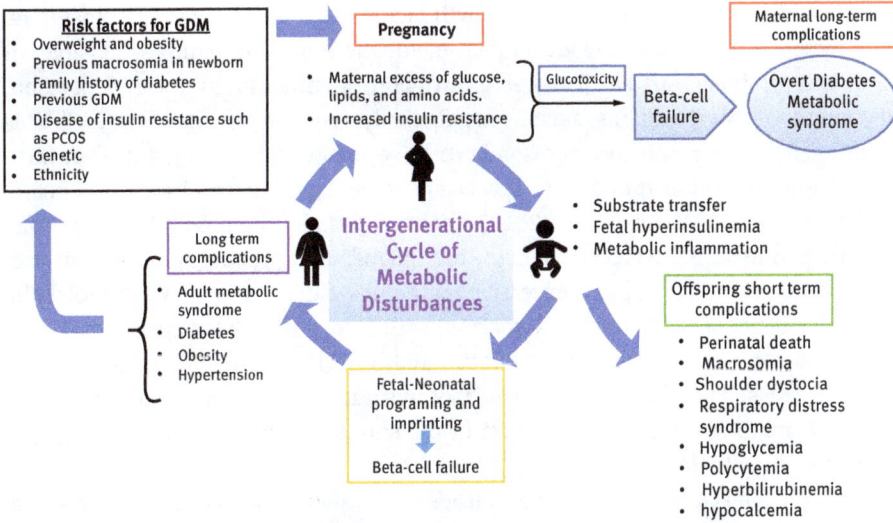

Figure 24.1: Schematic representation of the intergenerational cycle of hyperglycemia in pregnancy.

hyperglycemia and other fetal b-cell secretagogue substrates induce fetal hyperinsulinemia that is responsible for the immediate neonatal adverse outcome and result in fetal metabolic programming, childhood obesity, and long-term metabolic abnormalities that may reflect on the next generation.

24.4 The Offspring Point of View

The effects of maternal hyperglycemia on the offspring start in utero and can linearly lead to adverse outcomes both for short- and long-term period [40, 41]. It is believed that increased maternal glucose levels reach the fetal circulation leading to fetal hyperglycemia which stimulate the fetal pancreas resulting in pancreatic hypertrophy and an exaggerated fetal response to insulin. Consequently, there is more transfer and consumption of glucose to fetal tissue, increasing the glucose gradient between the mother and the fetus, thereby driving more glucose from mother circulation to fetal circulation. This process is termed the "fetoplacental glucose steal phenomenon" and can even explain why some women with fetuses with all the characteristics of diabetic fetopathy are often found to have "normal" glucose tolerance [42, 43]. The fetal pancreas of women with diabetes is sensitive to glucose from early pregnancy [43]. Maternal excess of circulating glucose and other fetal β-cell secretagogues such as lipids and amino acids transports the placenta and stimulates endogenous production of insulin and insulin-like growth factor 1 that start the cascade of the offspring complications [44]. Insulin is both a growth factor and anabolic hormone; therefore, fetal hyperinsulinemia can result in fetal metabolic reprogramming responsible for short-term problems such as fetal overgrowth and/or adiposity due to fat deposition, and long-term complications, such as metabolic dysfunction later in life [13, 43]. This phenomenon can result in macrosomia or large for gestational age (LGA) at birth [45]. One study demonstrated that the accelerated fetal growth could start even before the diagnosis of GDM, as early as 20–28 weeks of gestation [46]. Both hyperglycemia severity and maternal weight at delivery are independent predictors for LGA or macrosomic infant [4, 40, 47] and excessive maternal weight gain (>18 kg) doubles the risk [48]. Macrosomia, in turn, is associated with increased risk for operative vaginal and caesarean delivery, shoulder dystocia, and birth injury [49–51]. These risks are further increased in offspring of diabetic mothers due to disproportionate distribution of the fat mass favoring accumulation in the shoulder and abdomen, resulting in truncal asymmetry [4, 52, 53].

Chronic fetal hyperinsulinemia also leads to elevated metabolic rates that result in increased oxygen consumption and fetal hypoxemia as the placenta is unable to meet the increased metabolic demands [54]. Fetal hypoxemia is the reason for increased risk of morbidity, metabolic acidosis, birth asphyxia, and stillbirth [5, 44, 55]. Fetal hypoxia also increases erythropoietin production, which is the precursor to known complications in neonates born to mothers with GDM, i.e., polycythemia and hyperbilirubinemia [56]. In turn, fetal polycythemia may cause blood hyperviscosity that further alters oxygen delivery. As the fetal red cell mass increases, iron redistribution results in iron deficiency in developing organs, which may contribute to cardiomyopathy and altered neurodevelopment [44, 55, 56]. Once delivered, hyper-insulinemic neonates, who were dependent on maternal hyperglycemia, rapidly eliminate glucose into the tissues, and without additional substrate are prone to develop hypoglycemia. Although hypoglycemia is self-limited and resolves as the hyperinsulinemia resolves, it can contribute to brain injury if not properly managed [43, 52, 57]. Increased amounts of insulin in the fetal circulation can alter lung surfactant synthesis, leading to delayed lung maturation which can result in a life-threatening condition in the neonatal period, termed respiratory distress syndrome [57, 58].

Long-term metabolic effects have been observed in offspring of mothers with GDM and the underlying pathogenetic mechanisms have been a subject of interest for many years. In addition to genetic predisposition, the intrauterine environment and nutritional status of GDM mothers are involved in fetal programming that eventually leads to metabolic-related diseases later in life (Figure 24.1). Although the underlying mechanism for fetal programing is still under discussion, the concept of epigenetic imprinting has been widely accepted, as it brings new insights into the molecular pathogenesis of human diseases. Maternal hyperglycemia can induce changes in DNA methylation and microRNA of genes found in fetal blood, skeletal muscle, and adipose tissue. These genes are known to be involved in energy metabolism, anti-inflammatory processes, insulin resistance, and β-cells apoptosis, which therefore could partially explain the increased risk for cardiometabolic morbidities later in life [59–64]. In addition, hyperglycemia has been linked with altered expressions of angiogenesis associated molecules in the trophoblast [65] and in overexpression of proinflammation factors such as IL-6 and TNF-α [66], which adversely affect the intrauterine environment.

In a more clinical perspective, maternal hyperglycemia during pregnancy was found to be associated with many adverse metabolic outcomes during the offspring childhood and even adult life. Offspring of GDM as compared to non-diabetes mothers show evidence of an adverse cardiovascular phenotype, including increase in adiposity, BMI, insulin resistance, overt diabetes, systolic blood pressure, and associated metabolic diseases [8, 67–76], which were all demonstrated to be independent of maternal and childhood BMI [70, 77]. In turn, the adult offspring females are more likely to experience diabetes in their own pregnancies, contributing to a vicious intergenerational cycle of this pathology (see Figure 24.1) [78].

24.5 Prevention of Long-Term Effects on the Offspring

The hyperglycemia and adverse pregnancy outcome (HAPO) study has clearly demonstrated that the natural history of untreated GDM mothers have substantial long-term risks for both mother and child [41]. Although GDM treatment can reduce immediate maternal and fetal complications [4, 79], its effect on the long-term offspring prognosis is still unknown. Animal models documented that hyperglycemia, diabetes, obesity, cardiovascular disease, and structural hypothalamic changes in offspring of GDM mother can be prevented by normalization of maternal blood glucose levels during pregnancy [80, 81]. One observational study [82] demonstrated association between worsening hyperglycemia in pregnancy and increased risk of obesity at ages 5–7. In this study, there was a small group of mothers that were treated for GDM and association with childhood obesity disappeared. However, in follow-up studies of the offspring of women treated for GDM, there seem to be no improvement in the long-term prognosis of offspring [83–85]. However, postpartum follow-up studies are still of relatively short duration (4–10 years) and long-term results are awaited. Yet, these data mandate closer follow-up for these neonates.

24.6 Screening and Diagnosis for GDM

The history of GDM screening and diagnosis began about six decades ago when O'Sullivan and Mahan described the first criteria for GDM diagnosis that were focused on identifying women at high risk for the development of T2D after pregnancy [86]. In earlier times, it was common that screening for GDM was based on patient's medical history, focusing on past obstetric outcomes such as bearing a child with macrosomia, and family history of T2D. Those high-risk women then performed 3-h 100-g oral glucose tolerance test (OGTT), and a diagnosis of GDM was made when at least two of the four glucose values met or exceeded threshold levels. The cutoff values were estimated based on the mean plus two standard deviations for prediction later development of T2D [86]. Screening for GDM based on risk factors, rather than universal screening, was thought to be cost-effective and, more importantly, saved the burden of unnecessary OGTT in low risk women. In practice, this approach has complicated the detection process and failed to identify half of women with GDM who did not have any risk factors [87–90]. Realizing the insensitivity of the selective screening, it was suggested first by O'Sullivan et al. [91] in 1973 and later adopted by the US task force [92] to screen all pregnant women for GDM by non-fasting 1-h 50-g glucose challenge test (GCT) at or beyond 24 gestational weeks. They recommended that only pregnant women who did not pass the GCT should proceed to the second-step 100-g OGTT. Later, by 1979 the diagnostic criteria cutoffs, proposed by O'Sullivan and Mahan [86], were modified to account for changes in laboratory methodology by the National Diabetes Data Group (NDDG) in 1979 [2] and Carpenter and Coustan (C&C) in 1982 [93], which are the commonly used thresholds (Table 26.1). Consecutive studies discovered that lesser degrees of hyperglycemia were associated with an increased risk of adverse perinatal outcome, including LGA fetuses, shoulder dystocia, neonatal hypoglycemia, caesarean delivery, and hypertensive disorders [94–97]. Consequently, in 1999 the WHO recommended that GDM diagnosis should be similar as for the detection of T2D and 2-h 75 g OGTT test should be applied instead of the former 3-h 100-g OGTT. These criteria were not evidence-based, as their cutoff values were selected arbitrarily according to expert opinion and consensus [31]. However, the validity of this test as screening tool was only evidenced after being used in the HAPO) study in 2008 [40]. The HAPO study was designed to evaluate the development of adverse pregnancy outcomes rather than future development of T2D. It was a prospective multinational cohort study of more than 23,000 pregnant women, and has demonstrated that risk of adverse maternal, fetal, and neonatal outcomes linearly correlated with maternal glycemia, even within ranges previously considered normal for pregnancy. They have determined maternal glucose level at 24–32 weeks of gestation by a 2-h 75-g OGTT and reported that all three maternal plasma glucose values (fasting, 1 h, and 2 h) correlated with adverse outcomes. However, for most complications there was not a glucose inflection point above which the incidence of adverse outcomes increases, but rather a continuum of risk [40]. The evidence provided by the HAPO study formed the basis of the International Association of Diabetes in Pregnancy Study Groups (IADPSG) criteria for GDM screening and diagnosis in 2010 [98]. The IADPSG recommended a "one-step" method involving 75-g 2-h oral OGTT at 24–28 weeks of gestation and proposed that only one value needs to be abnormal in order to diagnose GDM. The diagnostic thresholds were based on an adjusted odds ratio threshold of 1.75 of delivering an infant affected by key fetal complications of maternal hyperglycemia, namely, increased size at birth, increased adiposity, and elevated cord blood C-peptide levels, a marker for hyperinsulinemia [98]. A secondary analysis of HAPO data using IADPSG diagnostic cutoffs confirmed that women diagnosed with GDM by IADPSG criteria had significantly increased odds ratios for birth weight >90th percentile (OR 1.87), cord blood C peptide >90th percentile (OR 2.00), and primary caesarean delivery (OR 1.31) compared to women with no GDM [99]. Using these criteria and one abnormal value for diagnosis, the incidence of GDM notably increases from 5–6% to 15–20% [100].

Over a decade following the IADPSG recommendation, the debate and disagreement about screening and diagnostic criteria still go on, especially due to inconsistency of available data. There is no consensus regarding the optimal strategy for GDM diagnosis, and the main diabetes and obstetric societies still struggle to find the ideal algorithm. Table 24.1 shows the major differences in guidelines in controversies between societies.

24.6.1 "Two-Step" Method for Screening

The two-step method for GDM screening consists of a first-step GCT and a second-step OGTT. GCT test is based on oral intake of 50-g glucose solution, given to the non-fasting women followed by venous glucose examination 1 h later. A positive result is defined as a blood glucose value higher than 130–140 mg/dL. Only women whose glucose levels meet or exceed screening threshold undergo a 100-g, 3-h diagnostic OGTT, a test found to be associated with increased maternal stress and dissatisfaction [103, 104]. In this approach, GDM is diagnosed in women who have two or more abnormal values [1]. Table 26.1 outlines the diagnostic cutoffs. Recently, a systematic review demonstrated increased risks for the same poor outcomes for women with one abnormal value as women with two abnormal values [105]. Consequently, ACOG accepted GDM diagnosis to be based on only one abnormal value, but the benefit from treatment in this approach is still unclear [1].

The two-step approach is considered superior by some organizations because there is a lack of evidence that the one-step strategy, which increases the prevalence of GDM diagnosis, leads to improved maternal or fetal outcomes but is associated with increased healthcare costs, life disruption, and psychosocial burdens. Even more, "over diagnosing" may lead to "medicalized" pregnancies previously categorized as normal, which means more frequent prenatal visits, fetal and maternal surveillance, and interventions, including induction of labor without clear benefit of improvements in the most clinically important health- and patient-centered outcomes [106, 107].

24.6.2 "One-Step" Method for Screening

This one-step strategy requires **all** pregnant women to perform the fasting 75-g OGTT. For GDM diagnosis, at least one of the three glucose values must meet or exceed the recommended thresholds (see Table 24.1) [98].

Societies supporting this approach believe it to be simpler diagnostic method as it omits the screening test. It is a more evidence-based strategy, which the expected benefits are inferred from intervention trials that focused on women with lower levels of hyperglycemia than identified using older GDM diagnostic criteria. Those trials have shown a reduction of macrosomia, preeclampsia, and shoulder dystocia with treatment of mild GDM [4, 79]. Furthermore, although the IADPSG cutoffs will diagnose more women with GDM [108], a majority (80–90%) of mild GDM cases can be managed with diet alone [4, 79]. Moreover, many experts justify the criteria and the increase in workload in the background of the globally mounting burden of T2D [109]. Existing data reveal that woman with GDM based on the IADPSG criteria have a similarly increased risk for glucose intolerance postpartum compared to women with GDM based on other diagnostic criteria [110]. Recently, the HAPO follow-up study demonstrated that women who would have been diagnosed with GDM by the one-step approach, as compared with those without, were at 3.4-fold higher risk of developing prediabetes and T2D and had children with a higher risk of obesity and increased body fat [41, 70]. In light of these findings, experts in favor of the one-step approach see a window of opportunity to identify a large group of women at increased risk of glucose intolerance later in life that would benefit from timely implement strategies to prevent the further development of T2D. Indeed, a cost-benefit estimation comparing the two strategies concluded that the one-step approach is cost-effective only if patients with GDM receive postdelivery counseling and care to prevent T2D [111].

24.6.3 Optimal Diagnostic Approach – Evidence-Based

Several retrospective studies that compared pregnancy outcome of one-step approach using IADPSG criteria versus two-step ACOG C&C criteria found that the one-step approach identified more women at increased risk of adverse outcomes associated with GDM [112–119], in particular LGA and macrosomia [115, 116] and exhibited improved outcomes due to diagnosis and treatment [115–118]. However, available data are not all consistent; some studies didn't find statistical significant differences between the two approaches on pregnancy outcomes [120–123], and one study reported the one-step approach is associated with increasing both the diagnosis and caesarean delivery rate, without decreasing the rate of LGA or macrosomic neonates or improving maternal or neonatal morbidity [124].

Currently there are few RCTs directly comparing the one-step to the two-step approach [125–128]. However, one did not report pregnancy outcomes [125] and another only evaluated the feasibility of randomization and screening [127]. Sevket et al. showed significantly higher GDM prevalence and better pregnancy outcomes in women with normal glucose tolerance that were diagnosed by the one-step method as compared to the women with normal glucose tolerance with the two-step method [126]. However, they did not report the effect of women diagnosed with GDM by these two methods on pregnancy outcomes. In the most recent RCT 249 pregnant women were recruited and randomized to either the one-step or the two-step method. The authors did not find significant differences in GDM incidence and adverse pregnancy outcomes between the one-step method using the IADPSG criteria and the two-step approach using C&C criteria. However, as the trial was underpowered, the findings are not conclusive [128].

At present, no RCT has compared the long-term maternal and perinatal outcomes in women diagnosed with GDM by the one-step versus two-step approach. It is not clear if increased identification of patients with mild GDM would require the same intensity of glucose monitoring, fetal testing, and intervention as those with GDM diagnosed by more stringent criteria [129]. Data are also lacking on how the treatment of lower levels of hyperglycemia will affect a mother's future risk for T2D development and her offspring's risk for obesity, diabetes, and other metabolic disorders [77, 85]. The limited information contributes to the ongoing discussion on whether implementing the IADPSG screening strategy will be cost-effective. Concerns related to the benefit of treatment in the additionally diagnosed women and the increased cost of the health care services impede its wide use, and the inconsistent current literature supports use of each strategy.

24.6.4 Early Pregnancy Testing

It is agreed by professional societies that women with risk factors for T2D should be tested at their initial prenatal visit for overt diabetes [1, 31, 32, 37, 98, 102], but the best test is not clear (see Table 26.1). Several strategies have been proposed, including the nonpregnancy recommended screening tests: fasting plasma glucose (FPG), 75-g OGTT, random plasma glucose (RPG), and A1C, or the typical 24–28 weeks of GDM diagnostic tests (50-gram GCT followed by OGTT). It should be noted that testing for FPG or A1C could lead to an underdiagnosis of women with preexisting diabetes as they both decrease early in pregnancy, and the typical 24–28 weeks of diagnostic testing have not been validated for diagnosis in early pregnancy [130]. Therefore, negative OGTT before 24 weeks should be repeated between 24 and 28 weeks [1].

Will early diagnosis of GDM result in an improved outcome? As there are no RCTs, extensive debate continues regarding the benefit of diagnosing hyperglycemia less severe than overt diabetes early in pregnancy and whether treatment will improve outcome. Earlier presentation with hyperglycemia, as compared to typical diagnosis at 24–28 weeks, may be more likely to have adverse outcomes and a need for insulin or other glucose-lowering medications [131, 132]. In fact, women with GDM diagnosis prior to 12 weeks of gestation may have similar pregnancy outcomes to women with preexisting or overt diabetes [133], and hyperglycemia early in pregnancy may result in unfavorable fetal metabolic imprinting [82]. However, data showing benefit of early treatment of GDM are lacking.

24.6.5 Repeat Testing

In most protocols, a negative OGTT at 24–28 weeks is not repeated later in pregnancy. However, several studies have shown that repeating the test after an initially normal OGTT will identify 4–29% additional [134–137]. Diagnosis of GDM, even at late pregnancy, has consequences for both the pregnant woman and her offspring, as it results in a set of actions, including intensified monitoring during pregnancy and labor, and postpartum screening for neonatal hypoglycemia, which is common in infants born from diabetic mothers [138]. Therefore, as there are no clear guidelines, repeat testing can be considered on an individualized basis in women with sonographic findings suggestive of a diagnosis of gestational diabetes, such as fetal overgrowth or polyhydramnios, or in those with a past history of gestational diabetes [134].

24.7 Non-pharmacologic Management

24.7.1 Prevention of Gestational Diabetes

The most important treatment modality is preventing GDM. High glucose levels may lead to disturbances in construction, function, and development of the fetus; therefore, maintaining normal levels of glucose from the very beginning of pregnancy is utmost important. To date, evidence from RCTs is limited [102], but findings from observational studies suggest that approximately 45% of GDM cases might be preventable by adoption of a healthy diet before pregnancy, maintaining a BMI <25 kg/m^2, exercising for ≥30 min/day and avoiding cigarette smoking [139–141].

24.7.2 Lifestyle Intervention

Once diagnosed, early intervention for GDM is essential to prevent subsequent damage in both mother and fetus [142]. The primary goal is preventing fetal overgrowth and pregnancy complications by controlling maternal hyperglycemia [6, 13]. Lifestyle modification is the cornerstone of treatment and should be initiated shortly after diagnosis [101]. For about 70–80% of women diagnosed with GDM, lifestyle measures such as changing dietary intake and engaging in physical activity are sufficient to achieve glycemic control [101, 143, 144]. It is anticipated that this proportion will be even higher if the lower diagnostic thresholds are used [119]. Excessive gestational weight gain is also associated with fetal overgrowth in both healthy and GDM pregnancies [144, 145]. In that respect, the IOM published recommendations for weekly gestational weight gain goals that are dependent on maternal prepregnancy BMI [144].

24.7.3 Glucose Monitoring and Targets

Although the optimal approach to glucose monitoring has not been determined [146], women with GDM are encouraged to self-monitor blood glucose levels initially at least four times daily: fasting and 1 or 2 h after beginning of each main meal [1, 147–149]. Postprandial glucose monitoring is associated with better glycemic control and lower risk of preeclampsia as compared to preprandial monitoring [4–6, 150]. Based on results of a randomized trial [151], when glycemic goals are easily obtained within 2 weeks of initiating lifestyle interventions many providers recommend that women may reduce the frequency of glucose measurements to every other day or twice weekly if the values are within target.

Glycemic targets include fasting glucose value <95 mg/dL and either 1-h postprandial glucose <140 mg/dL or 2-h postprandial glucose <120 mg/dL [1, 101, 152, 153]. Based on studies reporting association between increasing fasting maternal glucose levels and increasing neonatal adiposity/size that is LGA [154–156], some societies proposed that threshold of fasting glucose should be lowered to <90 mg/dL if achieved without hypoglycemia [152, 153]. Nevertheless, it was emphasized that if fasting threshold is maintained at <87 mg/dL, there is an increased likelihood of small-for-gestational-age infants [152].

Little guidance is available as to what proportion of measurements exceeding these thresholds should trigger intervention. However, most would agree that when glycemia remains elevated after ≥1–2 weeks of lifestyle interventions, daily glucose testing should be continued, and pharmacological treatment should be initiated. A recent retrospective cohort study suggested that advanced age or BMI by themselves are already indicators of medical requirement [157]. Ultrasonography assessment of fetal growth may also assist in guiding the intensity of glucose control that is needed in an individual woman. Appropriately growing baby, with fetal abdominal circumference <75th percentile, can be a reassuring sign of maternal glucose control and it may be safe to postpone initiation of pharmacological treatment. Conversely, excessive fetal growth may lead to intensification of treatment with lower glycemia goals [158–161]. Indeed, it was concluded in a meta-analysis from 2014, that ultrasound-based management of women with a broad severity-spectrum of gestational diabetes reduced the occurrence of LGA infants compared with conventional management, but increased ultrasound examination frequency and the number of women requiring insulin treatment [162].

24.8 Pharmacological Treatment

During medical treatment, the goals for glucose control and weight gain are the same as those for lifestyle interventions alone. Table 26.1 describes the different recommendations for pharmacological treatment by societies.

24.8.1 Insulin

Traditionally, insulin has been the primary medical treatment if the glycemic treatment goals are not achieved with lifestyle intervention. Insulin lowers blood glucose by stimulating peripheral glucose uptake and inhibiting glucose production release by the liver and is effective and safe for the fetus, as it does not cross the placenta. However, it requires multiple daily injections and subsequently the need to train the patients in the technical aspect of treatment, resulting in more weight gain and higher medical cost [163–165]. In addition, hypoglycemia occurs in approximately 70% of women who use insulin sometime during their pregnancy [166]. Human insulin and several insulin analogues (for example, insulin aspart, insulin lispro, and insulin detemir) have been formally tested and are considered safe to use in pregnancy [143].

24.8.2 Oral Antidiabetic Medication

Oral glucose-lowering medications, such as metformin and the sulfonylurea (commonly glyburide), have been extensively studied in women with GDM as they are both affordable and simple to take but cross the placenta, thus potentially affecting developing fetus. Systematic reviews comparing treatment with oral antihyperglycemic agents or insulin in GDM women found both approaches to be effective [167–169]. However, it is difficult to draw firm conclusions about the optimal approach because of inconsistencies in criteria for GDM, glucose targets, patient adherence to treatment, and clinical outcome measures across studies, as well as lack of data regarding long-term outcomes in offspring [169]. Therefore, all major international guidelines recommend lifestyle interventions and insulin as the gold standard for pharmacotherapy when needed but differ regarding the possible use of metformin or glyburide [1, 37, 101, 102, 170].

24.8.2.1 Metformin

Metformin is a biguanide that acts mainly by suppressing hepatic glucose production and promotes glucose uptake by peripheral tissues which result in reduction in FPG levels, improving insulin resistance and lowering A1C [171]. In RCTs, metformin seems to be comparable to insulin in glycemic control and immediate neonatal outcomes [172, 173] with less episodes of hypoglycemia [174] and less maternal weight gain [164]. Up to 50% of patients initially treated with metformin ultimately require insulin for glycemic control [172]. Predictors for failing metformin treatment include early detection of GDM, high BMI, baseline A1C, and FPG at diagnosis [172, 175, 176].

Several studies found that compared with insulin, metformin lowered birth weight and risks for macrosomia and LGA infants without increasing risk for small for gestational infants [174, 177, 178]. However, metformin-exposed children appear to experience accelerated postnatal growth, resulting in heavier infants and higher BMI by mid-childhood compared to children whose mothers were treated with insulin.

24.8.2.2 Sulfonylureas

Glyburide, a second-generation sulfonylurea, acts to increase insulin secretion from the pancreatic β-cell and improve peripheral insulin sensitivity. The resulting hyperinsulinemia leads to a decline in plasma glucose levels and A1C [13], and can cause weight gain, and maternal hypoglycemia, particularly if taken without food. In one RCT, glyburide was as effective as insulin in achieving glycemic control, rates of LGA and overall perinatal outcomes were similar [179]. However, a meta-analysis of 18 RCTs comparing the efficacy and safety of insulin, metformin and glyburide [164] observed higher infant birth weight, increased incidence of macrosomia and neonatal hypoglycemia with glyburide. Therefore, despite the rise in use of glyburide in pregnancy, it is generally not recommended as a first-line therapy in guidelines (Table 26.1).

24.9 Obstetric Considerations

Antenatal fetal testing is recommended and should be initiated at 32 weeks in women with GDM and poor glycemic control or those treated medically with insulin or oral agents due to suboptimal glycemic control at some time earlier in pregnancy [1]. Typical surveillance includes twice weekly nonstress test and amniotic fluid index, a strategy which has been shown to reduce stillbirth in pregnancies with pregestational or GDM [180]. For women with GDM well controlled on nutritional therapy alone, no increase in stillbirth has been observed and additional antenatal screening may not be necessary [181, 182]. The specific time to initiate surveillance and frequency of monitoring have not been studied and vary by institution. Many practitioners perform third trimester ultrasound in all women with GDM to assess fetal weight and identify cases where elective induction or caesarean delivery may be indicated to prevent birth complications. While this approach may be beneficial in reducing rates of shoulder dystocia and brachial plexus injury, current ultrasound measurement techniques have poor sensitivity and specificity for identifying macrosomic infants [51, 183, 184]. ACOG recommends incorporating serial measures of amniotic fluid as polyhydramnios can result from fetal hyperglycemia [1, 185].

Timing of delivery in pregnancies affected by GDM must weigh the risks of later delivery (stillbirth and delivery complications from excessive fetal growth) versus the potential disadvantage of earlier induction (risks of prematurity, longer labor, and possible increase in caesarean delivery). Studies examining the impact of early delivery versus expectant management have yielded conflicting results [186–189]. Increasing evidence suggests that induction of labor in women with GDM does not lead to higher caesarean delivery rates than expectant management [186, 188] with one study demonstrating reduction in caesarean section rate when labor is induced before 40 weeks [190]. Moreover, older studies and a 2008 meta-analysis reported reduced rates of macrosomia and shoulder dystocia with elective induction of labor at 38–39 weeks versus expectant management [187, 191]. However, a recent multicenter RCT found no difference in incidence of caesarean delivery or maternal or fetal complications (though intended sample size was not achieved) [188]. Table 26.1 lists the recommendations for labor induction for different societies.

24.10 Postpartum Management and Long-Term Maternal Health

Immediately after delivery pharmacotherapy for GDM treatment can be stopped, although glucose monitoring for a few days to exclude marked ongoing hyperglycemia is recommended. There is universal recognition that GDM identifies future risk of T2D with affected women exhibiting more than sevenfold increased risk compared with women with normoglycemic pregnancies and that the cumulative incidence of T2D is as high as 70% [12, 192, 193]. Higher fasting glucose level on OGTT was the factor found to associate most closely with risk of progression of GDM to T2D [192]. Older age, obesity, and family history were suggested as well [194]. This risk of overt diabetes is related both to preexisting (often undiagnosed) baseline abnormalities and to further progressive β-cell dysfunction and insulin resistance after the index GDM pregnancy associated mainly with weight gain postpartum [13]. Emerging evidence also suggests that the vasculature of women with a prior GDM is permanently altered, predisposing them to cardiovascular disease (CVD) [7, 195, 196].

Diagnosing women with GDM provides a unique opportunity to identify those with future risk of vascular disease in young age at an early point in the disease's natural history, when risk modification and primary prevention may potentially be feasible. As effective prevention interventions are available, women diagnosed with GDM should receive lifelong screening for glucose intolerance to allow interventions to reduce diabetes risk and to allow treatment at the earliest time possible [32]. Therefore, all women with GDM should undergo postpartum OGTT at 4–12 weeks to identify persistent glucose intolerance or over diabetes [1, 101]. If postpartum OGTT is normal, routine screening should continue every 1–3 years or more frequently depending on their other risk factors [143]. Due to higher recurrence rate of GDM of 41.3%, compared to 4.2% in women without previous GDM [197], early screening in subsequent pregnancies is indicated [101]. Unfortunately, less than a fifth of mothers with GDM undergo postpartum glucose screening [198], and the opportunity to prevent or delay T2D by lifestyle interventions and medical treatments may be lost [199, 200].

Women should be encouraged to breastfeed has it been shown to reduce the risk of T2D [201, 202]. Breastfeeding was also found to have additional short- and long-term beneficial effects on offspring metabolic health [203]. Moreover, returning to prepregnancy body weight is of paramount importance because it is associated with a substantial improvement in the overall metabolic condition [204]. The American Diabetes Association recommends considering metformin for women with prediabetes and a prior history of GDM because it has been found to be particularly effective for preventing T2D in this population [205].

References

[1]   Committee on Practice B-O. ACOG Practice Bulletin No. 190: Gestational Diabetes Mellitus. Obstet Gynecol 2018;131(2):e49–e64.
[2]   Classification and diagnosis of diabetes mellitus and other categories of glucose intolerance. National Diabetes Data Group. Diabetes 1979;28(12):1039–1057.
[3]   Jarrett RJ. Gestational diabetes: A non-entity?. BMJ 1993;306(6869):37–38.
[4]   Crowther CA, Hiller JE, Moss JR et al. Effect of treatment of gestational diabetes mellitus on pregnancy outcomes. N Engl J Med 2005;352(24):2477–2486.
[5]   Langer O, Yogev Y, Most O et al. Gestational diabetes: The consequences of not treating. Am J Obstet Gynecol 2005;192(4):989–997.
[6]   Hartling L, Dryden DM, Guthrie A et al. Benefits and harms of treating gestational diabetes mellitus: A systematic review and meta-analysis for the U.S. Preventive Services Task Force and the National Institutes of Health Office of Medical Applications of Research. Ann Intern Med 2013;159(2):123–129.
[7]   Daly B, Toulis KA, Thomas N et al. Increased risk of ischemic heart disease, hypertension, and type 2 diabetes in women with previous gestational diabetes mellitus, a target group in general practice for preventive interventions: A population-based cohort study. PLoS Med 2018;15(1):e1002488.

[8]   Clausen TD, Mathiesen ER, Hansen T et al. High prevalence of type 2 diabetes and pre-
      diabetes in adult offspring of women with gestational diabetes mellitus or type 1 diabetes:
      The role of intrauterine hyperglycemia. Diabetes Care 2008;31(2):340–346.
[9]   Dabelea D, Hanson RL, Lindsay RS et al. Intrauterine exposure to diabetes conveys risks for
      type 2 diabetes and obesity: A study of discordant sibships. Diabetes 2000;49(12):
      2208–2211.
[10] Dabelea D, Snell-Bergeon JK, Hartsfield CL et al. Increasing prevalence of gestational
      diabetes mellitus (GDM) over time and by birth cohort: Kaiser Permanente of Colorado GDM
      Screening Program. Diabetes Care 2005;28(3):579–584.
[11] Kim SY, Saraiva C, Curtis M et al. Fraction of gestational diabetes mellitus attributable to
      overweight and obesity by race/ethnicity, California, 2007-2009. Am J Public Health
      2013;103(10):e65–72.
[12] Zhu Y, Zhang C. Prevalence of Gestational Diabetes and Risk of Progression to Type 2
      Diabetes: A Global Perspective. Curr Diab Rep 2016;16(1):7.
[13] McIntyre HD, Catalano P, Zhang C et al. Gestational diabetes mellitus. Nat Rev Dis Primers
      2019;5(1):47.
[14] Bardenheier BH, Elixhauser A, Imperatore G et al. Variation in prevalence of gestational
      diabetes mellitus among hospital discharges for obstetric delivery across 23 states in the
      United States. Diabetes Care 2013;36(5):1209–1214.
[15] Lao TT, Ho LF, Chan BC et al,. Maternal age and prevalence of gestational diabetes mellitus.
      Diabetes Care 2006;29(4):948–949.
[16] Okosun IS, Chandra KM, Boev A et al. Abdominal adiposity in U.S. adults: Prevalence and
      trends, 1960-2000. Prev Med 2004;39(1):197–206.
[17] Zhang C, Ning Y. Effect of dietary and lifestyle factors on the risk of gestational diabetes:
      Review of epidemiologic evidence. Am J Clin Nutr 2011;94(6Suppl):1975S–9S.
[18] King JC. Maternal obesity, metabolism, and pregnancy outcomes. Annu Rev Nutr 2006;26:
      271–291.
[19] Kahn BB, Flier JS. Obesity and insulin resistance. J Clin Invest 2000;106(4):473–481.
[20] Sathyapalan T, Mellor D, Atkin SL. Obesity and gestational diabetes. Semin Fetal Neonatal
      Med 2010;15(2):89–93.
[21] Durnwald C. Gestational diabetes: Linking epidemiology, excessive gestational weight gain,
      adverse pregnancy outcomes, and future metabolic syndrome. Semin Perinatol 2015;39(4):
      254–258.
[22] Jenum AK, Morkrid K, Sletner L et al. Impact of ethnicity on gestational diabetes identified
      with the WHO and the modified International Association of Diabetes and Pregnancy Study
      Groups criteria: A population-based cohort study. Eur J Endocrinol 2012;166(2):317–324.
[23] Anghebem-Oliveira MI, Martins BR, Alberton D et al. Type 2 diabetes-associated genetic
      variants of FTO, LEPR, PPARg, and TCF7L2 in gestational diabetes in a Brazilian population.
      Arch Endocrinol Metab 2017;61(3):238–248.
[24] Teh WT, Teede HJ, Paul E et al. Risk factors for gestational diabetes mellitus: Implications for
      the application of screening guidelines. Aust N Z J Obstet Gynaecol 2011;51(1):26–30.
[25] Levy A, Wiznitzer A, Holcberg G et al. Family history of diabetes mellitus as an independent
      risk factor for macrosomia and cesarean delivery. J Matern Fetal Neonatal Med 2010;23(2):
      148–152.
[26] Ben-Haroush A, Yogev Y, Hod M. Epidemiology of gestational diabetes mellitus and its
      association with Type 2 diabetes. Diabet Med 2004;21(2):103–113.
[27] Plows JF, Stanley JL, Baker PN et al. The Pathophysiology of Gestational Diabetes Mellitus. Int
      J Mol Sci 2018;19(11).

[28]   Edey LF, Georgiou H, O'Dea KP et al. Progesterone, the maternal immune system and the onset of parturition in the mouse. Biol Reprod 2018;98(3):376–395.

[29]   Carter AM. Evolution of placental function in mammals: The molecular basis of gas and nutrient transfer, hormone secretion, and immune responses. Physiol Rev 2012;92(4): 1543–1576.

[30]   Musial B, Fernandez-Twinn DS, Vaughan OR et al. Proximity to Delivery Alters Insulin Sensitivity and Glucose Metabolism in Pregnant Mice. Diabetes 2016;65(4):851–860.

[31]   Diagnostic Criteria and Classification of Hyperglycaemia First Detected in Pregnancy. WHO Guidelines Approved by the Guidelines Review Committee. Geneva 2013.

[32]   American Diabetes A. 2. Classification and Diagnosis of Diabetes: Standards of Medical Care in Diabetes-2020. Diabetes Care 2020;43(Suppl 1):S14–S31.

[33]   Rieck S, Kaestner KH. Expansion of beta-cell mass in response to pregnancy. Trends Endocrinol Metab 2010;21(3):151–158.

[34]   Barbour LA, McCurdy CE, Hernandez TL et al. Cellular mechanisms for insulin resistance in normal pregnancy and gestational diabetes. Diabetes Care 2007;30(Suppl 2):S112–9.

[35]   Johns EC, Denison FC, Norman JE et al. Gestational Diabetes Mellitus: Mechanisms, Treatment, and Complications. Trends Endocrinol Metab 2018;29(11):743–754.

[36]   Buchanan TA. Pancreatic B-cell defects in gestational diabetes: Implications for the pathogenesis and prevention of type 2 diabetes. J Clin Endocrinol Metab 2001;86(3): 989–993.

[37]   Hod M, Kapur A, Sacks DA et al. The International Federation of Gynecology and Obstetrics (FIGO) Initiative on gestational diabetes mellitus: A pragmatic guide for diagnosis, management, and care. Int J Gynaecol Obstet 2015;131(Suppl 3):S173–211.

[38]   Ashcroft FM, Rohm M, Clark A et al. Is Type 2 Diabetes a Glycogen Storage Disease of Pancreatic beta Cells?. Cell Metab 2017;26(1):17–23.

[39]   Kleinberger JW, Maloney KA, Pollin TI. The Genetic Architecture of Diabetes in Pregnancy: Implications for Clinical Practice. Am J Perinatol 2016;33(13):1319–1326.

[40]   Group HSCR Be M, Lp L et al. Hyperglycemia and adverse pregnancy outcomes. N Engl J Med 2008;358(19):1991–2002.

[41]   Lowe WL Jr., Scholtens DM, Lowe LP et al. Association of gestational diabetes with maternal disorders of glucose metabolism and childhood adiposity. JAMA 2018;320(10):1005–1016.

[42]   Pedersen J, Bojsen-Moller B, Poulsen H. Blood sugar in newborn infants of diabetic mothers. Acta Endocrinol (Copenh) 1954;15(1):33–52.

[43]   Desoye G, Nolan CJ. The fetal glucose steal: An underappreciated phenomenon in diabetic pregnancy. Diabetologia 2016;59(6):1089–1094.

[44]   Mitanchez D, Yzydorczyk C, Siddeek B et al. The offspring of the diabetic mother—short- and long-term implications. Best Pract Res Clin Obstet Gynaecol 2015;29(2):256–269.

[45]   Schwartz R, Gruppuso PA, Petzold K et al. Hyperinsulinemia and macrosomia in the fetus of the diabetic mother. Diabetes Care 1994;17(7):640–648.

[46]   Sovio U, Murphy HR, Smith GC. Accelerated fetal growth prior to diagnosis of gestational diabetes mellitus: a prospective cohort study of nulliparous women. Diabetes Care 2016;39(6):982–987.

[47]   Ben-Haroush A, Hadar E, Chen R et al. Maternal obesity is a major risk factor for large-for-gestational-infants in pregnancies complicated by gestational diabetes. Arch Gynecol Obstet 2009;279(4):539–543.

[48]   Hillier TA, Pedula KL, Vesco KK et al. Excess gestational weight gain: Modifying fetal macrosomia risk associated with maternal glucose. Obstet Gynecol 2008;112(5):1007–1014.

[49]   Stotland NE, Caughey AB, Breed EM et al. Risk factors and obstetric complications associated with macrosomia. Int J Gynaecol Obstet 2004;87(3):220–226.

[50]   Gascho CL, Leandro DM, Ribeiro EST et al. Predictors of cesarean delivery in pregnant women with gestational diabetes mellitus. Rev Bras Ginecol Obstet 2017;39(2):60–65.

[51]   Scifres CM, Feghali M, Dumont T et al. Large-for-gestational-age ultrasound diagnosis and risk for cesarean delivery in women with gestational diabetes mellitus. Obstet Gynecol 2015;126(5):978–986.

[52]   Metzger BE, Persson B, Lowe LP et al. Hyperglycemia and adverse pregnancy outcome study: Neonatal glycemia. Pediatrics 2010;126(6):e1545–52.

[53]   Cohen BF, Penning S, Ansley D et al. The incidence and severity of shoulder dystocia correlates with a sonographic measurement of asymmetry in patients with diabetes. Am J Perinatol 1999;16(4):197–201.

[54]   Philips AF, Dubin JW, Matty PJ et al. Arterial hypoxemia and hyperinsulinemia in the chronically hyperglycemic fetal lamb. Pediatr Res 1982;16(8):653–658.

[55]   Nold JL, Georgieff MK. Infants of diabetic mothers. Pediatr Clin North Am 2004;51(3): 619–637viii.

[56]   Salvesen DR, Brudenell JM, Snijders RJ et al. Fetal plasma erythropoietin in pregnancies complicated by maternal diabetes mellitus. Am J Obstet Gynecol 1993;168(1 Pt 1):88–94.

[57]   Jovanovic L, Pettitt DJ. Gestational diabetes mellitus. JAMA 2001;286(20):2516–2518.

[58]   Moore TR. A comparison of amniotic fluid fetal pulmonary phospholipids in normal and diabetic pregnancy. Am J Obstet Gynecol 2002;186(4):641–650.

[59]   West NA, Kechris K, Dabelea D. Exposure to maternal diabetes in utero and DNA methylation patterns in the offspring. Immunometabolism 2013;1:1–9.

[60]   El Hajj N, Pliushch G, Schneider E et al. Metabolic programming of MEST DNA methylation by intrauterine exposure to gestational diabetes mellitus. Diabetes 2013;62(4):1320–1328.

[61]   Cheng X, Chapple SJ, Patel B et al. Gestational diabetes mellitus impairs Nrf2-mediated adaptive antioxidant defenses and redox signaling in fetal endothelial cells in utero. Diabetes 2013;62(12):4088–4097.

[62]   Houshmand-Oeregaard A, Hansen NS, Hjort L et al. Differential adipokine DNA methylation and gene expression in subcutaneous adipose tissue from adult offspring of women with diabetes in pregnancy. Clin Epigenetics 2017;9:37.

[63]   Houshmand-Oeregaard A, Hjort L, Kelstrup L et al. DNA methylation and gene expression of TXNIP in adult offspring of women with diabetes in pregnancy. PLoS One 2017;12(10): e0187038.

[64]   Hjort L, Martino D, Grunnet LG et al. Gestational diabetes and maternal obesity are associated with epigenome-wide methylation changes in children. JCI Insight 2018;3(17).

[65]   Chang SC, Vivian Yang WC. Hyperglycemia induces altered expressions of angiogenesis associated molecules in the trophoblast. Evid Based Complement Alternat Med 2013;2013:457971.

[66]   Yu J, Zhou Y, Gui J et al. Assessment of the number and function of macrophages in the placenta of gestational diabetes mellitus patients. J Huazhong Univ Sci Technolog Med Sci 2013;33(5):725–729.

[67]   Clausen TD, Mathiesen ER, Hansen T et al. Overweight and the metabolic syndrome in adult offspring of women with diet-treated gestational diabetes mellitus or type 1 diabetes. J Clin Endocrinol Metab 2009;94(7):2464–2470.

[68]   Kim SY, England JL, Sharma JA et al. Gestational diabetes mellitus and risk of childhood overweight and obesity in offspring: A systematic review. Exp Diabetes Res 2011;2011:541308.

[69]   Bianco ME, Josefson JL. Hyperglycemia during pregnancy and long-term offspring outcomes. Curr Diab Rep 2019;19(12):143.

[70] Scholtens DM, Kuang A, Lowe LP et al. Hyperglycemia and adverse pregnancy outcome follow-up Study (HAPO FUS): maternal glycemia and childhood glucose metabolism. Diabetes Care 2019;42(3):381–392.

[71] Ehrlich SF, Rosas LG, Ferrara A et al. Pregnancy glucose levels in women without diabetes or gestational diabetes and childhood cardiometabolic risk at 7 years of age. J Pediatr 2012;161(6):1016–1021.

[72] Nehring I, Chmitorz A, Reulen H et al. Gestational diabetes predicts the risk of childhood overweight and abdominal circumference independent of maternal obesity. Diabet Med 2013;30(12):1449–1456.

[73] Aceti A, Santhakumaran S, Logan KM et al. The diabetic pregnancy and offspring blood pressure in childhood: A systematic review and meta-analysis. Diabetologia 2012;55(11): 3114–3127.

[74] Kelstrup L, Damm P, Mathiesen ER et al. Insulin resistance and Impaired pancreatic beta-cell function in adult offspring of women with diabetes in pregnancy. J Clin Endocrinol Metab 2013;98(9):3793–3801.

[75] Grunnet LG, Hansen S, Hjort L et al. Adiposity, dysmetabolic traits, and earlier onset of female puberty in adolescent offspring of women with gestational diabetes mellitus: a clinical study within the danish national birth cohort. Diabetes Care 2017;40(12):1746–1755.

[76] Wu CS, Nohr EA, Bech BH et al. Long-term health outcomes in children born to mothers with diabetes: A population-based cohort study. PLoS One 2012;7(5):e36727.

[77] Tam WH, Ma RCW, Ozaki R et al. In utero exposure to maternal hyperglycemia increases childhood cardiometabolic risk in offspring. Diabetes Care 2017;40(5):679–686.

[78] Lambrinoudaki I, Vlachou SA, Creatsas G. Genetics in gestational diabetes mellitus: Association with incidence, severity, pregnancy outcome and response to treatment. Curr Diabetes Rev 2010;6(6):393–399.

[79] Landon MB, Spong CY, Thom E et al. A multicenter, randomized trial of treatment for mild gestational diabetes. N Engl J Med 2009;361(14):1339–1348.

[80] Harder T, Aerts L, Franke K et al. Pancreatic islet transplantation in diabetic pregnant rats prevents acquired malformation of the ventromedial hypothalamic nucleus in their offspring. Neurosci Lett 2001;299(1-2):85–88.

[81] Aerts L, Van Assche FA. Animal evidence for the transgenerational development of diabetes mellitus. Int J Biochem Cell Biol 2006;38(5-6):894–903.

[82] Hillier TA, Pedula KL, Schmidt MM et al. Childhood obesity and metabolic imprinting: The ongoing effects of maternal hyperglycemia. Diabetes Care 2007;30(9):2287–2292.

[83] Gillman MW, Oakey H, Baghurst PA et al. Effect of treatment of gestational diabetes mellitus on obesity in the next generation. Diabetes Care 2010;33(5):964–968.

[84] Landon MB, Mele L, Varner MW et al. The relationship of maternal glycemia to childhood obesity and metabolic dysfunction(double dagger). J Matern Fetal Neonatal Med 2020;33(1): 33–41.

[85] Landon MB, Rice MM, Varner MW et al. Mild gestational diabetes mellitus and long-term child health. Diabetes Care 2015;38(3):445–452.

[86] O'Sullivan JB, Mahan CM. Criteria for the oral glucose tolerance test in pregnancy. Diabetes 1964;13:278–285.

[87] Idris N, Hatikah CC, Murizah M et al. Universal versus selective screening for detection of gestational diabetes mellitus in a malaysian population. Malays Fam Physician 2009;4(2-3): 83–87.

[88] Miailhe G, Kayem G, Girard G et al. Selective rather than universal screening for gestational diabetes mellitus?. Eur J Obstet Gynecol Reprod Biol 2015;191:95–100.

[89] Cosson E, Benbara A, Pharisien I et al. Diagnostic and prognostic performances over 9 years of a selective screening strategy for gestational diabetes mellitus in a cohort of 18,775 subjects. Diabetes Care 2013;36(3):598–603.

[90] Farrar D, Simmonds M, Bryant M et al. Risk factor screening to identify women requiring oral glucose tolerance testing to diagnose gestational diabetes: A systematic review and meta-analysis and analysis of two pregnancy cohorts. PLoS One 2017;12(4):e0175288.

[91] O'Sullivan JB, Mahan CM, Charles D et al. Screening criteria for high-risk gestational diabetic patients. Am J Obstet Gynecol 1973;116(7):895–900.

[92] Va M. Force USPST. Screening for gestational diabetes mellitus: U.S. Preventive Services Task Force recommendation statement. Ann Intern Med 2014;160(6):414–420.

[93] Carpenter MW, Coustan DR. Criteria for screening tests for gestational diabetes. Am J Obstet Gynecol 1982;144(7):768–773.

[94] Yang X, Hsu-Hage B, Zhang H et al. Women with impaired glucose tolerance during pregnancy have significantly poor pregnancy outcomes. Diabetes Care 2002;25(9): 1619–1624.

[95] Vambergue A, Nuttens MC, Verier-Mine O et al. Is mild gestational hyperglycaemia associated with maternal and neonatal complications? The Diagest Study. Diabet Med 2000;17(3):203–208.

[96] Langer O, Brustman L, Anyaegbunam A et al. The significance of one abnormal glucose tolerance test value on adverse outcome in pregnancy. Am J Obstet Gynecol 1987;157(3): 758–763.

[97] Sermer M, Naylor CD, Gare DJ et al. Impact of increasing carbohydrate intolerance on maternal-fetal outcomes in 3637 women without gestational diabetes. The Toronto Tri-Hospital Gestational Diabetes Project. Am J Obstet Gynecol 1995;173(1):146–156.

[98] International Association of D, Pregnancy Study Groups Consensus P Metzger BE et al. International association of diabetes and pregnancy study groups recommendations on the diagnosis and classification of hyperglycemia in pregnancy. Diabetes Care 2010;33(3):676–682.

[99] Waters TP, Dyer AR, Scholtens DM et al. Maternal and neonatal morbidity for women who would be added to the diagnosis of GDM using iadpsg criteria: a secondary analysis of the hyperglycemia and adverse pregnancy outcome study. Diabetes Care 2016;39(12): 2204–2210.

[100] Sacks DA, Hadden DR, Maresh M et al. Frequency of gestational diabetes mellitus at collaborating centers based on IADPSG consensus panel-recommended criteria: The Hyperglycemia and Adverse Pregnancy Outcome (HAPO) Study. Diabetes Care 2012;35(3): 526–528.

[101] American Diabetes A. 14. Management of diabetes in pregnancy: standards of medical care in diabetes-2019. Diabetes Care 2019;42(Suppl1):S165–S72.

[102] Diabetes Canada Clinical Practice Guidelines Expert C Feig DS, Berger H et al,. Diabetes and pregnancy. Can J Diabetes 2018;42(Suppl 1):S255–S82.

[103] Rumbold AR, Crowther CA. Women's experiences of being screened for gestational diabetes mellitus. Aust N Z J Obstet Gynaecol 2002;42(2):131–137.

[104] Dalfra MG, Nicolucci A, Bisson T et al. Quality of life in pregnancy and post-partum: A study in diabetic patients. Qual Life Res 2012;21(2):291–298.

[105] Roeckner JT, Sanchez-Ramos L, Jijon-Knupp R et al. Single abnormal value on 3-hour oral glucose tolerance test during pregnancy is associated with adverse maternal and neonatal outcomes: A systematic review and metaanalysis. Am J Obstet Gynecol 2016;215(3):287–297.

[106] Vandorsten JP, Dodson WC, Espeland MA et al. NIH consensus development conference: Diagnosing gestational diabetes mellitus. NIH Consens State Sci Statements 2013;29(1): 1–31.

[107] Saade GR. Expanding the screening for diabetes in pregnancy: Overmedicalization or the right thing to do?. Obstet Gynecol 2013;122(2 Pt 1):195–197.

[108] Brown FM, Wyckoff J. Application of One-Step IADPSG Versus two-step diagnostic criteria for gestational diabetes in the real world: impact on health services, clinical care, and outcomes. Curr Diab Rep 2017;17(10):85.

[109] Sacks DB, Coustan DR, Cundy T et al. Gestational diabetes mellitus: why the controversy?. Clin Chem 2018;64(3):431–438.

[110] Benhalima K, Lens K, Bosteels J et al. The risk for glucose intolerance after gestational diabetes mellitus since the introduction of the IADPSG criteria: a systematic review and meta-analysis. J Clin Med 2019;8(9).

[111] Werner EF, Pettker CM, Zuckerwise L et al. Screening for gestational diabetes mellitus: Are the criteria proposed by the international association of the Diabetes and Pregnancy Study Groups cost-effective?. Diabetes Care 2012;35(3):529–535.

[112] O'Sullivan EP, Avalos G, O'Reilly M et al. Atlantic Diabetes in Pregnancy (DIP): The prevalence and outcomes of gestational diabetes mellitus using new diagnostic criteria. Diabetologia 2011;54(7):1670–1675.

[113] Ethridge JK Jr., Catalano PM, Waters TP. Perinatal outcomes associated with the diagnosis of gestational diabetes made by the international association of the diabetes and pregnancy study groups criteria. Obstet Gynecol 2014;124(3):571–578.

[114] Benhalima K, Hanssens M, Devlieger R et al. Analysis of Pregnancy Outcomes Using the New IADPSG Recommendation Compared with the Carpenter and Coustan Criteria in an Area with a Low Prevalence of Gestational Diabetes. Int J Endocrinol 2013;2013:248121.

[115] Duran A, Saenz S, Torrejon MJ et al. Introduction of IADPSG criteria for the screening and diagnosis of gestational diabetes mellitus results in improved pregnancy outcomes at a lower cost in a large cohort of pregnant women: The St. Carlos Gestational Diabetes Study Diabetes Care 2014;37(9):2442–2450.

[116] Hung TH, Hsieh TT. The effects of implementing the International Association of Diabetes and Pregnancy Study Groups criteria for diagnosing gestational diabetes on maternal and neonatal outcomes. PLoS One 2015;10(3):e0122261.

[117] Kuo CH, Li HY. Diagnostic strategies for gestational diabetes mellitus: review of current evidence. Curr Diab Rep 2019;19(12):155.

[118] Wu ET, Nien FJ, Kuo CH et al. Diagnosis of more gestational diabetes lead to better pregnancy outcomes: Comparing the International Association of the Diabetes and Pregnancy Study Group criteria, and the Carpenter and Coustan criteria. J Diabetes Investig 2016;7(1):121–126.

[119] Mayo K, Melamed N, Vandenberghe H et al. The impact of adoption of the international association of diabetes in pregnancy study group criteria for the screening and diagnosis of gestational diabetes. Am J Obstet Gynecol 2015;212(2):224e1-9.

[120] Fuller KP, Borgida AF. Gestational diabetes mellitus screening using the one-step versus two-step method in a high-risk practice. Clin Diabetes 2014;32(4):148–150.

[121] Oriot P, Selvais P, Radikov J et al. Assessing the incidence of gestational diabetes and neonatal outcomes using the IADPSG guidelines in comparison with the Carpenter and Coustan criteria in a Belgian general hospital. Acta Clin Belg 2014;69(1):8–11.

[122] Wei YM, Yang HX, Zhu WW et al. Effects of intervention to mild GDM on outcomes. J Matern Fetal Neonatal Med 2015;28(8):928–931.

[123] Kong JM, Lim K, Thompson DM. Evaluation of the International Association of the Diabetes In Pregnancy Study Group new criteria: Gestational diabetes project. Can J Diabetes 2015;39(2): 128–132.

[124] Feldman RK, Tieu RS, Yasumura L. Gestational diabetes screening: the international association of the diabetes and pregnancy study groups compared with carpenter-coustan screening. Obstet Gynecol 2016;127(1):10–17.

[125] Meltzer SJ, Snyder J, Penrod JR et al. Gestational diabetes mellitus screening and diagnosis: A prospective randomised controlled trial comparing costs of one-step and two-step methods. BJOG 2010;117(4):407–415.

[126] Sevket O, Ates S, Uysal O et al. To evaluate the prevalence and clinical outcomes using a one-step method versus a two-step method to screen gestational diabetes mellitus. J Matern Fetal Neonatal Med 2014;27(1):36–41.

[127] Scifres CM, Abebe KZ, Jones KA et al. Gestational diabetes diagnostic methods (GD2M) pilot randomized trial. Matern Child Health J 2015;19(7):1472–1480.

[128] Khalifeh A, Eckler R, Felder L et al. One-step versus two-step diagnostic testing for gestational diabetes: A randomized controlled trial. J Matern Fetal Neonatal Med 2020;33(4): 612–617.

[129] Mendez-Figueroa H, Daley J, Lopes VV et al. Comparing daily versus less frequent blood glucose monitoring in patients with mild gestational diabetes. J Matern Fetal Neonatal Med 2013;26(13):1268–1272.

[130] McIntyre HD, Sacks DA, Barbour LA et al. Issues with the diagnosis and classification of hyperglycemia in early pregnancy. Diabetes Care 2016;39(1):53–54.

[131] Immanuel J, Simmons D. Screening and treatment for early-onset gestational diabetes mellitus: a systematic review and meta-analysis. Curr Diab Rep 2017;17(11):115.

[132] Bartha JL, Martinez-Del-Fresno P, Comino-Delgado R. Early diagnosis of gestational diabetes mellitus and prevention of diabetes-related complications. Eur J Obstet Gynecol Reprod Biol 2003;109(1):41–44.

[133] Sweeting AN, Ross GP, Hyett J et al. Gestational diabetes mellitus in early pregnancy: evidence for poor pregnancy outcomes despite treatment. Diabetes Care 2016;39(1):75–81.

[134] De Wit L, Bos DM, Van Rossum AP et al. Repeated oral glucose tolerance tests in women at risk for gestational diabetes mellitus. Eur J Obstet Gynecol Reprod Biol 2019;242:79–85.

[135] Seshiah V, Balaji V, Balaji MS et al. Gestational diabetes mellitus manifests in all trimesters of pregnancy. Diabetes Res Clin Pract 2007;77(3):482–484.

[136] Kurtbas H, Keskin HL, Avsar AF. Effectiveness of screening for gestational diabetes during the late gestational period among pregnant Turkish women. J Obstet Gynaecol Res 2011;37(6): 520–526.

[137] Boriboonhirunsarn D, Sunsaneevithayakul P. Abnormal results on a second testing and risk of gestational diabetes in women with normal baseline glucose levels. Int J Gynaecol Obstet 2008;100(2):147–153.

[138] Voormolen DN, De Wit L, Van Rijn BB et al. Neonatal hypoglycemia following diet-controlled and insulin-treated gestational diabetes mellitus. Diabetes Care 2018;41(7):1385–1390.

[139] Zhang C, Tobias DK, Chavarro JE et al. Adherence to healthy lifestyle and risk of gestational diabetes mellitus: Prospective cohort study. BMJ 2014;349:g5450.

[140] Tobias DK, Zhang C, Van Dam RM et al. Physical activity before and during pregnancy and risk of gestational diabetes mellitus: A meta-analysis. Diabetes Care 2011;34(1):223–229.

[141] Catalano P, deMouzon SH. Maternal obesity and metabolic risk to the offspring: Why lifestyle interventions may have not achieved the desired outcomes. Int J Obes (Lond) 2015;39(4): 642–649.

[142] Sexton H, Heal C, Banks J et al. Impact of new diagnostic criteria for gestational diabetes. J Obstet Gynaecol Res 2018;44(3):425–431.

[143] American Diabetes A. 13. Management of Diabetes in Pregnancy: Standards of Medical Care in Diabetes-2018. Diabetes Care 2018;41(Suppl 1):S137–S43.

[144] Rasmussen KM, Catalano PM, Yaktine AL. New guidelines for weight gain during pregnancy: What obstetrician/gynecologists should know. Curr Opin Obstet Gynecol 2009;21(6):521–526.

[145] Kurtzhals LL, Norgaard SK, Secher AL et al. The impact of restricted gestational weight gain by dietary intervention on fetal growth in women with gestational diabetes mellitus. Diabetologia 2018;61(12):2528–2538.

[146] Raman P, Shepherd E, Dowswell T et al. Different methods and settings for glucose monitoring for gestational diabetes during pregnancy. Cochrane Database Syst Rev 2017(10): CD011069.

[147] Weisz B, Shrim A, Homko CJ et al. One hour versus two hours postprandial glucose measurement in gestational diabetes: A prospective study. J Perinatol 2005;25(4):241–244.

[148] Moses RG, Lucas EM, Knights S. Gestational diabetes mellitus. At What Time Should the Postprandial Glucose Level Be Monitored? Aust N Z J Obstet Gynaecol 1999;39(4):457–460.

[149] Sivan E, Weisz B, Homko CJ et al. One or two hours postprandial glucose measurements: Are they the same?. Am J Obstet Gynecol 2001;185(3):604–607.

[150] De Veciana M, Major CA, Morgan MA et al. Postprandial versus preprandial blood glucose monitoring in women with gestational diabetes mellitus requiring insulin therapy. N Engl J Med 1995;333(19):1237–1241.

[151] Mendez-Figueroa H, Schuster M, Maggio L et al. Gestational diabetes mellitus and frequency of blood glucose monitoring: a randomized controlled trial. Obstet Gynecol 2017;130(1): 163–170.

[152] Metzger BE, Buchanan TA, Coustan DR et al. Summary and recommendations of the Fifth International Workshop-Conference on Gestational Diabetes Mellitus. Diabetes Care 2007;30(Suppl 2):S251–60.

[153] Blumer I, Hadar E, Hadden DR et al. Diabetes and pregnancy: An endocrine society clinical practice guideline. J Clin Endocrinol Metab 2013;98(11):4227–4249.

[154] Durnwald CP, Mele L, Spong CY et al. Glycemic characteristics and neonatal outcomes of women treated for mild gestational diabetes. Obstet Gynecol 2011;117(4):819–827.

[155] Uvena-Celebrezze J, Fung C, Thomas AJ et al. Relationship of neonatal body composition to maternal glucose control in women with gestational diabetes mellitus. J Matern Fetal Neonatal Med 2002;12(6):396–401.

[156] Catalano PM, Thomas A, Huston-Presley L et al. Increased fetal adiposity: A very sensitive marker of abnormal in utero development. Am J Obstet Gynecol 2003;189(6):1698–1704.

[157] Ali A, Shastry S, Nithiyananthan R et al. Gestational diabetes-Predictors of response to treatment and obstetric outcome. Eur J Obstet Gynecol Reprod Biol 2018;220:57–60.

[158] Kjos SL, Schaefer-Graf UM. Modified therapy for gestational diabetes using high-risk and low-risk fetal abdominal circumference growth to select strict versus relaxed maternal glycemic targets. Diabetes Care 2007;30(Suppl 2):S200–5.

[159] Kjos SL, Schaefer-Graf U, Sardesi S et al. A randomized controlled trial using glycemic plus fetal ultrasound parameters versus glycemic parameters to determine insulin therapy in gestational diabetes with fasting hyperglycemia. Diabetes Care 2001;24(11):1904–1910.

[160] Bonomo M, Cetin I, Pisoni MP et al. Flexible treatment of gestational diabetes modulated on ultrasound evaluation of intrauterine growth: A controlled randomized clinical trial. Diabetes Metab 2004;30(3):237–244.

[161] Rossi G, Somigliana E, Moschetta M et al. Adequate timing of fetal ultrasound to guide metabolic therapy in mild gestational diabetes mellitus. Results from a Randomized Study Acta Obstet Gynecol Scand 2000;79(8):649–654.

[162] Balsells M, Garcia-Patterson A, Gich I et al. Ultrasound-guided compared to conventional treatment in gestational diabetes leads to improved birthweight but more insulin treatment: Systematic review and meta-analysis. Acta Obstet Gynecol Scand 2014;93(2):144–151.

[163] Norman RJ, Wang JX, Hague W. Should we continue or stop insulin sensitizing drugs during pregnancy?. Curr Opin Obstet Gynecol 2004;16(3):245–250.

[164] Jiang YF, Chen XY, Ding T et al,. Comparative efficacy and safety of OADs in management of GDM: Network meta-analysis of randomized controlled trials. J Clin Endocrinol Metab 2015;100(5):2071–2080.

[165] Lv S, Wang J, Xu Y. Safety of insulin analogs during pregnancy: A meta-analysis. Arch Gynecol Obstet 2015;292(4):749–756.

[166] Refuerzo JS. Oral hypoglycemic agents in pregnancy. Obstet Gynecol Clin North Am 2011;38(2):227–234ix.

[167] Dhulkotia JS, Ola B, Fraser R et al. Oral hypoglycemic agents vs insulin in management of gestational diabetes: A systematic review and metaanalysis. Am J Obstet Gynecol 2010;203(5):457e1-9.

[168] Balsells M, Garcia-Patterson A, Sola I et al. Glibenclamide, metformin, and insulin for the treatment of gestational diabetes: A systematic review and meta-analysis. BMJ 2015;350: h102.

[169] Brown J, Grzeskowiak L, Williamson K et al. Insulin for the treatment of women with gestational diabetes. Cochrane Database Syst Rev 2017(11):CD012037.

[170] Society of Maternal-Fetal Medicine Publications Committee. Electronic address pso. SMFM Statement: Pharmacological treatment of gestational diabetes. Am J Obstet Gynecol 2018;218(5):B2–B4.

[171] Rena G, Hardie DG, Pearson ER. The mechanisms of action of metformin. Diabetologia 2017;60(9):1577–1585.

[172] Rowan JA, Hague WM, Gao W et al. Metformin versus insulin for the treatment of gestational diabetes. N Engl J Med 2008;358(19):2003–2015.

[173] Ijas H, Vaarasmaki M, Morin-Papunen L et al. Metformin should be considered in the treatment of gestational diabetes: A prospective randomised study. BJOG 2011;118(7):880–885.

[174] Rowan JA, Rush EC, Plank LD et al. Metformin in gestational diabetes: The offspring follow-up (MiG TOFU): Body composition and metabolic outcomes at 7-9 years of age. BMJ Open Diabetes Res Care 2018;6(1):e000456.

[175] Corbould A, Swinton F, Radford A et al. Fasting blood glucose predicts response to extended-release metformin in gestational diabetes mellitus. Aust N Z J Obstet Gynaecol 2013;53(2): 125–129.

[176] Priya G, Kalra S. Metformin in the management of diabetes during pregnancy and lactation. Drugs Context 2018;7:212523.

[177] Battin MR, Obolonkin V, Rush E et al. Blood pressure measurement at two years in offspring of women randomized to a trial of metformin for GDM: Follow up data from the MiG trial. BMC Pediatr 2015;15:54.

[178] Tarry-Adkins JL, Aiken CE, Ozanne SE. Neonatal, infant, and childhood growth following metformin versus insulin treatment for gestational diabetes: A systematic review and meta-analysis. PLoS Med 2019;16(8):e1002848.

[179] Langer O, Conway DL, Berkus MD et al. A comparison of glyburide and insulin in women with gestational diabetes mellitus. N Engl J Med 2000;343(16):1134–1138.

[180] Kjos SL, Leung A, Henry OA et al. Antepartum surveillance in diabetic pregnancies: Predictors of fetal distress in labor. Am J Obstet Gynecol 1995;173(5):1532–1539.

[181] Gabbe SG, Mestman JG, Freeman RK et al. Management and outcome of class A diabetes mellitus. Am J Obstet Gynecol 1977;127(5):465–469.

[182] Casey BM, Lucas MJ, McIntire DD et al. Pregnancy outcomes in women with gestational diabetes compared with the general obstetric population. Obstet Gynecol 1997;90(6): 869–873.

[183] Humphries J, Reynolds D, Bell-Scarbrough L et al. Sonographic estimate of birth weight: Relative accuracy of sonographers versus maternal-fetal medicine specialists. J Matern Fetal Neonatal Med 2002;11(2):108–112.

[184] Johnstone FD, Prescott RJ, Steel JM et al. Clinical and ultrasound prediction of macrosomia in diabetic pregnancy. Br J Obstet Gynaecol 1996;103(8):747–754.

[185] Nobile De Santis MS, Radaelli T, Taricco E et al. Excess of amniotic fluid: Pathophysiology, correlated diseases and clinical management. Acta Biomed 200475 Suppl;1:53–55.

[186] Feghali MN, Caritis SN, Catov JM et al. Timing of delivery and pregnancy outcomes in women with gestational diabetes. Am J Obstet Gynecol 2016;215(2):243e1-7.

[187] Lurie S, Insler V, Hagay ZJ. Induction of labor at 38 to 39 weeks of gestation reduces the incidence of shoulder dystocia in gestational diabetic patients class A2. Am J Perinatol 1996;13(5):293–296.

[188] Alberico S, Erenbourg A, Hod M et al. Immediate delivery or expectant management in gestational diabetes at term: The GINEXMAL randomised controlled trial. BJOG 2017;124(4): 669–677.

[189] Peled Y, Perri T, Chen R et al. Gestational diabetes mellitus–implications of different treatment protocols. J Pediatr Endocrinol Metab 2004;17(6):847–852.

[190] Melamed N, Ray JG, Geary M et al. Induction of labor before 40 weeks is associated with lower rate of cesarean delivery in women with gestational diabetes mellitus. Am J Obstet Gynecol 2016;214(3):364e1-8.

[191] Witkop CT, Neale D, Wilson LM et al. Active compared with expectant delivery management in women with gestational diabetes: A systematic review. Obstet Gynecol 2009;113(1):206–217.

[192] Kim C, Newton KM, Knopp RH. Gestational diabetes and the incidence of type 2 diabetes: A systematic review. Diabetes Care 2002;25(10):1862–1868.

[193] Bellamy L, Casas JP, Hingorani AD et al. Type 2 diabetes mellitus after gestational diabetes: A systematic review and meta-analysis. Lancet 2009;373(9677):1773–1779.

[194] Casagrande SS, Linder B, Cowie CC. Prevalence of gestational diabetes and subsequent Type 2 diabetes among U.S. Women Diabetes Res Clin Pract 2018;141:200–208.

[195] Retnakaran R. Hyperglycemia in pregnancy and its implications for a woman's future risk of cardiovascular disease. Diabetes Res Clin Pract 2018;145:193–199.

[196] Kramer CK, Campbell S, Retnakaran R. Gestational diabetes and the risk of cardiovascular disease in women: A systematic review and meta-analysis. Diabetologia 2019;62(6): 905–914.

[197] Getahun D, Fassett MJ, Jacobsen SJ. Gestational diabetes: Risk of recurrence in subsequent pregnancies. Am J Obstet Gynecol 2010;203(5):467e1-6.

[198] Rayanagoudar G, Hashi AA, Zamora J et al. Quantification of the type 2 diabetes risk in women with gestational diabetes: A systematic review and meta-analysis of 95,750 women. Diabetologia 2016;59(7):1403–1411.

[199] Knowler WC, Barrett-Connor E, Fowler SE et al. Reduction in the incidence of type 2 diabetes with lifestyle intervention or metformin. N Engl J Med 2002;346(6):393–403.

[200] Diabetes Prevention Program Research G. Long-term Effects of Metformin on Diabetes Prevention: Identification of Subgroups That Benefited Most in the Diabetes Prevention Program and Diabetes Prevention Program Outcomes Study. Diabetes Care 2019;42(4): 601–608.

[201] Stuebe AM, Rich-Edwards JW, Willett WC et al. Duration of lactation and incidence of type 2 diabetes. JAMA 2005;294(20):2601–2610.

[202] Nam GE, Han K, Kim DH et al. Associations between breastfeeding and type 2 diabetes mellitus and glycemic control in parous women: a nationwide, population-based study. Diabetes Metab J 2019;43(2):236–241.

[203] Horta BL, De Lima NP. Breastfeeding and Type 2 Diabetes: Systematic Review and Meta-Analysis. Curr Diab Rep 2019;19(1):1.
[204] Berggren EK, Presley L, Amini SB et al. Are the metabolic changes of pregnancy reversible in the first year postpartum?. Diabetologia 2015;58(7):1561–1568.
[205] American Diabetes A. 3. Prevention or delay of type 2 diabetes: standards of medical care in diabetes-2019. Diabetes Care 2019;42(Suppl1):S29–S33.

Haitham Baghlaf, Cynthia Maxwell

25 Obesity and Pregnancy

25.1 Introduction and Epidemiology

The World Health Organization (WHO) defines obesity as an abnormal or excessive adipose deposition that might affect an individual's health [1]. Worldwide, overweight and obesity rates have been rising steadily over the last four decades, with the most recent data reporting an estimated 14% and 9% of people considered overweight and obese, retrospectively [1]. In the United States (US), this is even more profound than other industrialized countries. It is estimated that two-thirds of the US population over the age of 20 are overweight, and more than one third are obese [2]. Forty percent of women in reproductive age were obese in 2017–2018 based on the National Health and Nutrition Examination Surveys (NHANES) [3]. Moreover, this increasing trend in prevalence was persistent across all races but more profound in the black African American women with an obesity prevalence of 56.9%. Women with Asian non-Hispanic race had the lowest prevalence of obesity at 17.2%. Also, the prevalence of morbid obesity, defined as body mass index (BMI) >40 kg/m^2, increased from 4.7% to 9.2% in the last two decades [3]. Efforts to reduce rates of obesity is of paramount importance as it is associated with long-lasting health implications such as cancers, diabetes mellitus (DM), hypertension (HTN), and dyslipidemia, with the last three contributing to coronary heart disease and stroke in the long term [4, 5]. Osteoarthritis is also more prevalent among obese women, and it is the leading cause of disability in adults [6]. It is estimated that the US annual health expenditure on obesity-related disorders is almost 240billion USD [7]. Lastly, maternal obesity complicates 24.8% of pregnancies in the US [8]. It poses a significant risk not only to the mother but also to the fetus. Infants to obese women were more likely to encounter obesity in childhood, and DM and coronary heart disease in adulthood [9].

Obesity can be assessed by different anthropometric measures such as waist circumference more than 88 cm and waist-to-hip ratio of >0.85. BMI is one of the most commonly used methods because it is simple and replicable in clinical settings. It was first introduced in the 1830s by Lambert Quetelet, a mathematician, and it was called the Quetelet index. It is calculated by dividing the individual's weight in kilograms by the height in meters squared. WHO divides BMI into categories, and they are presented in Table 25.1. Obesity measured as BMI of 30 kg/m^2 or more has an increased risk of mortality [10–12]. This was true even after adjusting for preexisting diseases [13, 14]. Although adopting BMI as the used method to assess obesity in pregnancy does not differentiate between lean and fat body mass or take into account the distribution of body adipose tissue, it is the most practical method during pregnancy. It does not rely on measuring skin folds. In this chapter, we will be using the term "high BMI" interchangeably with "obesity".

https://doi.org/10.1515/9783110615258-025

Table 25.1: WHO categorization of body mass index.

Prepregnancy weight category	Body mass index (BMI), kg/m²
Underweight	<18.5
Normal	18.6–24.9
Overweight	25–29.9
Obese	≥30
Obese class I	30–34.9
Obese class II	35–39.9
Obese class III (morbidly obese)	≥40

25.2 Preconception

Obesity has a direct relationship to morbidity and mortality. Adjusted rate difference per 10,000 women calculated an increased risk of severe maternal morbidity or mortality of 24.9 (95% CI 15.7–34.6) for obesity class I, 35.8 (95% CI 23.1–49.5) for obesity class II, and 61.1 (95% CI 44.8–78.9) for obesity class III, compared to normal BMI [15]. Women with high BMI planning pregnancy would benefit from preconception counseling to minimize adverse maternal and neonatal outcomes.

Micronutrient deficiency is more common in the obese population. This might be explained by their high-calorie diet intake, rich in carbohydrates, and deficient in micronutrients [16, 17]. Vitamin D and folic acid are both deficient in obese patients compared to patients with normal BMI [18, 19]. A Cochrane review included 15 trials assessing the benefit of vitamin D supplements during pregnancy. They found that vitamin D supplementation might reduce the rate of preeclampsia, preterm birth, and low birth weight [20]. Women with a high BMI may benefit from vitamin D supplementation during pregnancy.

Folic acid supplementation reduces the risk of congenital malformations, such as neural tube defect (NTD) and congenital heart defect (CHD) [21–23]. It has been proven that in women with a history of previous pregnancy affected by NTD, folic acid supplementation has decreased the risk of recurrence by 71% [24]. In this study, patients were not stratified based on their BMI. A systematic review and meta-analysis reported a threefold increased risk of NTD in women with morbid obesity [25]. Moreover, women with high BMI were found to have lower serum folate levels even after controlling for folate intake [18]. Although supplementation with folic acid would appear to be important in women with high BMI, studies are lacking in assessing NTD reduction in high folic acid supplementation groups. International societies recommend starting folic acid of 0.4–5 mg supplementation at least three months prior to pregnancy [26, 27].

Patients should be encouraged to start lifestyle modifications before pregnancy. Dietitian referral should be obtained, especially in class II obesity or more. Physical activity has been shown to decrease the inflammatory process and increase insulin sensitivity, promoting weight loss, and decreasing the risk of DM [28, 29]. Moreover, exercis can normalize a preexisting HTN or lower the doses of hypertensive medications to control the blood pressure [30]. The American Heart Association (AHA) recommends all adults perform at least 150 min of moderate-intensity exercise per week [31]. Obese women with a sedentary lifestyle should start at 60–90 min of low- to moderate-intensity exercise weekly and increase the interval as they progress.

Women with morbid obesity or BMI 35 kg/m^2 with comorbidities in whom lifestyle modifications have failed are considered candidates for bariatric surgeries [32]. Bariatric surgery is subcategorized into restrictive and bypass surgeries. Patients lose weight at a rapid rate following these surgeries. Usually, any abnormality in the menstrual cycle or fertility leads to an increased rate of unplanned pregnancy in this population [33]. In the medical literature, pregnancies post-bariatric surgeries were matched to the control group based on prepregnancy BMI, presurgery BMI, or even they were compared to the general population [34–37]. A recent systematic review and meta-analysis subdivided their results based on the type of control group [38]. The authors reported 79%, 61%, 41%, and 69% reduction rates in gestational diabetes (GDM), gestational HTN, preeclampsia, and large for gestational age (LGA), respectively, in women who underwent bariatric surgery compared to women who had similar presurgery BMI. However, this group was more likely to carry small for gestational age (SGA) fetus compared to its control with an odds ratio (OR) of 2.18 (CI 1.41–3.38). This might be due to the micronutrient deficiency seen after the surgery. These outcomes are essential to outline to bariatric surgery candidates who might consider pregnancy in the near future. Bariatric surgery patients should be aware that their risk of SGA persisted even when compared to the control group based on their prepregnancy BMI. Again, this is most likely due to malnutrition and malabsorption effects seen after bariatric surgery. However, their risk of GDM, preeclampsia, and gestational HTN would be based solely on their prepregnancy BMI. The optimal waiting period between bariatric surgery and pregnancy has not been identified. There is controversy in pregnancy and neonatal outcomes in patients who conceived earlier than two years. Few studies showed an increased risk of neonatal adverse outcomes, and others failed to show any difference [39–41]. The majority of health care providers will advocate for at least 1–2 years' interval to avoid pregnancy during the weight-loss period.

Obesity is associated with an increased risk of obstructive sleep apnea (OSA) and obesity hypoventilation syndrome. The further increase in chest adiposity, neck soft tissue, and neck edema during pregnancy will have a marked impact on OSA. Patients can be screened for OSA by the Berlin questionnaire, and if it is positive, they should undergo laboratory polysomnography testing. Berlin questionnaire sensitivity and specificity were reported to be only 35% and 65%, respectively [42]. OSA increases the risks of cardiomyopathy and preeclampsia and can be challenging to manage during the postpartum period [43]. Treatment consists of continuous positive airway pressure (CPAP), weight loss prior to pregnancy, and minimizing gestational weight gain (GWG) during pregnancy. In light of the unknown optimal screening method, we tend to refer all patients with DM or HTN and history of snoring for in-laboratory polysomnography.

25.3 First Trimester

25.3.1 Maternal Considerations

The first visit to prenatal care is of paramount importance in establishing a superb physician–patient relationship. The health care provider should avoid stigmatizing language and use a high BMI term instead of "obesity." If a preconception visit was not done previously, it is crucial to discuss the potential complications encountered in pregnancy and screen for all the health conditions mentioned in the previous section. Moreover, clinics, labor and delivery ward, and operating rooms should be established in a way to accommodate women with high BMI and to ensure patients and health care providers' safety. These include but are not limited to bariatric OR beds, appropriate hospital gowns, weighing scales, wheelchairs, and waiting area seats to accommodate this population. Moreover, large blood pressure cuff sizes should be available in the clinic, and the labor and delivery room.

GWG plays an important role not only in regard to pregnancy and neonatal outcomes but also in terms of weight retention after delivery [44–46]. The Institute of Medicine (IoM) has published a guideline on the optimal weight gain during pregnancy (Table 25.2), and it takes into account the prepregnancy BMI [47]. However, there is no consensus on the optimal GWG in women with high BMI. Women with high GWG are at higher risk of GDM, gestational HTN, preeclampsia, LGA, and operative delivery [44]. Although weight loss during pregnancy decreases the risk of LGA, pregnancy-induced hypertension disorders, and cesarean section rates, it increases the risk of SGA by three-quarters, and it should be avoided [44].

Table 25.2: Optimal weight gain in pregnancy [47].

Prepregnancy BMI	Total weight gain (lbs)	Weight gain in second and third trimesters (lbs/week): Mean (range)
Underweight	28–40	1 (1–1.3)
Normal	25–35	1 (0.8–1)
Overweight	15–25	0.6 (0.5–0.7)
Obese	11–20	0.5 (0.4–0.6)

Women with high BMI usually start pregnancy with comorbidities, such as HTN, DM, and dyslipidemia [4, 5]. We recommend obtaining baseline assessment of renal function (i.e., serum creatinine and random urinary protein/creatinine ratio) to differentiate between preexisting kidney disease and pregnancy-induced hypertension disorders with acute kidney failure in the second or third trimester of pregnancy. Women with high BMI are at higher risk of DM type 2 and GDM; screening with random blood sugar and hemoglobin A1c in the first prenatal visit would help set them apart [5, 48, 49]. There is an increased risk of nonalcoholic steatohepatitis (NASH) in obese women [50]. Baseline liver enzymes and function tests (i.e., serum transaminases, bilirubin, albumin and coagulation profile) will play an essential role in differentiating chronic liver diseases from an acute cause occurring in the second half of the pregnancy. Furthermore, blood volume increases by 40–50% during pregnancy resulting in a 30–50% increase in cardiac output [51]. Obesity increases cardiac output even more. It has been reported that for every kilogram of fat, there is an increase of almost 500 ml/min in cardiac output [52]. We recommend performing an echocardiogram for patients with BMI >40 and in those with BMI >30 in addition to chronic HTN to assess for any preexisting cardiac dysfunction.

Adiposity is associated with ovulatory cycle abnormalities, leading to prolonged follicular and shorter luteal phases, causing inaccuracy in estimating the due date using the last menstrual period [53]. Estimated due date based on ultrasound measurement of the crown-rump length in the first trimester is the most accurate method.

25.3.2 Fetal Considerations

Maternal serum screening for aneuploidy and open neural tube defect are affected by adiposity. Alpha-fetoprotein, human chorionic gonadotropin, and unconjugated estriol levels are inversely correlated to maternal weight [54]. Thus, maternal weight adjustment is required in first- or second-trimester screening [55]. Moreover, noninvasive prenatal testing (NIPT) is hindered by high maternal BMI. Adiposity increases maternal DNA to fetal DNA fraction, leading to failure rate in NIPT ranging from 5.4% to 70% in women with morbid obesity [56–60]. This raises the question if NIPT should be offered to women with morbid obesity. Furthermore, obesity affects ultrasound quality and accuracy of nuchal translucency (NT) measurement [61, 62]. Despite advancements in ultrasound imaging quality, it poses a challenge in attaining good quality images [61, 63–65]. The operator has to trade resolution for depth to obtain better fetal images in women with high BMI. Also, adiposity increases the sound waves' traveling area [63]. These result in poor ultrasound visualization with unattainable or inaccurately measured NT, leading to an increased risk of undetected chromosomal anomalies [61, 62]. The FaSTER trial reported a dose–response relationship between unattainable NT and BMI [61]. However, Gandhi and colleagues did not find such a relationship, though combining transabdominal and transvaginal ultrasound exams was required [66].

25.4 Second Trimester

25.4.1 Maternal Considerations

The risk of GDM is related to BMI, with some studies reporting up to a threefold increased risk [48, 49]. Many societies recommend early screening for diabetes [67–69]. The most recommended screening method is the 50 g glucose challenge test. Others use hemoglobin A1c, fasting plasma glucose, or random plasma glucose level [70]. Adopting one of the above methods will result in early diagnosis of GDM and the early start of insulin treatment [71]. However, none of the above-mentioned methods improved short-term maternal or fetal outcomes [70]. Studies addressing long-term outcomes are lacking. Women with prior bariatric surgery may not tolerate the glucose challenge test due to dumping syndromes; seven-point daily capillary blood glucose (CBG) or continuous glucose monitoring is recommended.

25.4.2 Fetal Considerations

Fetuses to mothers with high BMI are more likely to have congenital anomalies than their normal BMI counterparts [72]. Spina bifida risk is more than doubled in obese women [72]. Other congenital anomalies including congenital cardiac defects, cleft lip and palate, limb reduction, and anorectal atresia are increased [72]. However, obesity was associated with a reduction of gastroschisis by 83% [72]. Incomplete single anatomy scan and the need for repeat ultrasound exams are more likely to be encountered in women with high BMI [73–75]. Eastwood and coauthors reported 44% of morbidly obese women requiring more than one ultrasound exam to complete fetal anatomy [64]. In their cohort, 11.1% had incomplete anatomy scans despite repeat exams. In conclusion, obese women, especially BMI >40kg/m^2, are more likely to encounter undetected prenatal congenital anomalies due to a higher background risk of congenital defects and the likelihood of suboptimal or incomplete anatomy scans.

25.5 Third Trimester

25.5.1 Maternal Considerations

The third trimester is the highest period for the diagnosis of hypertensive disorders in pregnancy. Wang and colleagues performed a systematic review and meta-analysis, including 29 prospective cohort studies [76]. Obesity class I, II, and III were more likely to be complicated with preeclampsia compared to women with normal BMI with an odds ratio of 1.70 (95% CI 1.60–1.81), 2.93 (95% CI 2.58–3.33), and 4.14 (95% CI 3.61–4.75), respectively. Moreover, the risk of recurrence of preeclampsia was more common in women with high BMI [77]. The Society of Obstetricians & Gynecologists of Canada (SOGC) and the National Institute for Health and Care Excellence (NICE) recognize obesity as a risk factor for preeclampsia and recommend starting aspirin 81–162 mg between 12 and 16 weeks of gestation and until 36 weeks of gestation in the presence of an additional risk factor for preeclampsia [27, 78].

Hormonal changes and increased blood flow seen in pregnancy lead to hyperemic airway [79]. Moreover, the enlarged uterus exerts an elevation of the diaphragm [79]. Also, the anteroposterior diameter of the thoracic cage expands outward by 2 cm [80]. As a result, respiratory reserved volume, the residual volume, and the functional residual capacity are reduced in pregnancy [81]. Obesity exerts an additive effect to pregnancy on the respiratory function due to the enlarged neck circumference, enlarged breasts, and increased adiposity in the chest wall [82, 83]. Altogether, there is a decrease in both chest compliance and total lung capacity; these factors lead to difficulty with intubation in obese women. It has to be noted that women with high BMI are more prone to ventilation-perfusion mismatch, atelectasis, and hypoxia in the supine position. This should be noted by the obstetrics and anesthesia team in preparation for the cesarean section [84]. Also, hypoxemia is more likely to occur in these patients during intubation [80]. This, among other numerous causes, shows the importance of anesthesia consult during pregnancy.

Pregnancy and obesity combined heighten the risk of developing venous thromboembolism (VTE), especially during the third and postpartum periods, through different mechanisms. Pregnancy itself places women at a fivefold higher risk of VTE in the antepartum period compared to nonpregnant women [85]. It is estimated that VTE complicates 5.4, 7.2, and 4.3 per 10,000 pregnancies in the antepartum, peripartum, and postpartum periods, respectively [86]. Obesity doubles these risks of VTE in pregnant women [87]. This is influenced by the increase in abdominal adiposity exacerbating the venous stasis in pregnancy [88]. Also, mobility difficulties occur more commonly in women with high BMI, and it exaggerates VTE's risk even more [88]. Lastly, an increase in adiposity releases more inflammatory markers such as interleukin-6 and tumor necrosis factor-alpha, creating a prothrombotic effect [89]. Low molecular weight heparin (LMWH) is the first line of treatment during pregnancy [90, 91]. It is recommended that doses should be calculated based on the patient's weight. However, there is controversy about dose frequency, with some studies suggesting that twice-daily dosing is more effective, considering the changes in blood volume, glomerular filtration rate, and protein-binding pharmacokinetics in pregnancy [90]. However, Patel and his colleagues found that the half-life of LMWH is prolonged with the advancing gestational age, proposing daily dosage [92].

25.5.2 Fetal Considerations

Symphysis-fundus height, abdominal palpitation, and clinical judgment are the used methods to assess fetal growth in the low-risk population. These methods are insensitive in evaluating fetal growth in obese patients due to adiposity. Although ultrasound is the best mode of assessment available to rule out LGA or SGA fetuses, it is not without limitations, mentioned in the previous sections. It has been reported that obesity decreases the accuracy of calculating the estimated fetal weight by ultrasound [93, 94]. However, more recent studies did not find this correlation [95, 96]. This might be due to the advancements in ultrasound technology and the acquired operators' skills as the obesity rate increased over the past few decades.

Maternal BMI is proportionally related to the risk of intrauterine fetal demise (IUFD). In a Danish cohort, the calculated hazard ratios (HR) for fetal demise in obese women compared to women with normal BMI were 3.5 (95% CI 1.9–6.4) and 4.6 (95% CI 1.6–13.4) at 37–39 weeks' gestation and ≥40 weeks' gestation, respectively [97]. The mechanism underlying the risk of IUFD is unknown.

25.5.3 Intrapartum

The time for spontaneous labor to start is usually delayed in obese patients, resulting in prolonged pregnancy [98]. Even in the event of spontaneous labor, women with high BMI usually exercise an altered labor curve requiring a longer time to achieve full dilatation [99]. Furthermore, they have a different response to induction agents than nonobese women [100]. This might be secondary to decreased calcium influx in the myometrium, resulting in less frequent and forcefully contractions in obese women than counterparts with normal BMI [101]. This increases their likelihood of requiring augmentation in labor and delivery by cesarean section due to failed induction or arrested labor. Initiating labor is a challenging and difficult process in women with high BMI, and most of the time, different mechanical and pharmacological methods might be required to achieve labor [100, 102]. Continuous fetal heart rate monitoring is not required unless comorbidity or obstetrical compilations are present. Obesity imposes challenges to monitor uterine contractions adequately and/or fetal heart rate activity during labor. The health care provider should be familiar with the use of intrauterine pressure catheter and electronic fetal heart rate scalp monitoring during labor.

High maternal BMI is associated with difficulty inserting an epidural catheter due to increased fat deposition around the spine area, making it difficult to palpate the intervertebral spaces and requiring longer needles [103–105]. The failure rate of the initial epidural was as high as 42% in morbidly obese women compared to 6% in nonobese parturients [106]. Utilizing ultrasound to assess intervertebral spaces has doubled the epidural placement success rate in obese women [105].

Vaginal delivery is associated with particular risks to women with high BMI, such as shoulder dystocia and postpartum hemorrhage [107–110]. Women should be counseled about these risks, and healthcare providers should anticipate them, be prepared, and manage them in a timely fashion. Moreover, one should be patient before making the diagnosis of obstructed labor in this population to decrease the cesarean section rate.

The cesarean section imposes challenges to the obstetrical, anesthesia, and nursing teams. As mentioned above, special equipment should be available, and anesthesia consult in the second or third trimester should have already been made. A systematic review and meta-analysis of 11 studies showed that the cesarean section rate is increased in women with high BMI, and the rate is doubled in women with class II obesity [111]. Surgical site infection (SSI) is one of the devastating complications of cesarean sections. There is a three- to five-fold increase in the rate of SSI in women with high BMI [112]. Multiple efforts are made at different levels to decrease this risk, including but not limited to prophylactic antibiotics regimen with their optimal dosing, skin incision placement, and subcutaneous tissue closure. These will be addressed in more detail in the following paragraphs.

Prophylactic antibiotics are given 15–60 min prior to skin incision has shown to reduce the risk of SSI by 50% [113]. It is unclear whether women with high BMI should receive 3 g of cefazolin instead of 2 g. Obese women receiving 3 g of cefazolin achieved higher adipose concentration of cefazolin compared to 2 g [114]. However, in a retrospective cohort study at two tertiary hospitals in the US, the SSI rate did not differ between 3 g and 2 g of cefazolin in morbidly obese women [115]. A recent randomized clinical trial reported that the use of cephalexin 500 mg combined with metronidazole 500 mg every 8 h for 48 h after the cesarean section reduced the SSI rate by almost 60% to placebo in obese patients [116].

In low-risk populations, low abdomen (Pfannenstiel) incision is preferred in cesarean sections. It provides adequate exposure during the procedure and cosmetic result to the patient. It is controversial to determine which type of skin incision in the obese population is associated with low risk to the mother and her neonate. In light of the absence of randomized clinical trials, most obstetricians prefer Pfannenstiel incision to vertical incision in women with morbid obesity [117]. Although the vertical incision is associated with an increased risk of wound complications, it has been associated with a lower risk of low 5-min Apgar score and low umbilical artery PH in morbidly obese women [118]. In their cohort of morbidly obese women, Tixier and colleagues found that supraumbilical transverse incision was associated with easy access to the lower uterine segment and deliver the baby compared to other techniques without other significant differences [119]. At our institution, we tend to perform a transverse supraumbilical when the panniculus displaces the umbilicus caudally to the level of the symphysis pubis. Intraoperative ultrasound can also be used to assess the thinnest layer of subcutaneous tissue to determine the best level of the cesarean section incision [120].

Subcutaneous tissue in obese women is suboptimally perfused with oxygen and is more susceptible to infection and seroma development. Systematic review and meta-analysis looking at the closure of subcutaneous tissue with a depth exceeding 2 cm reported a 34% reduction of wound complications [121]. Even more, closure of the subcutaneous tissue with multiple layers might be required in some patients. In multiple studies, retrospective and randomized clinical trials, subcutaneous drain placement did not show any benefit compared to subcutaneous tissue closure [122, 123].

Prophylactic negative pressure wound therapy (NPWT) has gained popularity as a method to decrease the risk of SSI in the obese population. Two recent systematic reviews and meta-analyses studies were published to assess the use of NPWT and the reduced risk of SSI [124, 125]. The first systematic review and meta-analysis included only randomized clinical trials in their meta-analysis, and it did not show a reduction in the SSI rate [125]. However, the second meta-analysis included RCT and non-RCT in their analysis and reported a reduced risk of 32% in the NPWT group [124]. There are two new RCT since the publication of these systematic reviews and meta-analyses, and neither found a reduction of SSI with the use of NPWT in obese women [126, 127].

25.6 Postpartum

Breastfeeding is encouraged in women with obesity. A systematic review found that obese women have more difficulty initiating breastfeeding, tend to breastfeed for a shorter period, and have impaired lactogenesis due to excessive adipose tissue resulting in less milk supply [128–130]. An Ontario study compared breastfeeding in 4,676 obese women to 11,327 women with normal BMI. They reported a reduction rate in intention to breastfeed and exclusive breastfeeding on discharge in obese women by 16% and 32%, respectively [131]. Breastfeeding interventional programs will be beneficial in optimizing the rates of initiation and continuation of breastfeeding. Furthermore, breastfeeding is associated with less postpartum weight retention, and this reduction is even higher in obese women [131].

Weight retention is a devastating sequela of excessive gestational weight gain. A meta-analysis of nine observational studies reported increased weight retention in the excessive gestational weight gain group compared to appropriate gestational weight gain based on IOM [132]. Women who lose weight in between pregnancies were less likely to encounter GDM, cesarean section, or failed trial of labor after cesarean section [133–136]. Interventional methods to modify lifestyle should be applied. If it has not been done before, women who meet the criteria for bariatric surgery will benefit from a referral in the postpartum period.

Depression disorders are common during pregnancy [137]. Up to 19.2% of women encounter at least one event of major depressive episodes in the 12-week postpartum period [138]. As mentioned in the previous sections, obese women are more likely to have complicated pregnancies, gain more weight than they intend, lead to poor self-image perception, fail to achieve spontaneous labor, and achieve vaginal delivery. Moreover, their neonates are more likely to be admitted to the neonatal intensive care unit and have delayed breastfeeding initiation or continuation. These all result in an increased risk of major depressive disorders in the postpartum period. Few studies have looked at postpartum depression in women with high BMI, and the majority reported a positive association [139–142]. This group of patients would need a low threshold to diagnose postpartum depression, especially if they had a complicated pregnancy or labor.

25.7 Conclusion

Women who are obese have higher medical and surgical risks in pregnancy. As such, they should be evaluated prior to pregnancy to screen for associated medical conditions, and require close monitoring during pregnancy and postpartum to ensure optimal maternal and fetal outcome.

References

[1] World Health Organization. Obesity and overweight 2020, April 1. Available from: https://www.who.int/news-room/fact-sheets/detail/obesity-and-overweight

[2] Worldometer. Obese people in the world: Retrieving data 2020. Available from: https://www.worldometers.info/obesity/

[3] Hales CM, Carroll MD, Fryar CD, et al. Prevalence of obesity and severe obesity among adults: united states, 2017–2018. NCHS Data Brief. 2020;(360):1–8.

[4] Strumpf E The obesity epidemic in the United States: Causes and extent, risks and solutions. Issue Brief (Commonw Fund). 2004;(713):1–6.

[5] Bloomgarden ZT. Third annual world congress on the insulin resistance syndrome: associated conditions. Diabetes Care 200629(9):2165–2174.

[6] Hunter DJ, Bierma-Zeinstra S. Osteoarthritis. Lancet 2019;393(10182):1745–1759.

[7] Schlosser E. Fast Food Nation, 1st, Mariner Books, 2012.

[8] Branum AM, Kirmeyer SE, Gregory EC. Prepregnancy body mass index by maternal characteristics and state: data from the birth certificate, 2014. Natl Vital Stat Rep 2016;65(6):1–11.

[9] Leddy MA, Power ML, Schulkin J. The impact of maternal obesity on maternal and fetal health. Rev Obstet Gynecol 2008;1(4):170–178.

[10] Kayem G, Kurinczuk J, Lewis G et al. Risk factors for progression from severe maternal morbidity to death: A national cohort study. PLoS One 2011;6(12):e29077.

[11] Mariona FG. Does maternal obesity impact pregnancy-related deaths? Michigan experience. J Matern Fetal Neonatal Med 2017;30(9):1060–1065.

[12] Goffman D, Madden RC, Harrison EA et al. Predictors of maternal mortality and near-miss maternal morbidity. J Perinatol 2007;27(10):597–601.

[13] Katzmarzyk PT, Ardern CI. Overweight and obesity mortality trends in Canada, 1985–2000. Can J Public Health 2004;95(1):16–20.

[14] Adams KF, Schatzkin A, Harris TB et al. Overweight, obesity, and mortality in a large prospective cohort of persons 50 to 71 years old. N Engl J Med 2006;355(8):763–778.

[15] Lisonkova S, Muraca GM, Potts J et al. Association between prepregnancy body mass index and severe maternal morbidity. Jama 2017Nov 14;318(18):1777–1786.

[16] Cedergren MI, Källén BA. Maternal obesity and infant heart defects. Obes Res 2003;11(9): 1065–1071.

[17] Racusin D, Stevens B, Campbell G et al. Obesity and the risk and detection of fetal malformations. Semin Perinatol 2012;36(3):213–221.

[18] Mojtabai R. Body mass index and serum folate in childbearing age women. Eur J Epidemiol 2004;19(11):1029–1036.

[19] Gangloff A, Bergeron J, Lemieux I et al. Changes in circulating vitamin D levels with loss of adipose tissue. Curr Opin Clin Nutr Metab Care 2016;19(6):464–470.

[20] De-Regil LM, Palacios C, Lombardo LK et al. Vitamin D supplementation for women during pregnancy. Cochrane Database Syst Rev 2016;14(1):Cd008873.

[21] Ingrid Goh Y, Bollano E, Einarson TR et al. Prenatal multivitamin supplementation and rates of congenital anomalies: A meta-analysis. J Obstet Gynaecol Can 2006;28(8):680–689.

[22] Shaw GM, O'Malley CD, Wasserman CR et al. Maternal periconceptional use of multivitamins and reduced risk for conotruncal heart defects and limb deficiencies among offspring. Am J Med Genet 1995;59(4):536–545.

[23] LI X, Li S, Mu D et al. The association between periconceptional folic acid supplementation and congenital heart defects: A case-control study in China. Prev Med 2013;56(6):385–389.

[24] Prevention of neural tube defects: results of the Medical Research Council Vitamin Study. MRC vitamin study research group. Lancet 1991;338(8760):131–137.

[25] Rasmussen SA, Chu SY, Kim SY et al. Maternal obesity and risk of neural tube defects: A metaanalysis. Am J Obstet Gynecol 2008;198(6):611–619.

[26] Royal college of obstetricians & gynecologists. Being overweight in pregnancy and after birth 2018, November 11. Available from: https://www.rcog.org.uk/en/patients/patient-leaflets /being-overweight-pregnancy-after-birth/

[27] Maxwell C, Gaudet L, Cassir G et al. Guideline No. 391-pregnancy and maternal obesity part 1: pre-conception and prenatal care. J Obstet Gynaecol Can 2019;41(11):1623–1640.

[28] Dimitrov S, Hulteng E, Hong S. Inflammation and exercise: Inhibition of monocytic intracellular TNF production by acute exercise via β(2)-adrenergic activation. Brain Behav Immun 2017;61:60–68.

[29] Borghouts LB, Keizer HA. Exercise and insulin sensitivity: A review. Int J Sports Med 2000;21(1):1–12.

[30] Kane JA, Mehmood T, Munir I et al. Cardiovascular risk reduction associated with pharmacological weight loss: a meta-analysis. Int J Clin Res Trials 2019;4:1.

[31] American Heart Association. American heart association recommendations for physical activity in adults and kids, 2018, April 18. Available from: https://www.heart.org/en/healthy-living/fitness/fitness-basics/aha-recs-for-physical-activity-in-adults

[32] Lau DC, Douketis JD, Morrison KM et al. 2006 Canadian clinical practice guidelines on the management and prevention of obesity in adults and children [summary]. Cmaj 2007;176(8): S1–13.

[33] Maggard MA, Yermilov I, Li Z et al. Pregnancy and fertility following bariatric surgery: A systematic review. Jama 2008;300(19):2286–2296.

[34] Wax JR, Cartin A, Wolff R et al. Pregnancy following gastric bypass surgery for morbid obesity: Maternal and neonatal outcomes. Obes Surg 2008;18(5):540–544.

[35] Adams TD, Hammoud AO, Davidson LE et al. Maternal and neonatal outcomes for pregnancies before and after gastric bypass surgery. Int J Obes (Lond) 2015;39(4):686–694.

[36] Dell'Agnolo CM, Carvalho MD, Pelloso SM. Pregnancy after bariatric surgery: Implications for mother and newborn. Obes Surg 2011;21(6):699–706.

[37] Kjær MM, Lauenborg J, Breum BM et al. The risk of adverse pregnancy outcome after bariatric surgery: A nationwide register-based matched cohort study. Am J Obstet Gynecol 2013;208(6):464.e1–5.

[38] Kwong W, Tomlinson G, Feig DS. Maternal and neonatal outcomes after bariatric surgery; a systematic review and meta-analysis: Do the benefits outweigh the risks?. Am J Obstet Gynecol 2018;218(6):573–580.

[39] Parent B, Martopullo I, Weiss NS et al. Bariatric surgery in women of childbearing age, timing between an operation and birth, and associated perinatal complications. JAMA Surg 2017;152(2):128–135.

[40] Kjær MM, Nilas L. Timing of pregnancy after gastric bypass-a national register-based cohort study. Obes Surg 2013;23(8):1281–1285.

[41] Dolin C, Ude Welcome AO, Caughey AB. Management of pregnancy in women who have undergone bariatric surgery. Obstet Gynecol Surv 2016;71(12):734–740.

[42] Olivarez SA, Maheshwari B, McCarthy M et al. Prospective trial on obstructive sleep apnea in pregnancy and fetal heart rate monitoring. Am J Obstet Gynecol 2010;202(6):552.e1–7.

[43] Louis JM, Mogos MF, Salemi JL et al. Obstructive sleep apnea and severe maternal-infant morbidity/mortality in the United States, 1998–2009. Sleep 2014;37(5):843–849.

[44] Kapadia MZ, Park CK, Beyene J et al. Weight loss instead of weight gain within the guidelines in obese women during pregnancy: a systematic review and meta-analyses of maternal and infant outcomes. PLoS One 2015;10(7):e0132650.

[45] Catalano PM, Mele L, Landon MB et al. Inadequate weight gain in overweight and obese pregnant women: What is the effect on fetal growth?. Am J Obstet Gynecol 2014Aug;211(2):137.e1–7.

[46] Siegel AM, Tucker A, Adkins LD et al. Postpartum Weight Loss in Women with Class-III Obesity: Do They Lose What They Gain?. Am J Perinatol 2020;37(1):53–58.

[47] Institute of M, National Research Council Committee to Reexamine IOMPWG. The National Academies Collection: Reports funded by National Institutes of Health. In: Rasmussen KM, Yaktine AL, editors. Weight Gain during Pregnancy: Reexamining the Guidelines, Washington (DC): National Academies Press (US) Copyright © 2009, National Academy of Sciences., 2009.

[48] Weiss JL, Malone FD, Emig D et al. Obesity, obstetric complications and cesarean delivery rate–a population-based screening study. Am J Obstet Gynecol 2004Apr;190(4):1091–1097.

[49] Sebire NJ, Jolly M, Harris JP et al. Maternal obesity and pregnancy outcome: A study of 287,213 pregnancies in London. Int J Obes Relat Metab Disord 2001;25(8):1175–1182.

[50] Jarvis H, Craig D, Barker R et al. Metabolic risk factors and incident advanced liver disease in non-alcoholic fatty liver disease (NAFLD): A systematic review and meta-analysis of population-based observational studies. PLoS Med 2020;17(4):e1003100.

[51] Capeless EL, Clapp JF. Cardiovascular changes in early phase of pregnancy. Am J Obstet Gynecol 1989;161(6 Pt 1):1449–1453.

[52] Vasan RS. Cardiac function and obesity. Heart 2003Oct;89(10):1127–1129.

[53] Santoro N, Lasley B, McConnell D et al. Body size and ethnicity are associated with menstrual cycle alterations in women in the early menopausal transition: The Study of Women's Health across the Nation (SWAN) Daily Hormone Study. J Clin Endocrinol Metab 2004;89(6):2622–2631.

[54] Palomaki GE, Bradley LA, McDowell GA et al. Technical standards and guidelines: Prenatal screening for Down syndrome: This new section on "Prenatal Screening for Down

Syndrome," together with the new section on "Prenatal Screening for Open Neural Tube Defects," replaces the previous Section H of the American College of Medical Genetics Standards and Guidelines for Clinical Genetics Laboratories. Genetics in Medicine 20052005/05/01;7(5):344–354.

[55] Chitayat D, Langlois S, Wilson RD. No. 261-prenatal screening for fetal aneuploidy in singleton pregnancies. J Obstet Gynaecol Can 2017;39(9):e380–e394.

[56] Ashoor G, Syngelaki A, Poon LC et al. Fetal fraction in maternal plasma cell-free DNA at 11–13 weeks' gestation: Relation to maternal and fetal characteristics. Ultrasound Obstet Gynecol 2013;41(1):26–32.

[57] Canick JA, Palomaki GE, Kloza EM et al. The impact of maternal plasma DNA fetal fraction on next generation sequencing tests for common fetal aneuploidies. Prenat Diagn 2013;33(7): 667–674.

[58] Hudecova I, Sahota D, Heung MM et al. Maternal plasma fetal DNA fractions in pregnancies with low and high risks for fetal chromosomal aneuploidies. PLoS One 2014;9(2):e88484.

[59] Yared E, Dinsmoor MJ, Endres LK et al. Obesity increases the risk of failure of noninvasive prenatal screening regardless of gestational age. Am J Obstet Gynecol 2016;215(3):370.e1–6.

[60] Juul LA, Hartwig TS, Ambye L et al. Noninvasive prenatal testing and maternal obesity: A review. Acta Obstet Gynecol Scand 2020;99(6):744–750.

[61] Aagaard-Tillery KM, Flint Porter T, Malone FD et al. Influence of maternal BMI on genetic sonography in the FaSTER trial. Prenat Diagn 2010;30(1):14–22.

[62] Thornburg LL, Mulconry M, Post A et al. Fetal nuchal translucency thickness evaluation in the overweight and obese gravida. Ultrasound Obstet Gynecol 2009;33(6):665–669.

[63] Paladini D. Sonography in obese and overweight pregnant women: Clinical, medicolegal and technical issues. Ultrasound Obstet Gynecol 2009;33(6):720–729.

[64] Eastwood KA, Daly C, Hunter A et al. The impact of maternal obesity on completion of fetal anomaly screening. J Perinat Med 2017;45(9):1061–1067.

[65] Dashe JS, McIntire DD, Twickler DM. Effect of maternal obesity on the ultrasound detection of anomalous fetuses. Obstet Gynecol 2009;113(5):1001–1007.

[66] Gandhi M, Fox NS, Russo-Stieglitz K et al. Effect of increased body mass index on first-trimester ultrasound examination for aneuploidy risk assessment. Obstet Gynecol 2009;114(4):856–859.

[67] ACOG. Practice Bulletin No 156: Obesity in Pregnancy. Obstet Gynecol 2015;126(6):e112–26.

[68] Berger H, Gagnon R, Sermer M. Guideline No. 393-Diabetes in Pregnancy. J Obstet Gynaecol Can 2019;41(12):1814–1825e1.

[69] Feig DS, Berger H, Donovan L et al. Diabetes and pregnancy. Can J Diabetes 2018;42(Suppl 1):S255–s282.

[70] Shinar S, Berger H. Early diabetes screening in pregnancy. Int J Gynaecol Obstet 2018;142(1): 1–8.

[71] Bianchi C, De Gennaro G, Romano M et al. Early vs. standard screening and treatment of gestational diabetes in high-risk women – An attempt to determine relative advantages and disadvantages. Nutr Metab Cardiovasc Dis 2019;29(6):598–603.

[72] Stothard KJ, Tennant PW, Bell R et al. Maternal overweight and obesity and the risk of congenital anomalies: A systematic review and meta-analysis. JAMA 2009;301(6):636–650.

[73] Hendler I, Blackwell SC, Bujold E et al. The impact of maternal obesity on midtrimester sonographic visualization of fetal cardiac and craniospinal structures. Int J Obes Relat Metab Disord 2004;28(12):1607–1611.

[74] Hendler I, Blackwell SC, Bujold E et al. Suboptimal second-trimester ultrasonographic visualization of the fetal heart in obese women: Should we repeat the examination?. J Ultrasound Med 2005;24(9):1205–1209.quiz 1210–1.

[75] Hunsley C, Farrell T. The influence of maternal body mass index on fetal anomaly screening. Eur J Obstet Gynecol Reprod Biol 2014;182:181–184.

[76] Wang Z, Wang P, Liu H et al. Maternal adiposity as an independent risk factor for preeclampsia: A meta-analysis of prospective cohort studies. Obes Rev 2013;14(6):508–521.

[77] Mostello D, Kallogjeri D, Tungsiripat R et al. Recurrence of preeclampsia: Effects of gestational age at delivery of the first pregnancy, body mass index, paternity, and interval between births. Am J Obstet Gynecol 2008;199(1):55.e1–7.

[78] Redman CW. Hypertension in pregnancy: The NICE guidelines. Heart 2011;97(23):1967–1969.

[79] Munnur U, De Boisblanc B, Suresh MS. Airway problems in pregnancy. Crit Care Med 2005;33(10 Suppl):S259–68.

[80] Honarmand A, Safavi MR. Prediction of difficult laryngoscopy in obstetric patients scheduled for Caesarean delivery. Eur J Anaesthesiol 2008;25(9):714–720.

[81] LoMauro A, Aliverti A. Respiratory physiology of pregnancy: Physiology masterclass. Breathe (Sheff) 2015;11(4):297–301.

[82] Brodsky JB, Lemmens HJ, Brock-Utne JG et al. Morbid obesity and tracheal intubation. Anesth Analg 2002;94(3):732–736.table of contents.

[83] Gonzalez H, Minville V, Delanoue K et al. The importance of increased neck circumference to intubation difficulties in obese patients. Anesth Analg 2008;106(4):1132–1136. table of contents.

[84] Damia G, Mascheroni D, Croci M et al. Perioperative changes in functional residual capacity in morbidly obese patients. Br J Anaesth 1988;60(5):574–578.

[85] Heit JA, Kobbervig CE, James AH et al. Trends in the incidence of venous thromboembolism during pregnancy or postpartum: A 30-year population-based study. Ann Intern Med 2005;143(10):697–706.

[86] Liu S, Rouleau J, Joseph KS et al. Epidemiology of pregnancy-associated venous thromboembolism: A population-based study in Canada. J Obstet Gynaecol Can 2009;31(7): 611–620.

[87] Ageno W, Becattini C, Brighton T et al. Cardiovascular risk factors and venous thromboembolism: A meta-analysis. Circulation 2008;117(1):93–102.

[88] Allman-Farinelli MA. Obesity and venous thrombosis: A review. Semin Thromb Hemost 2011;37(8):903–907.

[89] Braekkan SK, Siegerink B, Lijfering WM et al. Role of obesity in the etiology of deep vein thrombosis and pulmonary embolism: Current epidemiological insights. Semin Thromb Hemost 2013;39(5):533–540.

[90] Chan WS, Rey E, Kent NE et al. Venous thromboembolism and antithrombotic therapy in pregnancy. J Obstet Gynaecol Can 2014;36(6):527–553.

[91] James A. Practice bulletin no. 123: Thromboembolism in pregnancy. Obstet Gynecol 2011;118(3):718–729.

[92] Patel JP, Green B, Patel RK et al. Population pharmacokinetics of enoxaparin during the antenatal period. Circulation 2013;128(13):1462–1469.

[93] Aksoy H, Aksoy Ü, Karadağ Ö et al. Influence of maternal body mass index on sonographic fetal weight estimation prior to scheduled delivery. J Obstet Gynaecol Res 2015;41(10):1556–1561.

[94] Fox NS, Bhavsar V, Saltzman DH et al. Influence of maternal body mass index on the clinical estimation of fetal weight in term pregnancies. Obstet Gynecol 2009;113(3):641–645.

[95] Manzanares S, Gonzalez-Escudero A, Gonzalez-Peran E et al. Influence of maternal obesity on the accuracy of ultrasonography birth weight prediction. J Matern Fetal Neonatal Med 2019;28:1–6.

[96] O'Brien CM, Louise J, Deussen A et al. In overweight and obese women, fetal ultrasound biometry accurately predicts newborn measures. Aust N Z J Obstet Gynaecol 2020;60(1): 101–107.

[97] Nohr EA, Bech BH, Davies MJ et al. Prepregnancy obesity and fetal death: A study within the Danish National Birth Cohort. Obstet Gynecol 2005;106(2):250–259.

[98] Arrowsmith S, Wray S, Quenby S. Maternal obesity and labour complications following induction of labour in prolonged pregnancy. Bjog 2011;118(5):578–588.

[99] Norman SM, Tuuli MG, Odibo AO et al. The effects of obesity on the first stage of labor. Obstet Gynecol 2012;120(1):130–135.

[100] Ellis JA, Brown CM, Barger B et al. Influence of maternal obesity on labor induction: a systematic review and meta-analysis. J Midwifery Womens Health 2019;64(1):55–67.

[101] Zhang J, Bricker L, Wray S et al. Poor uterine contractility in obese women. Bjog 2007;114(3): 343–348.

[102] Pevzner L, Powers BL, Rayburn WF et al. Effects of maternal obesity on duration and outcomes of prostaglandin cervical ripening and labor induction. Obstet Gynecol 2009;114(6):1315–1321.

[103] Lamon AM, Habib AS. Managing anesthesia for cesarean section in obese patients: Current perspectives. Local Reg Anesth 2016;9:45–57.

[104] Grau T, Leipold RW, Horter J et al. The lumbar epidural space in pregnancy: Visualization by ultrasonography. Br J Anaesth 2001;86(6):798–804.

[105] Sahin T, Balaban O, Sahin L et al. A randomized controlled trial of preinsertion ultrasound guidance for spinal anaesthesia in pregnancy: Outcomes among obese and lean parturients: Ultrasound for spinal anesthesia in pregnancy. J Anesth 2014Jun;28(3):413–419.

[106] Hood DD, Dewan DM. Anesthetic and obstetric outcome in morbidly obese parturients. Anesthesiology 1993;79(6):1210–1218.

[107] Cedergren MI. Maternal morbid obesity and the risk of adverse pregnancy outcome. Obstet Gynecol 2004;103(2):219–224.

[108] Zhang C, Wu Y, Li S et al. Maternal prepregnancy obesity and the risk of shoulder dystocia: A meta-analysis. Bjog 2018;125(4):407–413.

[109] Mwanamsangu AH, Mahande MJ, Mazuguni FS et al. Maternal obesity and intrapartum obstetric complications among pregnant women: Retrospective cohort analysis from medical birth registry in Northern Tanzania. Obes Sci Pract 2020Apr;6(2):171–180.

[110] Fallatah AM, Babatin HM, Nassibi KM et al. Maternal and neonatal outcomes among obese pregnant women in king abdulaziz university hospital: a retrospective single-center medical record review. Med Arch 2019;73(6):425–432.

[111] Poobalan AS, Aucott LS, Gurung T et al. Obesity as an independent risk factor for elective and emergency caesarean delivery in nulliparous women–systematic review and meta-analysis of cohort studies. Obes Rev 2009;10(1):28–35.

[112] Ayres-de-campos D. Obesity and the challenges of caesarean delivery: Prevention and management of wound complications. Best Pract Res Clin Obstet Gynaecol 2015;29(3):406–414.

[113] Costantine MM, Rahman M, Ghulmiyah L et al. Timing of perioperative antibiotics for cesarean delivery: A metaanalysis. Am J Obstet Gynecol 2008;199(3):301.e1–6.

[114] Swank ML, Wing DA, Nicolau DP et al. Increased 3-gram cefazolin dosing for cesarean delivery prophylaxis in obese women. Am J Obstet Gynecol 2015;213(3):415.e1–8.

[115] Ahmadzia HK, Patel EM, Joshi D et al. Obstetric surgical site infections: 2 grams compared with 3 grams of cefazolin in morbidly obese women. Obstet Gynecol 2015Oct;126(4):708–715.

[116] Valent AM, DeArmond C, Houston JM et al. Effect of post-cesarean delivery oral cephalexin and metronidazole on surgical site infection among obese women: a randomized clinical trial. Jama 2017Sep 19;318(11):1026–1034.

[117] Smid MC, Smiley SG, Schulkin J et al. The problem of the pannus: physician preference survey and a review of the literature on cesarean skin incision in morbidly obese women. Am J Perinatol 2016;33(5):463–472.

[118] Sutton AL, Sanders LB, Subramaniam A et al. Abdominal Incision Selection for Cesarean Delivery of Women with Class III Obesity. Am J Perinatol 2016;33(6):547–551.

[119] Tixier H, Thouvenot S, Coulange L et al. Cesarean section in morbidly obese women: Supra or subumbilical transverse incision?. Acta Obstet Gynecol Scand 2009;88(9):1049–1052.

[120] Kingdom JC, Baud D, Grabowska K et al. Delivery by caesarean section in super-obese women: beyond pfannenstiel. J Obstet Gynaecol Can 2012May;34(5):472–474.

[121] Chelmow D, Rodriguez EJ, Sabatini MM. Suture closure of subcutaneous fat and wound disruption after cesarean delivery: A meta-analysis. Obstet Gynecol 2004;103(5 Pt 1): 974–980.

[122] Gates S, Anderson ER. Wound drainage for caesarean section. Cochrane Database Syst Rev 2013;13(12):CD004549.

[123] Ramsey PS, White AM, Guinn DA et al. Subcutaneous tissue reapproximation, alone or in combination with drain, in obese women undergoing cesarean delivery. Obstet Gynecol 2005;105(5 Pt 1):967–973.

[124] Yu L, Kronen RJ, Simon LE et al. Prophylactic negative-pressure wound therapy after cesarean is associated with reduced risk of surgical site infection: A systematic review and meta-analysis. Am J Obstet Gynecol 2018Feb;218(2):200–210.e1.

[125] Smid MC, Dotters-Katz SK, Grace M et al. Prophylactic negative pressure wound therapy for obese women after cesarean delivery: a systematic review and meta-analysis. Obstet Gynecol 2017;130(5):969–978.

[126] Wihbey KA, Joyce EM, Spalding ZT et al. Prophylactic negative pressure wound therapy and wound complication after Cesarean delivery in women with Class II or III Obesity: A Randomized Controlled Trial. Obstet Gynecol 2018;132(2):377–384.

[127] Hussamy DJ, Wortman AC, McIntire DD et al. Closed incision negative pressure therapy in morbidly obese women undergoing Cesarean delivery: A randomized controlled trial. Obstet Gynecol 2019;134(4):781–789.

[128] Turcksin R, Bel S, Galjaard S et al. Maternal obesity and breastfeeding intention, initiation, intensity and duration: A systematic review. Matern Child Nutr 2014;10(2):166–183.

[129] Bever Babendure J, Reifsnider E, Mendias E et al. Reduced breastfeeding rates among obese mothers: A review of contributing factors, clinical considerations and future directions. Int Breastfeed J 2015;10:21.

[130] Nazlee N, Bilal R, Latif Z et al. Maternal body composition and its relationship to infant breast milk intake in rural Pakistan. Food Nutr Sci 2011;2(9):932–937.

[131] Visram H, Finkelstein SA, Feig D et al. Breastfeeding intention and early post-partum practices among overweight and obese women in Ontario: A selective population-based cohort study. J Matern Fetal Neonatal Med 2013;26(6):611–615.

[132] Nehring I, Schmoll S, Beyerlein A et al. Gestational weight gain and long-term postpartum weight retention: A meta-analysis. Am J Clin Nutr 2011;94(5):1225–1231.

[133] Getahun D, Kaminsky LM, Elsasser DA et al. Changes in prepregnancy body mass index between pregnancies and risk of primary cesarean delivery. Am J Obstet Gynecol 2007;197(4):376.e1–7.

[134] Getahun D, Ananth CV, Peltier MR et al. Changes in prepregnancy body mass index between the first and second pregnancies and risk of large-for-gestational-age birth. Am J Obstet Gynecol 2007;196(6):530.e1–8.

[135] Glazer NL, Hendrickson AF, Schellenbaum GD et al. Weight change and the risk of gestational diabetes in obese women. Epidemiology 2004;15(6):733–737.

[136] Callegari LS, Sterling LA, Zelek ST et al. Interpregnancy body mass index change and success of term vaginal birth after cesarean delivery. Am J Obstet Gynecol 2014;210(4):330. e1–330.e7.

[137] Bennett HA, Einarson A, Taddio A et al. Prevalence of depression during pregnancy: Systematic review. Obstet Gynecol 2004Apr;103(4):698–709.

[138] Gavin NI, Gaynes BN, Lohr KN et al. Perinatal depression: A systematic review of prevalence and incidence. Obstet Gynecol 2005;106(5 Pt 1):1071–1083.

[139] Mina TH, Denison FC, Forbes S et al. Associations of mood symptoms with ante- and postnatal weight change in obese pregnancy are not mediated by cortisol. Psychol Med 2015;45(15):3133–3146.

[140] Salehi-Pourmehr H, Mohammad-Alizadeh S, Jafarilar-Agdam N et al. The association between pre-pregnancy obesity and screening results of depression for all trimesters of pregnancy, postpartum and 1 year after birth: A cohort study. J Perinat Med 2018;46(1):87–95.

[141] Gould Rothberg BE, Magriples U, Kershaw TS et al. Gestational weight gain and subsequent postpartum weight loss among young, low-income, ethnic minority women. Am J Obstet Gynecol 2011;204(1):52.e1–11.

[142] LaCoursiere DY, Barrett-Connor E, O'Hara MW et al. The association between prepregnancy obesity and screening positive for postpartum depression. Bjog 2010;117(8):1011–1018.

Vivian Huang, Geoffrey C. Nguyen

26 Managing Inflammatory Bowel Disease During Pregnancy

26.1 Background

Inflammatory bowel disease (IBD) is a group of chronic inflammatory conditions of the digestive tract that include Crohn's disease (CD) and ulcerative colitis (UC). Patients with IBD are often in their young adult years of life, during the time when they are considering pregnancy or are pregnant. In this review, we will cover the important medical and surgical aspects of IBD and IBD therapy that could influence pregnancy and pregnancy outcomes.

26.2 Prepregnancy and Inflammatory Bowel Disease

The prepregnancy time period with respect to IBD is important for setting the stage for pregnancy. Women with IBD were previously thought to have decreased fertility relating to their IBD diagnosis. In more recent years, we have come to understand that women with uncomplicated IBD in remission have similar fertility as the general population, and that the perceived increased infertility may in part be related to voluntary childlessness [1].

26.2.1 Voluntary Childlessness

Voluntary childlessness refers to the choice a patient makes to not become pregnant, because of either medical advice or personal choice. This choice may be based on advice or decisions based on inaccurate knowledge, misperceptions, or from fears and concerns about IBD and IBD medications [2–4]. Thus, it is important that any clinician involved in the management of IBD in a woman of child-bearing potential be knowledgeable regarding IBD, IBD medications, and interaction with reproduction. The clinician should be open to discussion of the topic with their patient, and refer to experts for further education and counselling or to educational sessions [5, 6].

26.2.2 IBD Disease Activity

Active disease preconception reduces fertility, likely due to the inflammatory burden, although possibly may be related to the increased risk of miscarriage with

https://doi.org/10.1515/9783110615258-026

active IBD. Therefore, it is extremely important to optimize management of IBD in the preconception time period.

26.2.2.1 IBD Medications

Except for two IBD therapies, specifically methotrexate and tofacitinib (both will be further discussed in the 'Medication' Section 26.4), IBD medications that are required to maintain disease remission should be continued in the preconception time period. Since many patients are known to stop their IBD medication when attempting to conceive and even when pregnant, women with IBD may benefit from specific preconception education about medication safety [7]. Preconception care has been shown to reduce the risk of IBD relapse during pregnancy and increase medication adherence and smoking cessation [8].

26.2.2.2 IBD-Related Surgeries

The impact of surgery for IBD on fertility remains controversial, with some studies reporting reduced fertility or longer time to conception after surgery, and others reporting no differences [7–9]. With the ileal pouch anal anastomosis (IPAA) surgery, infertility rates have been reported as high as 69% [10]. However, recent studies suggest that the laparoscopic approach may reduce infertility rate [11] or time to conceive compared to the open approach [10]. The type of surgery a woman has had may also affect their future delivery methods, as those who have had the IPAA surgery are often advised toward caesarean section, in order to avoid any potential damage to the anal sphincter or pouch. Therefore, any woman with IBD who may require surgery to treat their IBD should have the discussion with their surgeon and gynecologist regarding potential impact on fertility and delivery methods.

26.3 Pregnancy with Inflammatory Bowel Disease

If a woman with IBD conceives during a time of IBD disease remission, they are more likely to remain in remission, but they still have a small risk (estimated approximately one-third) of experiencing a disease flare during pregnancy. On the other hand, if they conceive during a time of IBD disease activity, they are more likely to remain in their current disease state or experience a worsening of their flare [12]. A small proportion of patients who conceived at time of disease activity will enter remission in pregnancy. Women with ulcerative colitis may have up to two times risk of flaring during pregnancy, especially in the first and second trimesters [13].

Most women with IBD will have good pregnancy outcomes, similar to general healthy population. Some studies reported increased risk of congenital abnormalities, although the general consensus is that this overall risk is no higher than that reported in the general population, and that individual study observations may be related to disease activity, older age of the mothers, or possibly exposure to certain medications [14, 15]. Women with active IBD during pregnancy are more likely to have infants of low birth weight and preterm birth with higher risk among women with active ulcerative colitis [16]. Recent literature suggests that women with IBD may be at increased risk for gestational diabetes (OR 2.96 (CI: 1.47–5.98)) and preterm prelabor rupture of membranes (OR 12.20 (CI 2.15–67.98)) [17]. It is thought that some of this increased risk is related to disease activity, especially if leading to steroid use or inflammation associated risk of premature labor. In addition, adverse pregnancy outcomes are associated with inadequate gestational weight gain among women with IBD, and special attention to nutrition should be made [18].

Close monitoring and management of the IBD by their gastroenterologist is highly recommended, in conjunction with obstetrical monitoring and management. Apart from two of the current IBD therapies, methotrexate and tofacitinib (both will be further discussed in the 'Medication' Section 26.4), IBD medications that are required to achieve and maintain disease remission should be continued in the gestational period to reduce the risk of disease flare and associated complications.

26.4 IBD Medications

As with most maternal chronic diseases, expert opinion and guidelines recommend achieving and maintaining disease remission throughout pregnancy for optimal maternal and neonatal outcomes. This recommendation applies to IBD as well, with specific caveats and nuances related to the rapidly growing armamentarium of IBD therapies approved for general use. The main categories of IBD therapies that we will discuss include (1) sulfasalazine and 5-aminosalicylates, (2) immunomodulators (azathioprine, methotrexate), (3) biologics (anti-TNF, anti-IL12/23, anti-integrin), (4) small molecule (tofacitinib), and (5) corticosteroids.

26.4.1 Sulfasalazine and 5-Aminosalicylates

Sulfasalazine and 5-aminosalicylates are common maintenance medications for ulcerative colitis (and in some cases for Crohn's disease) that can be continued throughout pregnancy. Since sulfasalazine inhibits folate synthesis, if a woman is on sulfasalazine they should take additional folate supplementation [19, 20]. Of note, certain Asacol® brand medications contain the dibutylphthalate chemical which has been shown to cause teratogenicity in animal models and thus it is recommended to avoid this 5-aminosacylate, if possible, during pregnancy [21, 22]. 5-Aminosalicylates may be taken orally or rectally, and there is no contraindication to using rectal therapy during pregnancy.

26.4.2 Immunomodulators

Thiopurines used for treating IBD include azathioprine (Imuran®) and 6-mercaptopurine (Purinethol®). There is no increase in adverse outcomes of spontaneous abortion, adverse birth outcomes, or adverse infant outcomes (up to 1 year) [23], or in long-term development or immune function in children up to 6 years [24]. Small case series had reported increased risk of anemia in infants exposed to maternal thiopurines [25], although a recent comparative observational study reported no impact [26]. Routine monitoring of blood counts and liver tests with appropriate adjustment of maternal thiopurine dose in pregnancy is recommended. There is no evidence regarding monitoring of thiopurine metabolites or the therapeutic range in pregnancy, and thus, it is not routinely recommended.

Methotrexate is a teratogenic medication and should be stopped at least three months before conception. Women with IBD who discover they have conceived while on methotrexate should be referred to a high-risk obstetrician for counseling and management.

26.4.3 Biologics

Anti-tumor necrosis factor biologics (anti-TNF) are monoclonal antibodies designed to inhibit tumor necrosis factor and are broadly effective for the induction and maintenance of remission for both CD and UC. Anti-TNF agents include infliximab, adalimumab, golimumab, certolizumab, and their respective biosimilars. There is a high rate of transfer of these biologics across the placenta especially in the third trimester, except for certolizumab which lacks the F_c portion of IgG1 that facilitates placental transfer [27]. Anti-TNF biologics can be detected in infants up to 12 months following birth [28]. However, the PIANO registry of over 1,000 pregnant women with IBD has reassured that treatment with anti-TNF agents during pregnancy did not increase risk of adverse pregnancy outcomes or outcomes in early childhood [29]. Given this safety data, anti-TNF therapy can be started during pregnancy, preferably with certolizumab if available. If a woman is on anti-TNF therapy, it should be continued during pregnancy to prevent disease relapse. For biologics that are administered every eight weeks, it is common practice to time the last dose prior to delivery around 30–32 weeks and to resume immediately after delivery. However, even with this practice, there are detectable levels of these biologics in the infant's blood following delivery and live vaccines should be avoided in the first 12 months of life.

There is less safety data on the newer biologics, ustekinumab and vedolizumab. The former is an IL-12/IL-23 antagonist, while the latter is an anti-integrin monoclonal antibody that impedes lymphocyte trafficking to intestinal endothelium. There do not appear to be any concerning safety signals among women with IBD exposed to these biologics during pregnancy. In addition, there has been more experience with the use of ustekinumab during pregnancy for rheumatological and dermatologic conditions indications [30]. In general, women who have achieved disease remission on these agents should continue them as maintenance therapy during pregnancy. Their use as an inducing agent during pregnancy should be considered on an individual basis, especially among biologic-naïve patients in whom anti-TNF therapy may be a safer alternative.

26.4.4 Small Molecules

While there are many small molecule drugs in development for IBD, tofacitinib, which is a JAK kinase inhibitor, is the only one currently approved for the treatment of IBD and is effective for both induction and maintenance of remission. Tofacitinib, however, has been shown to demonstrate teratogenicity in animal studies [31]. Therefore, tofacitinib is contraindicated in pregnancy. Women of childbearing age should be counselled to use contraception, and those who inadvertently become pregnant while on tofacitinib should stop the medication and should immediately notify their obstetric and IBD providers.

26.4.5 Corticosteroids

Systemic steroids are highly effective in achieving disease remission for UC and CD, though they are not effective in maintaining remission. During pregnancy, they may play a role in inducing remission for patients who are newly diagnosed or those with breakthrough symptoms while on maintenance therapy. Because of a possible link with cleft palate, alternative therapies should be considered in the first trimester. However, the priority is to control disease activity, and if steroids are necessary to achieve remission, they should be administered. Budesonide, with its limited systemic absorption due to first-pass effect, may result in less corticosteroid exposure to the fetus.

26.5 Delivery and Postpartum

Though women with IBD, especially CD, are more likely to undergo cesarean delivery than the general population, that decision should generally be based on obstetrical indications. The only IBD-related indication for cesarean delivery is the presence of active perianal CD because perineal lacerations during labor may exacerbate perianal disease and may be more difficult to heal in the presence of the latter. Women who have a history of perianal fistula but have documented closure of the fistula and no active perianal symptoms usually do not require cesarean delivery. Whether to consider cesarean delivery in women with a pelvic pouch should be an individualized decision after discussion with the obstetrician, IBD provider, and ideally with the surgeon who constructed the pouch if possible. It is helpful for patients to have discussions regarding mode of delivery and the indications for having cesarean delivery early on in the pregnancy to manage expectations. Women who undergo cesarean delivery should receive prophylaxis against venous thromboembolism.

In general, medical therapy for IBD should not influence the decision to breastfeed. Conversely, women who decide to breastfeed should not stop their IBD medications as that may increase the risk of a disease flare. The majority of medications, including 5-ASA, corticosteroids, thiopurines, and biologics (anti-TNF, anti IL-12/IL-23, anti-integrin), are considered safe for breastfeeding. The one exception may be methotrexate, which should not be initiated in the postpartum period, which is usually not an issue because it is contraindicated in pregnancy.

26.6 Conclusion

Pregnancy is an often exciting and anxiety-provoking time for women with IBD. Many have concerns that their IBD medications may harm their fetus. Women should be counseled that optimizing control of IBD disease activity is one of the primary determinants of IBD pregnancy outcomes. With the exception of methotrexate and tofacitinib, women with IBD are generally advised to continue medications that have enabled them to achieve and maintain remission. A multidisciplinary approach to managing IBD during pregnancy that involves a gastroenterology and obstetrics or medical obstetrics can be helpful to navigate the journey especially if IBD flares occur during pregnancy.

References

[1]   Tavernier N, Fumery M, Peyrin-Biroulet L, Colombel JF, Gower-Rousseau C. Systematic review: fertility in non-surgically treated inflammatory bowel disease. Aliment Pharmacol Ther 2013;38(8):847–853. doi: 10.1111/apt.12478. Epub 2013 Sep 4.

[2]   Walldorf J, Brunne S, Gittinger FS, Michl P. Family planning in inflammatory bowel disease: childlessness and disease-related concerns among female patients. Eur J Gastroenterol Hepatol 2018;30(3):310–315.

[3]   Selinger CP, Ghorayeb J, Madill A. What factors might drive voluntary childlessness (VC) in women with IBD? Does IBD-specific pregnancy-related knowledge matter?. J Crohns Colitis 201610(10):1151–1158.

[4]   Ellul P, Zammita SC, Katsanos KH et al. Perception of reproductive health in women with inflammatory bowel disease. J Crohns Colitis 2016;10(8):886–891.

[5]   Huang VW, Chang HJ, Kroeker KI et al. Does the level of reproductive knowledge specific to inflammatory bowel disease predict childlessness among women with inflammatory bowel disease?. Can J Gastroenterol Hepatol 2015;29(2):95–103.

[6]   Mountifield R, Andrews JM, Bampton P. It IS worth the effort: patient knowledge of reproductive aspects of inflammatory bowel disease improves dramatically after a single group education session. J Crohns Colitis 2014;8(8):796–801.

[7]   Lee S, Crowe M, Seow CH et al. The impact of surgical therapies for inflammatory bowel disease on female fertility. Cochrane Database Syst Rev 2019;23(7):CD012711.

[8]   De Lima A, Zelinkova Z, Mulders AG, van der Woude CJ. Preconception care reduces relapse of inflammatory bowel disease during pregnancy. Clin Gastroenterol Hepatol 2016;14(9): 1285–1292.

[9]   Gorgun E, Cengiz TB, Aytac E et al. Does laparoscopic ileal pouch-anal anastomosis reduce infertility compared with open approach?. Surgery 2019;166(4):670–677.

[10]   Gorgun E, Remzi FH, Goldberg JM et al. Fertility is reduced after restorative proctocolectomy with ileal pouch anal anastomosis: A study of 300 patients. Surgery 2004;136(4):795–803.

[11]   Beyer-Berjot L, Maggiori L, Birnbaum D, Lefevre JH, Berdah S, Panis Y. A total laparoscopic approach reduces the infertility rate after ileal pouch-anal anastomosis: a 2-center study. Ann Surg 2013;258(2):275–282.

[12]   Abhyankar A, Ham M, Moss AC. Meta-analysis: the impact of disease activity at conception on disease activity during pregnancy in patients with inflammatory bowel disease. Aliment Pharmacol Ther 2013;38(5):460–466.

[13]   Pedersen N, Bortoli A, Duricova D et al. European Crohn-Colitis Organisation-ECCO-Study group of epidemiology committee-EpiCom. The course of inflammatory bowel disease during pregnancy and postpartum: a prospective European ECCO-EpiCom Study of 209 pregnant women. Aliment Pharmacol Ther 2013;38(5):501–512.

[14]   Ban L, Tata LJ, Fiaschi L, Card T. Limited risks of major congenital anomalies in children of mothers with IBD and effects of medications. Gastroenterology 2014;146(1):76–84.

[15]   Nørgård B, Puho E, Pedersen L, Czeizel AE, Sørensen HT. Risk of congenital abnormalities in children born to women with ulcerative colitis: a population-based, case-control study. Am J Gastroenterol 2003;98:2006–2010.

[16]   Kammerlander H, Nielsen J, Kjeldsen J, Knudsen T, Friedman S, Nørgård B. The effect of disease activity on birth outcomes in a Nationwide cohort of Women with moderate to severe inflammatory bowel disease. Inflamm Bowel Dis 2017Jun;23(6):1011–1018.

[17]   Tandon P, Govardhanam V, Leung K, Maxwell C, Huang V. Systematic review with meta-analysis: risk of adverse pregnancy-related outcomes in inflammatory bowel disease. Alimentary Pharm Ther 2020;51(3):320–333.

[18] Bengtson MB, Martin CF, Aamodt G, Vatn MH, Mahadevan U. Inadequate gestational weight gain predicts adverse pregnancy outcomes in mothers with inflammatory bowel disease: results from a prospective US pregnancy cohort. Dig Dis Sci 2017;62(8):2063–2069.

[19] Van Der Woude CJ, Kolacek S, Dotan I, Oresland T et al. European evidenced-based consensus on reproduction in inflammatory bowel disease. J Crohns Colitis 2010;4:493–510.

[20] Nielsen OH, Maxwell C, Hendel J. IBD medications during pregnancy and lactation. Nat Rev Gastroenterol Hepatol 2014;11:116–127.

[21] Hernández-Díaz S, Su YC, Mitchell AA, Kelley KE, Calafat AM, Hauser R. Medications as a potential source of exposure to phthalates among women of childbearing age. Reprod Toxicol 2013;37:1–5.

[22] Nguyen GC, Seow CH, Maxwell C et al. IBD in pregnancy consensus group; Canadian association of gastroenterology. The toronto consensus statements for the management of inflammatory bowel disease in pregnancy. Gastroenterology 2016;150(3):734–757.

[23] Kanis SL, De Lima-karagiannis A, De Boer NKH, Van Der Woude CJ. Use of thiopurines during conception and pregnancy is not associated with adverse pregnancy outcomes or health of infants at one year in a prospective study. Clin Gastroenterol Hepatol 2017;15(8):1232–1241.

[24] De Meij TG, Jharap B, Kneepkens CM, Van Bodegraven AA, De Boer NK. Dutch Initiative on Crohn and Colitis. Long-term follow-up of children exposed intrauterine to maternal thiopurine therapy during pregnancy in females with inflammatory bowel disease. Aliment Pharmacol Ther 2013;38(1):38–43.

[25] Jharap B, De Boer NK, Stokkers P et al. Dutch Initiative on Crohn and Colitis. Intrauterine exposure and pharmacology of conventional thiopurine therapy in pregnant patients with inflammatory bowel disease. Gut 2014 Mar;63(3):451–457.

[26] Koslowsky B, Sadeh C, Grisaru-Granovsky S, Miskin H, Goldin E, Bar-Gil Shitrit A. Thiopurine therapy for inflammatory bowel disease during pregnancy is not associated with anemia in the infant. Dig Dis Sci 2019;64(8):2286–2290.

[27] Chaparro M, Jisbert JP. Transplacental transfer of immunosuppressants and biologics used for the treatment of inflammatory bowel disease. Curr Pharm Biotechnol. 2011 May;12 (5):765–73.

[28] Mahadevan U, Wolf DC, Dubinsky M. Placental transfer of anti-tumor necrosis factor agents in pregnant patients with inflammatory bowel disease. Clin Gastroenterol Hepatol 2013;11:286–92.

[29] Mahadevan U, Long MD, Kane SV, et al. Pregnancy and Neonatal Outcomes After Fetal Exposure to Biologics and Thiopurines Among Women With Inflammatory Bowel Disease. Gastroenterology. 2021 Mar;160(4):1131–113.

[30] Kimball BA, Guenther L, Kalia S et al. Pregnancy Outcomes in Women With Moderate-to-Severe Psoriasis From the Psoriasis Longitudinal Assessment and Registry (PSOLAR). JAMA Dermatol. 2021;157(3):301–306.

[31] Pfizer Inc. Xeljanz prescribing information. 2014. http://labeling.pfizer.com/ShowLabeling. aspx?id=959. Accessed 26 Mar 2016.

[32] Nielsen OH, Maxwell C, Hendel J. IBD medications during pregnancy and lactation. Nat Rev Gastroenterol Hepatol. 2014 Feb;11(2):116–27.

Homero Flores-Mendoza, Harrison Banner, John W. Snelgrove

27 Intrahepatic Cholestasis of Pregnancy

27.1 Introduction

Intrahepatic cholestasis of pregnancy (ICP) is a pregnancy-specific liver disorder, presenting usually in the late second to third trimester, that is characterized by pruritus and elevation in serum bile acids and, occasionally, liver enzymes. ICP is diagnosed in the absence of other causes and generally resolves following delivery. A relationship with adverse fetal outcomes, including stillbirth and perinatal death, has been reported [1].

ICP is the most common liver disease in pregnancy and incidence varies worldwide [2]. Reported incidence of ICP in different countries and ethnic groups has been found to vary between 0.07% and 27.6% [3–5]. The reason for such striking incidence variations is complex and unknown but is more than likely related to differences in diagnostic criteria, genetics, ethnicity, hormonal influence, multiple gestations, geographical and environmental factors, and maternal age and history of liver disease. Interestingly, a higher incidence of ICP has been reported in higher and lower latitudes of Earth and in winter months, further supporting the theory of multifactorial etiology of the disease [6].

27.2 Etiology

Bile flow is interrupted in ICP such that bile acids, which would ordinarily leave the hepatocytes via the bile ducts, instead accumulate in the liver and ultimately in the serum. The etiology of ICP is not completely understood, but likely includes a combination of genetic, hormonal, environmental, and maternal health history factors [7].

27.2.1 Genetics

Genetic susceptibility is supported by evidence of mutations in *ABCB4*, *ABCB11*, *ABCC2*, and related genes in different ethnic groups with increased risk, and in familial cases of cholestasis with a high recurrence rate. These mutations have been found in different population studies including European and South American populations and also have a role in diseases characterized by cholestasis in childhood that can lead to fulminant liver failure and death in the absence of liver transplantation [8]. These gene mutations lead to a deficient cannalicular and basolateral export of bile acids. Bile acid transporters are critical for maintenance enterohepatic

https://doi.org/10.1515/9783110615258-027

circulation, stimulation of bile flow, intestinal absorption of lipophilic nutrients, solubilization and excretion of cholesterol, as well as antimicrobial and metabolic effects [9].

27.2.2 Hormonal

The role of hormones, particularly estrogen, and its relationship with the development of ICP are supported by several theories. First, ICP occurs mainly in the late second to third trimesters when estrogen levels reach their peak. Second, ICP occurs more commonly in multiple gestation pregnancies where estrogen levels are higher as compared to singleton pregnancies [10]. A Canadian retrospective study of all multiple gestation deliveries found an incidence of ICP of 4.2%, which is significantly higher than the incidence reported in singleton pregnancies in other population-based cohort studies [11]. Third, a higher incidence and earlier presentation of cholestasis have been reported following in vitro fertilization (IVF) in the context of ovarian hyperstimulation, with presentation as early as in the first trimester of pregnancy [12]. The role of progesterone, both endogenous and exogenous, and its role in the development of ICP have also been proposed, though these theories are still under study [13].

27.2.3 Environmental

A higher incidence of ICP has been reported in higher and lower latitudes of Earth. ICP is more common in the winter months in Finland, Sweden, Chile, and Portugal. In the Chilean Araucanian indigenous population, ICP incidence has been reported to be the highest in the world, with an incidence rate of 22.1% [14]; interestingly, incidence levels in Chile and other Scandinavian region have decreased since their original description in the late 1970s, with a current prevalence in Chile ranging from 1.5% to 4% of all pregnancies [15]. Geographical location and its relationship with exposure to sunlight and vitamin D levels, diet, and genetic predisposition within isolated ethnic populations have been proposed as causal factors but are yet to be proven.

27.2.4 History of Prior Liver Disease

A relationship between the development of ICP and a history of gallstones and primary hepatic disease, particularly viral hepatitis, has been reported. In a population-based study that analyzed the occurrence of these diseases in women with ICP and in controls, a significant association of ICP with hepatitis C and non-alcoholic liver fibrosis was found. Furthermore, some patients with ICP were found to be at a significant risk of development of cirrhosis and other severe chronic diseases after delivery [16].

27.3 Clinical Manifestations

The cardinal manifestation of ICP is pruritus of distinct severity, which does not spare the palms and soles of feet and is often worse in the nighttime. Other manifestations of severe liver dysfunction such as severe right upper quadrant pain, nausea, hypoglycemia, jaundice, steatorrhea, and encephalopathy have been reported but are rare, and should prompt an investigation for diagnoses related to other causes of hepatobiliary disease. Physical examination is usually normal, but excoriation stigmata are often encountered [17]. Pruritus accompanied by skin lesions, particularly with normal laboratory findings, are often primary dermatologic conditions related to pregnancy, such as pruritic urticarial papules and plaques of pregnancy, or coexisting dermatological or infectious disorders unrelated to pregnancy.

The hallmark laboratory findings encountered in ICP is a rise in serum bile acids above normal range levels. A mild-to-moderate rise in liver enzymes, alkaline phosphatase, and bilirubin levels can also be encountered. Other direct or indirect markers for liver dysfunction such as coagulation screen, gamma-glutamyl transpeptidase, and glucose are usually within normal ranges [18]. Any severe disturbance in liver function parameters should prompt an investigation of other causes.

27.4 Diagnosis

Diagnosis of ICP is made clinically with the new onset of pruritus, typically in the mid- to late trimester of pregnancy, that is accompanied with an elevation in serum bile acid levels (>10 μmol/L). Occasionally, a rise in liver enzymes in the absence of primary hepatobiliary disease can occur.

Differential diagnosis, as always, should be based on thorough history taking, physical examination, and present and past laboratory evaluation. As a diagnosis of exclusion, preexisting causes of pruritus, hepatic impairment, or both should be investigated. Other pregnancy-specific causes of pruritus, such as pruritus gravidarum, atopic eruptions of pregnancy, polymorphic eruptions of pregnancy, pemphigoid gestationis, prurigo of pregnancy, and pruritic folliculitis of pregnancy, have to be investigated and ruled out; these are dermatologic eruptions, which differentiate them from ICP. Special consideration should be placed in ruling out previous primary or acquired hepatobiliary disease and pregnancy-related disorders that affect the liver, such as hyperemesis gravidarum, preeclampsia, HELLP syndrome, and acute fatty liver of pregnancy. A complete list of differential diagnosis with typical clinical presentation and distinguishing features can be found in Table 27.1 [19].

Table 27.1: Comparison between ICP and other dermatologic and hepatic disorders in pregnancy.

Differential diagnosis	Typical clinical presentation	Distinguishing features
Pregnancy-specific causes of pruritus		
Pruritus gravidarum	Pruritus, usually in the third trimester	Similar presentation to intrahepatic cholestasis of pregnancy, but normal liver function tests and bile acids.
Atopic eruption of pregnancy	Pruritus, usually in the third trimester	Dry, red rash with or without small blisters. Typically affects trunk and limb flexures.
Polymorphic eruption of pregnancy	Pruritus, usually in the third trimester	Typically affects lower abdominal striae with umbilical-sparing; Urticarial papules or plaques, vesicles, and target lesions.
Pemphigoid gestationis	Itchy rash, usually in the second or third trimester	Rare autoimmune condition characterized by complement-fixing immunoglobulin G antibodies. Rash develops into large, tense blisters associated with increased risk of preterm delivery and SG. Recurs in subsequent pregnancies and with combined oral contraceptive.
Prurigo of pregnancy	Pruritus, usually in the third trimester	Groups of red-brown papules on the abdomen and extensor surfaces of the limbs. Papules may persist postpartum.
Pruritic folliculitis of pregnancy	Pruritus, usually in the third trimester	Acneiform eruption on the shoulders, upper back, thighs, and arms; Follicular papules and pustules, which may be filled with pus, but culture is typically sterile; rash usually improves with advancing gestation.
Preexisting causes of pruritus		
Atopic dermatitis	Pruritus, any gestation	History of atopy.
Allergic or drug reaction	Pruritus, any gestation	History of exposure to allergen or drug. Maculopapular rash.

Table 27.1 (continued)

Differential diagnosis	Typical clinical presentation	Distinguishing features
Systemic disease	History of liver, renal, or thyroid disease	Signs and symptoms of systemic disease; History of pruritus before conception.
Pregnancy-specific causes of hepatic impairment		
Acute fatty liver of pregnancy	Nausea, vomiting, headache, abdominal pain, polyuria, polydipsia in the third trimester	New nausea and vomiting in the third trimester are not caused by hyperemesis gravidarum; Women with AFLP are more unwell and often have associated renal impairment, coagulopathy, hypoglycemia, and preeclampsia.
HELLP syndrome	Hypertension, proteinuria, headache, epigastric pain, visual disturbance in the second or third trimester	Hypertension and proteinuria are predominant features.
Hyperemeis gravidarum	Nausea and vomiting in the first trimester	Presentation in early pregnancy, abnormal liver function test resolves with successful treatment.
Preexisting causes of hepatic impairment		
Viral hepatitis	Jaundice, nausea, vomiting, abdominal pain	Systemic symptoms, generally unwell, contacts.
Primary biliary cirrhosis or primary sclerosing cholangitis	Pruritus, jaundice, lethargy, other autoimmune disorders	Symptoms before pregnancy; associated autoantibodies.
Autoimmune hepatitis	Nausea, lethargy, jaundice, other autoimmune disorders	Symptoms before pregnancy; associated autoantibodies.
Drug-induced liver injury	Pruritus, jaundice	Ingestion of drugs before onset of symptoms or biochemical abnormalities.
Biliary obstruction	Abdominal pain, pale stools, dark urine	Liver ultrasound scan abnormalities.
Venoocclusive disease	Abdominal pain, distension (ascites), jaundice, gastrointestinal bleeding	Thrombosis demonstrated on imaging, thrombophilia.

From Williamson and Geenes [1].

27.5 Maternal and Fetal Implications

Aside from maternal discomfort due to potentially significant symptoms, there is usually complete resolution of the disease after delivery. As previously mentioned, there is evidence from a population-based study that some patients with ICP were found to be at a significant risk of developing cirrhosis and other severe chronic diseases after delivery. The authors propose increased follow-up in patients with ICP [16].

The main concern regarding ICP is the potential for fetal morbidity and mortality. The potential risks associated with ICP are stillbirth, preterm birth, iatrogenic preterm birth, preterm or term meconium-stained amniotic fluid, and admission to NICU. Severity of the disease is thought to be related to serum bile acid levels; a previous guideline by the Royal College of Obstetrics and Gynecologists [20] defined severe ICP when total serum bile acid levels were over 40 µmol/L, while mild ICP was defined as bile acid levels under 20 µmol/L, based on studies which showed elevated risk of adverse pregnancy outcomes for patients in the severe group but not in the mild group [21]. A recent individual patient data meta-analysis aimed to quantify the adverse perinatal effects of ICP in women with increased bile acid concentrations and determine whether elevated bile acid concentrations were associated with the risk of stillbirth and preterm birth. These authors found that the risk of stillbirth in singleton pregnancies is increased at 3.44% in women with ICP when serum bile acids concentrations are 100 mmol/L or higher. For women in this high-risk category, the rate of stillbirth increased with gestational age. There was no statistically significant difference in stillbirth rates with bile acid levels <100 mmol/L compared to background population risk. This study also demonstrated that preterm birth rates, particularly due to iatrogenic preterm birth, were higher in women with ICP irrespective of total serum bile acid levels [22].

Patients should be counseled that, in the vast majority of patients with bile acid levels <100 mmol/L, poor fetal outcome cannot be predicted by laboratory results, and that decisions regarding delivery timing should not be based on these results alone. Aside from continuous fetal monitoring during labor, no specific method of antenatal fetal monitoring, including ultrasound and cardiotocography, has been proven to be a reliable method for preventing stillbirth in patients with ICP [20].

27.6 Treatment

Upon diagnosis of ICP, ursodeoxycholic acid (UDCA) should be offered for the treatment of cholestatic symptoms to all patients. UDCA has also shown to decrease bile acid levels and transaminase levels. Dosing should be started at the minimal level possible (8–10 mg/kg per day) and titrated up to relieve symptoms at a maximum dose of 20 mg/kg per day [23]. A meta-analysis found a statistically significant reduction in pruritus and improvement in hepatic function in ICP patients with UDCA treatment [24]. Ideal frequency of follow-up is unknown, but some guidelines recommend it reasonable to repeat laboratory tests weekly until delivery and 10 days postnatally until laboratory testing returns to normal [20]. If poor or partial response to therapy, additional testing should be performed to rule out other causes of hepatobiliary dysfunction.

Despite significantly improving maternal symptoms, evidence regarding fetal benefits is not as encouraging. A Cochrane systematic review on this topic concluded that there were fewer instances of fetal distress/asphyxia events in the UDCA groups as compared to placebo; however, the difference was not statistically significant [25]. A recent large randomized placebo-controlled trial aimed to evaluate whether UDCA reduced adverse perinatal outcomes in women with ICP and found that UDCA use in ICP patients did not reduce a composite of outcomes that included perinatal death, preterm birth, and NICU admission [26].

In refractory cases where maximal UDCA dosages are reached and symptoms are still present, second-line therapies can be considered. Second-line agents available include rifampin, cholestyramine, and S-adenosyl-methionine (SAM) [27–29]. Although efficacy and safety have been proven with these medications, they have not been proven to be more effective than UDCA alone and should be used as an add-on therapy or for patients unable to take UDCA. Therapies such as hydroxyzine, chlorpeniramine, and dexamethasone have not been studied sufficiently to be able to provide recommendations regarding their standardized use [25].

For refractory cases to medications, therapies such as plasmapheresis have been piloted with successful results. Plasmapheresis is an extracorporeal exchange technique used to remove large-molecular-weight substances from plasma. The mechanism whereby plasmapheresis decreases pruritus is unknown, but may be through removal of bile salts. Although no randomized controlled trials or systematic reviews are available to compare plasmapheresis with other pharmacological therapies, successful results from case reports conclude that given the potential for rare but serious adverse effects, plasmapheresis should be reserved for severe cases of ICP that are refractory to medical therapy [30].

27.7 Delivery

One of the most challenging decisions faced by a clinician caring for a patient with ICP is the timing of delivery. Timing of delivery should be individualized on a case-by-case basis. Decision making and counseling regarding recommended timing of delivery should include risks and benefits of iatrogenic preterm delivery versus unexplained late stillbirth. Unfortunately, no fetal well-being antenatal test has proven effective in reducing adverse fetal outcomes and because of that, there is no trial evidence to guide timing of delivery in pregnancies complicated by ICP. Most guidelines advocate delivery between 36 and 38 weeks of gestation or at diagnosis if diagnosis is made later in gestation, though these recommendations predate the publication of the Ovadia et al. meta-analysis which did not show a significantly elevated risk of stillbirth in patients with bile acids <100 mmol/L [22]. Because of the linear relationship with adverse fetal outcomes at bile acid levels >100 μmol/L, delivery before 36 weeks may occasionally be indicated depending on laboratory and clinical circumstances [31]. As previously mentioned, continuous fetal monitoring during labor is recommended and cesarean section should be reserved for usual obstetrical indications. The first timing-of-delivery trial in women with intrahepatic cholestasis of pregnancy concluded that a randomized trial was unlikely to be feasible because of the rarity of stillbirth as a pregnancy outcome [32].

References

[1]   Williamson C, Geenes V. Intrahepatic cholestasis of pregnancy Obstet Gynecol 2014;124: 120–133.
[2]   Clinical updates in women's health care summary: liver disease: reproductive considerations. Obstet Gynecol 2017;129:236.
[3]   Lee RH, Goodwin TM, Greenspoon J, Incerpi M. The prevalence of intrahepatic cholestasis of pregnancy in a primarily Latina Los Angeles population J Perinatol 2006;26:527.
[4]   Reyes H, Gonzalez MC, Ribalta J et al. Prevalence of intrahepatic cholestasis of pregnancy in Chile. Ann Intern Med 1978;88:487.
[5]   Laifer SA, Stiller RJ, Siddiqui DS et al. Ursodeoxycholic acid for the treatment of intrahepatic cholestasis of pregnancy. J Matern Fetal Med 2001;10:131.
[6]   Geenes V, Williamson C. Intrahepatic cholestasis of pregnancy World J Gastroenterol 2009;15:2049.
[7]   Dixon PH, Williamson C. The pathophysiology of intrahepatic cholestasis of pregnancy Clin Res Hepatol Gastroenterol 2016;40:141.
[8]   Pataia V, Dixon PH, Williamson C. Pregnancy and bile acid disorders Am J Physiol Gastrointest Liver Physiol 2017;313:G1.
[9]   Halilbasic E, Claudel T, Traunder M. Bile acid transporters and regulatory nuclear receptors in the liver and beyond. J Hepatol 2013;58(1):155–168.
[10]   Gonzalez MC, Reyes H, Arrese M et al. Intrahepatic cholestasis of pregnancy in twin pregnancies. J Hepatol 1989;9:84.
[11]   Lausman AY, Al-Yaseen E, Sam D, Nitsch R, Barrett JF. Intrahepatic cholestasis of pregnancy in women with a multiple pregnancy: an analysis of risks and pregnancy outcomes. J Obstet Gynaecol Can 2008;30(11):1008–1013.
[12]   Zamah AM, El-Sayed YY, Milki AA. Two cases of cholestasis in the first trimester of pregnancy after ovarian hyperstimulation. Fertil Steril 2008;90(4):1202 e7–10.
[13]   Abu-Hayyeh S, Ovadia C, Lieu T et al. Prognostic and mechanistic potential of progesterone sulfates in intrahepatic cholestasis of pregnancy and pruritus gravidarum. Hepatology 2016;63:1287.

[14] Reyes H, Gonzalez MC, Ribalta J et al. Prevalence of intrahepatic cholestasis of pregnancy in chile. Ann Intern Med 1978;88:487.

[15] Germain AM, Carvajal JA, Glasinovic JC, Kato CS, Williamson C. Intrahepatic cholestasis of pregnancy: an intriguing pregnancy-specific disorder. JSoc GynecolInvestig 2002;9:10–14.

[16] Ropponen A, Sund R, Riikonen S et al. Intrahepatic cholestasis of pregnancy as an indicator of liver and biliary diseases: a population-based study. Hepatology 2006;43:723.

[17] Kondrackiene J, Kupcinskas L. Intrahepatic cholestasis of pregnancy-current achievements and unsolved problems World J Gastroenterol 2008;14:5781.

[18] Heikkinen J, Mäentausta O, Ylöstalo P, Jänne O. Changes in serum bile acid concentrations during normal pregnancy, in patients with intrahepatic cholestasis of pregnancy and in pregnant women with itching Br J Obstet Gynaecol 1981;88:240.

[19] Williamson C, Geenes V. Intrahepatic cholestasis of pregnancy Obstet Gynecol 2014;124:120.

[20] Royal college of obstetricians and gynaecologists. Obstetric Cholestasis. 2011; Available at: https://www.rcog.org.uk/globalassets/documents/guidelines/gtg_43.pdf

[21] Glantz A, Marschall H-U, Mattsson L-A. Intrahepatic cholestasis of pregnancy: relationships between bile acid levels and fetal complication rates. Hepatology 2004;40(2):467–474.

[22] Ovadia C, Seed PT, Sklavounos A et al. Association of adverse perinatal outcomes of intrahepatic cholestasis of pregnancy with biochemical markers: results of aggregate and individual patient data meta-analyses. Lancet 2019;393:899.

[23] Pusl T, Beuers U. Intrahepatic cholestasis of pregnancy Orphanet J Rare Dis 2007;2:26.

[24] Grand'Maison S, Durand M, Mahone M. The effects of ursodeoxycholic acid treatment for intrahepatic cholestasis of pregnancy on maternal and fetal outcomes: a meta-analysis including non-randomized studies. J Obstet Gynaecol Can 2014;36(7):632–641.

[25] Gurung V, Middleton P, Milan SJ et al. Interventions for treating cholestasis in pregnancy. Cochrane Database Syst Rev 2013;CD000493.

[26] Chappell LC, Bell JL, Smith A et al. Ursodeoxycholic acid versus placebo in women with intrahepatic cholestasis of pregnancy (PITCHES): a randomised controlled trial. Lancet 2019;394:849.

[27] Saleh MM, Abdo KR. Consensus on the management of obstetric cholestasis: national UK survey BJOG 2007;114:99.

[28] Liu J, Murray AM, Mankus EB et al. Adjuvant use of Rifampin for refractory intrahepatic cholestasis of pregnancy. Obstet Gynecol 2018;132:678.

[29] Zhang Y, Lu L, Victor DW et al. Ursodeoxycholic acid and S-adenosylmethionine for the treatment of intrahepatic cholestasis of pregnancy: a meta-analysis. Hepat Mon 2016;16: e38558.

[30] Warren JE, Blaylock RC, Silver RM. Plasmapheresis for the treatment of intrahepatic cholestasis of pregnancy refractory to medical treatment. Am J Obstet Gynecol 2005;192(6): 2088–2089.

[31] ACOG committee opinion No. 764: medically indicated late-lreterm and early-Term deliveries. Obstet Gynecol 2019;133:e151.

[32] Chappell LC, Gurung V, Seed PT et al. Ursodeoxycholic acid versus placebo, and early term delivery versus expectant management, in women with intrahepatic cholestasis of pregnancy: semifactorial randomised clinical trial. BMJ 2012;344:e3799.

Ghaydaa Aldabie, Karen A. Spitzer, Carl A. Laskin
28 Pregnancy and the Rheumatic Diseases

28.1 Introduction

When dealing with any disease in pregnancy, one should always consider the effect of the disease on pregnancy and the effect of pregnancy on the disease. Rheumatic diseases have multisystemic effects and may manifest differently during pregnancy and the postpartum period. This can add a significant challenge to the management of such patients. Furthermore, the use of certain antirheumatic medications during pregnancy may complicate the situation, as many of these medications may influence pregnancy outcomes. Ideally, a preconception assessment should be undertaken for every woman with a rheumatic disease as she contemplates a pregnancy. The patient must be assessed regarding her disease activity status and the antirheumatic treatment she is receiving. Once pregnancy is confirmed, it is crucial to have a multidisciplinary approach and collaboration between the rheumatologist and the obstetrician. Where other medical specialists may be involved, a "lead internist" must be designated to coordinate the medical side of management.

Although there are many rheumatic diseases, this chapter will focus on systemic lupus erythematosus (SLE), antiphospholipid syndrome (APS), and rheumatoid arthritis (RA).

28.2 Rheumatoid Arthritis

Rheumatoid arthritis (RA) is a systemic autoimmune disorder of unknown etiology that affects primarily the synovial joints. RA can occur at any age, but the peak onset is between the ages of 30 and 50. It affects 1–2% of the population, with a female to male ratio of 2:1. RA classically presents as symmetric polyarthritis that involves the small- and medium-sized joints and may cause chronic inflammation, erosion of cartilage, and joint deformities. Extra-articular manifestations may include the skin, eye, heart, lungs, renal, nervous, and gastrointestinal systems [1].

Women of childbearing age and RA should undergo appropriate family planning with prepregnancy counseling annually.

28.2.1 Effects of RA on Pregnancy

Pregnancy outcomes are generally similar to that seen in the general population, with no significant increase in maternal or fetal morbidity observed [2].

https://doi.org/10.1515/9783110615258-028

28.2.2 Effects of Pregnancy on RA

Several studies showed a spontaneous improvement in 60–80% of RA during pregnancy [3,4]. The improvement usually starts in the first trimester and lasts through the duration of pregnancy. However, 25% of the pregnant women with RA may have active disease during pregnancy, requiring further therapeutic intervention [2, 3].

There are no clear predictors for RA improvement during pregnancy. Some studies suggest that pregnant women with RA, who lack both rheumatoid factor (RF) and anti-citrullinated peptide antibodies (anti-CCP), are more likely to improve during pregnancy than patients with either or both autoantibodies. However, the duration of disease does not seem to be a predictor of disease activity or remission during pregnancy [4].

Studies have shown that often the majority of women with RA may have a postpartum flare of their disease particularly within the first 3–4 months [5–8]. A recent systematic review of 10 studies, which included 237 patients, reported that RA improved in 60% of patients during pregnancy and flared in 46.7% of cases after delivery [5]. Ostensen et al. reported that 75% of pregnant women with RA went into remission, while 62% developed postpartum exacerbation [8].

28.3 Management of Rheumatoid Arthritis During Pregnancy

Exercise, physiotherapy, and occupational therapy are important tools to maintain function for the pregnant patient with RA. Prepregnancy assessment regarding the status of disease activity and the counseling regarding the importance of being on a treatment regimen that is known to be safe in pregnancy are crucial.

28.3.1 Nonsteroidal Anti-inflammatory Drugs

Nonsteroidal anti-inflammatory drugs (NSAIDs) are commonly used in the treatment of the rheumatic diseases including RA, seronegative arthritis, and systemic lupus erythematosus (SLE). In circumstances where a pregnant woman has active inflammatory disease, the use of nonselective NSAIDs such as naproxen or ibuprofen may be considered. However, the use of these medications should be restricted to the first and second trimesters up to 32 weeks of gestation because of concerns regarding premature closure of the ductus arteriosus, fetal intracranial hemorrhage during labor and delivery, and an observed decrease in amniotic fluid volume [9].

Selective COX-2 inhibitors such as celecoxib should be avoided during pregnancy due to the insufficient data regarding safety of this type of NSAID during pregnancy [10].

Breastfeeding on NSAIDs appears to be safe. The American Academy of Pediatrics (AAP) considers ibuprofen, naproxen, and celecoxib to be compatible with breastfeeding [11].

28.3.2 Glucocorticoids

Glucocorticoids have been widely used in most of the rheumatological diseases. Although dexamethasone, prednisone, and prednisolone all cross the placenta, the rate of the placental passage of prednisone and prednisolone is much lower compared with dexamethasone [12]. In the case of both prednisone and prednisolone, 18% of the maternal dose crosses the placenta, whereas 50% of the maternal dose of dexamethasone will cross the placenta. Glucocorticoid use during pregnancy may increase the risk of premature rupture of the membranes [13] and preterm labor and delivery. Additionally, it may increase the maternal risk of pregnancy-induced hypertension, gestational diabetes, and infection [14, 15].

Some observational studies suggested an association regarding glucocorticoid exposure in the first trimester of pregnancy with the risk of fetal cleft lip and palate formation [16, 17]. However, in a 2011 nationwide cohort study of patients in Denmark, there was no increased orofacial clefts identified among 51,973 infants exposed to glucocorticoids during the first trimester of pregnancy compared with unexposed infants [18].

The AAP, the British Society of Rheumatology (BSR), and the British Health Professionals in Rheumatology (BHPR) consider the use of glucocorticoids to be compatible with nursing. The European League Against Rheumatism (EULAR) agrees with these recommendations. However, women who are receiving more than 50 mg of prednisone daily are advised to delay breastfeeding for 4 h after receiving this dose [10].

28.3.3 Conventional Disease-Modifying Antirheumatic Drugs

Conventional disease-modifying antirheumatic drugs (cDMARDS), including methotrexate, leflunomide, hydroxychloroquine, and sulfasalazine, are frequently used to treat many rheumatic diseases. Not all are considered safe in pregnancy.

28.3.4 Methotrexate

Methotrexate (MTX) is a folate antagonist that has been used to treat a number of rheumatological diseases such as RA, seronegative spondyloarthritis (SPA), and, to a lesser extent, in SLE patients.

MTX is teratogenic and an abortifacient. Ideally, it should be withdrawn 3 months before pregnancy, although EULAR recommends stopping it 1–3 months before conception. The exposure to MTX during pregnancy can cause many congenital anomalies, including cleft palate, hydrocephalus, anencephaly, meningoencephalocele, congenital stenosis of tubular long bones, abnormal facial features, and delayed ossification [10, 19, 20].

Patients should be followed on their new pregnancy-safe medications for 3–6 months prior to conception to ensure good disease control before advising pregnancy.

Although the current evidence suggests that a breastfeeding infant would receive less than 1% of the mother's dose [21], the data regarding fetal safety are limited and, subsequently BSR, BHPR, and EULAR guidelines suggest avoiding MTX in breastfeeding mothers [10, 22]. Furthermore, the American Academy of Pediatrics considers MTX to be incompatible with breastfeeding.

28.3.5 Leflunomide

Leflunomide (LEF) is a pyrimidine synthesis inhibitor that is used in the treatment of RA. LEF should be avoided in women who will be pursuing pregnancy even if delayed for multiple years, as there is a theoretical concern regarding possible fetal teratogenic effect based on animal models. Although the half-life of LEF is approximately 15 days, its major metabolite (teriflunomide) undergoes extensive enterohepatic circulation and stays detectable in the serum for up to two years.

If women on LEF contemplate a pregnancy, a cholestyramine washout procedure (8 g orally three times daily for 11 days) should be considered [10, 22]. The washout can be confirmed by measurement of drug levels less than 0.02 mg/L on two tests performed two weeks apart. Unfortunately, this washout protocol may be clinically ineffective when women are already pregnant. However, there is no definitive data that LEF is actually teratogenic.

No data exits regarding safety of breastfeeding while receiving LEF, therefore the use of LEF among nursing mothers should be discouraged [10, 22].

28.3.6 Sulfasalazine

Sulfasalazine (SSZ) has an anti-inflammatory effect mediated by its 5-aminosalicylic acid moiety and antibacterial characteristics associated with its sulfapyridine moiety. It has been used in the treatment of RA and inflammatory bowel disease.

SSZ appears to be a safe treatment option during pregnancy, as large administrative database linkage studies and meta-analyses showed no increase in fetal loss or congenital malformations associated with the use of SSZ in pregnancy [23].

In general, SSZ should be given concomitantly with folate supplementation of 5 mg daily throughout pregnancy [22], as SSZ inhibits absorption and metabolism of folic acid, which may increase the fetal risk of developing neural tube defects.

28.3.7 Tumor Necrosis Factor Inhibitors (anti-TNF)

Anti-TNF such as adalimumab, etanercept, infliximab, golimumab, and certolizumab have been used in the treatment of many inflammatory joint diseases, including RA and spondyloarthropathies (SPA). Passive placental passage occurs when a drug molecule has a molecular weight of 500 daltons or less. All of the above agents are IgG molecules with molecular weighs ranging from 91 kDa (certolizumab) and about 150 kDa to the other agents noted above. Placental passage is through active transport via the neonatal Fc receptor transport molecule in the placenta. It is maximal in the late second to early third trimesters [24]. Since certolizumab lacks an Fc receptor since it is a pegylated Fab'2 molecule, placental passage is minimal. Based on these facts, the Food and Drug Administration (FDA) in 2018 approved the use of certolizumab throughout pregnancy and during breastfeeding.

28.3.8 Injectable Anti-TNF Agents

Infliximab, etanercept, and adalimumab can be used throughout pregnancy, but some will stop the drugs around 30–32 weeks to minimize placental passage. In the case of infliximab, recommendations have varied from stopping the drug at 16–32 weeks. Regardless, no major side effects have yet to be described using these agents throughout pregnancy [10, 22].

28.3.9 Janus Kinase Pathway Inhibitors

Janus kinase (JAK) pathway inhibitors such as tofacitinib, baricitinib, upadacitinib, and filgotinib are small molecules, around 300 daltons, that inhibit the activity of one or more of the Janus kinase family of enzymes (JAK1, JAK2, JAK3, TYK2), thereby interfering with the JAK-STAT signaling pathway. They can be used in many rheumatological diseases, including RA and psoriatic arthritis (PSA). However, as this class of treatment was created and developed recently, there is very limited data regarding the safety of using it during pregnancy. In addition, considering the small molecular size, placental passage will be passive, likely leading to a higher concentration in the fetal circulation.

The only clear formulated recommendation established so far is for tofacitinib, with EULAR recommending withdrawing tofacitinib at least 2 months prior to conception [10].

28.4 Systemic Lupus Erythematosus

Systemic lupus erythematosus (SLE) is a chronic, multisystem, autoimmune disease that affects predominately females with the highest incidence reported during childbearing years.

SLE can affect many organ systems of the body. Patients with SLE present with variable clinical features ranging from skin and mild joint involvement to life-threatening renal, hematologic, cardiac, or central nervous system disease.

Pregnancy in a woman with SLE can be complicated by SLE disease activity and adverse maternal/fetal outcomes. This is likely attributed to the hormonal shifts required to maintain pregnancy [25]. Disease flares in pregnancy can be challenging to distinguish from physiologic changes observed in pregnancy and having a multidisciplinary team involved in prenatal care may be necessary [26].

28.4.1 Prepregnancy Assessment

A preconception evaluation should be done for every woman with SLE contemplating pregnancy. This assessment should include symptoms at initial diagnosis, current disease activity, timing of last flare of the disease, disease-related organ damage, medications, and serologic evaluation for autoantibodies associated with disease activity and adverse pregnancy outcomes.

28.4.2 Disease Activity

Ideally, women with SLE should conceive when their disease is inactive, as conception within 6 months of having lupus activity is associated with a 4-fold increase in pregnancy loss rate and an increase in risk of flare during pregnancy [25]. Precise definition of active disease varies among different studies. In the PROMISSE study, which is a large prospective observational study, SLE disease activity was measured using Physician's Global Assessment and the Systemic Lupus Erythematosus Pregnancy Disease Activity Index [27].

In routine practice, most rheumatologists may not apply formal instruments. However, having increased disease manifestations, new organ involvement, and adding or adjusting the dose of the immunosuppressive medications are general indicators of SLE flares.

28.4.3 Medication Review

It is crucial to review SLE medications before planning pregnancy, as some may be contraindicated for use in pregnancy requiring a change to pregnancy-safe medications. This change should be followed by clinical and serological observation for 4–6 months to ensure disease stability. This also should be applied in cases of tapering or stopping current medications [22].

28.4.4 Assessment of Autoantibodies

Assessing certain autoantibodies, including antiphospholipid antibodies (APLs) and anti-Ro/SSA and anti-La/SSB antibodies, helps to determine specific pregnancy risks, specific pregnancy monitoring, and whether there is a need to consider additional therapy.

28.5 The Effects of Pregnancy on SLE

28.5.1 SLE Flare

Studies have reported that approximately 25–70% of women with SLE may experience a flare of disease at any point during pregnancy and up to 3 months after delivery [28, 29].

The increased risk of SLE flare can be attributed to many factors, including having active disease during the 6 months prior to conception, a history of lupus nephritis, discontinuation of hydroxychloroquine before or during pregnancy, and being a primigravida [30–32].

In a prospective observational study, an SLE Disease Activity Index (SLEDAI) score of 4 or more at 6 months prior to conception predicted the development of adverse outcomes such as preeclampsia and lupus flares [33].

28.5.2 Renal Disease

Generally, renal blood flow and the glomerular filtration rates increase by more than 50% during pregnancy to accommodate the increased blood volume; this causes a transient decline in the serum creatinine level. However, a permanent reduction in renal function may occur in up to 10% of pregnant women with glomerular filtration rates initially normal or mildly low (serum creatinine less than 132 µmol/L) [34].

Renal involvement is a common manifestation of SLE, as up to 60% of lupus patients may experience focal or diffuse renal involvement at some point during the disease course [35]. Women with SLE and active lupus nephritis should be advised against pregnancy until their disease is in remission for at least 6–12 months to reduce the risk of having maternal and fetal complications. In an observational study of 104 women with SLE having a total of 193 pregnancies, active renal disease was observed in 81 patients and low birth weight was more common in pregnancies with renal disease. The presence of active renal disease during pregnancy was also associated with the risk of developing pregnancy-induced hypertension and lupus flares [30]. A retrospective evaluation of 90 pregnancies among 58 lupus patients showed that women with lupus nephritis in remission had significantly lower rates of preeclampsia, pregnancy loss, and preterm birth compared with women with active lupus nephritis [36].

28.5.3 Preeclampsia

Preeclampsia (PET) is defined as blood pressure over 140/90 or the rise of 30 mmHg systolic or 15 mmHg diastolic in combination with proteinuria (>300 mg/24 h) and edema at greater than 20 weeks of gestation. The risk of developing preeclampsia in lupus pregnancies is higher among patients with underlying renal disease, patients with APLs, diabetes mellitus, or prior history of preeclampsia [37].

It is important to distinguish preeclampsia from a renal lupus flare during pregnancy, as the treatment will differ depending on the diagnosis. In general, both preeclampsia and lupus nephritis may manifest as thrombocytopenia, hypertension, worsening proteinuria, edema, and renal impairment. Lupus nephritis is more likely to be suspected if there is a high anti-ds DNA titer and/or active urinary sediment (hematuria, urinary casts). PET is more likely to be present if there are features suggestive of HELLP syndrome (hemolysis, elevated liver enzymes, low platelets). While up to 25% of pregnant women with active lupus nephritis will have a reduction of C3 and C4 complement levels, 10–15% of patients with PET may demonstrate a rise of these complement components [38].

Although the beneficial role of low-dose aspirin (81–162 mg) in preventing preterm and severe preeclampsia has been documented in non-autoimmune patients, women with SLE at higher risk of PET, including those with lupus nephritis, may also benefit from receiving low-dose aspirin [39–43].

28.5.4 The Effects of SLE on Pregnancy

Pregnancy in the setting of SLE is associated with a higher rate of overall pregnancy complications compared to healthy women. In a recent study which evaluated 13,555 pregnancies in women with SLE, it was observed that those with SLE had a 2- to 4-fold increased rate of obstetric complications including preterm labor, unplanned cesarean delivery, fetal growth restriction, preeclampsia, and eclampsia. This study also demonstrated that maternal mortality was 20-fold higher among pregnant women with SLE [44].

Many predictors of adverse pregnancy outcomes among women with SLE have been identified, including having active disease, a prior history of lupus nephritis, use of antihypertensives, the presence of APLs, thrombocytopenia, and being a primigravida [27, 32, 45].

28.5.5 Neonatal Lupus

Anti-Ro/SSA and anti-La/SSB antibodies are present in 25–30% of women with SLE, particularly those with secondary Sjogren's syndrome. In general, the transplacental passage of anti-Ro (SSA) and/or anti-La (SSB) antibodies has been linked to the risk of developing congenital complete heart block in the fetus and neonatal lupus. However, having these antibodies has not been absolutely associated with unfavorable pregnancy complications or outcomes [46].

Congenital complete heart block (CCHB) can occur in 0.7–2% of neonates which may require a permanent pacemaker [47]. In contrast, the recurrence rate of CCHB in subsequent pregnancies is 16–20% [48].

Women with SLE who have these antibodies should be monitored with fetal echocardiography and ultrasounds weekly or biweekly between 16 and 26 weeks gestation and less frequently afterward [48].

While dexamethasone and IVIG have been used in many studies as treatment for CCHB, the efficacy of these therapeutic interventions has not been established in large cohorts [49]. In addition, there is growing evidence that the administration of hydroxychloroquine during pregnancy may reduce the occurrence of CCHB in a fetus exposed to these maternal antibodies, especially in mothers who already had a child with CCHB [50, 51].

28.5.6 Antiphospholipid Antibodies and Pregnancy

Antiphospholipid syndrome is defined by the presence of (antiphospholipid antibodies (APLs) in association with vascular thrombosis (arterial and/or venous) and/or recurrent pregnancy losses in women. APLs include three types of antibodies: the lupus anticoagulants (LAC), anticardiolipin antibody (aCL) IgG and IgM, and β2 glycoprotein-I (β2GP-I) IgG and IgM [52]. These antibodies can be detected in 35–40% of lupus patients at any point of their disease course [53].

Women with SLE who have APLs are prone to have adverse pregnancy outcomes, including recurrent pregnancy losses (three or more consecutive losses before 10 weeks gestation), fetal death after 10 weeks gestation, or premature birth prior to 34 weeks gestation due to preeclampsia, or placental insufficiency. Many factors can be associated with pregnancy loss in such a group of patients. The PROMISSE study demonstrated that LAC, but not aCL or aβ2GPI, is the main APL antibody that is linked with poor pregnancy outcomes [54]. Other predictors include high-titer aPLs and/or a previous fetal loss [55].

The presence of APLs was also linked to an increased risk of maternal thromboembolism and early onset of preeclampsia during pregnancy. APLs can cause placental vasculopathy leading to placental insufficiency that, in turn, may lead to fetal intrauterine growth restriction and fetal demise [56, 57].

In women with definite obstetric APS, where adverse pregnancy outcomes have occurred in the past, combination treatment with low molecular weight heparin and low-dose aspirin is recommended to decrease the risk of adverse pregnancy outcomes [58].

28.5.7 Advise Against Pregnancy/Early Therapeutic Termination

There are situations where women with SLE are advised against conception and, if pregnant, would be advised to consider termination of the pregnancy. Conditions falling into these special circumstances include severe lupus flare within the previous 6 months [59], pulmonary hypertension, severe heart failure, severe valvopathy [60], severe restrictive lung disease, chronic kidney disease, stroke within the past 6 months, uncontrolled hypertension, a history of previous severe early-onset preeclampsia (<28 weeks), or HELLP syndrome despite receiving aspirin and heparin, or women who are receiving medications that are known to be teratogenic are at high risk for medical and obstetric complications [61, 62]. Appropriate prepregnancy counseling might discourage or delay conception. Once pregnant with active disease, counseling to advise termination might be necessary [60].

28.5.8 Contraception

Many contraceptive methods are available for women with SLE who are advised to avoid pregnancy. The choice of contraception varies depending on the status of SLE activity and the presence or absence of APLs.

Women with inactive SLE or stable SLE and negative APLs can use combined hormonal contraceptive (estrogen and progestin) pills [63]. This was supported by the results of two recent studies, which found no association between the combined oral contraceptive use and the risk of SLE flare [63, 64].

On the other hand, the use of combined contraception in women with SLE and positive APLs should be avoided owing to an increased risk of thromboembolism and cardiovascular risk [48, 65].

Although current data suggest that SLE patients with or without APLs can receive progestin-only contraception as an alternative, as the risk of thromboembolic events with this type of contraception seems to be low [66], a careful interpretation of this data is needed, since different generations of progestins have differing risks of thromboembolism.

A recent meta-analysis of eight observational studies, two of which were in populations at elevated risk for thrombosis, found that the use of progestin-only contraception was not correlated with an increased risk of thromboembolism compared with nonusers [66].

The same conflict regarding the risk of thromboembolism among progestin contraception users is also obvious when we review the international recommendations. The American College of Obstetricians and Gynecologists guidelines for contraceptive use in patients suggested that progestin-only contraceptive may be a safer alternative than estrogen-progestin contraceptives for women with SLE plus APLs and vascular disease [65]. This concern of thromboembolism seems to be correlated with the generation of progestin used. Many studies showed previously that risk of thromboembolic events is the highest among the third-generation progestin users compared to the first- and second-generation users. Emergency contraception can be considered for all SLE patients, including APL-positive patients.

28.6 Specific Medication Use in the Management of SLE During Pregnancy

28.6.1 Antimalarials

Antimalarial drugs such as hydroxychloroquine (HCQ), and chloroquine have been used extensively in the treatment of rheumatologic diseases, due to their immuno-regulatory and anti-inflammatory effects. HCQ is the most widely used antimalarial drug. It is recommended in women with RA and SLE. Additionally, as mentioned previously, receiving HCQ during pregnancy may reduce the risk of CCHB in a fetus exposed to anti-Ro and anti-La maternal antibodies, especially in mothers who already had a child with CCHB [44]. Current data indicate that HCQ can be used safely during pregnancy, with no increased risk of congenital malformations [10, 22, 30, 65]. Pregnant women with SLE should be advised to continue HCQ throughout pregnancy, as many studies showed that the lack of adherence to HCQ during pregnancy correlated with risk of disease flare [30, 67].

Women with SLE can continue HCQ while they are nursing, as approximately only 2% of the maternal dose will be excreted in the breast milk [68]. This is consistent with the AAP recommendation that HCQ is compatible with breastfeeding.

28.6.2 Azathioprine

Azathioprine (AZA) is a purine metabolism antagonist that is used as a steroid-sparing agent in the treatment of the more severe manifestations of certain rheumatologic diseases including SLE. Based on the current evidence, AZA can be continued safely during pregnancy at doses up to 2mg/kg/day, with no increased risk of fetal anomalies [10, 22]. In addition, EULAR, BSR, and BHPR showed that AZA can be continued in breastfeeding, as a minimal amount of this drug will be excreted in breast milk [10, 22, 48].

28.6.3 Mycophenolate Mofetil

Mycophenolate mofetil (MMF) is an inhibitor of purine biosynthesis. It has been used commonly in SLE, systemic sclerosis and vasculitis. Women in childbearing ages should be counseled regarding the possible teratogenic effect of MMF. Women should also be advised to use effective contraception or even two forms of contraception while they are using MMF, especially since MMF can decrease the effectiveness of oral contraceptives. In the case of pregnancy planning, MMF should be discontinued at least six weeks prior to conception [22].

Once MMF is stopped, women should be followed on their new pregnancy-safe medications for 4–6 months prior to conception to ensure good disease control on the new regimen.

MMF use should be avoided while women are breastfeeding, as the data are limited regarding MMF excretion into breast milk [10, 22].

28.6.4 Cyclophosphamide

Cyclophosphamide (CYC) is a cytotoxic, alkylating agent used in the treatment of life-threatening and severe manifestations of SLE and vasculitis. Women of child-bearing age should receive counseling before receiving CYC regarding the risk of irregularity of the menstrual cycle, premature ovarian failure, and infertility [69]. As studies showed that using CYC during pregnancy was associated with the development of congenital anomalies, CYC should be avoided for at least eight weeks before contemplating a pregnancy, and women in childbearing age should use an effective method of contraception while they are receiving CYC [10, 22]. The likelihood of embryotoxicity resulting from CYC use during pregnancy differs according to the stage of pregnancy at which time the medication was given. The risk of teratogenicity from CYC is highest when it is used during the first trimester [14]. EULAR therefore recommends against using CYC in the first trimester. However, the use of this medication can be considered in the second and third trimesters if there is a life-threatening or refractory major organ involvement in certain rheumatic diseases such as SLE or vasculitis [48, 70].

Women on CYC should avoid nursing, as there are limited data regarding the excretion of CYC into breast milk [22].

28.7 Conclusion

Pregnancy is a safe option for most women with a rheumatic disease. Preparing the patient for a pregnancy is readily accomplished through frequent and thorough counseling involving the woman and her partner. A prepregnancy clinical and laboratory assessment is an important step in the preparation for pregnancy. The disease should be under excellent control for ideally 6 months on pregnancy-safe medications. Close follow-up prior to conception will assist in patient compliance and understanding. During pregnancy, the rheumatologist or "lead internist" works closely with the obstetrician in managing the patient medically. Where necessary, other medical specialists may be consulted. In most cases, both maternal and fetal outcomes should occur with minimal or no adverse events.

References

[1]   Young A, Koduri G. Best Pract Res Clin Rheumatol 2007;21(5):907–927.

[2]   Tandon VR, Sharma S, Mahajan A, Khajuria V, Kumar A. Pregnancy and rheumatoid arthritis. Indian J Med Sci 2006;60(8):334–344.

[3]   De Man YA, Dolhain RJ, Van De Geijn FE, Willemsen SP, Hazes JM. Disease activity of rheumatoid arthritis during pregnancy: Results from a nationwide prospective study. Arthritis Rheum 2008;59(9):1241–1248.

[4]   De Man YA, Bakker-Jonges LE, Goorbergh CM et al. Women with rheumatoid arthritis negative for anti-cyclic citrullinated peptide and rheumatoid factor are more likely to improve during pregnancy, whereas in autoantibody-positive women autoantibody levels are not influenced by pregnancy. Ann Rheum Dis 2010;69(2):420–423. Epub 2009 Mar 11.

[5]   Jethwa H, Lam S, Smith C, Giles I. Does rheumatoid arthritis really improve during pregnancy? a systematic review and metaanalysis. J Rheumatol 2019;46(3):245–250.

[6]   Nelson JL, Ostensen M. Pregnancy and rheumatoid arthritis. Rheum Dis Clin North Am 1997;23(1):195–212.

[7]   Persellin RH. The effect of pregnancy on rheumatoid arthritis. Bull Rheum Dis 1976–1977;27(9):922.

[8]   Ostensen M, Aune B, Husby G. Effect of pregnancy and hormonal changes on the activity of rheumatoid arthritis. Scand J Rheumatol 1983;12:69–72.

[9]   Campbell S, Clohessy A, O'Brien C, Higgins S, Higgins M, McAuliffe F. Fetal anhydramnios following maternal non-steroidal anti-inflammatory drug use in pregnancy. Obstet Med 2017;10(2):93–95.

[10] Götestam Skorpen C, Hoeltzenbein M, Tincani A et al. The EULAR points to consider for use of antirheumatic drugs before pregnancy, and during pregnancy and lactation. Ann Rheum Dis 2016;75(5):795–810.

[11] Sachs HC and COMMITTEE ON DRUGS. American academy of pediatrics, the transfer of drugs and therapeutics into human breast milk: an update on selected topics. Pediatrics 2013;132 (3):e796–e809.

[12] Beitins IZ, Bayard F, Ances IG, Kowarski A, Migeon CJ. The transplacental passage of prednisone and prednisolone in pregnancy near term. J Pediatr 1972;81(5):936.

[13] Guller S, Kong L, Wozniak R, Lockwood CJ. Reduction of extracellular matrix protein expression in human amnion epithelial cells by glucocorticoids: A potential role in preterm rupture of the fetal membranes. J Clin Endocrinol Metab 1995;80(7):2244.

[14] Østensen M, Khamashta M, Lockshin M et al. Anti-inflammatory and immunosuppressive drugs and reproduction. Arthritis Res Ther 2006;8(3):209. Epub 2006 May 11.

[15] Laskin CA, Bombardier C, Hannah ME et al. Prednisone and Aspirin in Women with Autoantibodies and Unexplained Recurrent Fetal Loss. N Engl J Med 1997;337:148–154.

[16] Park-Wyllie L, Mazzotta P, Pastuszak A et al. Birth defects after maternal exposure to corticosteroids: Prospective cohort study and meta-analysis of epidemiological studies. Teratology 2000;62(6):385.

[17] Carmichael SL, Shaw GM. Maternal corticosteroid use and risk of selected congenital anomalies. Am J Med Genet 1999;86(3):242–244.

[18] Hviid A, Mølgaard-Nielsen D. Corticosteroid use during pregnancy and risk of orofacial clefts. CMAJ 2011;183(7):796–804. Epub 2011 Apr 11.

[19] Buckley LM, Bullaboy CA, Leichtman L, Marquez M. Multiple congenital anomalies associated with weekly low-dose methotrexate treatment of the mother. Arthritis Rheum 1997;40(5):971.

[20] Milunsky A, Graef JW, Gaynor MF Jr. Methotrexate-induced congenital malformations. J Pediatr 1968;72(6):790.

[21] Thorne JC, Nadarajah T, Moretti M, Ito S. Methotrexate use in a breastfeeding patient with rheumatoid arthritis. J Rheumatol 2014;41(11):2332.

[22] Flint J, Panchal S, Hurrell A et al. BSR and BHPR guideline on prescribing drugs in pregnancy and breastfeeding – Part I: Standard and biologic disease modifying anti-rheumatic drugs and corticosteroids. Rheumatology 2016;55:1693–1697.

[23] Viktil K, Engeland A, Furu K. Outcomes after anti-rheumatic drug use before and during pregnancy: A cohort study among 150 000 pregnant women and expectant fathers. Scand J Rheumatol 2012;41:196e201.

[24] Griffiths SK, Campbell JP. Placental structure, function and drug transfer. Continuing Educ Anaesth Crit Care Pain 2015;15(Issue 2):84–89.

[25] Clowse ME. Lupus activity in pregnancy. Rheum Dis Clin N Am 2007;33(2):237–252.

[26] Lateef A, Petri M. Managing lupus patients during pregnancy. Best Pract Res Clin Rheumatol 2013;27:3.

[27] Buyon JP, Kim MY, Guerra MM et al. Predictors of pregnancy outcomes in patients with lupus: a cohort study. Ann Intern Med 2015;163(3):153.

[28] Smyth A, Oliveira GH, Lahr BD, Bailey KR, Norby SM, Garovic VD. A systematic review and meta-analysis of pregnancy outcomes in patients with systemic lupus erythematosus and lupus nephritis. Clin J Am Soc Nephrol 2010;5(11):2060–2068. Epub 2010 Aug 5.

[29] Tedeschi SK, Massarotti E, Guan H et al. Specific systemic lupus erythematosus disease manifestations in the six months prior to conception are associated with similar disease manifestations during pregnancy. Lupus 2015;24:1283e92.

[30] Clowse ME, Magder L, Witter F, Petri M. Hydroxychloroquine in lupus pregnancy. Arthritis Rheum 2006;54(11):3640.

[31] Gladman DD, Tandon A, Ibañez D, Urowitz MB. The effect of lupus nephritis on pregnancy outcome and fetal and maternal complications. J Rheumatol 2010;37(4):754–758. Epub 2010 Mar 15.

[32] Saavedra MA, Sánchez A, Morales S, Navarro-Zarza JE, Ángeles U, Jara LJ. Primigravida is associated with flare in women with systemic lupus erythematosus. Lupus 2015;24(2):180. Epub 2014 Sep 24.

[33] Kwok LW, Tam LS, Zhu T et al. Predictors of maternal and fetal outcomes in pregnancies of patients with systemic lupus erythematosus. Lupus 2011;20:829–836.

[34] Jungers P, Houillier P, Forget D, Henry-Amar M. Specific controversies concerning the natural history of renal disease in pregnancy. Am J Kidney Dis 1991;17:116.

[35] Houssiau FA. Management of lupus nephritis: An update. J Am Soc Nephrol 2004;15: 2694–2704. (Cameron JS: Lupus nephritis. J Am Soc Nephrol 10: 413–424, 1999).

[36] Wagner SJ, Craici I, Reed D et al. Maternal and foetal outcomes in pregnant patients with active lupus nephritis. Lupus 2009;18(4):342.

[37] Ruiz-Irastorza G, Khamashta MA. Lupus and pregnancy: Ten questions and some answers. Lupus 2008;17:416.

[38] Buyon JP, Cronstein BN, Morris M, Tanner M, Weissmann G. Serum complement values (C3 and C4) to differentiate between systemic lupus activity and pre-eclampsia. Am J Med 1986;81:194–200.

[39] Porter F, Gyamfi-Bannerman C, Manuck T. ACOG committee opinion: low-dose aspirin use during pregnancy. Obstet Gynecol 2018;132(1):e 44–52.

[40] Schramm AM, Clowse ME. Aspirin for prevention of preeclampsia in lupus pregnancy. Autoimmune Dis 2014;2014:920467.

[41] LeFevre ML. U.S. preventive services task force. low-dose aspirin use for the prevention of morbidity and mortality from preeclampsia: U.S. preventive services task force recommendation statement. Ann Intern Med 2014;161(11):819.

[42] Rolnik DL, Wright D, Poon LC et al. Aspirin versus placebo in pregnancies at high risk for preterm preeclampsia. N Engl J Med 2017;377(7):613Epub 2017 Jun 28.

[43] MacDonell KL, Moutquin JM, Sebbag I. Society of obstetricians and gynaecologists of Canada. SOGC clinical practice guideline. Diagnosis, evaluation, and management of the hypertensive disorders of pregnancy. J Obstet Gynaecol Can 2014;36(5):416–438.

[44] Clowse ME, Jamison M, Myers E, James AH. A national study of the complications of lupus in pregnancy. Am J Obstet Gynecol 2008;199(2):127. e1–6. Epub 2008 May 5.

[45] Borella E, Lojacono A, Gatto M et al. Predictors of maternal and fetal complications in SLE patients: A prospective study. Immunol Res 2014;60(2–3):170–176.

[46] Mecacci F, Pieralli A, Bianchi B, Paidas MJ. The impact of autoimmune disorders and adverse pregnancy outcome. Semin Perinatol 2007;31:223–226.

[47] Brucato A, Frassi M, Franceschini F et al. Congenital heart block risk to newborns of mothers with anti-Ro/SSA antibodies detected by counter immunoelectrophoresis. A prospective study of 100 women. Arthritis Rheum 2001;44:1832–5.

[48] Andreoli L, Bertsias GK, Agmon-Levin N et al. Eular recommendations for women's health and the management of family planning, assisted reproduction, pregnancy and menopause in patients with systemic lupus erythematosus and/or antiphospholipid syndrome. Ann Rheum Dis 2017;76:476–485.

[49] Friedman DM, Llanos C, Izmirly PM et al. Evaluation of fetuses in a study of intravenous immunoglobulin as preventive therapy for congenital heart block: Results of a multicenter, prospective, open-label clinical trial. Arthritis Rheum 2010;62(4):1138–1146.

[50] Tunks RD, Clowse ME, Miller SG et al. Maternal autoantibody levels in congenital heart block and potential prophylaxis with anti inflammatory agents. Am J Obstet Gynecol 2013;208(64): e1–7.

[51] Izmirly P, Kim M, Costedoat-Chalumeau N, et al. The Prospective Open Label Preventive Approach to Congenital Heart Block with Hydroxychloroquine (PATCH) Study Demonstrates a Reduction in the Recurrence Rate of Advanced Block. ACR/ARP Abstract 2019.

[52] Khamashta MA. Management of thrombosis and pregnancy loss in antiphospholipid syndrome. Lupus 1998;7:S162–S16.

[53] Kutteh WH. Antiphospholipid antibodies and reproduction. J Reprod Immunol 1997;35:1.

[54] Yelnik CM, Laskin CA, Porter TF et al. Lupus anticoagulant is the main predictor of adverse pregnancy outcomes in aPL-positive patients: Validation of PROMISSE study results. Lupus Sci Med 2016;3(1):e000131.

[55] Lockshin MD. Pregnancy loss and antiphospholipid antibodies. Lupus 1998;7:S86–S8.

[56] Magid MS, Kaplan S, Sammaritano LR et al. Placental pathology in SLE: A prospective study. Am J Obstet Gynecol 1998;79:226–23.

[57] Levy RA, Avaad E, Oliviera J et al. Placental pathology in antiphospholipid syndrome. Lupus 1998;7:S81–S8.

[58] Mak A, Cheung MW, Cheak AA et al. Combination of heparin and aspirin is superior to aspirin alone in enhancing live births in patients with recurrent pregnancy loss and positive anti-phospholipid antibodies: A meta-analysis of randomized controlled trials and meta-regression. Rheumatology (Oxford) 2010;49:281–288.

[59] Hoeper MM, Bogaard HJ, Condliffe R et al. Definitions and diagnosis of pulmonary hypertension. J Am Coll Cardiol 2013;62:D42e50.

[60] Regitz-Zagrosek V, Roos-Hesselink JW, Bauersachs J et al. ESC guidelines for the management of cardiovascular diseases during pregnancy: the task force for the management of cardiovascular diseases during pregnancy of the European Society of Cardiology (ESC). Eur Heart J 2018 September 07;39(34):3165–3241.

[61] Ruiz-Irastorza G, Khamashta M. Lupus and pregnancy: integrating clues from the bench and bedside. Eur J Clin Invest 2011;41(6):672–678.

[62] Ateka-Barrutia O, Nelson-Piercy C. Management of rheumatologic diseases in pregnancy. Int J Clin Rheumtol 2012;7(5):541–558.

[63] Sánchez-Guerrero J, Uribe AG, Jiménez-Santana L et al. A trial of contraceptive methods in women with systemic lupus erythematosus. N Engl J Med 2005;353:2539–2549.

[64] Petri M, Kim MY, Kalunian KC et al. Combined oral contraceptives in women with systemic lupus erythematosus. N Engl J Med 2005;353:2550–2558.

[65] ACOG. Practice Bulletin No. 206: use of hormonal contraception in women with coexisting medical conditions. Obstet Gynecol 2019;133(2):e128.

[66] Mantha S, Karp R, Raghavan V, Terrin N, Bauer KA, Zwicker JI. Assessing the risk of venous thromboembolic events in women taking progestin-only contraception: a meta-analysis. BMJ 2012;345:e4944. Epub 2012 Aug 7.

[67] Ioannidis JP, Katsifis GE, Tzioufas AG et al. Predictors of sustained amenorrhea from pulsed intravenous cyclophosphamide in premenopausal women with systemic lupus erythematosus. J Rheumatol 2002;29:2129–2135.

[68] Parke A, West B. Hydroxychloroquine in pregnant patients with systemic lupus erythematosus. J Rheumatol. 1996;23(10):1715.

[69] Luisiri P, Lance NJ, Curran JJ. Wegener's granulomatosis in pregnancy. Arthritis Rheum 1997;40:1354–1360.

[70] Canadian rheumatology association. Canadian oroquine. J Rheumatol 2000;27(12):2919.

Tadeu A. Fantaneanu, Esther Bui

29 Epilepsy and Pregnancy

29.1 Introduction

Worldwide, approximately 15 million women with epilepsy (WWE) are of childbearing age [1]. In the event of pregnancy, these women face several concerns, including the impact of a pregnancy on their seizures, as well as the impact of seizures and antiepileptic drugs (AEDs) on their developing fetus. Reassuringly 65–80% of women with epilepsy will either have no change in their baseline seizure frequency or have an improvement in their seizures. Only a minority of women will experience worsening of their seizures [2, 3]. Despite these reassuring statistics one of the biggest challenges in the management of WWE is AEDs, as AEDs should be continued throughout pregnancy. This is distinct from other common neurological diseases such as migraine, peripheral neuropathy and multiple sclerosis where women may have a choice to lower or discontinue their medications.

In this chapter we will explore issues in the management of WWE in the context of pregnancy. This is a three-tiered model of care, divided into key phases: preconception care, intra-partum care, and postpartum care.

29.2 Preconception

Preconception counselling is one of the most important aspects of care for WWE. It improves the rate of periconceptional folate use as well as decreases the risk AED exposure and seizures in pregnancy [4, 5]. This counselling should begin in adolescence and continue regularly as part of routine epilepsy care. Despite the established risks of fetal malformations and AEDs, 50–65% of all pregnancies are unplanned among WWE [6, 7]. This is not significantly different from that of the general population. Given these risks, preconception counselling and planned pregnancy are a cornerstone of care for WWE.

29.2.1 Contraception

Emphasis should be on the importance of a planned pregnancy, and the use of effective contraception until a woman is ready for pregnancy, from both a personal and a medical perspective. Currently many options are available, including oral contraceptive pills (OCP), topical patches, intramuscular (IM) depot injections, implants, and intrauterine devices. Unfortunately, many commonly used AEDs interact

https://doi.org/10.1515/9783110615258-029

with these hormonal contraceptives by inducing cytochrome P450 enzymes or uridine-diphosphate-glucuronosyltransferase (UGT) enzymes. This results in inducing the metabolism (and hence clearance) of estrogen and progesterone. By doing so, women are at risk for contraceptive failure. Contraceptive failure is estimated to be 3–6% among WWE, a three- to six-fold increase compared to the general population [8]. This is especially relevant for newer OCPs with the lowest estrogen and progesterone doses available on the market. For WWE, the intrauterine device (IUD) (either copper- or hormone-based) is the recommended contraceptive method due to the minimal drug–drug interactions with AEDs [9]. This is attributed to the local contraceptive effects of the IUD as compared to the more systemic hormonal effects of other hormonal contraceptives. Less data is known about IM medroxyprogesterone with a dose every 3 months reported to have a failure rate similar to the IUD. However, issues around decrease bone mineral density and a more delayed return to full fertility make this drug less attractive [10]. If neither an IUD nor IM medroxyprogesterone is used, then barrier methods combined with hormonal contraception are recommended [8].

OCPS can also interact with AEDs, specifically lamotrigine and to a lesser extent valproate (see Table 29.1). This occurs through the induction of UGT enzymes by the estrogen component of hormonal contraceptives; a common metabolic pathway shared by these drugs. Oxcarbazepine levels can also be lowered, but the mechanism with this drug is unclear. As such, OCPs can decrease drug levels, resulting in an increased risk for recurrent seizures [11].

Table 29.1: The interaction between antiepileptic drugs and oral contraceptive pills.

Enzyme-inducing AEDs that can lower oral contraceptive levels	AEDs that can be lowered by OCPs
Phenytoin	Lamotrigine
Carbamazepine	Valproic acid
Oxcarbazepine	Oxcarbazepine (mechanism unclear)
Eslicarbazepine	
Phenobarbital	
Topiramate (>200 mg/day)	
Primidone	
Felbamate	
Rufinamide	
Perampanel	
Clobazam	

29.2.2 Preconception Risk Stratification

Prior to conceiving, two important questions need to be answered: (1) are anticonvulsants still needed and (2) can the drug regimen be further simplified, or the drug dose(s) safely lowered? Many people who have been seizure free for >2 years may have a reasonable chance of remaining seizure free off AEDs in the right context. Factors that predict seizure recurrence after drug withdrawal include longer duration of epilepsy, shorter seizure free interval, adult onset of seizures, and epileptiform abnormalities on EEG [12]. A detailed reassessment as well as updated drug levels and a neurological consultation for individualized risk stratification are the first steps in preconception care. An online prediction tool is available to aid clinicians: http://epilepsypredictiontools.info/index [12].

The priority in the management of WWE is to have seizure control throughout pregnancy. Seizures, especially generalized convulsive seizures, have been associated with hypoxia, deceleration of fetal heart rate, acidosis, blunt trauma, preterm delivery, and low birth weight [8, 13, 14]. Recent studies have identified a ten times increased risk of maternal mortality attributed to epilepsy, including sudden unexpected death in epilepsy (SUDEP) [15, 16]. One of the most important predictors of seizure control in pregnancy is pre-pregnancy seizure frequency, especially in the 9–12 months prior to conception [2, 17]. Other predictors of seizures in pregnancy include a diagnosis of focal epilepsy, polytherapy, and decreased serum levels of AEDs [18]. Interestingly, women with catamenial epilepsy (i.e., related to menses) may experience an improvement in seizures during pregnancy [19]. This is postulated in part due to the stabilization in pregnancy of monthly hormonal fluctuations.

Seizure control is balanced by maintaining AEDs at the lowest possible therapeutic level to reduce fetal drug exposure. In choosing specific AEDs, broad-spectrum AEDs are preferred for both generalized and focal epilepsies. These include lamotrigine, levetiracetam, topiramate, valproic acid, and benzodiazepines. In contrast, narrow-spectrum drugs, which target specific channels such as sodium channels, are preferred for focal onset seizures. These drugs include carbamazepine, oxcarbazepine, eslicarbazepine, phenytoin, gabapentin, pregabalin, and lacosamide. Interestingly these narrow-spectrum drugs have the potential to worsen generalized onset seizures such as absence or myoclonic seizures [20].

Of all the available AEDs, valproate has the highest risk of major congenital malformations (MCM), estimated to be 6–10% based on pregnancy registry data [1]. Reported malformations with valproate include neural tube defects, cleft palate, and cardiac and urogenital malformations. Other AEDs have associated increased risks of MCMs, including phenytoin (2.9–6.4%), Carbamazepine (2.9–5.5%), topiramate (3.6%), phenobarbital (5.5%), and oxcarbazepine. Across multiple pregnancy registries lamotrigine (1.9–3.2%) and levetiracetam (0.7–2.4%) have been associated with the lowest risk of MCMs [1, 21]. This is summarized in Figure 29.1. Furthermore, there is evidence that the risk of MCMs increases with the dose of medication [45] (Figure 29.2). The specific MCMs associated with individual AEDs are outlined in Figure 29.3.

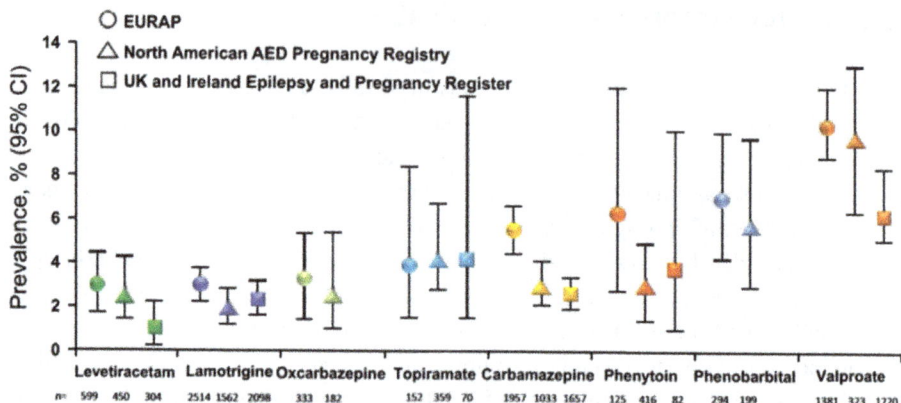

Figure 29.1: Risk of major congenital malformations associated with antiepileptic drugs (Tomson et al. Teratogenicity of antiepileptic drugs. April 2019;32(2) (Wolters Kluwer)).

Other important factors contributing to increasing the risk of major congenital malformation include drug dose (Figure 29.2) as well as polytherapy, particularly if polytherapy includes valproate or topiramate within the combination [1].

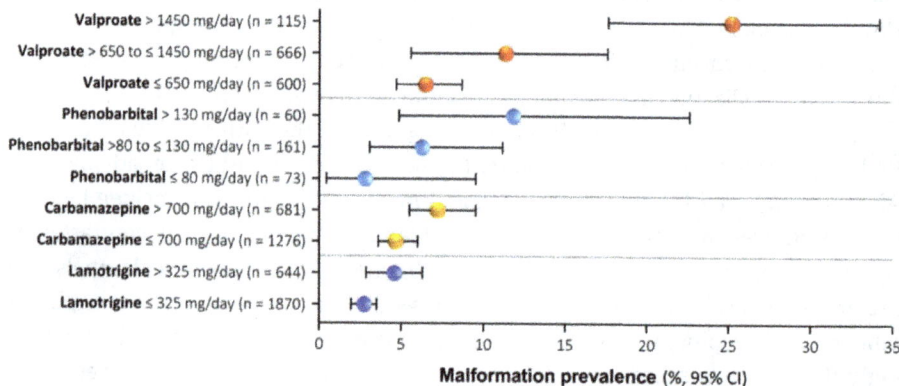

Figure 29.2: Dose dependency of major congenital malformations with anti-epileptic drugs (Tomson et al. Teratogenicity of antiepileptic drugs. April 2019;32(2) (Wolters Kluwer)).

In addition to MCMs there are cognitive and behavioral adverse effects associated with in utero AED exposure, specifically with valproate, especially at doses $\geq$ 1,000 mg/day [21]. Intelligence quotient (IQ) of these children were found to be 6–9 points lower compared to children exposed to lamotrigine, carbamazepine, or phenytoin particularly in verbal performance. Autism rates have also been found to be five times higher with valproate compared to the general population [22].

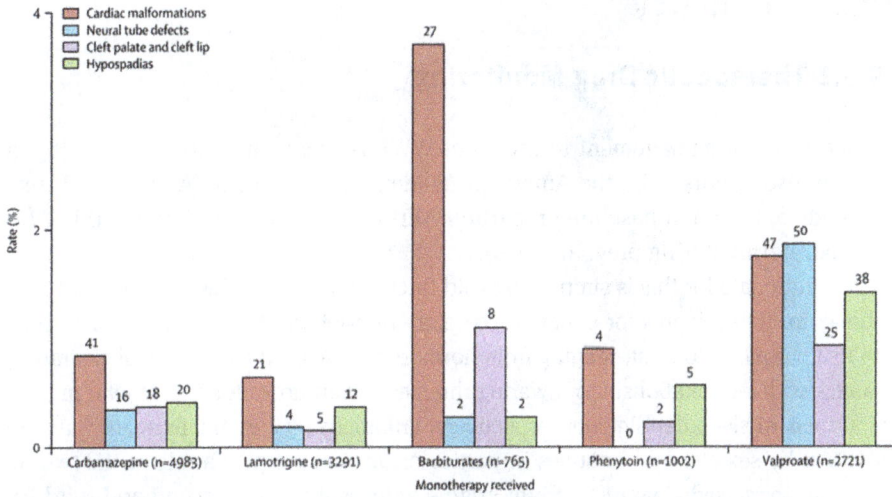

Figure 29.3: Types of major congenital malformations associated with anti-epileptic drugs (Tomson T, Battino D. Teratogenic effects of antiepileptic drugs. Lancet Neurol. 2012 Sep 1;11(9):803–13).

29.2.3 Folate Supplementation

All WWE of childbearing age should take folate supplementation at least 3 months prior to conception. The current recommended dose in the general population is 0.4 mg/day. However, some AEDs, including valproate, carbamazepine, oxcarbazepine, phenytoin, phenobarbital and primidone, alter folic acid metabolism, resulting in decreased folic acid levels [23, 24]. Folate supplementation was associated with higher IQ in a North American cohort study, and lower risk of autistic traits in a Norwegian population-based study [25, 26]. Concerns, however, have also been raised with folate over supplementation, including risk of cleft palate and cognitive and behavioral impairment [21, 27]. Thus, current consensus recommends the use of 1 to 4-5 mg folate with higher doses preferred for women taking AEDs with the highest risk of major congenital malformations including (1) high dose valproate, (2) polytherapy with valproate or topiramate or (3) women with a prior pregnancy, personal history or family history of major congenital malformation. Maternal age alone is not an indication for high dose folate [1, 28].

29.3 Pregnancy

29.3.1 Therapeutic Drug Monitoring

The mainstay of management in pregnant WWE is therapeutic drug monitoring, a practice also endorsed by the American Academy of Neurology (AAN), which recommends obtaining a baseline prepartum AED level and performing monthly AED level monitoring during pregnancy [29].

The rationale for this is simple: to avoid fluctuations in AED levels that could lead to breakthrough seizures for patients. There are physiologic and psychosocial reasons for this fluctuation to exist, ranging from hormonal changes, increased renal clearance, and altered liver metabolism to lowering the medication doses for fear of fetal malformation risk or sleep deprivation, respectively. Enhanced glucuronidation, attributed to induction by sex steroid hormones in particular, appears to play a role in the two- to three-fold increased clearance of lamotrigine with peaks in the second and third trimesters but beginning as early as the first gestational week [30]. Similar declines are observed for levetiracetam more significantly in the first trimesters and for oxcarbazepine (up to 40%) and topiramate by the second trimester [31]. Carbamazepine levels, on the other hand, seem to remain stable during pregnancy [32].

Overall, multiple studies have identified that AED concentrations falling below 65% of the preconception baseline levels result in seizure worsening [33]; this is particularly true of lamotrigine and levetiracetam, two of the most commonly prescribed AEDs for WWE. Commonly, these two drugs may need to be titrated up to two to three times their prepartum dose based on intrapartum seizure control and serum drug levels.

29.3.2 Vitamin K Administration

Historically, vitamin K supplementation was recommended in the third trimester for WWE taking enzyme-inducing (EI) AED (i.e. carbamazepine, phenytoin, phenobarbital, primidone) as they were thought to be at higher risk for vitamin K deficiency and associated bleeding. But recent evidence casts doubt on this. A study involving 662 WWE on enzyme-inducing AEDs failed to show any difference in newborn bleeding complications when both control groups and newborns of WWE received vitamin K administration at birth, in comparison to third trimester supplementation [34]. Another retrospective study involving 109 WWE did not show an increased risk of postpartum hemorrhage, including in women on enzyme-inducing AEDs, when compared to controls who did not have epilepsy [35]. The AAN 2009 practice guideline concludes that there is insufficient evidence for third trimester supplementation [29]. At present time, the data would not seem to support third trimester oral supplementation in WWE, though newborn administration of vitamin K remains a recommended practice in the USA and Canada.

29.3.3 Seizures and Emergencies in Pregnancy

On rare occasions, first time seizures can occur during pregnancy. Third trimester seizures should prompt an emergent evaluation in the hospital with particular attention to the possibility of eclampsia. If eclampsia is ruled out, a routine workup for a first episode seizure should be performed and include neuroimaging (particularly vascular imaging), electroencephalography, a toxicology screen, electrolytes and serum chemistries, liver function tests, and, if clinically indicated, a screen for infectious etiologies. Risk factors for seizure recurrence in a first episode seizure include an abnormal EEG, abnormal neuroimaging, a seizure out of sleep, or a prior history of a brain insult [36].

Status epilepticus (SE) refers to a state of uninterrupted seizure activity operationally defined as lasting more than 5 min. It may be subdivided into convulsive and non-convulsive forms, the former carrying the greatest morbidity and mortality, while the latter may be managed less aggressively in close collaboration with a neurologist. Convulsive status epilepticus (CSE) remains a rare entity in pregnancy, and few reports in the literature exist to give the reader a complete overview of its clinical course. The management remains somewhat controversial as teratogenic medications should preferentially be avoided in the first trimester, though they may be administered with few concerns in the third trimester. No published protocol during pregnancy exists, though the algorithm outlined by the American Epilepsy Society for CSE provides a reasonable approach with first-line agents benzodiazepines being subsequently complemented by second-line intravenous AED (i.e., phenytoin, levetiracetam, lacosamide) and third-line anesthetic agents (i.e., propofol, midazolam)[37]. Given the risks to the developing fetus and mother, and depending on stage of pregnancy, emergency delivery via C-section may be also required.

29.3.4 Labor and Delivery

During pregnancy, patients are encouraged to reflect on a delivery plan. Despite the lack of strong evidence, a number of steps are frequently suggested to ensure a safe and positive outcome for both mother and baby.

Ideally the birth would occur in a hospital setting to help ensure a rapid response time to possible adverse events such as generalized tonic-clonic seizures. An epidural should be considered especially in the event of a prolonged labor to address prolonged sleep deprivation and physiological stress, which can lower seizure threshold. IV lorazepam should be present at the bedside and quickly available if needed. For relaxation techniques such as use of a soaker tub, we recommend that patients are supervised.

While in hospital the patient should bring their own medication supply to avoid changes between their usual anti-seizure drug formulations and hospital formulations which could bring about fluctuations in AED levels that could risk trigger a seizure.

We recommend a minimum of 6–8 h of sleep per 24 h cycle which usually entails introducing a bottle early to allow at least one bottle feeding of pumped breastmilk (or formula) which can be administered by a family member to help ensure a less-interrupted sleeping cycle. The 3 days following delivery are usually the highest risk for seizure breakthroughs and helping mitigate this with adequate sleep is paramount [28].

29.4 Postpartum

Given the almost immediate return to pharmacokinetic baseline once the baby is delivered, early consideration to a postpartum AED tapering regimen should be given to avoid toxicity. This especially applies to glucuronidated AEDs where the taper should begin on postpartum day 3 (i.e., lamotrigine). Previously, an empiric postpartum tapering regimen was highlighted recommending sequential dose reductions of lamotrigine on days 3, 7, and 10 with a return to preconception baseline dose with an added 50–100 mg to mitigate the effects of sleep deprivation [28]. Renally excreted drugs such as levetiracetam, oxcarbazepine, eslicarbazepine, lacosamide, gabapentin, and pregabalin may also require a dose reduction in the first week postpartum, aiming for a prepartum dose with an additional 10–25% dose. For other AEDs, titration back closer to the prepartum dose should be done over a 6- to 10-week period with ongoing close monitoring for seizure recurrence and symptoms of drug toxicity [38].

29.4.1 Breastfeeding

The Canadian Pediatrics Society and the American Academy of Pediatrics recommend breastfeeding as the sole form of nutrition for the first 6 months of life [39]. Breastfeeding is associated with many advantages for the infant, including decreased risk of asthma, acute otitis media, childhood leukemias as well as beneficial cognitive effects to name but a few [40, 41]. Even though the amount of AED exposure for the child through breastmilk is uncertain for most compounds, physicians are often uncomfortable recommending breastfeeding to WWE on AEDs. Adequate studies assessing antiepileptic drug exposure to newborns were lacking, though recent data suggest that AED concentrations in infant serum samples of breastfed babies are lower than their maternal concentrations [42]. In general, the amounts of AEDs transmitted to breastmilk are lower than those transmitted via placental passage in utero. A number of studies have also shown that neurocognitive outcomes of children who were breastfed by WWE exposed to AEDs were no worse than non-breastfed children at 3 years and actually better by 6 years [25, 43, 44]. Overall, the data would suggest that WWE can safely choose to breastfeed and should be supported in this decision by their treating team. We do recommend, however, that for WWE on potentially sedating AEDs such as benzodiazepines or barbiturates, the baby be closely monitored for withdrawal symptoms and sedation.

29.4.2 Safety in the Postpartum period

In the initial and mid-term postpartum months continuing with proper sleep hygiene and maximizing undisturbed sleep are paramount. As previously suggested one option to ensure uninterrupted 4 hour stretches of sleep for the mom would be to bottle an aliquot of pumped breastmilk (or formula) and have a partner or relative administer one or more nighttime feeds. Other general safety precautions for patients with epilepsy remain in effect at this time, including avoiding taking baths, changing the baby on the floor, or bathing the baby while supervised. Co-sleeping is also discouraged to prevent injury to the baby [10].

Particular attention should be paid to mood changes in the postpartum period, especially for mothers who are on mood-negative AEDs such as levetiracetam, perampanel, or, to a lesser extent, topiramate and brivaracetam, as the risks of postpartum blues and depression remain a concern. WWE should have adequate social and familial supports in place to help them cope with the potentially daunting changes experienced in the first few months of motherhood.

29.5 Conclusion

The management of WWE in pregnancy is very rewarding as most women do well. Individualized care for WWE is targeted at three important stages: preconception, intrapartum, and postpartum care. Each of these stages has their unique challenges. Health professionals need to co-navigate the important decisions made during the preconception stage as well as close and careful management of AEDs to minimize the risks to mother and fetus. Postpartum care is focused primarily on maternal and infant safety.

References

[1]   Tomson T, Battino D, Bromley R et al. Management of epilepsy in pregnancy: a report from the international league against epilepsy task force on women and pregnancy. Epileptic Disord 2019;21(6):497–517.

[2]   Thomas SV, Syam U, Devi JS. Predictors of seizures during pregnancy in women with epilepsy. Epilepsia 2012;53(5):e85–8.

[3]   Battino D, Tomson T, Bonizzoni E et al. Seizure control and treatment changes in pregnancy: observations from the EURAP epilepsy pregnancy registry. Epilepsia 2013;54(9): 1621–1627.

[4]   Baishya J, Jose M, A S R, Sarma PS, Thomas SV. Do women with epilepsy benefit from epilepsy specific pre-conception care?. Epilepsy Res 2020;160:106260. doi: 10.1016/j. eplepsyres.2019.106260. Epub 2019 Dec 23.

[5]   Abe K, Hamada H, Yamada T, Obata-Yasuoka M, Minakami H, Yoshikawa H. Impact of planning of pregnancy in women with epilepsy on seizure control during pregnancy and on maternal and neonatal outcomes. Seizure 2014;23(2):112–116.

[6]   Herzog AG, Mandle HB, Cahill KE, Fowler KM, Hauser WA. Predictors of unintended pregnancy in women with epilepsy. Neurology 2017;88(8):728–733.

[7]   Johnson EL, Burke AE, Wang A, Pennell PB. Unintended pregnancy, prenatal care, newborn outcomes, and breastfeeding in women with epilepsy. Neurology 2018;91(11):e1031–e1039. doi: 10.1212/WNL.0000000000006173. Epub 2018 Aug 10.

[8]   Sazgar M. Treatment of Women With Epilepsy. Continuum (Minneap Minn) 2019;25(2): 408–430. doi: 10.1212/CON.0000000000000713.

[9]   Reimers A1. 2016 Apr 19;7:69–76. doi: 10.2147/OAJC.S85541. eCollection 2016. Contraception for women with epilepsy: counselling, choices, and concerns.

[10]   Bui E, Klein A, editors. Women with Epilepsy: a Practical Management HandbookPublished July 31st 2014 by, Cambridge University Press.

[11]   Herzog AG, Blum AS, Farina EL et al. Valproate and lamotrigine level variation with menstrual cycle phase and oral contraceptive use. Neurology 2009;72(10): 911–914.

[12]   Lamberink HJ, Otte WM, Geerts AT et al. Individualised prediction model of seizure recurrence and long-term outcomes after withdrawal of antiepileptic drugs in seizure-free patients: a systematic review and individual participant data meta-analysis. Lancet Neurol 2017;16(7): 523.

[13]   Hiilesmaa V, Teramo K. Fetal and maternal risks with seizures. In: Harden C, Thomas SV, Tomson T, Hoboken NJ, editors. Epilepsy in Women, Wiley-Blackwell, 2013;115–127.

[14]   Chen YH, Chiou HY, Lin HC, Lin HL. Affect of seizures during gestation on pregnancy outcomes in women with epilepsy. Arch Neurol 2009;66(8):979–984.

[15]   Edey S, Moran N, Nashef L. SUDEP and epilepsy-related mortality in pregnancy. Epilepsia 2014;55(7):e72–4.

[16]   MacDonald SC, Bateman BT, McElrath TF, Hernández-Díaz S. Mortality and Morbidity During Delivery Hospitalization Among Pregnant Women With Epilepsy in the United States. JAMA Neurol 2015;72(9):981–988.

[17]   Vajda FJ, Hitchcock A, Graham J, O'brien T, Lander C, Eadie M. Seizure control in antiepileptic drug-treated pregnancy. Epilepsia 2008;49(1):172–176.

[18]   Reisinger TL, Newman M, Loring DW, Pennell PB, Meador KJ. Antiepileptic drug clearance and seizure frequency during pregnancy in women with epilepsy. Epilepsy Behav 2013;29(1):13–18.

[19]   Cagnetti C, Lattanzi S, Foschi N, Provinciali L, Silvestrini M. Seizure course during pregnancy in catamenial epilepsy. Neurology 2014;83(4):339–344.

[20]   Glauser T, Ben-Menachem E, Bourgeois B et al. ILAE Subcommission on AED Guidelines. Updated ILAE evidence review of antiepileptic drug efficacy and effectiveness as initial

monotherapy for epileptic seizures and syndromes. Epilepsia 2013;54(3): 551–563. Epub 2013 Jan 25.

[21] Murray LK, Smith MJ, Jadavji NM. Maternal oversupplementation with folic acid and its impact on neurodevelopment of offspring. Nutr Rev 2018;76(9):708–721. ilepsy Behav 2013; 29(1): 13–8.

[22] Christensen J, Grønborg TK, Sørensen MJ et al. Prenatal valproate exposure and risk of autism spectrum disorders and childhood autism. JAMA 2013;309(16):1696–1703. doi: 10.1001/jama.2013.2270.

[23] Wegner C, Nau H. Alteration of embryonic folate metabolism by valproic acid during organogenesis: implications for mechanism of teratogenesis. Neurology 1992;42((4 Suppl 5)):17.

[24] Dansky LV, Rosenblatt DS, Andermann E. Mechanisms of teratogenesis: folic acid and antiepileptic therapy. Neurology 1992;42(4 suppl 5):32–42.

[25] Meador KJ, Baker GA, Browning N et al. Fetal antiepileptic drug exposure and cognitive outcomes at age 6 years (NEAD study): a prospective observational study. Lancet Neurol 2013;12:244–252.

[26] Bjørk M, Riedel B, Spigset O et al. Association of Folic Acid Supplementation During Pregnancy With the Risk of Autistic Traits in Children Exposed to Antiepileptic Drugs In Utero. JAMA Neurol 2018;75(2):160.

[27] Rozendaal AM, Van Essen AJ, Te Meerman GJ et al. Periconceptional folic acid associated with an increased risk of oral clefts relative to non-folate related malformations in the Northern Netherlands: a population based case-control study. Eur J Epidemiol 2013;28(11):875–887.

[28] Pennell PB, McElrath T, Uptodate Topic: management of epilepsy during preconception, pregnancy and postpartum period.

[29] Harden CL, Pennell PB, Koppel BS et al. Practice parameter update: management issues for women with epilepsy – Focus on pregnancy (an evidence-based review): Vitamin K, folic acid, blood levels, and breastfeeding: report of the quality standards subcommittee and therapeutics and technology assessment subcommittee of the American Academy of Neurology and American Epilepsy Society. Neurology 2009;73(2):142–149.

[30] Polepally AR, Pennell PB, Brundage RC, Stowe ZN, Newport DJ, Viguera AC et al. Model-based lamotrigine clearance changes during pregnancy: clinical implication. Ann Clin Transl Neurol 2014;1(2):99–106.

[31] Voinescu PE, Pennell PB. Delivery of a Personalized Treatment Approach to Women with Epilepsy. Semin Neurol 2017;37(6):611–623.

[32] Johnson EL, Stowe ZN, Ritchie JC et al. Carbamazepine clearance and seizure stability during pregnancy. Epilepsy Behav 2014;33:49–53.

[33] Pennell PB, Peng L, Newport DJ et al. Lamotrigine in pregnancy: clearance, therapeutic drug monitoring, and seizure frequency. Neurology 2008;70(22 Pt 2):2130–2136.

[34] Kaaja E, Kaaja R, Matila R, Hiilesmaa V. Enzyme-inducing antiepileptic drugs in pregnancy and the risk of bleeding in the neonate. Neurology 2002;58(4):549–553.

[35] Sveberg L, Vik K, Henriksen T, Taubøll E. Women with epilepsy and post partum bleeding – Is there a role for vitamin K supplementation?. Seizure 2015;28:85–87.

[36] Krumholz A, Wiebe S, Gronseth GS et al. Evidence-based Guideline: management of an Unprovoked First Seizure in Adults. Vol. 84, Neurology, Lippincott Williams and Wilkins; 2015, 1705–1713.

[37] Glauser T, Shinnar S, Gloss D et al. Evidence-based guideline: treatment of convulsive status epilepticus in children and adults: report of the guideline committee of the American Epilepsy Society. Epilepsy Curr 2016;16(1):48–61.

[38] Vélez-Ruiz N, Pennell PB. Issues for women with epilepsy neurol clin. Neurol Clin 2016;34(2): 411–ix.

[39] Critch JN. Nutrition for healthy term infants, birth to six months: an overview. Paediatr Child Heal 2013;18(4):206–207.

[40] Ip S, Chung M, Raman G, Trikalinos TA, Lau J. A summary of the agency for healthcare research and quality's evidence report on breastfeeding in developed countries. Vol. 4, Breastfeeding Medicine. Breastfeed Med 2009.

[41] Binns C, Lee M, Low WY. The Long-Term Public Health Benefits of Breastfeeding. Asia-Pacific J Public Heal 2016;28(1):7–14.

[42] Birnbaum AK, Meador KJ, Karanam A et al. Antiepileptic Drug Exposure in Infants of Breastfeeding Mothers with Epilepsy. JAMA Neurol 2019;55414:1–10.

[43] Meador KJ, Baker GA, Browning N et al. Cognitive function at 3 years of age after fetal exposure to antiepileptic drugs. N Engl J Med 2009;360(16):1597–1605.

[44] Veiby G, Engelsen BA, Gilhus NE. Early child development and exposure to antiepileptic drugs prenatally and through breastfeeding: a prospective cohort study on children of women with epilepsy. JAMA Neurol 2013;70(11):1367–1374.

[45] Tomson T, Battino D, Bonizzoni E et al. EURAP study group. Dose-dependent risk of malformations with antiepileptic drugs: an analysis of data from the EURAP epilepsy and pregnancy registry. Lancet Neurol 2011;10(7):609.

Arieh Ingber

30 Specific Dermatoses of Pregnancy

30.1 Introduction

In this chapter we will provide an up-to-date review of dermatologic diseases which are specific to pregnancy. The nomenclature of these diseases has changed several times, which can make things challenging for the clinician [1, 2]. This chapter aims to use terms that are considered more accurate.

30.2 Polymorphic Eruption of Pregnancy (PEP)

30.2.1 Epidemiology

This is also commonly known as Pruritic Urticarial Papules and Plaques of Pregnancy (PUPPP). This is the most common dermatosis specific to pregnancy, occurring in about 1 in every 160–200 pregnancies. It is more common among Caucasians, and in 80% of the cases it presents in primigravid women. It was previously reported to occur more often in multiple gestation pregnancies and in overweight women; however, this may not be the case. It usually occurs in the third trimester of pregnancy, from week 35 and onward. One study [3] suggested a male-to-female infant ratio of 2:1. It rarely recurs in subsequent pregnancies, unless they are multiple gestations, and then it is generally less severe than the first episode [4–7].

30.2.2 Pathogenesis

The pathogenesis of PEP is not clear. Conventional theory is that the distension of the abdominal skin during pregnancy causes an alteration of the epidermal skin, and generation of a new antigen. PEP is a reaction to this antigen. This theory is supported by studies revealing that PEP is more common in multiple gestation, or in overweight/obese women [8].

In a study fetal DNA was found in the skin of mothers with PEP, suggesting that chimerism may be the basic pathogenesis of this dermatosis [9].

Recently it was postulated that mast cells (MCs) have a role in the pathogenesis of PEP. During pregnancy, there are many endocrine as well as immunological changes as an adaptation to the developing fetus. MCs are known for their susceptibility to hormones. While physiological numbers of MCs were shown to positively influence pregnancy outcome, at least in mouse models, uncontrolled augmentations in quantity

https://doi.org/10.1515/9783110615258-030

and/or activation can lead to pregnancy complications. It is tempting to speculate that MCs are involved in the onset of PEP, although no studies are existing showing a direct link between MCs and this disease. There are several lines of evidence that clearly suggest a role for MCs. First, as in urticaria, antihistamines are the first-line option in the treatment of PEP and are effective in most patients. Second, even though PEP and urticaria are different diseases, there are several similarities in terms of the clinical symptoms, including pruritic erythema and urticarial lesions. Third, autologous whole blood injections have been reported as an effective treatment option in PEP [10, 11].

30.2.3 Clinical Presentation

The rash usually appears in the third trimester. In 90% of the cases, the disease starts in the abdomen, buttocks, and thighs, and then spreads to the upper limbs and trunk, sparing the face, neck, and hands and feet. Significantly it appears in the abdominal skin and inside and around the striae distensae. As a rule, an important clue to the diagnosis of this disease is the sparing of the navel. In the vast majority of cases the rash is urticarial and edematous and is very itchy. Rarely, the rash may have associated blisters and target-like lesions [4, 12, 13], and purpura is not typically seen [14].

30.2.4 Laboratory Tests

Laboratory tests are normal except eosinophilia in some cases. Direct and indirect immunofluorescence tests are negative [4].

30.2.5 Histopathology

Skin biopsy is rarely necessary. The histology of PEP is not specific. Two patterns have been described: superficial (early) and deep (late). In the early superficial pattern, the findings are epidermal: edema of the papillary dermis, focal parakeratosis, exocytosis of eosinophils, hyperkeratosis, and perivascular lymphohistiocytic infiltration. In the late deeper pattern, the infiltrate is interstitial scattered with eosinophils. The papillary dermis is edematous occasionally with blister formation [15].

30.2.6 Treatment

In mild cases, antihistamines and weak-to-moderate potent steroid creams are recommended. Both are considered safe in pregnancy.

In severe refractory cases, a short course of oral prednisone at a dose of 0.5 mg/kg/day is needed [16] at least until delivery, with a rapid taper. In some cases, this treatment is necessary even after delivery.

Several investigational approaches include phototherapy by narrowband UVB, reported to be effective in some cases [14]; autologous whole blood (AWB) injection was reported to be effective in three cases of PEP unresponsive to therapy [11]; and omalizumab. The latter should theoretically work in cases with urticarial predominance, but information regarding its safety in pregnancy is still under evaluation. Our recommendation would be to proceed with systemic steroids in cases refractory to antihistamines and topical steroids.

30.2.7 Prognosis

The prognosis of PEP is usually excellent. No fetal or maternal complications have been reported. In the most of cases PEP dramatically improves within hours after delivery. In some cases, the disease can last longer, even several weeks postpartum. The disease usually does not recur in subsequent pregnancies [4, 17].

30.3 Pemphigoid Gestationis (PG)

For many years, the disease was known as herpes gestationis, likely due to the herpetiform appearance of the eruption. However, this led to the misunderstanding of it being an infectious rash. The new term of "pemphigoid gestationis" more accurately captures the underlying pathogenesis of this being an autoimmune and vesicular/bullous lesion.

30.3.1 Epidemiology

PG is a rare disease and the least common of the specific dermatoses of pregnancy. The incidence varies in different parts of the world and is estimated at 1:7,000–50,000 births. The disease is more common in Caucasians [18, 19]. There is a higher frequency of HLA-DR3 and HLA-DR4 in patients with the disease. All these facts suggest a genetic background of the disease [20].

30.3.2 Pathogenesis

PG is an autoimmune, usually blistering, disease. Most patients develop antibodies against two hemidesmosome proteins, BP180 (BPAG2, collagen XVII), and less frequently BP230. These circulating antibodies belong to immunoglobulin G1 subclass (occasionally and/or to G3). Immunoglobulin G1 is binding to the extracellular NC16A domain of BP 180 and/or BP 230 antigen at the basal layer inducing the formation of PG lesions. These antibodies have a very strong complement activation ability, and at the end of the road inducing C3 deposition at basement membrane zone along the upper part of lamina lucida [21].

Recently it was demonstrated that there is a strong association between MHC class II molecules and PG, indicating a pivotal role of MHC class II in the pathogenesis of the disease.MHC class II molecules are aberrantly expressed on amniochorion stromal cells and on the trophoblast. Consequently, BP 180, which is expressed in the amniotic epithelium of the placenta and the umbilical cord, is presented to maternal MHC class II in the presence of paternal MHC class II and is recognized as a foreign antigen, resulting in the formation of IgG autoantibodies, predominantly of the IgG_1 and IgG_3 subclasses, directed to BP 180 [22].

For years, PG was considered as a bullous pemphigoid variant of pregnancy. A recent study suggested different pathogenesis between PG and bullous pemphigoid [23].

30.3.3 Clinical Presentation

PG usually begins in the second trimester of pregnancy at week 21 of gestation. The eruption presents as periumbilical erythematous urticarial lesions that later spread to limbs, abdomen, and chest and develop into tense vesicles or blisters. Pruritus is severe in most cases. Palms and soles involvement may occur. Rarely the rash may appear on face and neck. At the early stage of the disease, differentiating it from PEP may be difficult. Involvement of the umbilicus is an important clue to diagnosis of PG. The lesions are arranged in a grouped pattern (resembling dermatitis herpetiformis) around the umbilicus. Occasionally, striae distensae are involved. Rarely vesicles and blisters do not develop, and mucosal lesions are very rare. In most of cases, an exacerbation of the diseases can be seen close to delivery and immediately after [24, 25].

30.3.4 Laboratory Tests

Most hematologic studies are within normal limits. Eosinophilia is not uncommon and may correlate with disease severity. Laboratory values that may be elevated include immunoglobulin levels, erythrocyte sedimentation rates, acute phase reactant levels, and antithyroid antibodies [26].

30.3.5 Histopathology and Immunofluorescence

Skin biopsy is very beneficial for the immunofluorescence. Histopathology will reveal sub-epidermal blister formation with eosinophilic infiltrate. Perivascular inflammatory reaction at the dermo-epidermal junction is present. Edema in the dermis is often prominent [27]. In most patients, direct immunofluorescence (DIF) exhibits a linear band of C3 deposition with or without immunoglobulin G (present in 20–25% of patients) along the basement membrane. Indirect immunofluorescence may detect circulating antibodies for basement membrane zone (HG factor) [21]. Recognition of the bullous pemphigoid antigen (BP 180) by ELISA was reported and was used to determine the severity of the disease [28]. HLA-DR3/DR4 is present in half of patients with PG, as compared with 3% of the general population [20].

30.3.6 Treatment

Most patients suffer from widespread vesicles and severe pruritus. Usually, systemic treatment with prednisone 0.5 mg/kg/day is mandatory. This treatment may be limited by the gestational age of pregnancy. In early pregnancy, steroid exposure is associated with an increased risk of cleft lip/palate. As always, physicians must consider the risks and benefits for the mother and fetus. Second-line agents include dapsone, cyclosporine, and intravenous immunoglobulin [29–31]. Recently, azathioprine combined with intravenous immunoglobulin was found to be effective in a 37-year-old pregnant woman who failed on prednisone treatment [32].

30.3.7 Prognosis

There is often a postpartum flare, and so disease control in the peripartum period is important. Ultimately, the disease regresses a few weeks or months after delivery. Some studies revealed higher rates of premature deliveries and small for gestational age babies. As a result, they may benefit from follow-up in high-risk pregnancy units [33, 34]. In 5–10% of infants born to mothers with PG, a transient rash is seen postpartum, which resolves after a few weeks [34], due to the transplacental transfer of antibodies. The existence of a second autoimmune disease in PG patients, Hashimoto thyroiditis, Graves' disease, and others has been reported [35], and women should be evaluated for underlying autoimmunity.

30.4 Impetigo Herpetiformis, also Known as Generalized Pustular Psoriasis of Pregnancy

30.4.1 Nomenclature

This rare disease of pregnancy is in a long debate if it is a disease sui generis or a variant of generalized pustular psoriasis of Von Zumbusch. The term "impetigo her-petiformis" originated due to the pustules which are the main features of this illness; however, the term "impetigo" would suggest a bacterial contagious disease, and this disease is not bacterial and not contagious. On the other hand, the name "generalized pustular psoriasis of pregnancy" would indicate that this disease is pustular psoriasis. It is still controversial if the disease is specific to pregnancy or general pustular psoriasis exacerbated by pregnancy [36, 37]. As long as the debate continues, it makes sense to keep the historical name.

30.4.2 Epidemiology

This is a very rare disease, with less than 200 cases were reported in the literature [38]. Surprisingly, it has reported in nonpregnant women and even in men. It is clear that in these patients the disease is classical pustular psoriasis of Von Zumbusch, while in pregnant women it may be a different illness specific to pregnancy [39].

30.4.3 Pathogenesis

The cause of this disease is unknown. Since hypocalcemia and hypoparathyroidism were reported in some patients, some authors have related this illness to hypopara-thyroidism. The increased consumption of calcium at the last trimester of the pregnancy causes hypocalcemia in patients with latent hypoparathyroidism. It has been shown that hypocalcemia may induce general pustular psoriasis [39–41].

Recently, new data were published on the pathogenesis of impetigo herpetiformis following a study on different genetic profiles of psoriasis vulgaris and general pustular psoriasis. The majority of general pustular psoriasis that is not accompanied by psoriasis vulgaris is caused by homozygous or compound heterozygous mutations of *IL36RN*, which encodes IL-36 receptor antagonist (IL-36RN, a part of the IL-36 signaling system that is thought to be present in epithelial barriers and to take part in local inflammatory response). Only a small number of cases with general pustular psoriasis preceding or accompanied by psoriasis vulgaris were found to have *IL36RN* mutations. These findings further support the idea that general pustular psoriasis with psoriasis vulgaris differs genetically from general pustular psoriasis alone. Till now there have been no reports of impetigo herpetiformis with *IL36RN* mutations. A recent publication reported on two cases of impetigo herpetiformis with homozygous and heterozygous *IL36RN* mutations. These findings support the view that impetigo herpetiformis is not related to psoriasis vulgaris but may be related to general pustular psoriasis [42, 43].

30.4.4 Clinical Presentation

Impetigo herpetiformis is a dramatic disease, occasionally with systemic symptoms. It may present in any stage of pregnancy, but usually appears in the last trimester of pregnancy. Most patients do not have a personal or familial history of psoriasis and do not subsequently develop chronic plaque psoriasis. We have seen a case of impetigo herpetiformis in a young pregnant patient, with no history of psoriasis, who years later developed widespread plaque psoriasis [37].

The onset is acute, occasionally with a prodrome of high fever, chills, and malaise. The rash is present on lower abdomen, navel, inframammary folds, armpits, and the neck. The primary lesions are red papules and patches and numerous pin-size sterile pustules. Slight scales often present on the patches. The lesions are arranged in a peculiar pattern: rings and serpentine distribution. Sometimes the pustules create a "lakes" of pus [44].

30.4.5 Laboratory Investigations

Leukocytosis, neutrophilia, and relative lymphopenia are the common findings in the acute stage. Hypocalcemia and hyperphosphatemia due to hypoparathyroidism are relatively common. In some cases hypoalbuminemia, high levels of urea, and high uric acid were reported. Immunofluorescence tests, direct and indirect, are negative [39, 40].

30.4.6 Histopathology

Sub-corneal neutrophilic pustules and neutrophilic influx into the upper epidermis (forming Kogoj micro-abscesses) are the common findings along with parakeratosis. There is also chronic perivascular infiltrate in the upper dermis [45].

30.4.7 Treatment

Impetigo herpetiformis is a severe illness. Careful treatment and follow-up are required. Electrolytes, particularly calcium and albumin levels, must be followed. Systemic prednisone 0.5–1.0 mg/kg/day is the treatment of choice. Antibiotic treatment usually is necessary to prevent secondary infection. Cyclosporine, narrowband UVB, and methotrexate (at late pregnancy) were reported as potential therapies [46–48]. Recently a case which was complicated by intrauterine growth restriction was successfully treated with granulocyte and monocyte apheresis [49].

30.4.8 Prognosis

Before the era of steroids and antibiotics, the prognosis of this disease was very poor with high maternal mortality. Nowadays the maternal prognosis is good, but the fetal prognosis may be occasionally still poor. Stillbirths may happen. The fetal prognosis is in correlation to the disease severity. Proper control of the maternal illness is mandatory. Cesarean section should be done if possible, in case of disease exacerbation [38, 39, 50].

30.5 Prurigo of Pregnancy (Besnier)

This disease was introduced in 1904 by Ernest Besnier, a French dermatologist [51]. Many authors consider it as a variant of atopic dermatitis of pregnancy and it's often cataloged in the basket of atopic eruption of pregnancy [25].

30.5.1 Epidemiology

The reported incidence is 1:300–400 pregnancies [52], although it may in fact occur more frequently. It's more common among Caucasians. The disease typically develops beyond the 20th week of pregnancy but may appear at any gestational age [52, 53]. The cause of prurigo of pregnancy (Besnier) and the severe pruritus is not known.

30.5.2 Clinical Presentation

The rash appears predominantly on the extensor parts of the limbs and dorsal aspects of the hand and feet. Rarely the papules can also occur on the abdomen and trunk. Prurigo defined as papules with erosions on the top. Occasionally, nodules can be seen resembling prurigo nodularis, but they are much smaller and in lighter color than prurigo nodularis. The skin around the papules is normal. The lesions do not merge and do not form plaques. Typically they are arranged in longitudinal pattern. The lesions are extremely itchy, resulting in excoriated lesions, sometimes associated with secondary infection [19, 53, 54].

30.5.3 Laboratory Investigations

The laboratory tests are within the normal limits. Direct and indirect immunofluorescence tests are negative.

30.5.4 Histopathology

Chronic superficial perivascular inflammatory cell infiltrate with eosinophils, histiocytes, and neutrophils [14].

30.5.5 Treatment

Moderate-to-potent steroid creams and antihistamines are the common treatment. In my experience, the best treatment is phototherapy by narrowband UVB [53].

30.5.6 Prognosis

The prognosis is excellent with no effect on the pregnancy and the newborn. The disease resolves after delivery and usually does not return in subsequent pregnancies [14, 55].

30.6 Pruritic Folliculitis of Pregnancy

This is another unique disease of pregnancy and occurs much more frequently than appreciated by clinicians. It is commonly misdiagnosed as atopic dermatitis, acne, bacterial folliculitis, or PEP [54, 55].

30.6.1 Epidemiology

In the UK, it was estimated to happen in 1 of 3,000 pregnancies [56].

30.6.2 Pathogenesis

It is commonly thought that the cause of the disease is hormonal changes in pregnancy [57]. The exact mechanism of the disease is unknown. In one study, high levels of serum androgens were detected, but this finding was not confirmed by others [58, 59]. Some authors noted similarities between this disease and PEP. Indeed, folliculitis may be seen in some cases of PEP, but it is easy to differentiate between these two diseases which in many ways are not alike.

30.6.3 Clinical Presentation

The disease begins in the second to the third trimesters of pregnancy in healthy women with no personal or familial background of atopic dermatitis. The disease is usually widespread, mainly on the back and abdomen. Occasionally, it appears also on the limbs. The primary lesions are follicular red papules and sterile pustules. The rash is monomorphic resembling papulo-pustular acne or steroid acne [53, 60]. Contrary to the disease name the disease is usually not pruritic [55, 61].

30.6.4 Laboratory Tests and Histopathology

The laboratory tests are within the normal limits. The pathological findings are usually not specific. Perifollicular neutrophilic infiltrate is common [62]. Direct and indirect immunofluorescence tests are negative [12].

30.6.5 Treatment

Steroid creams and antihistamines are not effective and usually not needed. Anti-acne topical medication was reported to have some benefit [53, 60].

30.6.6 Prognosis

The prognosis is excellent with no effect on the pregnancy and the newborn. The disease resolves usually in 1 month after delivery and does not recur in subsequent pregnancies [55, 63]. In one study of 14 patients small for date babies were born [59].

30.7 Linear IgM Dermatosis of Pregnancy

A very rare dermatosis was reported in two pregnant women in Israel. Both of them were reported from the Department of Dermatology, Rabin Medical Center, Campus Beilinson – one case by us [64] and the other case by another group [65]. Although this is a rare disease, I decided to introduce it. It is likely the disease is more common, but overlooked.

30.7.1 Pathogenesis

Some authors considered the diseases as a variant of prurigo of pregnancy or PEP [14], but it is more resembling pruritic folliculitis of pregnancy. The presence of IgM at the basal membrane zone may suggest an autoimmune background. In one of the patients the disease appeared one week after beginning of nifedipine treatment for premature contractions. Three days after cessation of the drug much improvement was noticed. The patient decided to take again nifedipine and the rash exacerbated quickly. They concluded that this disease may be drug related [65]. IgM was detected in the serum of healthy persons by indirect immunofluorescence technique. It was also reported in association with many dermatological conditions like urticaria, Grover's disease, and vasculitis [66, 67]. IgM deposits at the basement membrane zone by direct immunofluorescence test are rare in other dermatological conditions, indicating the uniqueness of these patients.

30.7.2 Clinical Presentation

In both cases, the disease appeared late in pregnancy: one at 30 weeks gestation, and the other at 37 weeks. The primary lesions were red follicular papules and sterile pustules on the abdomen and limbs. The rash was intensely pruritic.

30.7.3 Laboratory Tests

Laboratory tests were within the normal limits. Direct immunofluorescence test revealed linear IgM deposits at the basement membrane zone in both patients. Indirect immunofluorescence was negative in both cases. In one patient after the resolution of the rash the direct immunofluorescence test turned negative.

30.7.4 Histopathology

In biopsies, folliculitis was observed.

30.7.5 Treatment

Treatment was reassurance and local comfort measures. The disease did not respond to topical nonsteroidal creams and oral antihistamines.

30.7.6 Prognosis

The prognosis was excellent; the rash resolved in a few weeks. The disease had no effect on mother and newborn.

References

[1]   Danesh M, Pomeranz MK, McMeniman E, Murase JE. Dermatoses of pregnancy: nomenclature, misnomers, and myths. Clin Dermatol 2016;34:314–319.
[2]   Holmes RC, Black MM. The specific dermatoses of pregnancy: a reappraisal with special emphasis on a proposed simplified clinical classification. Clin Expt Dermatol 1982;7:65–73.
[3]   Vaughan Jones SA, Hern S, Nelson-Piercy C, Seed PT, Black MM. A prospective study of 200 women with dermatoses of pregnancy correlating clinical findings with hormonal and immunopathological profiles. Br J Dermatol 1999;141:71–81.
[4]   Lawley TJ, Hertz KC, Wade TR, Ackerman AB, Katz SI. Pruritic urticarial papules and plaques of pregnancy. JAMA 1979;241:1969–9.
[5]   Dehdashti AL, Wikas SM. Pruritic urticarial papules and plaques of pregnancy occurring postpartum. Cutis 2015;95:344–347.
[6]   Ghazeeri G, Kibbi AG, Abbas O. Pruritic urticarial papules and plaques of pregnancy: epidemiological, clinical, and histopathological study of 18 cases from Lebanon. Int J Dermatol 2012;51:1047–1053.
[7]   Thurston A, Grau RH. An update on the dermatoses of pregnancy. J Okla State Med Assoc 2008;101:7–11.
[8]   Rudolph CM, Al-Fares S, Vaughan-Jones SA, Müllegger RR, Kerl H, Black MM. Polymorphic eruption of pregnancy: clinicopathology and potential trigger factors in 181 patients. Br J Dermatol 2006;154:54–60.
[9]   Aractingi S, Berkane N, Bertheau P, et al. Fetal DNA in skin of polymorphic eruptions of pregnancy. Lancet 1998;352:1898–1901.
[10]   Woidacki K, Zenclussen AC, Siebenhaar F . Mast cell-mediated and associated disorders in pregnancy: a risky game with an uncertain outcome?. Front Immunol 2014;19(5):231.
[11]   Jeon IK, On HR, Oh SH, Hann SK. Three cases of pruritic urticarial papules and plaques of pregnancy (PEP) treated with intramuscular injection of autologous whole blood. J Eur Acad Dermatol Venereol 2015;29:797–800.

[12] Brandão P, Sousa-Faria B, Marinho C, Vieira-Enes P, Melo A, Mota L. Polymorphic eruption of pregnancy: review of literature. See comment in PubMed Commons below J Obstet Gynaecol 2017;37:137–140.

[13] Taylor D, Pappo E, Aronson IK. Polymorphic eruption of pregnancy. See comment in PubMed Commons below Clin Dermatol 2016;34:383–391.

[14] Kraumpouzos G, Cohen LM. Dermatoses of pregnancy. J Am Acad Dermatol 2003;45:1–19.

[15] Callen JP, Hanno R. Pruritic urticarial papules and plaques of pregnanacy. a clinicopathologic study. J Am Acad Dermatol 1981;5:401–405.

[16] Shornik JK. Dermatoses of pregnancy. Sem Cutan Med Surg 1988;17:172–181.

[17] Schmidt E, Zillikens D. Pemphigoid diseases. Lancet 2013;381:320–332.

[18] Kroumpouzos G, Zillikens D. Pemphigoid gestationis. In: Kroumpouzos G, eds. Text Atlas of Obstetric Dermatology. Philadelphia, PA: Lippincott Williams & Wilkins; 2013, 180–193.

[19] Shornick JK, Stastny P, Gilliam JN. High frequency of histocompatibility antigens HLA-DR3 and DR4 in herpes gestations. J Clin Invest 1981;68:553–555.

[20] Chimanovitch I, Schmidt E, Messer G, et al. IGG1 and IGG3 are the major immunoglobulin subclasses targeting epitopes within the NC16 A domain of BP180 in pemphigoid gestationis. J Invest Dermatol 1999;113:140–142.

[21] Sadik CD, Lima AL, Zillikens D. Pemphigoid gestationis: toward a better understanding of the etiopathogenesis. Clin Dermatol 2016;34(3):378–382.

[22] Tani N, Kimura Y, Koga H, et al. Clinical and immunological profiles of 25 patients with pemphigoid gestationis. Br J Dermatol 2015;172:120–129.

[23] Jenkins RE, Hern S, Black MM. Clinical features and management of 87 patients with pemphigoid gestationis. Clin Exp Dermatol 1999;24:255–259.

[24] Ambros-Rudolph CM, Mullegger RR, Vaughan-Jones SA, et al. The specific dermatoses of pregnancy revisited and reclassified: results of a retrospective two-center study on 505 pregnant patients. J Am Acad Dermatol 2006;54:395–404.

[25] Lawley TJ, Stingl G, Katz SI. Fetal and maternal risk factors in herpes gestationis. Arch Dermatol 1978;114:552–555.

[26] Hertz KC, Katz SI, Maize J, et al. Herpes gestationis: A clinicopathologic study. Arch Dermatol 1976;112:1543–1548.

[27] Barnadas MA, Rubiales MV, Gonzalez MJ, et al. Enzyme-linked immunosorbent assay (ELISA) and indirect immunofluorescence testing in a bullous pemphigoid and pemphigoid gestationis. Int J Dermatol 2008;47:1245–1249.

[28] Rodrigues Cdos S, Filipe P, Solana Mdel M, et al. Persistent herpes gestationis treated with high-dose intravenous immunoglobulin. Acta Derm Venereol 2007;87:184–186.

[29] Kreuter A, Harati A, Breuckmann F, et al. Intravenous immune globulin in the treatment of persistent pemphigoid gestationis. J Am Acad Dermatol 2004;51:1027–1028.

[30] Hern S, Harman K, Bhogal BS, et al. A severe persistent case of pemphigoid gestationis treated with intravenous immunoglobulins and cyclosporin. Clin Exp Dermatol 1998;23: 185–188.

[31] Gan DC, Welsh B, Webster M. Successful treatment of a severe persistent case of pemphigoid gestationis with antepartum and postpartum intravenous immunoglobulin followed by azathioprine. Australas J Dermatol 2012;53:66–69.

[32] Shornick JK, Black MM. Fetal risks in herpes gestationis. J Am Acad Dermatol 1992;26:63–68.

[33] Al-Mutairi N, Sharma AK, Zaki A, et al. Maternal and neonatal pemphigoid gestationis. Clin Exp Dermatol 2004;29:202–204.

[34] Shornick JK, Black MM. Secondary autoimmune diseases in herpes gestationis (pemphigoid gestationis). J Am Acad Dermatol 1992;26:563–566.

[35] Chang SE, Kim HH, Choi JH, Sung KJ, Moon KC, Koh JK. Impetigo herpetiformis followed by generalized pustular psoriasis: more evidence of same disease entity. Int J Dermatol 2003;42 (9):754–755.

[36] Lotem M, Katzenelson V, Rotem A, Hod M, Sandbank M. Impetigo herpetiformis: a variant of pustular psoriasis or a separate entity?. J Am Acad Dermatol 1989;20:338–341.

[37] Winton GB, Lewis CW. Dermatoses of pregnanacy. J Am Acad Dermatol 1982;6:977–998.

[38] Hellreich P. The skin changes of pregnancy. Cutis 1974;13:82–86.

[39] Sasseville D, Wilkinson RD, Schnader JY. Dermatoses of pregnancy. Int J Dermatol 1981;20: 223–241.

[40] Baker H, Ryan TJ. Generalized pustular psoriasis. a clinical and epidemiological study of 104 cases. Br J Dermatol 1968;80:771–793.

[41] Sugiura K, Nakasuka A, Kono H, Kono M, Akiyama M. Impetigo herpetiformis with IL36RN mutations in a Chinese patient: a founder haplotype of c.115+6T>C in East Asia. J Dermatol Sci 2015;79:319–320.

[42] Sugiura K, Oiso N, Linuma S, et al. IL36RN mutations underlie impetigo herpetiformis. J Invest Dermatol 2014;134:2472–2474.

[43] Soutou B, Aractingi S. Skin disease in pregnancy. Best Pract Res Clin Obstet Gynaecol 2015;29:732–740.

[44] Eudy SF, Baker GF. Dermatopathology for the obstetrician. Clin Obstet Gynecol 1990;33: 728–737.

[45] Bozdag K, Ozturk S, Ermete M. A case of recurrent impetigo herpetiformis treated with systemic corticosteroids and narrowband UVB. Cutan Ocul Toxicol 2012;31:67–69.

[46] Shaw CJ, Wu P, Sriemevan A. First trimester impetigo herpetiformis in multiparous female successfully treated with oral cyclosporine. BMJ Case Rep 2011;12;2011.

[47] Luewan S, Sirichotiyakul S, Tongsong T. Recurrent impetigo herpetiformis successfully treated with methotrexate: a case report. J Obstet Gynecol Res 2011;37:661–663.

[48] Saito-Sasaki N, Izu K, Sawada Y, et al. Impetigo herpetiformis complicated with intrauterine growth restriction treated successfully with granulocyte and monocyte apheresis. Acta Derm Venereol 2017;10:97:410–411.

[49] Hayashi RH. Bullous dermatoses and prurigo of pregnancy. Clin Obstet Gynecol 1990;33: 746–753.

[50] Ernest Besnier BB 1831–1909. Arch Derm Syphilol 1929;20:95–99.

[51] Nurse DS. Prurigo of pregnancy. Australas J Dermatol 1968;9:258–267.

[52] Cohen LM. Dermatoses of pregnancy. West J Med 1998;169:223–224.

[53] Black MM. Prurigo of pregnancy, papular dermatitis of pregnancy, and pruritic folliculitis of pregnancy. Semin Dermatol 1997;8:23–25.

[54] Personal communication.

[55] Roger D, Vaillant L, Fignon A, et al. Specific pruritic diseases of pregnancy. A prospective study of 3192 pregnant women. Arch Dermatol 1994;130:744–749.

[56] Black MM, Stephens C. The specific dermatoses of pregnancy, the British perspective. Adv Dermatol 1989;7:105–127.

[57] Wilkinson SM, Buckler H, Wilkinson N. (1995). Androgen levels in pruritic folliculitis of pregnancy. Clin Exp Dermatol 1995;20:234–236.

[58] Vaughan Jones SA, Hern S, Nelson-Piercy C, et al. A prospective study of 200 women with dermatoses of pregnancy correlating clinical findings with hormonal and immunopathological profiles. Br J Dermatol 1999;141:71–81.

[59] Dacus JV. Pruritus in pregnancy. Clin Obstet Gynecol 1990;33:738–745.

[60] Tunzi M, Gray GR. Common skin conditions during pregnancy. Am Fam Physician 2007;75: 211–218.

[61] Al-Fares SI, Jones SV, Black MM. The specific dermatoses of pregnancy: a re-appraisal. J Eur Acad Dermatol Venereol 2001;15:197–206.

[62] Zoberman E, Farmer ER. Pruritic folliculitis of pregnancy. Arch Dermatol 1981;117:20–22.

[63] Alcalay J, Ingber A, Hazaz B, et al. Linear IgM dermatosis of pregnancy. J Am Acad Dermatol 1988;18:412–415.

[64] Unpublished data.

[65] Helm TN, Valenzuela R. Continuous dermoepidermal junction IgM detected by immunofluorescence: a report of nine cases. J Am Acad Dermatol Venereol 1992;26:203–206.

[66] Dahdah MI, Kibbi AG. Less well-defined dermatoses of pregnancy. Clin Dermatol 2006;24: 118–121.

Christoph Wohlmuth, Taymaa May

31 Gynecologic Cancer in Pregnancy

31.1 Introduction

Approximately 1 in 1,000 pregnancies is complicated by cancer, and the incidence has increased over the last few decades. This is likely attributable to the trend of delayed childbearing [1–3]. Risk factors for cancer in pregnancy include advanced maternal age, multiparity, and prior diagnosis of cancer [2–4]. Breast cancer, melanoma, cervical cancer, lymphoma, ovarian cancer, and leukemia represent the most common types (Figure 31.1) [2, 5].

Cancer in pregnancy poses an ethical dilemma with treatment of the mother for optimal oncological safety on the one hand, and the avoidance of harm to the fetus from treatment on the other hand [6]. Data on the optimal management of cancer in pregnancy are still limited. Management options include oncologic treatment during pregnancy, deferral of treatment until after delivery (with or without planned preterm delivery), and termination of pregnancy followed by cancer treatment. The risks and benefits for each option must be discussed with the patient taking into account the gestational age at diagnosis, tumor type, stage of disease, and prognosis [6, 7]. In principle, oncologic therapy should follow the same algorithm as for cancers diagnosed in nonpregnant women; however, the harmful effects of certain diagnostic modalities and the toxicities of some therapeutic agents must be taken into consideration when discussing treatment options. Supported by recent observations from multicenter registries, systemic treatment after the first trimester of pregnancy is feasible with acceptable toxicities and more pregnant patients now receive chemotherapy during pregnancy [5]. In many cases, termination of pregnancy does not improve maternal prognosis, but remains an option in cancers with poor maternal prognosis diagnosed before fetal viability or if treatment is indicated that is not compatible with continuation of pregnancy [6]. With optimal management, the oncologic outcome of women with cancer who are diagnosed during pregnancy appears to be similar to that of nonpregnant women [8].

31.2 Diagnosis

Awareness of the possibility of cancer in pregnancy among health care providers is critical as symptoms may be mistakenly attributed to physiologic changes during pregnancy. It has been shown that pregnant women have a 2.5-fold increased risk of being diagnosed with advanced-stage breast cancer compared to nonpregnant women [9]. A thorough physical examination and focused investigations are therefore

https://doi.org/10.1515/9783110615258-031

A

B

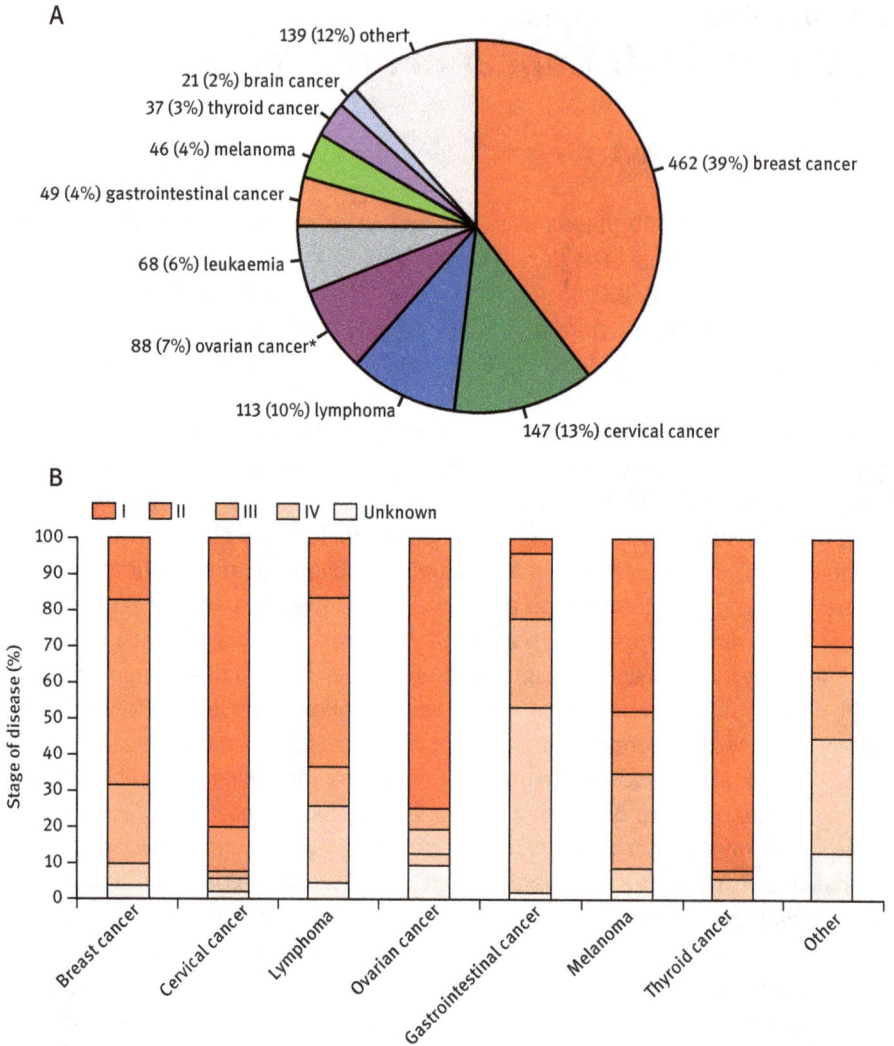

Figure 31.1: Distribution of cancers in pregnancy (A) and disease stage at diagnosis (B). Distribution and stage at diagnosis of cancers in pregnancy from 1,170 patients in the International Network on Cancer, Infertility and Pregnancy (INCIP) registry. Melanomas are underreported as not all patients are referred to the participating INCIP centers. *Ovarian cancers included borderline tumors; †consists of 25 different "other" cancer types. Reproduced with permission from de Haan et al. [5].

warranted to ensure early detection of malignancies. Adequate and comprehensive staging should be performed in pregnant patients with suspected malignancies. Whole-body diffusion-weighted MRI has recently been studied as a single-step staging modality in pregnant women with a clinical diagnosis of cancer. A good observer agreement and improved identification of nodal and distant metastases were seen with MRI compared to conventional multimodal staging, including ultrasound, X-ray, and CT [15].

For a full discussion of diagnostic imaging in pregnancy, please refer to Chapter 3.

31.3 Surgery

Surgery remains the primary treatment modality for most solid malignancies diagnosed at an early stage. Surgery can be performed throughout pregnancy, and current evidence does not support any teratogenic effects from surgery or anesthetic agents, even during the first trimester [16–18]. Data on the risk of miscarriage are conflicting. A study from an English database suggested an increased risk of spontaneous abortion associated with hospitalization for any non-obstetric surgery as compared to women who never had surgery during pregnancy (odds ratio 1.14, 95% CI 1.10–1.18). Conversely, a systematic review of over 12,000 women undergoing surgery during pregnancy has not found an increased risk when compared to baseline. In the largest study of obstetrical outcomes in women with cancer during pregnancy, the rate of spontaneous miscarriage was not increased compared to the baseline risk [5]. In pregnant women undergoing oncologic surgery, maternal hypotension and vena cava compression must be avoided, and adequate maternal oxygenation should be maintained. Intraoperative fetal monitoring is recommended in procedures with viable fetuses [6].

The type of surgery is determined by the underlying malignancy. Laparoscopy can be safely performed until 26–28 weeks of gestation depending on the type of procedure and the surgeon's experience. The open access is preferred over the Veress needle technique [6]. Studies have shown less fetal adverse events, shorter hospital stays, and fewer uterine contractions with laparoscopy compared to laparotomy [19, 20]. However, the same oncologic standards for the choice of open versus laparoscopic surgery must apply as in nonpregnant patients with similar malignancy [21, 22].

For suspicious ovarian masses, a frozen section should be obtained, and further surgical management tailored according to the histologic subtype. Staging may be performed until 22 weeks of gestation; however, if optimal visualization cannot be established with the gravid uterus, a restaging procedure may be performed after delivery [12]. In advanced stage epithelial ovarian cancer diagnosed in the first half of gestation, termination of pregnancy and surgical cytoreduction may be considered. If this is not an option or if the disease is diagnosed in the second half of pregnancy, neoadjuvant chemotherapy may be initiated with interval cytoreductive surgery planned after delivery [12]. Individualized treatment plans are important in these women, taking into account maternal and fetal health.

In cervical cancer, a cone biopsy may be performed to treat International Federation of Obstetrics and Gynecology [23] stage IA1 tumors without lymphovascular space invasion (LVSI). For stage IA1 with LVSI, IA2, and IB1 disease, a pelvic lymphadenectomy may be performed until 22 weeks of gestation for staging purposes [12]. Trachelectomy has been performed by some during pregnancy. However, a recent systematic review of 19 patients treated with radical trachelectomy between 7 and 22 weeks of gestation found a relatively high rate of pregnancy loss of 21% and high maternal blood loss with 50% of patients requiring blood transfusions [24]. Stage IB2 disease diagnosed prior to 22 weeks can be managed with lymph node staging followed by observation and completion surgery after delivery. Alternatively, patients with stage IB2 disease may be treated with neoadjuvant chemotherapy followed by fertility-preserving trachelectomy during pregnancy or definitive surgery after viability. For node-positive patients or patients with locally advanced disease, termination of pregnancy is often recommended as urgent adjuvant therapy including systemic chemotherapy and radiation therapy is warranted. In some cases, chemotherapy with continuation of pregnancy to reach viability may be considered. For women with stage IB3 cervical carcinoma diagnosed after 22 weeks gestation, neoadjuvant chemotherapy can be given, although data are limited in this subgroup. For cervical cancer diagnosed after 22 weeks of gestation, neoadjuvant chemotherapy or delayed definitive treatment after delivery may be considered depending on gestational age at diagnosis [12].

In women diagnosed with breast carcinoma, pregnancy is not an absolute indication for mastectomy [25]. However, the potential delay of adjuvant radiation therapy must be taken into account in the treatment planning. When chemotherapy is indicated, breast-conserving surgery may be performed in the second and third trimesters. Adjuvant radiation must be reserved until after delivery [25]. The sentinel nodal mapping technique can be used safely during pregnancy. The estimated absorbed dose using radiolabeled technetium for axillary sentinel technique in breast cancer is between 0.1 and 4.3 mGy and thus below the suggested threshold [26, 27]. Blue dye is generally not recommended due to the potential of anaphylactic reactions, but it has been used without complications in a case series of pregnant women undergoing sentinel mapping for breast cancer [28].

For pregnant women with gynecologic malignancies requiring nodal mapping, the use of indocyanine green (ICG) has been suggested as the preferred agent to due to concerns of high radiation exposure from radioactive technetium [29, 20]. Experience with ICG in pregnancy is limited; however, experimental studies using the standard clinical dose have shown that it does not cross the placenta [31].

Lastly, for melanoma diagnosed during pregnancy the same surgical principles apply as in nonpregnant women, and the sentinel mapping technique can be performed as in breast cancer [32, 33].

31.4 Systemic Treatment

31.4.1 Chemotherapy in Pregnancy

Cytotoxic chemotherapy interferes with cell growth and targets rapidly dividing cells. Although the fetal plasma concentrations of common cytotoxic drugs are lower compared to the maternal concentration, they can cross the placental barrier and are therefore potentially harmful to the fetus [34, 35]. This is especially critical during organogenesis in the first trimester. The risk for congenital malformations in the first trimester ranges between 8% and 25%, compared with 4% in the general population [36]. After the first trimester, the risk of malformations following chemotherapy is comparable to the general population [5, 37].

Fetal growth restriction complicates up to 25% of pregnancies after chemotherapy, and the risk appears highest for those receiving platinum-based drugs (OR 3.12, 95% CI 1.45–6.70) [5, 38]. This is supported by animal experiments that suggest a high placental passage of platinum-based agents [35]. The high rate of fetal growth restriction may, however, be multifactorial, and carboplatin represents a preferred agent for gynecologic malignancies during pregnancy. Apart from the direct cytotoxic effects, indirect effects from inflammation, maternal anemia, malnutrition, high concentrations of stress hormones, and the maternal illness itself may contribute to abnormal fetal growth [36].

Premature delivery and neonatal intensive care unit (NICU) admissions have been observed in 50–60% of pregnancies exposed to chemotherapy compared to 7–8% in the corresponding general population [5, 38]. In a multicenter registry, the rate of premature labor was 12.9% in pregnancies complicated with cancer compared to 4% in the normal population. In a retrospective study the rate of preterm premature rupture of membranes (PPROM) was 17% in patients receiving conventional chemotherapy and up to 30% with dose-dense regimens [37, 39]. Besides the suggested direct effects of chemotherapy on premature contractions and PPROM, the high rate of preterm birth is in part caused iatrogenically [5, 6]. Preterm birth increases the risk of perinatal morbidity and mortality, as well as neurodevelopmental delay, and the increased neonatal mortality observed in patients with cancer during pregnancy was attributed to prematurity in 89% of the cases in a large series [5, 40].

Furthermore, antenatal chemotherapy may cause serious neonatal hematologic toxicities. The treatment protocol should therefore be planned such that no chemotherapy is given within three weeks of delivery to allow metabolization of cytotoxic drugs and recovery of the fetal (and maternal) bone marrow [41]. Data on long-term outcome are still limited. Preliminary evidence suggests that developmental, cardiovascular, and neurologic outcomes are favorable [38, 42–45].

An overview of chemotherapeutic agents and the associated risks is shown in Table 31.1.

Table 31.1: Associated risks of common cytotoxic, endocrine, and biologic agents when used during pregnancy.

Drug class/function	Drug	Transplacental passage	Neonatal risks	Specific recommendations
Chemotherapy/cytotoxic drugs				
Platinum agents	Carboplatinum, Cisplatinum	60%	– SGA OR = 3.12 (1.45–6.70) – Ototoxicity: greater for cisplatin; carboplatin preferred – NICU admission OR = 1.66 (0.77–3.55)	Postnatal auditory test
Taxanes	Paclitaxel, Docetaxel	2%	– SGA OR = 2.07 (1.11–3.86) – NICU admission OR = 2.37 (1.31–4.28) – Accumulation in neonatal tissue possible due to immature metabolization by liver enzymes	
Alkylating agents	Cyclophosphamide	20%	– SGA OR=2.08 (0.88 to 4.91) – NICU admission OR=0.88 (0.46 to 1.70)	
Antimetabolites	5-Fluorouracil	28%	– SGA OR = 1.24 (0.70–2.22) – NICU admission OR = 1.03 (0.60–1.74)	
Antitumor antibiotics	Doxorubicin, Epirubicin	<10%	– SGA OR = 0.50 (0.21–1.22) – NICU admission OR = 1.21 (0.62–2.38) – Potential cardiotoxicity, not confirmed in a limited cohort followed postnatally	Postnatal echocardiography
Vinca alkaloids	Vinca alkaloids	20%	– SGA OR = 2.34 (1.04–5.25) – NICU admission OR = 1.63 (0.78–3.38)	

Endocrine agents

Selective estrogen receptor modulator (breast cancer)	Tamoxifen	n.a.	– Intrauterine fetal demise – Ambiguous genitalia – Goldenhar syndrome, Pierre-Robin sequence	Use NOT recommended

Biologic agents/targeted treatment

Her2-receptor inhibitor (Breast, gastric cancer)	Trastuzumab	n.a.	– Oligohy-dramnios, hypoplastic lungs and fetal death by its ligation to Her2-receptors that are present in the renal epithelium of the fetus	Use NOT recommended
Anti-CD20 antibody (NHL)	Rituximab	n.a.	– Neonatal cytopenia	To use with caution
Tyrosine kinase inhibitor (CML)	Imatinib	n.a.	– Exposure in first trimester associated with congenital malformations (11% of exposed fetuses) and spontaneous miscarriage. – Safety data for exposure in second or third trimester are limited but no major minor congenital malformations are reported	To use with caution
Pleiotropic cytokine (melanoma, CML, lymphoma, hairy cell leukemia and AIDS-related Kaposi sarcoma)	Interferon-α	n.a.	– Dose-dependent increased of miscarriage rate in animal models. Limited placental transfer. – One case reported with congenital malformations (exomphalos, right renal agenesis, and hemivertebrae)	Can be used on strict indication
Epidermal growth factor receptor inhibitors (lung cancer)	Erlotinib Gefitinib Afatinib Cetuximab	n.a.	– Increased risk of miscarriage in animal models – Three cases with erlotinib during pregnancy revealed no congenital malformations – Limited data	Use NOT recommended

(continued)

Table 31.1 (continued)

Drug class/function	Drug	Transplacental passage	Neonatal risks	Specific recommendations
Anti-angiogenic agents (epithelial ovarian cancer, renal cell cancer, thyroid cancer, hepatic cancer)	Bevacicumab Sorafenib Sunitinib	n.a.	– Miscarriage, fetal demise – Skeletal malformations in animal models – No human data for sorafenib and sunitinib – Intravitreal injections of bevacizumab was not associated with adverse events	Use NOT recommended
BRAF/MEK inhibitors (melanoma)	Vemurafenib Dabrafenib Trametinib Selumetinib	n.a.	– Limited data – No teratogenesis of vemurafenib reported in animal models. One case report of low birth weight and preterm delivery (administration after 25 weeks of gestation); one case of toxic epidermal necrolysis.	Use NOT recommended
Checkpoint inhibitors (melanoma, lung cancer, renal cancer)	Ipilimumab Nivolumab Pembrolizumab	n.a.	– Limited data – Increased risk of miscarriage in animal studies – Placental insufficiency and IUGR in two case reports – PD-L1 expression in syncytiotrophoblast and extravillous cytotrophoblasts in the human placenta	Use NOT recommended

31.4.2 Endocrine Therapy

Selective estrogen receptor modulators such as tamoxifen have been associated with miscarriage, congenital malformations, and fetal demise and are thus contraindicated during pregnancy [46, 47]. Similarly, aromatase inhibitors such as letrozole and anastrozole are contraindicated given their anti-estrogenic effects.

31.4.3 Targeted Therapies and Biologic Agents

Targeted therapies and biologic agents form integral parts in current cancer treatment protocols including breast cancer, melanoma, gynecologic cancers, and hematologic malignancies. To date, none of these agents are approved for use during pregnancy. Trastuzumab, a monoclonal antibody targeting Her2 expression that is used in breast cancer treatment, is associated with oligohydramnios, pulmonary hypoplasia, skeletal abnormalities, and neonatal death [48]. Data for other biologic agents are limited, and their use is discouraged during pregnancy [6]. An overview of biologic agents and the associated risks is shown in Table 33.1.

31.5 Radiation Therapy

The risk of fetal malformations and developmental delays increases after a cumulative radiation dose of 100–200 mGy, especially during the first trimester. Mental retardation and growth restriction may result from exposure to radiation during the second and third trimesters. Severe mental retardation is expected with fetal exposure to radiation exceeding 1 Gy, and miscarriage or fetal demise may occur following radiation exposures above 30 Gy [7, 49, 50]. Although curative radiation therapy doses are often below these levels and with proper uterine and the fetal shielding the fetus may not be exposed to these high radiation doses, the risk of future malignancies of the unborn child, especially leukemia, is increased with in utero radiation exposure [49]. Therefore, radiation therapy is generally not recommended during pregnancy [18].

31.6 Obstetric Management

Before and during treatment, fetal growth and Doppler assessment as well as measurement of cervical length should be performed to monitor fetal development and signs of preterm labor [6].

Prematurity is associated with significant neonatal morbidity and mortality and should be avoided whenever possible [6]. Delivery within 3 weeks of administration of chemotherapy should be avoided due to the risk of neonatal myelosuppression and infection. The delivery mode should be based on obstetric indications except for cervical and vulvar cancers, which are absolute indications for cesarean section to avoid episiotomy scar recurrence or major tumor bleeding [6, 12]. A corporeal uterine incision should be performed in cesarean section in cervical cancer to avoid tumor spillage from the lower uterine segment, and definitive surgical management can be performed at the time of delivery or shortly after delivery by an experienced gynecologic oncologist [12].

31.7 Conclusion

Symptoms suggestive of malignancies must not be attributed to "physiologic changes" in pregnancy and should prompt further investigations. During pregnancy, MRI and ultrasound represent the best imaging modalities of the abdomen, and mammograms and chest x-rays are considered safe modalities to image the breast and chest. Termination of pregnancy does not improve maternal outcome in many cases. Furthermore, iatrogenic preterm delivery adds neonatal morbidity and mortality. Therefore, oncologic treatment during pregnancy represents the best option in most cases. Surgery is safe during pregnancy, and chemotherapy with selected cytotoxic agents appears to be relatively safe after the first trimester. Radiation is usually deferred until after delivery. With the limited evidence available, all pregnancies complicated by cancer require individualized care in specialized centers providing multidisciplinary care by maternal–fetal medicine specialists, oncologists, and neonatologists.

References

[1]   Smith LH, Danielsen B, Allen ME, Cress R. Cancer associated with obstetric delivery: results of linkage with the California cancer registry. Am J Obstet Gynecol 2003;189:1128–1135.
[2]   Lee YY, Roberts CL, Dobbins T, et al. Incidence and outcomes of pregnancy-associated cancer in Australia, 1994–2008: a population-based linkage study. BJOG 2012;119:1572–1582.
[3]   Parazzini F, Franchi M, Tavani A, Negri E, Peccatori FA. Frequency of pregnancy related cancer: a population based linkage study in Lombardy, Italy. Int J Gynecol Cancer 2017;27: 613–619.
[4]   Yasmeen S, Cress R, Romano PS, et al. Thyroid cancer in pregnancy. Int J Gynaecol Obstet 2005;91:15–20.
[5]   De Haan J, Verheecke M, Van Calsteren K, et al. Oncological management and obstetric and neonatal outcomes for women diagnosed with cancer during pregnancy: a 20-year international cohort study of 1170 patients. Lancet Oncol 2018;19:337–346.

[6] Maggen C, Van Gerwen M, Van Calsteren K, Vandenbroucke T, Amant F. Management of cancer during pregnancy and current evidence of obstetric, neonatal and pediatric outcome: a review article. Int J Gynecol Cancer 2019; published online Jan 18. doi: 10.1136/ijgc-2018-000061.

[7] Zagouri F, Dimitrakakis C, Marinopoulos S, Tsigginou A, Dimopoulos M-A. Cancer in pregnancy: disentangling treatment modalities. ESMO Open 2016;1:e000016.

[8] Stensheim H, Møller B, Van Dijk T, Fosså SD. Cause-specific survival for women diagnosed with cancer during pregnancy or lactation: a registry-based cohort study. J Clin Oncol 2009;27:45–51.

[9] Zemlickis D, Lishner M, Degendorfer P, et al. Maternal and fetal outcome after breast cancer in pregnancy. Am J Obstet Gynecol 1992;166:781–787.

[10] Shaw P, Duncan A, Vouyouka A, Ozsvath K. Radiation exposure and pregnancy. J Vasc Surg 2011;53:28S–34S.

[11] Streffer C, Shore R, Konermann G, et al. Biological effects after prenatal irradiation (embryo and fetus). A report of the International Commission on Radiological Protection. Ann ICRP 2003;33:5–206.

[12] Amant F, Berveiller P, Boere IA, et al. Gynecologic cancers in pregnancy: guidelines based on a third international consensus meeting. Ann Oncol Off J Eur Soc Med Oncol 2019;30: 1601–1612.

[13] Moro F, Mascilini F, Pasciuto T, et al. Ultrasound features and clinical outcome of patients with malignant ovarian masses diagnosed during pregnancy: experience of a gynecological oncology ultrasound center. Int J Gynecol Cancer 2019;29:1182–1194.

[14] Ray JG, Vermeulen MJ, Bharatha A, Montanera WJ, Park AL. Association between MRI exposure during pregnancy and fetal and childhood outcomes. JAMA 2016;316:952–961.

[15] Han SN, Amant F, Michielsen K, et al. Feasibility of whole-body diffusion-weighted MRI for detection of primary tumour, nodal and distant metastases in women with cancer during pregnancy: a pilot study. Eur Radiol 2018;28:1862–1874.

[16] Cohen-Kerem R, Railton C, Oren D, Lishner M, Koren G. Pregnancy outcome following non-obstetric surgical intervention. Am J Surg 2005;190:467–473.

[17] ACOG Committee Opinion No. 775: nonobstetric Surgery During Pregnancy. Obstet Gynecol 2019;133:e285–6.

[18] Peccatori FA, Azim HA, Orecchia R, et al. Cancer, pregnancy and fertility: eSMO Clinical Practice Guidelines for diagnosis, treatment and follow-up. Ann Oncol Off J Eur Soc Med Oncol 2013;24(Suppl 6):vi160–70.

[19] Shigemi D, Aso S, Matsui H, Fushimi K, Yasunaga H. Safety of laparoscopic surgery for benign diseases during pregnancy: a nationwide retrospective cohort study. J Minim Invasive Gynecol;26:501–506.

[20] Webb KE, Sakhel K, Chauhan SP, Abuhamad AZ. Adnexal mass during pregnancy: a review. Am J Perinatol 2015;32:1010–1016.

[21] Colombo N, Sessa C, Du Bois A, et al. ESMO-ESGO consensus conference recommendations on ovarian cancer: pathology and molecular biology, early and advanced stages, borderline tumours and recurrent disease†. Ann Oncol Off J Eur Soc Med Oncol 2019;30:672–705.

[22] Ramirez PT, Frumovitz M, Pareja R, et al. Minimally invasive versus abdominal radical hysterectomy for cervical cancer. N Engl J Med 2018;379:1895–1904.

[23] Bhatla N, Berek JS, Cuello Fredes M, et al/ Revised FIGO staging for carcinoma of the cervix uteri. Int J Gynecol Obstet 2019;145:129–135.

[24] Douligeris A, Prodromidou A, Psomiadou V, Iavazzo C, Vorgias G. Abdominal radical trachelectomy during pregnancy: a systematic review of the literature. J Gynecol Obstet Hum Reprod 2019; published online July 2. doi: 10.1016/j.jogoh.2019.07.003.

[25] Toesca A, Gentilini O, Peccatori F, Azim HA, Amant F. Locoregional treatment of breast cancer during pregnancy. Gynecol Surg 2014;11:279–284.

[26] Keleher A, Wendt R, Delpassand E, Stachowiak AM, Kuerer HM. The safety of lymphatic mapping in pregnant breast cancer patients using Tc-99m sulfur colloid. Breast J 2004;10: 492–495.

[27] Pandit-Taskar N, Dauer LT, Montgomery L, St Germain J, Zanzonico PB, Divgi CR. Organ and fetal absorbed dose estimates from 99mTc-sulfur colloid lymphoscintigraphy and sentinel node localization in breast cancer patients. J Nucl Med 2006;47:1202–1208.

[28] Gropper AB, Calvillo KZ, Dominici L, et al. Sentinel lymph node biopsy in pregnant women with breast cancer. Ann Surg Oncol 2014;21:2506–2511.

[29] Rychlik A, Marin S, De Santiago J, Zapardiel I. Utility of laparoscopic indocyanine green-guided sentinel node biopsy in open cervical cancer surgery. Int J Gynecol Cancer 2016;26: 1288–1289.

[30] Papadia A, Mohr S, Imboden S, Lanz S, Bolla D, Mueller MD. Laparoscopic indocyanine green sentinel lymph node mapping in pregnant cervical cancer patients. J Minim Invasive Gynecol 2016;23:270–273.

[31] Robson SC, Mutch E, Boys RJ, Woodhouse KW. Apparent liver blood flow during pregnancy: a serial study using indocyanine green clearance. Br J Obstet Gynaecol 1990;97:720–724.

[32] Coit DG, Thompson JA, Algazi A, et al. NCCN guidelines insights: melanoma, version 3.2016. J Natl Compr Canc Netw 2016;14:945–958.

[33] Faries MB, Thompson JF, Cochran AJ, et al. Completion dissection or observation for sentinel-node metastasis in Melanoma. N Engl J Med 2017;376:2211–2222.

[34] Van Calsteren K, Verbesselt R, Beijnen J, et al. Transplacental transfer of anthracyclines, vinblastine, and 4-hydroxy-cyclophosphamide in a baboon model. Gynecol Oncol 2010;119: 594–600.

[35] Calsteren KV, Verbesselt R, Devlieger R, et al. Transplacental transfer of paclitaxel, docetaxel, carboplatin, and trastuzumab in a baboon model. Int J Gynecol Cancer 2010;20:1456–1464.

[36] Vandenbroucke T, Verheecke M, Fumagalli M, Lok C, Amant F. Effects of cancer treatment during pregnancy on fetal and child development. Lancet Child Adolesc Heal 2017;1:302–310.

[37] Van Calsteren K, Heyns L, De Smet F, et al. Cancer during pregnancy: an analysis of 215 patients emphasizing the obstetrical and the neonatal outcomes. J Clin Oncol 2010;28:683–689.

[38] Amant F, Vandenbroucke T, Verheecke M, et al. Pediatric outcome after maternal cancer diagnosed during pregnancy. N Engl J Med 2015;373:1824–1834.

[39] Cardonick E, Gilmandyar D, Somer RA. Maternal and neonatal outcomes of dose-dense chemotherapy for breast cancer in pregnancy. Obstet Gynecol 2012;120:1267–1272.

[40] Lu D, Ludvigsson JF, Smedby KE, et al. Maternal cancer during pregnancy and risks of stillbirth and infant mortality. J Clin Oncol 2017;35:1522–1529.

[41] Weisz B, Meirow D, Schiff E, Lishner M. Impact and treatment of cancer during pregnancy. Expert Rev Anticancer Ther 2004;4:889–902.

[42] Gziri MM, Amant F, Debiève F, Van Calsteren K, De Catte L, Mertens L. Effects of chemotherapy during pregnancy on the maternal and fetal heart. Prenat Diagn 2012;32:614–619.

[43] Avilés A, Neri N. Hematological malignancies and pregnancy: a final report of 84 children who received chemotherapy in utero. Clin Lymphoma 2001;2:173–177.

[44] Hahn KME, Johnson PH, Gordon N, et al. Treatment of pregnant breast cancer patients and outcomes of children exposed to chemotherapy in utero. Cancer 2006;107:1219–1226.

[45] Avilés A, Nambo M-J, Neri N. Treatment of early stages hodgkin lymphoma during pregnancy. Mediterr J Hematol Infect Dis 2018;10:e2018006.

[46] Isaacs RJ, Hunter W, Clark K. Tamoxifen as systemic treatment of advanced breast cancer during pregnancy–case report and literature review. Gynecol Oncol 2001;80:405–408.

[47] Tewari K, Bonebrake RG, Asrat T, Shanberg AM. Ambiguous genitalia in infant exposed to tamoxifen in utero. Lancet (London, England) 1997;350:183.

[48] Zagouri F, Sergentanis TN, Chrysikos D, Papadimitriou CA, Dimopoulos M-A, Bartsch R. Trastuzumab administration during pregnancy: a systematic review and meta-analysis. Breast Cancer Res Treat 2013;137:349–357.

[49] Kal HB, Struikmans H. Radiotherapy during pregnancy: fact and fiction. Lancet Oncol 2005;6:328–333.

[50] Fenig E, Mishaeli M, Kalish Y, Lishner M. Pregnancy and radiation. Cancer Treat Rev 2001;27:1–7.

Evangelia Vlachodimitropoulou Koumoutsea, Cynthia Maxwell

32 Maternal and Fetal Malignancies in Pregnancy

32.1 Epidemiology

A cancer diagnosis during pregnancy is indeed a relatively rare occurrence, thought to affect fewer than 1 in 1,000 pregnant women. A Danish registry has, however, shown that over a 30-year period this rate has been on the rise, reaching 8.3% in their population in 2006 [1]. This trend can be attributed partly to the increasing tendency of delaying pregnancy to the third and fourth decades of life, an improvement in diagnostic efficacy but also an increased incidence of certain types of cancers [2]. The malignancies most commonly noted in pregnancy are similar in incidence to those which develop outside pregnancy in this age group, and include cervical and breast cancer, melanoma, lymphomas, and acute leukemias.

Timely diagnosis is a pivotal aspect of successful treatment but unfortunately is often delayed in pregnancy. Since cancer is rare in this setting, it can often be low on the list of differential diagnoses, particularly since some of the presenting symptoms may be common in pregnancy or nonspecific. Regarding treatment, data from large clinical trials are often lacking due to the uniqueness of this clinical scenario and *best practice* is often limited to experience from small sample size studies or case reports.

Advances in cancer management in this unique setting have led to an overall rise in treatment uptake by 10% and an increase in the use of chemotherapy in pregnancy by 31% as evidenced by an Italian population-based study [3]. This increase in willingness to consider and undertake appropriate treatment has translated into an improvement in fetal outcomes, including an increase in the live birth rate and a reduction in the number of preterm births. Maternal survival in pregnancy appears to be the same as in nonpregnant women [3].

32.2 Diagnosing Cancer in Pregnancy

The detection of cancer in pregnancy may be delayed. The pregnancy often poses several challenges in establishing a diagnosis. For example, the symptoms of nausea and vomiting, abdominal discomfort, or painful breast changes that are often seen in malignancy are a common occurrence in pregnancy. Furthermore, there is often hesitation to submit the mother and fetus to diagnostic imaging, and the diagnostic accuracy of certain tumor markers in pregnancy is not fully established [4].

https://doi.org/10.1515/9783110615258-032

32.2.1 Imaging

There are a number of factors to consider when deciding upon the best imaging modality. Full staging of cancer may create a management conflict between fetal risk and maternal benefit, and factors to be taken into account include the safety of the fetus, the risk of cancer metastasis, and fetal viability. The diagnostic workup should always begin with a thorough physical examination followed by diagnostic interventions. If X-ray images are required, abdominal shielding should be provided. Mammography, which is used in the diagnosis of breast cancer, is increasingly difficult to accurately interpret owing to pregnancy-related breast vascular and density changes [5]. Imaging modalities include ultrasound, computed tomography (CT), and magnetic resonance imaging (MRI). For a full discussion of diagnostic imaging in pregnancy, please refer to Chapter 3.

32.2.2 Laboratory Markers

Pregnancy can be associated with a rise in several tumor markers, and thereby reduces their sensitivity and specificity in this setting [4], complicating the diagnosis of certain malignancies. CA-125, which is used in the diagnosis of epithelial ovarian cancer, and alpha-fetoprotein, used to diagnose germ cell malignancies, are both naturally elevated in pregnancy. Blood count parameters such as hemoglobin and hematocrit are usually lower, whereas the alkaline phosphatase (ALP) and lactate dehydrogenase (LDH), often used to aid cancer diagnosis, are increased during pregnancy [6, 7].

32.3 Specific Cancers in Pregnancy

Cancer can arise at any body location during pregnancy. However, the most common malignancies reported in pregnancy are breast, cervix, lymphoma, acute myeloid leukemia, ovarian cancer, and melanoma. It is beyond the scope of this review to discuss all cancer types and their pregnancy implications in detail.

32.3.1 Breast Cancer

Malignancy of the breast is the most commonly diagnosed cancer in pregnancy. Pregnancy-related physiological changes of the breast can cause a delay in the diagnosis ranging between 2 and 18 months, and occasionally leading to detection in the postpartum period [8]. In pregnancy, the most common histopathological findings of breast cancer tissue are estrogen receptor/progesterone receptor/HER2-negative [9]. The prognosis of these patients compared to nonpregnant women is a contentious issue due to a possible diagnostic delay leading to potentially more advanced disease as well as certain limitations to therapeutic options. However, pregnancy following completion of therapy is not thought to affect cancer prognosis adversely.

Symptomatology of breast cancer in pregnancy resembles that found in non-pregnant women and includes a palpable mass, bloody nipple discharge, and skin changes. First-line investigations for metastatic workup include mammography, ul-trasonography, and core needle biopsy, all of which can safely be utilized in pregnancy. Mammography has an 80% sensitivity in detecting malignancy in pregnancy [10]. Ultrasound evaluation is used to assess the breast tissue as well as stage lymph nodes and assist with performing biopsies [11]. The use of methylene blue dye is contraindicated; however, technetium-99m is known to be safe in pregnancy [8]. MRI has also been used to assist with the diagnosis and has been shown to have a 98% sensitivity in detection and may lead to a change in management in up to 28% of cases [12]. Chest radiographs to assist with staging should be obtained with abdominal shielding. In stages I and II breast cancer the incidence of bone metastasis is low, at 3% and 7% respectively, and thus a bone scan is usually unnecessary. However, for stage III disease evaluation bone scans can be performed postpartum or using a noncontrast skeletal MRI [10].

The goal of treatment is local disease control and prevention of metastasis. In the first trimester, chemotherapy is generally contraindicated for reasons of fetal toxicity, as first-line regimens are a combination of anthracycline-based regimens. Evidence is not strong to support taxanes such as paclitaxel, but they have been used after the first trimester. Radical mastectomy with axillary staging or breast-conserving surgery is a safe option throughout pregnancy. Adjuvant chemotherapy is usually reserved for the second trimester onward, and radiotherapy is reserved for the postpartum period. Hormonal therapies such as tamoxifen, aromatase inhibitors and gonadotropin-releasing hormone agonists are correlated with significant fetal malformations, and their use is contraindicated in pregnancy [13, 14].

Metastatic disease to the placenta is extremely rare, and the histopathological examination of the placenta is recommended in any pregnancy-associated malignancy. No affected fetuses have been described to date [15].

32.3.2 Lymphoma and Leukemia

Hodgkin lymphoma has a median presentation age of 32 years and an incidence of between 1 in 1,000 and 1 in 6,000 in pregnancy. The diagnosis is made using exci-sional lymph node biopsy, and if it is confirmed in the first trimester, termination of pregnancy is a strong consideration, especially in the presence of advanced/aggressive disease or B-symptoms. A delay in treatment can have grave implications to the mother's life. If a decision is made to continue with gestation, surveillance with no therapy intervention until the second trimester can be considered. The gold standard of treatment in the second and third trimesters is chemotherapy with ABVD (doxorubicin, bleomycin, vinblastine, dacarbazine) and has been associated with favorable outcomes for both mother and fetus. Infants are not considered to be at risk of intrauterine growth restriction or extreme prematurity [16].

Non-Hodgkin lymphoma occurs even more infrequently in pregnancy, and management involves chemotherapy, even in the first trimester. Fetal outcomes have previously been favorable in this setting [17]. Rituximab is a monoclonal antibody to the CD20 antigen expressed by normal and malignant B lymphocytes and is part of the standard of care chemotherapy regimens for the treatment of B-cell non-Hodgkin lymphoma as well as chronic lymphocytic leukemia. Experience in pregnancy ranges from treating lymphoma as well as other conditions such as immune thrombocytopenic purpura, and there have been no reports of significant harm to the fetus when used within 6 months of conception. Nevertheless, the neonate will be at higher risk of infections and B cells need to be monitored after birth [18]. The prognosis of non-Hodgkin lymphoma diagnosed in pregnancy is not different from that in the nonpregnant population [17].

One-third of acute leukemia cases in pregnancy comprise acute lymphoblastic leukemia and two-thirds acute myeloid leukemia. Initial symptomatology can be vague and overlap with pregnancy symptoms, leading to a delay in the diagnosis. In the majority of cases, treatment is required immediately following diagnosis. If the diagnosis takes place in the first trimester, termination of pregnancy should be considered. Chemotherapy regimens including cytarabine and daunorubicin are often adjusted in these cases to reduce toxicity to the fetus which can be as high as 50%. An alternate anthracycline, doxorubicin can be considered for induction chemotherapy for both types of leukemia in patients who wish to proceed with the pregnancy [19]. Leukemia and lymphoma, following melanoma, are the second most common malignancies that can metastasize to the placenta and affect the fetus [20].

32.3.3 Melanoma

Over the last few decades an increase in the incidence of melanoma has been recorded, now at an estimated lifetime risk of 1%. The mean age at diagnosis is 45 years of age, and an estimated one-third of affected women are of reproductive age. Furthermore, melanoma is thought to be one of the leading cancer diagnoses in pregnancy [21]. A number of reports have shown that melanoma tissue has a small number of estrogen, progesterone, and androgen receptors, perhaps increasing the risk of this disease in pregnancy [22, 23]. However, oral contraceptives have not shown to affect the incidence of the disease [24]. Previously, there was controversy regarding the survival from melanoma of pregnant as opposed to nonpregnant women; however, there does not appear to be any difference [25–27]. A number of studies have reported a shorter disease-free interval for pregnant women, which may be partially attributed to a shorter time to metastasis to the lymph nodes [28, 29].

Treatment in pregnancy is similar to nonpregnant women and pregnancy and is based on wide surgical excision with appropriately clear margins. This type of procedure poses very little risk to the fetus as it can commonly be performed under local anesthesia. In metastatic disease, resection of the involved lymph nodes is performed. Metastatic disease may be palliated using chemotherapy, and termination of pregnancy should be discussed in these cases. Dacarbazine containing chemotherapy has been administered to 28 women in the second and third trimesters, with one fetal death and one fetal malformation reported [30]. Interferon-α has occasionally also been used in this context, with significant maternal side effects such as joint pains and flulike symptoms. Interferon has been safely administered to pregnant women with hematological cancers, but it has not been extensively studied in this context [31, 32].

Malignant melanoma is responsible for half of the metastases noted in products of conception, and the fetus and the placenta should be carefully examined [20].

32.4 Targeted Therapies for Certain Malignancies in Pregnancy

In the last decade, important advances have been made in the field of cancer management. The experience with regard to the administration of targeted agents in pregnancy is still limited; however, it is important that more experience is obtained regarding the safety of these agents in terms of safety of the fetus. Compared to chemotherapy, monoclonal antibodies are large molecules and would require active transport to cross the placenta. Other molecules such as tyrosine kinase inhibitors (TKIs) are small molecules that can readily cross the placenta. The use of these "targeted" therapies is discouraged in pregnancy due to concern regarding potential interference with normal physiology required for fetal development. However, information regarding their use in pregnancy is gradually emerging.

32.4.1 Tamoxifen

Tamoxifen is a selective estrogen receptor modulator (SERM) used in the management of hormone receptor–positive breast cancer or following surgical intervention to reduce the risk of recurrence. To date, there have been 238 cases of tamoxifen use in pregnancy with 167 pregnancies with known outcomes. Twenty-one pregnancy outcomes with fetal abnormalities have been reported [33]. Some of these include ambiguous genitalia in the fetus [34], craniofacial malformations, Goldenhar syndrome, and Pierre-Robin sequence [35, 36]. This experience has led to the consensus guidance that tamoxifen is contraindicated during pregnancy. Furthermore, pregnancy is not advised for 3 months following discontinuation of treatment [37]. Despite this experience, however, the majority of fetuses born to women who have been exposed to tamoxifen do not have any abnormalities, and a direct causal relationship has not been established to date. The risk of fetal abnormalities is thought to be increased from 3.9% in the general population to 12.6% in women who receive tamoxifen during pregnancy [33].

32.4.2 Human Epidermal Growth Factor Receptor 2 (HER2)

Trastuzumab is a recombinant IgG1 monoclonal antibody used in the management of patients with HER2-positive breast and gastric cancer. The HER2 pathway plays a role in conception and implantation as well as fetal organogenesis and normal cardiac and neuronal development. In humans, its use is contraindicated in pregnancy as it has been linked to the development of severe oligohydramnios. The targeted HER2 oncogene is also expressed in the fetal kidney, and trastuzumab-related fetal renal impairment could be causal to fetal oligohydramnios. In a systematic review describing 18 pregnant women exposed to trastuzumab, the rate of oligohydramnios was 61% and a healthy live birth rate was reported in 53% [38]. Patients receiving trastuzumab as adjuvant therapy who became pregnant exposed the fetus to the drug in the first trimester. However, mothers who discontinued the drug all delivered healthy infants without any complications [38]. Thus, the administration of trastuzumab should be avoided during gestation, but if a woman undergoes an unplanned pregnancy, the drug should be stopped, and the pregnancy be allowed to continue.

32.4.3 Tyrosine Kinase Inhibitors

Currently in pregnancy, the molecule with the largest amount of data is imatinib. Imatinib is a tyrosine kinase inhibitor (TKI) that targets *BCR-ABL1*, encoding a mutant tyrosine kinase known as the Philadelphia chromosome balanced translocation (t9;22). Imatinib inhibits *BCR-ABL1* in a nonspecific fashion, and also other tyrosine kinases. It is used to manage diseases such as CML and ALL. Imatinib has been noted to cross the placenta into the fetal circulation in humans [39, 40]. Several reports have been published describing the use of imatinib in pregnancy, with all recorded malformations occurring in the first trimester, the rate of which is now thought to be 11%. One of the largest studies included 180 pregnant women exposed to imatinib and described 12 pregnancies with malformations following first-trimester exposure, more prevalently skeletal alterations [41]. Current recommendations support the avoidance of imatinib in the first trimester. First-trimester exposure is also associated with spontaneous miscarriage rates as high as 12% [42]. Second- and third-trimester exposure is considered safe. Dasatinib and nilotinib are second-generation TKIs approved for the management of Philadelphia-positive CML. Data on the use of TKI in pregnancy are limited, but these agents appear to have a similar safety profile to imatinib. It is advised that they are not used in pregnancy until further data becomes available [43].

32.4.4 All-Trans Retinoid Acid (ATRA)

ATRA, or otherwise known as tretinoin, is a naturally occurring derivative of vitamin A (retinol), and its use is indicated in the treatment of acute promyelocytic leukemia (APL). ATRA has been shown to cross the placenta and have teratogenic effects, including craniofacial malformation on the fetus in animal studies [44, 45]. In humans the toxicity is less evident with only 1 in 26 fetuses (4%) exposed to ATRA in one study being born with a congenital anomaly. This fetus was described as having Potter syndrome (renal agenesis and oligohydramnios), and this was diagnosed prior to administration of ATRA. A limited number of other complications have been reported in the literature, and these include two cases of cardiac arrhythmia and one case of right atrial and ventricular dilatation [46, 47]. Conversely, there are numerous reports of APL successfully treated in pregnancy with ATRA and no sequelae to the fetus [48]. Overall, current expert opinion does not discourage the use of ATRA following the first trimester of pregnancy.

32.4.5 CAR T-Cell Therapy

CAR T-cell therapy is a form of immunotherapy that uses specially altered T cells collected from the patient's blood, modified to produce special structures called chimeric antigen receptors, expanded and then re-infused to fight the patient's cancer or prevent a recurrence. Their use in the treatment of ALL, B-cell lymphoma, and metastatic melanoma is becoming more widespread. There are no data on transplacental/milk transfer of these engineered cells, but transgenic T cells in expectant mothers are expected to cross the placenta or be present in the breast milk. The CAR-T cells may shape the immune response in the fetus in unexpected ways which may be toxic or beneficial. Furthermore, their longevity and persistence in the patient have not been clearly described. Suggestions regarding the incorporation of a suicide gene that can be activated at conception may have an impact on disease relapse [49]. Studies looking at placental and milk transfer of these molecules in animals would provide valuable information regarding the future use of this revolutionary therapy in pregnancy.

32.5 Fetal Tumors

32.5.1 Sacrococcygeal Teratomas

These are the commonest forms of congenital tumors with an incidence of around 1 in 35,000 pregnancies. They appear to be more prevalent in female fetuses by four-fold. Sacrococcygeal teratomas (SCTs) are classified as per the Altman classification system which takes into account their specific location and extension; however, this classification does not appear to impact antenatal or postnatal surgical outcomes [50]. Initial diagnosis of SCT is usually made at the routine 20-week obstetric ultrasound. MRI evaluation can be used to characterize solid and cystic components, vascularity, obstruction, or deviation of internal structures, urinary and bowel complications, and aid surgical planning. Tumors with a solid component greater than 50% appear to have an up to 7 times poorer outcome compared to predominantly cystic masses (71% vs 9%) [51]. After 24 weeks of gestation, ultrasound surveillance every two weeks to monitor the growth of the tumor and assess for cardiac compromise and increasing vascularity is a popular approach. In utero therapies include radiofrequency ablation, vascular or interstitial laser, sclerosing therapies, and coiling of vessels. These interventions are offered only at highly specialized centers and in a single-center case series of 34 cases, survival appeared to be improved in the absence of heart failure (67% vs 30%) [52]. Prematurity was common in this case series with a mean delivery gestational age of 29.7 weeks. Complications from the interventions can include skin or muscle necrosis and leg palsy. Vascular techniques appear to offer better survival than interstitial ablation [53]. Open fetal surgery has been previously reported, but due to advances in in utero therapy this is not widely practiced. Delivery should be planned in a center with the required pediatric expertise. If the external component of the SCT exceeds 5 cm, a cesarean section is indicated. Postnatally, if the infant is stable an operation should be planned during the first week of life. α-fetoprotein and β-human chorionic gonadotropin levels should be obtained prior to surgery as they can be useful in detecting recurrence. In children undergoing SCT resection postnatally, 30% will present with issues such as constipation and incontinence in the future [54].

32.5.2 Neck Teratomas

Six percent of all teratomas are related to the neck, and 80% of these are benign. However, their rapid growth and mass effect can cause significant complications such as obstruction or deviation of the trachea and esophagus. Their origin is poorly understood. Their tertiary-level ultrasound assessment includes evaluation of solid and cystic components, calcification, vascularity, and invasion into or deviation of adjacent structures. After 24 weeks of gestation ultrasound assessment should be performed every 2 weeks. MRI assessment can provide detailed soft tissue views of the fetal head and neck [55]. Polyhydramnios can be significant in partial or total occlusion of the oropharynx, and amniotic fluid drainage may be indicated when there is significant maternal discomfort. The most important information from imaging antenatally is airway patency that will inform the mode of delivery and the need for an EXIT procedure. Most of the neck teratomas are managed postnatally with a very limited role for in utero therapy. If required, at delivery the ex utero intrapartum treatment (EXIT) procedure is performed to secure the fetal airway prior to interruption of perfusion by the placenta. Without this intervention, cervical neck masses are associated with mortality up to 50%, compared to 10% following an EXIT procedure [56]. Postnatal management options of the tumor include sclerotherapy and surgery. In general, the majority of lesions can be either reduced or fully removed, and the outcomes are favorable in the absence of other comorbidities.

32.6 Counseling for This and Future Pregnancy

Apart from the biological issues imposed on a patient with cancer, there are a number of psychological implications and dilemmas that require consideration. The woman has to make decisions taking into account her own life, and the fetus, as well as the rest of the family. Counseling in a multidisciplinary approach, often involving multiple physicians concurrently in one room, can help to avoid conflicting messages and reduce stress to the patient and the family. The team should commonly include an obstetrician-gynecologist, maternal-fetal medicine specialist, oncologist, neonatologist, pharmacist, social worker, and a psychological support worker. Counseling should include information on a number of aspects of the ongoing pregnancy, the potential impact on the mother and fetus as well as effects on future pregnancies. During this process, health care professionals should ensure privacy to the mother, and take all the time necessary for the counseling, provide accurate information with honesty and empathy, and give information on other support services available. It should always be clear that the patient has the final decision-making role regarding her care.

Once a maternal treatment plan is in place, assessment of the fetus at regular intervals using antenatal growth ultrasound scans should be undertaken. Fetal outcomes are highly dependent on the gestational age of investigations/treatment and the time of delivery. Chemotherapy during pregnancy is thought to be associated with growth restriction, but the incidence of congenital malformations is not increased [57]. Chemotherapy should not be administered after 35 weeks of gestation or within 3 weeks of delivery. When possible, surgery is delayed until the second trimester and should include fetal monitoring if the gestation is greater than 24 weeks.

It should be the primary goal of the treating physicians to avoid a preterm delivery; however, this is not always feasible. Steroid prophylaxis to aid lung maturation is common practice. Delivery should be based on obstetric indications. Nevertheless, induction of labor or cesarean section with malignancy as the indication is not uncommon [58]. Following delivery, the placenta is histologically evaluated to ensure there is no cancer involvement. Breastfeeding will often be contraindicated if hormonal cancer therapy or chemotherapy is required in the postpartum period. A common recommendation is to allow a 2-year period until the next pregnancy to monitor disease progression or recurrence. Education should also be provided on cancer risk during future pregnancies and on modalities and frequency of surveillance.

Contraception to prevent a future unplanned pregnancy should also be discussed, to prevent ethically challenging situations. Contraception selection in this patient cohort is complicated by the type of malignancy, disease status, and other medical comorbidities. Specific to breast cancer or other hormone-related malignancies, the use of combined contraception methods can adversely affect prognosis and recurrence risk. On the other hand, a levonorgestrel intrauterine device may be helpful to a patient on tamoxifen for breast cancer to counteract its effects on the endometrium [59]. Estrogen-containing contraception should also be avoided when hormone-sensitive cancer is active or the patient is within 6 months of treatment completion. Alternative contraception options include barrier methods or an intrauterine device [60].

32.7 Conclusion

Diagnosis and treatment of cancer in pregnancy is a rare occurrence, but it is complicated by the fact that it does not solely involve the mother but also the fetus. Management is often dependent on the extent of the disease, the required treatment options, and the gestational age of the pregnancy at diagnosis. The cornerstone of care for women in this situation is to be managed by a multidisciplinary team involving obstetrician–gynecologists, oncologists as well as neonatologists in order to provide the patient with enough information to empower her to make an informed decision regarding treatment for her, her family, and her pregnancy.

References

[1] Eibye S, Kjaer SK. Mellemkjaer. Obstet Gynecol 2012;122(3):607–617.

[2] Voulgaris EG, Pentheroudakis G, Pavlidis N. Cancer and Pregnancy: a comprehensive review. Surg Oncol 2011;20(4):e175–e185.

[3] Parazzine F, Franchi M, Tavani A, Negri E, Peccatori FA. Frequency of pregnancy related cancer: a population based linkage study in Lombardy, Italy. Int J Gynecol Cancer 2017;27(3):613–619.

[4] Han SN, Lotgerink A, Gziri MM, Van Calsteren K, Hanssens M, Amant F. Physiologic variations of serum tumor markers in gynecological malignancies during pregnancy: a systematic review. BMC Med 2012;10:86.

[5] Ayyappan AP, Kulkarni S, Crystal P. Pregnancy-associated breast cancer: spectrum of imaging appearances. Br J Radiol 2010;83:529–534.

[6] Sarandakou A, Protonotariou E, Rizos D. Tumor markers in biological fluids associated with pregnancy. Crit Rev Clin Lab Sci 2007;44:151–178.

[7] Moore RG, Miller MC, Eklund EE, Lu KH, Bast RC Jr, Lambert-Messerlian G. Serum levels of the ovarian cancer biomarker HE4 are decreased in pregnancy and increase with age. Am J Obstet Gynecol 2012;206:349.e1–349.e7.

[8] Botha MH, Rajaram S, Karunaratne K. Cancer in pregnancy. Obstet Gynecol 2018;143(S2): 137–142.

[9] Middleton LP, Amin M, Gwyn K, Theriault R, Sahin A. Breast carcinoma in pregnant women: assessment of clinicopathologic and immunohistochemical features. Cancer 2003;98: 1055–1060.

[10] Case AS. Pregnancy-associated breast cancer. Clin Obstet Gynecol 2016;59:779–788.

[11] Yang WT, Dryden MJ, Gwyn K, Whitman GJ, Theriault R. Imaging of breast cancer diagnosed and treated with chemotherapy during pregnancy. Radiology 2006;239:52–60.

[12] Myers KS, Green LA, Lebron L, Morris EA. Imaging appearance and clinical impact of preoperative breast MRI in pregnancy-associatedbreast cancer. AJR Am J Roentgenol 2017;209:W177–W183.

[13] Zagouri F, Dimitrakakis C, Marinopoulos S, Tsigginou A, Dimopoulos MA. Cancer in pregnancy: disentangling treatment modalities. ESMO Open 2016;1:e000016.

[14] National Comprehensive Cancer Network. NCCN Clinical Practice Guidelines in Oncology (NCCN guidelines). Breast Cancer 2017. https://www.nccn.org. Accessed February 1, 2018.

[15] Froehlich K, Schmidt A, Heger JI, et al. Breast cancer, placenta and pregnancy. Eur J Cancer 2019;115:68–78. doi: 10.1016/j.ejca.2019.03.021. Epub 2019 May 20.

[16] Hodby K, Fields PA. Management of lymphoma in pregnancy. Obstet Med 2009 Jun;2(2):46–51.

[17] Pinnix CC, Osborne EM, Chihara D, et al. Maternal and fetal outcomes after therapy for hodgkin or non-Hodgkin lymphoma diagnosed during pregnancy. Brief Report. 2016.

[18] Das G, Damotte V, Gelfand JM, et al. Rituximab before and during pregnancy. A Systematic Review, and A Case Series in MS and NMOSD 2018;5(3):1–11.

[19] Milojkovic M, Apperley JF. How I treat leukemia during pregnancy. Blood 2014;123(7): 974–984.

[20] Dildy 3rd GA, Moise Jr KJ, Carpenter Jr RJ, Klima T. Maternal malignancy metastatic to the products of conception: a review. Obstet Gynecol Surv 1989 Jul;44(7):535e40.

[21] Still R, Brennecke S. Melanoma in pregnancy. Obstet Med 2017 Sep;10(3):107–112.

[22] McCarty KS, Wortman J, Stowers S. Sex steroid receptor analysis in human melanoma. Cancer 1980;46:1463–1470.

[23] Kokoschka EM, Spona J, Knobler R. Sex steroid hormone receptor analysis in malignant melanoma. Br J Dermatol 1982;107(s23):54–59.

[24] Green A. Oral contraceptives and skin neoplasia. Contraception 1991;43:653–666.

[25] Stensheim H, Moller B, Van Dijk T, Fossa SD. Cause-specific survival for women diagnosed with cancer during pregnancy or lactation: a registry based cohort study. J Clin Oncol 2009;27(1):45e51.

[26] Lens MB, Rosdahl I, Ahlbom A, et al. Effect of pregnancy on survival in women with cutaneous malignant melanoma. J Clin Oncol 2004;22(21):4369e75.

[27] O'Meara AT, Cress R, Xing G, Danielsen B, Smith LH. Malignant melanoma in pregnancy: a population-based evaluation. Cancer 2005;103(6):1217–1226.

[28] Reintgen DS, McCarty Jr KS, Vollmer R, Cox E, Seigler HF. Malignant melanoma and pregnancy. Cancer 1985 Mar 15;55(6):1340e4.

[29] Slingluff Jr CL, Reintgen DS, Vollmer RT, Seigler HF. Malignant melanoma arising during pregnancy. A study of 100 patients. Ann Surg 1990;211(5):552–559.

[30] Pages C, Robert C, Thomas L, et al. Management and outcome of metastatic melanoma during pregnancy. Br J Dermatol 2010;162(2):274–281.

[31] Hiratsuka M, Minakami H, Koshizuka S, Sato I. Administration of interferonalpha during pregnancy: effects on fetus. J Perinat Med 2000;28(5):372–376.

[32] Baer MR, Ozer H, Foon KA. Interferon-alpha therapy during pregnancy in chronic myelogenous leukaemia and hairy cell leukaemia. Br J Haematol 1992 Jun;81(2):167–169.

[33] Schuurman TN, Witteveen PO, Van Der Wall E, et al. Tamoxifen and pregnancy: an absolute contraindication? Breast Cancer Res Treat 2019 May;175(1):17–25.

[34] Tewari K, Bonebrake RG, Asrat T, Shanberg AM. Ambiguous genitalia in infant exposed to tamoxifen in utero. Lancet 1997;350:183.

[35] Cullins SL, Pridjian G, Sutherland CM. Goldenhar's syndrome associated with tamoxifen given to the mother during gestation. JAMA 1994;271:1905–1906.

[36] Berger JC, Clericuzio CL. Pierre Robin sequence associated with first trimester fetal tamoxifen exposure. Am J Med Genet A 2008;146A:2141–2144.

[37] Barthelmes L, Gateley CA. Tamoxifen and pregnancy. Breast 2004;13:446–451.

[38] Azim HA Jr, Metzger-Filho O, De Azambuja E, et al. Pregnancy occurring during or following adjuvant trastuzumab in patients enrolled in the HERA trial (BIG 01-01). Breast Cancer Res Treat 2012;133:387–391.

[39] Russell MA, Carpenter MW, Akhtar MS, Lagattuta TF, Egorin MJ. Imatinib mesylate and metabolite concentrations in maternal blood, umbilical cord blood, placenta and breast milk. J Perinatol 2007;27:241–243.

[40] Ali R, Ozkalemkas F, Kimya Y, et al. Imatinib use during pregnancy and breast feeding: a case report and review of the literature. Arch Gynecol Obstet 2009;280:169–175.

[41] Pye SM, Cortes J, Ault P, et al. The effects of imatinib on pregnancy outcome. Blood 2008;111 (12):5505–5508.

[42] National Toxicology Program. NTP monograph: developmental effects and pregnancy outcomes associated with cancer chemotherapy use during pregnancy. NTP Monogr 2013;(2): i–214. PMID: 24736875.

[43] Barkoulas T, Hall PD. Experience with dasatinib and nilotinib use in pregnancy. J Oncol Pharm Pract 2018 Mar;24(2):121–128.

[44] Collins MD, Mao GE. Teratology of Retinoids. Annu Rev Pharmacol Toxicol 1999;39(1): 399–430.

[45] Berenguer, M., Darnaudery, M., Claverol, S., et al. Prenatal retinoic acid exposure reveals candidate genes for craniofacial disorders. Sci Rep 2018;8:17492.

[46] Takitani K, Hino N, Terada Y, et al. Plasma all-trans retinoic acid level in neonates of mothers with acute promyelocytic leukemia. Acta Haematol 2005;114:167–169.

[47] Siu BL, Alonzo, Vargo Ta, Fenrich AL. Transient dilated cardiomyopathy in a newborn exposed to idarubicin and all-trans-retinoic acid (ATRA) early in the second trimester of pregnancy. Int J Gynecol Cancer 2002;12:399–402.

[48] Valappil S, Kurkar M, Howell R. Outcome of pregnancy in women treated with all-*trans* retinoic acid; A case report and review of literature. Hematology 2007;12(5):415–418.

[49] Cosgrove C, Dellacecca ER, van den Berg JH, et al. Transgenerational transfer of gene-modified T cells. J Immuno Therapy of Cancer 2019;7:186.

[50] Derikx JP, De Backer A, Van De Schoot L, et al. Long-term functional sequelae of sacrococcygeal teratoma: a national study in the Netherlands. J Pediatr Surg 2007;42: 1122–1126.

[51] Akinkuotu AC, Coleman A, Shue E, et al. Predictors of poor prognosis in prenatally diagnosed sacrococcygeal teratoma: a multiinstitutional review. J Pediatr Surg 2015;50:771–774.

[52] Van Mieghem T, Al-Ibrahim A, Deprest J, et al. Minimally invasive therapy for fetal sacrococcygeal teratoma: case series and systematic review of the literature. Ultrasound Obstet Gynecol 2014;43:611–619.

[53] Sananes N, Javadian P, Schwach Werneck Britto I, et al. Technical aspects and effectiveness of percutaneous fetal therapies for large sacrococcygeal teratomas: cohort study and literature review. Ultrasound Obstet Gynecol 2016;47:712–719.

[54] Shalaby Ms, Walker G, O'Toole S, et al. The long-term outcome of patients diagnosed with sacrococcygeal teratoma in childhood. A study of a national cohort. Arch Dis Child 2014;99: 1009–1013.

[55] Ryan G, Somme S, Crombleholme TM. Airway compromise in the fetus and neonate: prenatal assessment and perinatal management. Semin Fetal Neonatal Med 2016;21:230–239.

[56] Laje P, Peranteau WH, Hedrick HL, et al. Ex utero intrapartum treatment (EXIT) in the management of cervical lymphatic malformation. J Pediatr Surg 2015;50:311–314.

[57] Cardonick E, Usmani A, Ghaffar S. Perinatal outcomes of a pregnancy complicated by cancer, including neonatal follow-up after in utero exposure to chemotherapy: results of an international registry. Am J Clin Onc 2010;33(3):221–228.

[58] Van Calsteren K, Heyns L, De Smet F, et al. Cancer during pregnancy: an analysis of 215 patients emphasizing the obstetrical and the neonatal outcomes. J Clin Oncol 2010;28: 683–689.

[59] Carlson RW, Allred DC, Anderson BO, et al. Invasive breast cancer. Clinical practice guidelines in oncology. JNCCN 2011;9:136–222.

[60] Patel A, Schwarz EB. Society of family planning. cancer and contraception. Release date May 2012. SFP guideline #20121. Contraception 2012;86:191–198.

Index

100-g oral glucose tolerance test 366
50-g glucose challenge test 366
5-aminosalicylates 407
6-mercaptopurine 408
6-minute walk testing 177
75 g OGTT 366
75-g OGTT 369

A1C 369
abdomen 454
abdominal X-ray 27
abnormal placentation 71, 76
abnormal vaginal discharge 317
abortifacient 426
abortion 336
abruption 69, 75, 79, 139
ABVD 486
ACE inhibitors 248
acquired immunodeficiency syndrome 261
active cardiac disease 105
active management of the third stage of
      labor 206
active renal disease 430
active urinary sediment 430
activity 371
acute chest syndrome 229, 245
acute coronary syndrome 216
acute fatty liver of pregnancy 52, 137, 416
acute fetal compromise 146
acute kidney injury 51, 138, 233–234
acute lymphoblastic leukemia 486
acute myeloid leukemia 486
acute myocardial infarction 216
acute promyelocytic leukemia 489
acute pulmonary edema 139
acute renal failure 317
acute respiratory distress syndrome 139, 233
acute tubular necrosis 52
acyclovir 287
adalimumab 408, 427
ADAMTS 13 234
adenosine 112
adherence 268
adjuvant chemotherapy 485
adult Hb 241
advanced age 371
advanced cardiac life support 124–125

advanced life support 122
advanced maternal age 109, 149, 159, 357, 469
adverse fetal outcomes 413
adverse fetal/neonatal outcomes 174
adverse maternal outcomes 193
adverse neurological 334
adverse perinatal outcomes 187, 189, 366
adverse pregnancy outcome 357
adverse pregnancy outcomes 264, 332, 369
agranulocytosis 336
AIDS 297
air embolism 149–150
airflow obstruction 187
airway hyperresponsiveness 187
airway management 124
ALARA 23
albumin/creatinine ratio 39
albuminuria 345, 350
aldosteronism 38
alkaline phosphatase 484
ALL 488–489
"all or none" period 6, 23
alloimmunization 250, 253
All-Trans retinoid acid 489
alpha-fetoprotein 391, 484
Alport's 60
Altman classification 490
ambulatory blood pressure monitoring
      device 81
amiodarone 329
amniocentesis 250, 268, 283, 298
amniotic fluid 147, 283
amniotic fluid drainage 491
amniotic fluid embolism 52, 121, 137, 145
amniotic fluid index 350, 373
amniotic fluid volume 251, 424
an IL-12/IL-23 antagonist 409
analgesia 17, 252
anaphylactic shock 150
anaphylactoid 147
anaphylactoid reaction 138
anaphylactoid syndrome of pregnancy 148
anaphylaxis 138, 149, 192
anastrozole 477
anatomy scan 268
anemia 104, 175, 177, 225, 230, 244, 247,
      408, 473

https://doi.org/10.1515/9783110615258-033

anencephaly 345, 426
anesthesia 140, 393
aneuploidy 391
angiogenic growth factors 71
angioplasty 103
angiotensin II antagonists 13
angiotensin receptor antagonists 45
angiotensin receptor blockers 113, 250
angiotensin-converting enzyme 113
angiotensin-converting enzyme inhibitors 13, 45, 250
anorectal atresia 392
anoxic brain injury 125
antepartum anticoagulation 104
antepartum management 103
antiarrhythmic 12, 13
antibiotics 9, 319, 395, 460
antibody avidity 283
anticholinergic agents 194
anti-citrullinated peptide antibodies 424
anticoagulant 166
anticoagulation 10, 106, 126, 168, 177, 183, 246
anti-ds DNA titer 430
antiepileptic drugs 9, 441
antifibrinolytics 151
antihistamines 454, 461–462, 464
antihypertensive 57
anti-IgE monoclonal antibody 192
anti-IL-5 monoclonal antibodies 192
anti-integrin monoclonal antibody 409
anti-La/SSB 429
antimalarial drugs 9, 433
antineoplastic 15
antioxidant 77
antiphospholipid antibody syndrome 75, 429, 432
antiproliferative effects 179
antiretrovirals 9
anti-Ro/SSA 429
antithrombin deficiency 160
antithyroid antibodies 457
antithyroid drugs 336
anti-TNF 427
anti-Toxoplasma therapies 302
anti-tumor necrosis factor biologics 408
anti-vascular endothelial growth factor 344
antiviral drugs 287
anxiety 10, 148

aortic and mitral regurgitation 107
aortic coarctation 108
aortic dissection 110, 121
aortic obstruction 132
aortic stenosis 102, 108
aortocaval compression 125
aortopathy 108–109
APACHE II 133
ARDS 317
aromatase inhibitors 477, 485
arrhythmias 99, 108, 112, 121, 177, 489
arterial blood gas measurements 193
arterial embolization 218
arthritis 243
artificial reproductive technologies 157
aspart 349
asphyxia 346
aspiration 135
aspirin 77, 251, 349, 393, 430, 432
asplenism 228
ASPRE 77
asthma 10
asthma exacerbations 193
asthma medications 193
atenolol 78
atopic dermatitis 461–462
atopic eruptions 415
atrial fibrillation 109, 112
atrial flutter 112
atrial septal defect 107
atrioventricular septal defects 107
atypical hemolytic uremic syndrome 52, 234
autoimmune 455–456
autoimmune thyroiditis 331
auto-infarction 247
autologous whole blood 455
autotransfusion 175
avascular necrosis 243
azathioprine 408, 434, 457
azithromycin 245
B1 gene 299
B2 phylogroup 318
bacteremia 318
bacterial folliculitis 461
bacteriuria 251
balloon intrauterine tamponade 200
balloon valvuloplasty 110
bariatric surgery 389, 392

baricitinib 427
basic life support 124
B-cell lymphoma 489
behavioral adverse effects 444
benzodiapines 134
Berlin questionnaire 389
beta-blockade 109, 140
beta-blockers 43, 140, 336
bicuspid aortic valve 108–110
bilateral cortical necrosis 53
bilateral pulmonary infiltrates 139
bilirubin 415
biologic agents 477
biophysical profile 251, 322, 350
bioprosthetic valves 105
biosimilars 408
birth injury 364
blindness 300
blisters 454
blood cultures 319
blood loss 226
blood pressure control 109
blood pressure measurement 40
blood pressure target 40
blood products 211
blood transfusion 208, 472
BMI 94, 371, 387
body mass index 387
bosentan 246
bowel hyperechogenicity 283
brachial plexus injury 374
brain natriuretic peptide 177, 180
breast cancer 469, 484
breast carcinoma 472
breast-conserving surgery 472, 485
breastfeed 375
breastfeeding 254, 272, 351, 396, 425–426,
    434, 448, 492
broad-spectrum antibiotics 319
bronchodilators 189, 194
bronchospasm 150
budesonide 192, 409
bullous 455
bullous pemphigoid antigen 457
bupropion 191

C1 esterase inhibitors 152
C3 and C4 complement 430
C3 deposition 457

CA-125 484
caesarean 364, 367, 374
Caesarean section 107, 270
Caesarian section 189
calcium 77, 231
calcium channel blockade 246
calcium channel blockers 44, 179
cancer 159, 387, 469, 483
capillary blood glucose 392
CAR T-cell therapy 489
carbamazepine 14, 443
carbetocin 206
carboplatin 473
carboprost 216
carcinogenicity 25
cardiac arrest 121, 126, 148
cardiac complications 104
cardiac computed tomography 103
cardiac disease in pregnancy 100
cardiac dysfunction 150
cardiac output 99, 111, 132, 175, 182, 208,
    244, 391
cardiomyopathy 113, 121, 230, 389
cardiopulmonary bypass 151
cardiorespiratory arrest 146
cardiovascular collapse 137
cardiovascular comorbidities 121
cardiovascular complications 107, 110
cardiovascular disease 69, 91, 99, 357
cardiovascular magnetic resonance 103
cardiovascular morbidity 93
cardiovascular physiology 99
cardiovascular resuscitation 138
cardiovascular system 131
cardioversion 112–113
CARPREG II 100
cART 262
catamenial epilepsy 443
catecholamines 134, 182, 183
Caucasians 453, 455
CD4 antigen 261
CD4 count 267
ceftriaxone 245
cell-mediated immunity 313
Centers for Disease Control and
    Prevention 261, 297
central hypothyroidism 331
central venous pressure catheters 104
cephalexin 395

cerebral injury 152
cerebral necrosis 300
cerebral venous thrombosis 28
cerebrovascular 91
certolizumab 408, 427
cervical cancer 469, 472
cervical incompetence 190
cervical length 477
cesarean 207, 393, 395–396, 410, 431,
    478, 490
cesarean section 189, 313
chemotherapy 469, 472, 485–486, 491
chest compressions 124
chest radiograph 27
chloroquine 433
chlorpeniramine 419
cholestyramine 419
cholestyramine washout 426
chorioamnionitis 205, 263, 316–317, 323
chorionic villus sampling 250
chorioretinitis 282, 301
chronic hypertension 36, 57, 149
chronic kidney disease 49, 75, 94, 248, 432
chronic lymphocytic leukemia 486
cigarette 75
CIPHER score 133
cirrhosis 230, 418
CKD 350
cleft lip and palate 392, 425
cleft palate 194, 409, 426, 443
clindamycin 319
club foot 345
CML 488
CMV hyperimmune globulin 286
CMV-IgM 282
coagulopathy 146, 150, 204
coarctation 109
cocaine 14
cognitive 444
cognitive impairment 332
coma 137
Combined antiretroviral therapy 261, 264
community-acquired pneumonia 317
compensated respiratory alkalosis 187
complement activation 147, 456
Complement associated TMA 234
compression duplex ultrasonography 161
computed tomography 27, 162

CONCEPTT trial 348
condomless timed intercourse 265
cone biopsy 472
congenital 107
congenital abnormalities 407
congenital anomalies 336, 392, 426, 435
congenital cardiac defects 392
congenital CMV infection 281, 290
congenital complete heart block 431
congenital heart defect 388
congenital heart disease 99, 121
congenital infection 298
congenital malformations 108, 134, 189, 192,
    343, 345, 388, 473, 477, 491
congenital mitral stenosis 108
congenital toxoplasma infection 301
congenital toxoplasmosis 297
congenital TTP 235
congenital tumors 490
congestive heart failure 99, 336
connective tissue diseases 174
constipation 490
continuous glucose monitoring 348
continuous glucose monitors 348
continuous positive airway pressure 390
contraception 230, 254, 273, 409, 433–434,
    441, 492
contraceptive failure 442
contractions 473
contrast reaction 31
Control of Hypertension in Pregnancy
    Study 40, 58
controlled cord traction 206
conventional disease-modifying antirheumatic
    drugs 425
cord blood C-peptide levels 367
cord drainage 209
Cordocentesis 284
core needle biopsy 485
coronary angiography 103
coronary artery disease 74
coronary heart disease 387
corticosteroids 80, 140, 152, 188, 409
corticsteroids 322
cost 372
cost-effective 362
cost-effectiveness 289
cough 245

coumarin 13
counsel 18
counseling 56, 264, 432, 491
creatinine 49, 250, 350
creatinine clearance 50
cretinism 334
critically ill pregnant patient 131
Crohn's disease 405, 407
crystalloids 211, 322
C-section 343, 346, 348
cyclophosphamide 435
cyclosporine 457, 460
cytarabine 486
cytochrome P450 enzymes 442
cytokines 152
cytomegalovirus 253, 281
cytotoxic chemotherapy 473

dapsone 457
dasatinib 489
daunorubicin 486
D-dimer 161–162
D-dimer level 158
death 137
decrease bone mineral density 442
decrease in functional residual capacity
    131, 187
decreased maternal bone mineral density 263
decreasing insulin requirements 350
defibrillation 124
dehydration 243, 251
delay in the rate of reduction of uterine
    size 317
delayed psychomotor development 282
Delivery 233
depression 11, 188, 396
dermatosis 453
detemir 349
developmental delay 300
dexamethasone 233, 419, 431
diabetes 57, 149, 343
diabetes insipidus 137
diabetes mellitus 74, 387
diabetic microvascular complications 343
diabetic nephropathy 59
diagnostic imaging 23
dialysis 61, 234
diarrhea 12
DIC 138, 146

diet 357, 370
dietary intake 371
diethylstilbestrol 7, 15
dietitian 389
dilated cardiomyopathy 113
dilated RV annulus 108
disability 387
disease activity 428
disease flares 406 ,428
disease remission 409
dissection 109
disseminated intravascular coagulation 52,
    140, 147, 282
disseminated intravascular coagulopathy 233
diuresis 183, 246
diuretics 46, 177
dobutamine 134
dolutegravir 265
dopamine 134
dual nonreverse transcriptase inhibitor 268
ductus arteriosus 424
dumping syndromes 392
dyslipidemia 387
dyspepsia 12

E. coli 318
early cord clamping 206
early goal-directed therapy 319
early intervention 370
early suckling 209
Ebstein 108
echocardiogram 250, 391
echocardiography 149, 177, 180, 246
eclampsia 78–79, 149, 431, 447
ECMO 183
eculizumab 53, 235
education 190
Ehlers–Danlos syndrome 109–110
Eisenmenger syndrome 105, 111
Elective cesarean section 182
electrocardiogram 100
electroencephalography 447
electrolytes 447
elemental iron 227
elevated transaminases 137
embolization 200
embryo cryopreservation 249
embryogenesis 23
embryonic 6

embryonic Hb 241
emergency delivery 107
emtricitabine 266
encephalopathy 137, 152, 415
endometritis 263
endomyometritis 323
endothelial dysfunction 91
endothelin 178
endothelin receptor antagonists 179
endotracheal intubation 131, 135, 183
end-stage renal disease 234, 345
environmental 413
eosinophilia 454, 456
epidermal 454
epidural 447
epidural anesthesia 104
epidural catheter 394
epilepsy 11
epinephrine 134, 194
episiotomy 211, 271
epithelial ovarian cancer 484
epoprostenol 246
ergonovine 271
ergot derivatives 206
erythrocyte sedimentation rates 457
erythropoietin 364
estrogen 414
etanercept 427
ethanol 7, 14
ethnic groups 413
ethnicity 357, 413
excessive fetal growth 371
excessive gestational weight gain 357, 396
exchange transfusion 245, 253
exercise 424
exercise testing 108
EXIT procedure 491
exophthalmos 335
expectant management 79–80
extra corporal membrane oxygenation 126
extracerebral ultrasound 300
extracorporeal life-support 138
extracorporeal membrane oxygenation 151
ex-utero intrapartum treatment 491

factor V Leiden 159
failed induction 394
falciparum malaria 242
false negative results 283

Family history 329
fasting glucose 371
fasting plasma glucose 369, 392
FDA 7
fentanyl 17, 134
ferritin 226
fertility 231
fertility-preserving 472
fetal abnormalities 488
fetal airway 491
fetal alcohol spectrum disorder 7, 14
fetal and neonatal death 102
fetal brain MRI 301
fetal cellular debris 145
fetal complications 111
fetal death 234, 432
fetal debris 147
fetal demise 127, 477
fetal distress 137
fetal DNA 453
fetal drug exposure 443
fetal echocardiography 102, 431
fetal electrodes 271
fetal goiter 336
fetal growth 477
fetal growth restriction 69, 283, 336, 431, 473
fetal Hb 241
fetal hemorrhage 141
fetal hyperinsulinemia 364
fetal hyperthyroidism 336–337
fetal hypoxemia 364
fetal hypoxia 193, 322
fetal infections 283, 285, 297, 301
fetal macrosomia 205, 346
fetal malformations 322, 336, 441, 477, 485
fetal monitoring 322
fetal morbidity 418, 423
fetal mortality 318
fetal MRI 285
fetal mucin 145
Fetal nervous system 330
fetal organogenesis 488
fetal overgrowth 370
fetal platelet counts 286
fetal programming 364
fetal radiation exposure 167
fetal shielding 477
fetal surgery 490
fetal tachycardia 322

fetal toxicity 7, 485
fetal weight 374
fetal–neonatal complications 99
fetoplacental glucose steal phenomenon 363
fever 234, 245, 317, 322, 459
fibrinogen 211
filgotinib 427
fixed outflow tract obstruction 108
flash glucose monitors 348
fluid and sodium restriction 177
fluid resuscitation 319, 322
fluticasone propionate 192
folate 441
folate levels 388
folate supplementation 407, 427, 445
folic acid 7, 231, 250–251, 264, 388
folic acid antagonists 15
folinic acid 302
folliculitis 462, 464
forced expiratory volume 131
forced expiratory volume in 1 second 187
forced vital capacity 187
foul-smelling amniotic fluid 317
free T3 330
free T4 330
fresh frozen plasma 151
functional class 177
fundoscopic eye examination 303
furosemide 177
future risk 374

gadolinium 30
gallstones 248, 414
gamma-glutamyl transpeptidase 415
gastrointestinal reflux disease 188
gastroschisis 392
GDM 392, 396
GDM screening 365
gene therapy 249
General anesthesia 183
generalized pustular psoriasis of
    pregnancy 458
generalized tonic-clonic seizures 447
genetic 455
genetic mutation 357
genetic susceptibility 413
genetic testing 255
genetics 413
genital tract 317

genital tract sepsis 313
genotype 242
geographical 413
gestational diabetes 189, 231, 389, 407, 425
gestational diabetes mellitus 94, 357
gestational hypertension 35, 37, 91–92, 104,
    343, 348, 389
gestational transient thyrotoxicosis 335
gestational trophoblastic disease 330
gestational trophoblastic neoplasm 140
gestational weight gain 407
glargine 349
globin chains 241
glomerular endotheliosis 74
glomerular hyperfiltration 49
glomerulonephritis 53
glomerulosclerosis 248
glucocorticoids 425
glucometer 348
glucose 415
glucose challenge test 392
glucose intolerance postpartum 368
glyburide 349, 372–373
glycemic control 373
glycemic targets 371
glycemic treatment 372
goiter 329, 335
golimumab 408, 427
graduated compression stockings 168
grand multiparity 205
Graves' disease 335, 457
gray 24
group A *Streptococcus* 313, 318
growth restriction 477
gynecologic malignancies 472

H_1N_1 influenza pandemic 313
HAPO 366
haptoglobin 233
Hashimoto thyroiditis 457
HbA1c 344
HbA1c >6.1% 348
HbA1c of <6.5% 347
headache 28, 81, 153
hearing loss 282, 290
heart failure 93, 108, 113–114, 121, 139, 183,
    231, 432
HELLP 37, 52, 69, 79–80, 137, 232, 234,
    415, 430

hematuria 248
heme iron polypeptide 226
hemodynamic adaptations 100
hemodynamic changes of pregnancy 176
hemodynamic collapse 183
hemodynamic peripartum monitoring 104
hemodynamic stress 110
hemofiltration 151
hemoglobin 225, 241
hemoglobin A1c 391–392
hemoglobin electrophoresis 228, 231
hemoglobin S 227
hemolysis 234, 242, 250
hemorrhage 121, 137, 140, 151
hemostatic system 158
heparin 177
heparin-induced thrombocytopenia 166
hepatic congestion 176
hepatic encephalopathy 137
hepatic failure 137
Hepatic rupture 233
hepatitis C 264, 414
hepatitis E 313
hepatopathy 248
hepcidin 226
hereditary kidney disease 60
heritable PAH 174
herpes gestationis 455
herpes simplex 313
herpesvirus 281
herpetiform 455
high CMV-IgM levels 286
high spinal anesthesia 149
higher heart rate levels 314
higher pulmonary pressures 176
high-risk behaviours 263
high-risk cardiac lesion 100
HIV genotyping 267
HIV testing 262
HIV viral load 267
HIV-1 261
HLA-DR3 455
HLA-DR4 455
Hodgkin lymphoma 485
Holt–Oram syndrome 102
hormonal fluctuations 188
hormone-mediated vasodilation 175
human chorionic gonadotropin 330, 391
human immunodeficiency viruses 261

humanized monoclonal antibody 235
hydantoin 14
hydralazine 41–42, 44, 78, 233
hydramnios 205
hydrocephalus 426
hydrops fetalis 283
hydroxychloroquine 429, 431, 433
hydroxyurea 229, 250
hydroxyzine 419
hyperbilirubinemia 346, 364
hypercholesterolemia 92
hypercoagulability 242
hyperemesis gravidarum 52, 415
hyperglycemia 344, 357, 365
hypertension 10, 73, 109–110, 336, 343,
    387, 430
hypertensive diseases of pregnancy 332
hypertensive disorders 91, 109, 392
hypertensive disorders of pregnancy 35, 69
hypertensive encephalopathy 207
hypertensive medications 389
hyperthermia 140, 322
hyperthyroidism 104, 335
hypertrophic cardiomyopathy 113
hypocalcemia 458
hypofibrinogenemia 151
hypoglycemia 372, 415
hypoparathyroidism 458
hypospadias 345
hypotension 176, 314
hypothyroidism 95, 331
hypoxemia 137, 139
hypoxia 189, 194, 245, 393
hysterectomy 138, 200, 323

IBD disease remission 406
ICSI 266
idiopathic PAH 174
idiopathic pulmonary arterial hypertension 111
idiopathic RV outflow tract tachycardia 112
IgA 303
IgG 282, 298
IgG autoantibodies 456
IgG avidity 298
IgG1 monoclonal antibody 488
IgM 282, 298, 303
ileal pouch anal anastomosis 406
iliac veins 161
imaging 23

imatinib 488
immune function 188, 408
immune thrombocytopenic purpura 486
immunization 247, 250, 266
immunocompromised 266
immunofluorescence 457, 459, 461–463
immunoglobulin 457
immunomodulating agents 281
immunosuppression 56, 235, 297
immunosuppressive therapies 297
immunotherapy 489
impaired immunity 261
impetigo herpetiformis 458
implantable cardioverter defibrillator 112
in vitro fertilization 414
Incentive spirometry 245
incidence of maternal cardiac arrest in
      pregnancy 121
increase in tidal volume 187
increased metabolic activity 358
increased metabolic requirements 329
increased preload 176
increased sympathetic activity 182
incurable condition 174
indocyanine green 472
induction 205, 346, 350, 374
infant birth weight 373
Infant cART prophylaxis 273
infant mortality rate 153
infections 12, 104, 159, 188, 243, 245, 253, 425
infective endocarditis 104
infertility 199, 249, 266, 329, 405, 435
inflammation 189, 473
inflammatory bowel disease 159, 405
inflammatory markers 393
infliximab 408, 427
influenza 313
inhaled corticosteroids 192
inotrope 208
insulin 372
insulin pump 348
insulin resistance 350
insulin sensitivity 351, 358, 389
intensive care unit 126
interferon-α 487
International Network of Obstetric Survey
      Systems 146
intra-aortic balloon pump 151
intracerebral hemorrhage 42

intracranial anomalies 285
intracranial hemorrhage 28
intracranial lesions 299
intrahepatic cholestasis 248
intrahepatic cholestasis of pregnancy 413
intratuterine growth restriction 229
intrauterine balloon devices 138
intrauterine device 442, 492
intrauterine fetal death 233, 282
intrauterine fetal demise 139, 228, 394
intrauterine growth restriction 49, 102, 189,
      233, 282, 300, 432, 486
intrauterine infection 281
intravenous immunoglobulin 457
intravenous insulin 350
Intravenous iron 227
in-utero fetal death 299
invasive monitoring 216
invasive obstetrical procedures 271
invasive ventilation 194
in-vitro fertilization 249
iodide 140
iodinated contrast 31
iodinated radiologic contrast 329
iodine 330, 334
iodine deficiency 331
iodine insufficiency 329
Iodine supplementation 334
ionizing radiation 23, 27
iron 177, 250–251
iron chelators 250
iron deficiency anemia 225
iron overload 230, 253
ischemic heart disease 93
isotretinoin 7
itchy 454
IVC compression 182, 322
IVF 266
IVIG 431

JAK kinase inhibitor 409
Janus kinase (JAK) pathway inhibitors 427
jaundice 415

Kleihauer–Betke test 141

labetalol 41–43, 78, 233
lacerations 204, 211
lactate 314, 319

lactate dehydrogenase 233, 484
lactation 32
lamotrigine 442, 448
laparoscopic 406
laparoscopy 471
laparotomy 471
large blood pressure cuff 390
large for gestational age 364, 389
large for gestational age infants 345
large-for-gestational age neonates 343
laser photocoagulation 344
last dose 408
late maternal age 121
late pregnancy 370
latent state 281
latent toxoplasma infection 297
L-CHAD deficiency 137
lead shielding 31
leflunomide 426
left lateral positioning 134, 141
LEFt score 162
left uterine displacement 125
left ventricular hypertrophy 113
left-to-right shunts 107
lenticulostriate vasculopathy 283
letrozole 477
leukemia 469, 477
leukocytosis 137, 317, 459
leukotriene receptor antagonists 192
levothyroxine 334
levothyroxine dose 334
lifestyle 389, 396
lifestyle modification 370
lipogenesis 358
lipolysis 358
lispro 349
listeriosis 313
lithium 329
live vaccines 409
liver 413
liver enzymes 413
liver function tests 391
liver transplantation 413
local anesthetics 149
Loeys–Dietz syndrome 109
long QT syndrome 112
long-acting beta-agonists 191
long-term development 408

long-term maternal and perinatal
    outcomes 369
lorazepam 448
low birth weight 189, 225, 388, 407, 430
low birthweight infants 189
low molecular weight heparin 106, 432
low-avidity CMV IgG 282
low-molecular-weight heparin 163
lung surfactant synthesis 364
lung volumes 131
lupus 57
lupus flares 430, 432
lupus nephritis 59, 429
lymph node biopsy 485
lymph nodes 487
lymphoma 469

macrocytosis 225
macrosomia 346, 348, 358, 364, 368, 373
magnesium sulfate 78, 81, 194
magnetic resonance imaging 26
magnetic resonance venography 161
major congenital malformations 192, 443
major depressive disorders 397
malaria 313
malformations 5–6, 23, 348
malignancies of the unborn child 477
malnutrition 473
mammography 484–485
manual removal 209
Marfan syndrome 102, 109, 110
massive PE 166
mast cells 453
mastectomy 472, 485
maternal and fetal risks 174
maternal antibodies 272
maternal burns 141
maternal code blue team 122
maternal death 99, 139, 157, 174, 199, 245, 313
maternal early warning 316
maternal hyperglycemia 364
maternal hypoglycemia 349–350
maternal hypotension 134
maternal infection 282, 297
maternal morbidity 69, 169, 199, 313, 388
maternal morbidity and mortality 102, 109
maternal mortality 111, 121, 145, 233, 235, 246,
    248, 253, 317, 324

maternal oxygen saturation 136
maternal seroconversion 298, 303
maternal serum screening 391
maternal severity index 133
maternal survival 127
maternal thromboembolism 432
mean blood glucose 348
measure blood loss 200
mechanical heart valves 106
mechanical hemostasis 204
mechanical ventilation 135, 139, 317
meconium-stained amniotic fluid 418
medical terminations 299
medication adherence 406
medications 5, 99, 250
melanoma 469, 472, 486, 489
meningoencephalocele 426
mental health 243
mental retardation 281, 285, 477
mental status 234
mental status changes 152
meperidine 17, 134
metastases 471
metastasis 485, 487
metastatic disease to the placenta 485
metformin 349, 372–373
methacholine challenge testing 190
Methimazole 336
methotrexate 406, 408, 410, 426
methyldopa 41, 43, 78
methylergometrine 207
methylergonovine 216
metronidazole 395
MHC class II molecules 456
microalbuminuria 248
microangiopathic hemolytic anemia 137, 232
microcephaly 282–283, 285
microcytic anemia 228
micronutrient 388–389
migraine 12, 441
mineralocorticoid receptor antagonists 113
minor malformations 345
minute ventilation 131, 187
miscarriage 102, 109, 332, 405, 471, 477
misoprostol 15, 206
misperceptions 405
mitral stenosis 102
mode of delivery 80
modified WHO 100

monitored postpartum 105
monoclonal antibodies 408, 486, 487
mononucleosis syndrome 281
mood 449
morbid obesity 387
morbidity 183
morphine 17, 134
morphological abnormalities 299
mortality 69, 105, 111, 152, 174, 387
mortality rates 111
mother-to-child transmission 301
mother-to-child transmission via breast
    milk 272
mother-to-fetus transmission 286
motor disability 285
moyamoya 247
MRI 109, 490–491
multidisciplinary 228, 231, 249, 251, 266, 272,
    336–337, 347, 410, 423, 428, 491
multidisciplinary approach 141, 190
multidisciplinary team 103, 177
multiparity 226, 469
multiple gestations 413, 414, 453
multiple pregnancy 205, 313, 330
multiple sclerosis 441
multivitamin 347
Mycophenolate mofetil 15, 434
myocardial infarction 149, 207
myocardial ischemia 138

nasal intubation 135
Neck Teratomas 490
negative pressure wound therapy 396
neoadjuvant chemotherapy 471
neonatal abstinence syndrome 135, 255
neonatal death 248, 345
neonatal hematologic toxicities 473
neonatal hyperthyroidism 336–337
neonatal hypoglycemia 194, 345–346, 348,
    350–351, 370
neonatal lupus 431
neonatal outcomes 373
nephropathy 247, 343–344
neural tube defect 388, 391
neural tube defects 265, 345, 443
neuraxial 17
neuraxial anesthesia 168
neurocognitive 449
neurodevelopment 330

neurodevelopmental delay 473
neurodevelopmental disorders 225
neuroimaging 447
neurological sequelae 282
neuropathic pain 243
neuropathy 344
nevirapine 263
New York Heart Association 100
nicotine replacement therap 191
nifedipine 41–42, 44, 78, 233, 463
nitric oxide 178
Nonadherence 193
non-alcoholic liver fibrosis 415
nonalcoholic steatohepatitis 391
Nondepolarizing neuromuscular blocking
    agents 134
non-Hodgkin lymphoma 486
noninvasive monitoring 211
noninvasive prenatal testing 391
noninvasive ventilation 135
nonproliferative retinopathy 344
nonsteroidal anti-inflammatory drugs 229, 424
Nonstress testing 322
nonstress tests 251, 350, 373
noradrenaline 322
norepinephrine 134
NPH 349
NSAIDs 248, 253
nuchal translucency 391
NYHA class III/IV 113, 104
NYHA functional class III or IV 179

obese 357
obesity 75, 149, 159, 188, 357, 365, 387
obesity hypoventilation 389
obstetric early warning score 133
obstetric emergency 145
obstetric hemorrhage 138
obstructive sleep apnea 389
occupational therapy 424
offspring's health 95
oligohydramnios 477, 488
omalizumab 455
oncogenesis 25
oncologic surgery 471
oncologic treatment 469
one-step strategy 368
oocysts 297
operative delivery 271

operative vaginal 364
ophthalmic disease 95
opiates 243, 252
opportunistic infection 261
oral contraceptive pills 441
oral contraceptives 486
organogenesis 473
osteoarthritis 387
osteopenia 231
OTC medications 5
ovarian cancer 469
ovarian hyperstimulation syndrome 159
ovarian masses 471
overt hypothyroidism 331–332
overweight 357, 453
ovulatory cycle 391
oxcarbazepine 443
oxygen 193, 246
oxygen consumption 131, 175
oxytocin 17, 138, 147, 183, 194, 199

pacemaker 431
paclitaxel 485
PAH-targeted therapy 174
palpitations 335
pancreatic β-cells 358, 373
pancreatitis 137
Pandemic 2009 influenza A (H_1N_1) 317
papillary dermis 454
papules 460, 462
paradoxical embolization 107
parakeratosis 454
parasite 297
paroxysmal supraventricular tachycardia 112
patent ductus arteriosus 107
PCR 283, 299, 303
peak expiratory flow measurements 193
pelvic arterial embolization 217
pelvic pain 317
pelvic pouch 410
pemphigoid gestationis 415, 455
percutaneous balloon valvuloplasty 108
perianal CD 410
perianal fistula 410
perimortem caesarian section
    delivery 124–125, 151
perinatal 13
perinatal antiretroviral therapy 262
perinatal death 348, 413

perinatal morbidity 233, 244, 350, 473
perinatal mortality 189, 253, 332, 343,
    345, 347
perinatal outcome 102, 332
perinatal outcomes 191, 329, 373
perinatal transmission 261–262, 270–271, 274
perinatal transmissions 262
peripartum cardiomyopathy 102, 112–113
peripartum hysterectomy 218
peripheral arterial disease 91
peripheral edema 176
peripheral neuropathy 441
peripheral vascular resistance 225
peritoneal lavage 141
periumbilical 456
periventricular echogenicity 283, 300
PET scan 27
Pfannenstiel 395
pharmacodynamics 9
pharmacokinetics 8, 393, 448
pharmacological treatment 371
pharmacotherapy 374
phenobarbital 443
phenylephrine 323
phenytoin 443
pheochromocytoma 38
phlegmasia alba dolens 167
phlegmasia cerulea dolens 167
phosphodiesterase type 5 inhibitors 179
photocoagulation 344
phototherapy 455, 461
physical activity 251, 389
physical examination 100
physiologic changes 131, 469
physiotherapy 424
PIANO registry 408
placenta 91, 487
placenta abruption 233
placental abruption 140, 233, 332
placental barrier 473
placental insufficiency 350, 432
placental retention 204
placental transfer 408
planned delivery 182
plasma exchange 235
plasma exchange transfusions 151
plasma infusion 235
plasma volume expansion 175
plasmapheresis 419

platinum-based drugs 473
PlGF 71–72, 82–83
pneumonia 245, 317
polycystic kidney disease 60
polycystic ovarian syndrome 358
polycythemia 364
polyhydramnios 370, 374, 491
polymorphic eruption of pregnancy 453
polysaccharide-iron complex 226
polysomnography 389
polytherapy 444
positive family history 160
posterior reversible encephalopathy
    syndrome 28
postpartum 157, 254
postpartum bleeding 234
postpartum flare 457
postpartum hemorrhage 102, 137, 189, 199,
    271, 395, 446
postpartum hypertension 45
postpartum OGTT 375
postpartum prophylaxis 271
postprandial glucose 348
postprandial glucose monitoring 371
post-thrombotic syndrome 168
prazosin 78
preconception 56, 390, 406
preconception assessment 423
preconception counseling 229, 231, 388, 441
preconception evaluation 99
predictors of seizures 443
prednisone 455, 457, 460
preeclampsia 36–37, 69–84, 91, 139, 159, 189,
    228, 232, 248, 251, 282, 333, 343–346,
    348, 368, 388–389, 392, 415, 430–432
preexisting diabetes 369
preexisting hypertension 91
preexisting medical conditions 313
pre-exposure prophylaxis 265
pregnancy loss 329, 430
pregnancy-induced hypertension 425, 430
preimplantation 23
premature deliveries 457
premature delivery 110, 473
premature ovarian failure 435
premature rupture of the membranes 189, 425
prematurity 336, 490
prenatal diagnosis 249
prenatal treatment 303

prenatal vitamin 226
preprandial glucose 348
prescription 5
preterm birth 189, 244, 253, 263, 343, 388,
    407, 418, 430
preterm delivery 189, 225, 248, 282, 329,
    332–333, 345–346
preterm labor 317, 425, 431
preterm premature rupture of membranes
    313, 473
prevent fetal transmission 289
prevent maternal CMV infection 289
prevent transmission 286
preventing perinatal transmission 263
prevention 206
primary hypothyroidism 331
primary maternal CMV 283
primary maternal infection 297
primiparity 313
procoagulant factors 147
progesterone 188, 414
progestins 433
prognosis 469
progressive RV dysfunction 173
proliferative remodeling 173
Proliferative retinopathy 344
prolonged life expectancy 274
promethazine 17
PROMISSE study 428, 432
prophylactic transfusion 253
prophylaxis 163, 273
propofol 134
propylthiouracil 336
prostacyclin 178
prostaglandin F_{2a} analogue 138
prostaglandins 194, 244
prostanoids 179
protamine 104
protease inhibitor 268
protein/creatinine ratio 39
proteinuria 37, 49–50, 69, 430
prothrombin complex 107
prothrombin mutation 160
prurigo 415
prurigo of pregnancy 463
pruritic erythema 454
pruritic folliculitis 415, 463
pruritic urticarial papules and plaques of
    pregnancy 415, 453

pruritus 413, 415, 456
pruritus gravidarum 415
psoriasis vulgaris 458
psychological 491
puerperal sepsis 316
pulmonary arterial lines 104
pulmonary edema 108–109, 233, 317
pulmonary embolism 30, 145, 149, 157
pulmonary function testing 190
pulmonary hypertension 102, 105, 111, 173,
    228–229, 246, 250, 432
pulmonary hypoplasia 477
pulmonary regurgitation 107
pulmonary stenosis 110
pulmonary vascular resistance 111
PUPPP 453
pustules 458, 462
pyelonephritis 317
pyrimethamine-sulfadiazine 301

quality of life 190
quickSOFA 315

radiation 103, 329, 472
radiation dose 477
radiation therapy 472
radioactive iodine 331
radioactive technetium 472
radiofrequency ablation 490
radiologic embolization 138
random plasma glucose 369, 392
rash 457
RBC transfusion 230
recent primary infection 283
recombinant human activated factor VII 218
recurrent pregnancy losses 432
red cell mass 175
reduce viral transmission 286
reduced pulmonary blood flow 176
Regional anesthesia 182
remission 406, 424
renal biopsy 51
renal disease 74
renal failure 137
renal function 49
renal function test 391
renal lupus flare 430
renal papillary necrosis 248
renal transplant 61

renal tubular dysgenesis 45
renin–angiotensin–aldosterone system 225
reproductive age 387
residual volume 187
respiratory alkalosis 131, 136
respiratory distress syndrome 346, 364
respiratory failure 194
respiratory function 393
restrictive lung disease 432
resuscitation 199, 208
retained placenta 209
retained products of conception 313
retinoic acid 15
retinopathy 250, 343–344, 350
reversible cerebral vasoconstriction
    syndrome 28
rheumatic 107
rheumatic diseases 423
rheumatic fever 108
rheumatoid arthritis 423
rheumatoid factor 424
rheumatological 409
rhinitis 188
rifampin 419
right heart failure 246
right upper quadrant pain 415
risk assessment 100
Risk stratification 180
rituximab 486
Ross operation 105
rupture of membranes 271
RV failure 176
RV overdistension 182

S. pneumoniae 317
sacrococcygeal teratomas 490
S-adenosyl-methionine 419
SAPS II 133
scheduled induction of labor 104
schistocytes 232–233
schizophrenia 11
screening 227, 298
screening for CMV 289
screening for HIV 262
secondary hypertension 38
secondary infection 281, 283
sedation 134
seizures 69, 137, 234, 247, 282, 300, 441
selective COX-2 inhibitors 425

selective estrogen receptor modulators 477,
    487
self-monitoring of blood glucose 348, 371
sensorineural hearing loss 281–282
sepsis 121, 149, 233, 313
septic abortion 52, 316, 323
septic shock 314
Sequential Operational Functionality
    Assessment Score 314
seroconversion 282, 297
serodifferent couples 264
Serological follow-up 303
serology testing 282
seronegative 281
seropositive individuals 264
seropositive patients 289
serum bile acid levels 418
serum bile acids 413, 415
serum B-type natriuretic peptide 100
serum creatinine level 430
severe asthma 187
severe hypertension 35, 42, 233
severe malformations 290
severe preeclampsia 91
sexual HIV transmissio 265
sFLt-1 37, 71–72, 74, 83
short-acting beta-agonists 191
short-acting bronchodilators 193–194
shoulder dystocia 364, 368, 395
sickle cell disease 228, 242
sickle cell trait 242
sickle Hb 241
sildenafil 246
Sjogren's syndrome 431
skeletal abnormalities 477
skin biopsy 457
sleep 448
small for gestational age 244, 263, 389, 457
small-for-gestational-age infants 371
smoking 149, 159, 191, 370, 406
socioeconomic 226
solid malignancies 471
soluble guanylate cyclase inhibitor 179
soluble transferrin receptor 226
source control 323
sperm washing 266
sphygmomanometer 40
spina bifida 392
Spinal anesthesia 182

spiramycin 301–302
spironolactone 177
spondyloarthropathies 427
spontaneous labor 394
stage 469
staging 470, 484
Staphylococcus 318
status epilepticus 447
stem-cell transplantation 249
steroid 492
steroid creams 455, 461–462
stillbirth 69, 75, 145, 159, 228, 248, 263, 336,
    347, 364, 373, 413, 418–419
Streptococcus 318
stress 243
striae distensae 456
stroke 29, 42, 207, 229, 234, 247, 387, 432
stroke volume 175
structural cardiac lesions 104
structural heart disease 112
subarachnoid hemorrhage 29
subclinical hyperthyroidism 330–332, 335
subtherapeutic levels 268
suction curettage 323
sudden cardiac death 113
sudden death 183
sudden infant death syndrome 18
sudden shock 145
sulfasalazine 407, 427
sulfonylurea 372
sulprostone 216
suppression of cell-mediated immunity 189
supraumbilical transverse incision 395
surgery 406, 471
surgical correction 110
surgical cytoreduction 471
surgical site infection 395
symmetric polyarthritis 423
symphysis-fundus height 394
syncytiotrophoblast 71
synovial joints 423
syntometrine 207
syphilis 263
systemic corticosteroids 193–194
systemic inflammatory response syndrome 314
systemic lupus erythematosus 75, 159, 428
systemic sclerosis 434
systemic vascular resistance 175, 182, 208

tachycardia 140, 317, 335
Takotsubo cardiomyopathy 113
tamoxifen 477, 485, 487
tenofovir 263, 266
teratogenic 5, 30, 113, 250, 345, 408, 426, 432,
    434, 489
teratogenicity 23, 231, 243, 246, 408–409
terminate the pregnancy 300
termination 246, 249, 469, 471, 485–487
termination of the pregnancy 432
tetracycline 14
tetraiodothyronine 329
tetralogy of Fallot 107
thalassemia 227, 230
thalassemia intermedia 231
thalassemia major 231
thalidomide 15
theophylline 192
therapeutic abortion 177, 183
therapeutic drug monitoring 446
therapeutic hypothermia 126
thionamide 140
thiopurines 408
third trimester 157, 454
thrombin 158
thrombocytopenia 232–234, 247, 430
thromboelastography 158
thromboelastometry 216
thromboembolectomy 151
thromboembolic 219
thromboembolic complications 100, 106, 199
thromboembolism 110, 183, 208, 433
thrombolysis 166
thrombophilia 74
thrombophilic defects 159, 169
thromboprophylaxis 81
thrombosis 228
thrombotic microangiopathy 232
thrombotic thrombocytopenic purpura 52, 234
thyroid antibody 329
Thyroid cancer 337
thyroid dysfunction 231, 329
thyroid hormones 329
thyroid nodules 337
thyroid stimulating hormone 330
thyroid storm 139, 336
thyroid surgery 331
thyroid ultrasound 337

Thyroidectomy 337
thyroiditis 335
thyrotoxicosis 335
thyroxine-binding globulin 329
tissue inflammation 358
tofacitinib 406, 409, 427
topiramate 443
total lung capacity 131, 187
total triiodothyronine 329
toxic adenoma 335
toxic multinodular goiter 335
toxic shock syndrome 317–318
toxicology 447
Toxoplasma gondii 297
trachelectomy 472
tranexamic acid 138, 208, 217
trans-esophageal echocardiography 103
transferrin saturation 226
transfusion 151, 199, 229, 246, 253
transfusion reactions 150
transplacental passage 298
transplacental transfer 457
transplacental transmission 281
transplant 114
transthoracic echocardiogram 100
trastuzumab 477, 488
trauma 140
tretinoin 489
tricuspid regurgitation 108, 176
truncal asymmetry 364
TSH 330
TSH receptor antibodies 336
TSH receptors 335
tumor markers 483–484
Turner syndrome 109–110
two-step method for GDM 367
type 1 diabetes 329, 331, 344
type 2 diabetes 343, 357
type 2 diabetes mellitus 94
tyrosine kinase inhibitors 487, 488

UK Obstetric Surveillance System 146
ulcerative colitis 405, 407
ultrasonography 161, 485
ultrasound 26, 29, 268, 283, 298–299, 374,
      391, 394, 490
ultrasounds 251, 431
unfractionated heparin 106, 163
universal screening 332

unknown HIV status 271
untreated GDM 365
upadacitinib 427
upper airways 131
uric acid 459
Urinary output 216
urinary tract infections 317
urine protein creatinine ratio 391
urogenital anomalies 345
urogenital malformations 443
ursodeoxycholic acid 418
urticaria 454, 463
urticarial 454
ustekinumab 409
uterine arterial blood flow 132
uterine artery blood flow 251
uterine atony 152, 199, 204
uterine balloon tamponade 217
uterine bleeding 153
uterine compression sutures 218
uterine contractions 175, 394
uterine gas gangrene 323
uterine manipulations 137
uterine massage 206
uterine rupture 140, 145
uterine tenderness 317
uterotonics 200
UVB 460

vaccination 289
Vaginal delivery 182
vaginal prostaglandins 147
valacyclovir 287
valproate 442–443
valproic acid 14
Valsalva 175, 182
valve thrombosis 106
valvular heart disease 121
varenicline 191
vascular disease 375
vascular thrombosis 432
vasculitis 434, 463
vaso- occlusive events 228
vasoconstriction 176
vasodilatory 179
vaso-occlusion 242
vaso-occlusive 251
vasopressors 134, 183, 319, 322
vedolizumab 409

VEGF 72, 74
vena caval compression 175, 471
venous access 125
venous stasis 393
venous thromboembolism 176–177, 393, 410
ventilation perfusion scintigraphy 31
ventilation/perfusion 162
ventilatory support 135
ventricular hypertrophy 245
ventricular septal defect 107
ventricular tachycardia 112
ventriculomegaly 283, 300
vertebral anomalies 345
vertical transmission 298, 302
vesicles 456
viral culture 283
viral suppression 264
visual impairment 282
vitamin A 489
vitamin C 226
vitamin D 78, 231, 388, 414
vitamin K 107, 446
vitamin K antagonist 168
vitamins C and E 77
voluntary childlessness 405
vomiting 267

waist circumference 387
waist-to-hip ratio 387

warfarin 106
warfarin embryopathy 106
weight gain 349, 372
weight loss 389–390
weight retention 396
wheelchairs 390
white blood cells 314
white coat hypertension 37
WHO classification of PH 173
with anti-factor Xa levels 167
Wolff–Parkinson–White 112
women with epilepsy 441
World Health Organization (WHO) 227, 297, 316
wound infection 263

younger women 174

ZAHARA 100
zidovudine 263, 270
zinc 78

α-fetoprotein 490
α-globin 227
α-thalassemia 230
β-agonist therapy 139
β-cell dysfunction 374
β-genes 227
β-human chorionic gonadotropin 490
β-thalassemia 230